RICKETTSIAE
AND RICKETTSIAL DISEASES

Academic Press Rapid Manuscript Reproduction

Based on the Conference on Rickettsiae and Rickettsial Diseases
Held at the Rocky Mountain Laboratories, Hamilton, Montana,
September 3–5, 1980

RICKETTSIAE
AND RICKETTSIAL DISEASES

Edited by

WILLY BURGDORFER
ROBERT L. ANACKER

Rocky Mountain Laboratories
National Institute of Allergy and Infectious Diseases
National Institutes of Health
Hamilton, Montana

ACADEMIC PRESS   1981

A Subsidiary of Harcourt Brace Jovanovich, Publishers
New York   London   Toronto   Sydney   San Francisco

ACADEMIC PRESS, INC.
111 Fifth Avenue, New York, New York 10003

United Kingdom Edition published by
ACADEMIC PRESS, INC. (LONDON) LTD.
24/28 Oval Road, London NW1 7DX

Library of Congress Cataloging in Publication Data
Main entry under title:

Rickettsiae and rickettsial diseases.

    Proceedings of the Conference on Rickettsiae and
Rickettsial Diseases, held at the Rocky Mountain
Laboratories in Hamilton, Montana, September 3-5, 1980.
    Includes index.
    1. Rickettsial diseases--Congresses. 2. Rickettsia--
Congresses. I. Burgdorfer, Willy, Date. II. Anacker,
Robert Leroy, Date. III. Conference on Rickettsiae and
Rickettsial Diseases (1980 : Rocky Mountain Laboratories)
[DNLM: 1. Rickettsiae--Congresses. 2. Rickettsial
infections--Congresses. WC 600 R539 1980]
RC114.7.R53   616.9'22   81-15058
ISBN 0-12-143150-9   AACR2

PRINTED IN THE UNITED STATES OF AMERICA

81 82 83 84   9 8 7 6 5 4 3 2 1

CONTENTS

BIOCHEMISTRY AND METABOLISM

CONTRIBUTORS AND PARTICIPANTS

Numbers in parentheses indicate the pages on which the authors' contributions begin.

Emmanuel T. Akporiaye (91), *Department of Biology, University of New Mexico, Albuquerque, New Mexico 87131*

Louise Albagli, *Orange County Health Department, Santa Ana, California 92701*

Cynthia C. Alley (631), *Center for Disease Control, Atlanta, Georgia 30333*

Richard H. Altieri (159), *Nassau County Department of Health, Hempstead, New York 11551*

Nina Amosenkova (335), *Pasteur Institute of Epidemiology and Microbiology, Leningrad, USSR*

Robert L. Anacker (159, 171, 179), *Laboratory of Microbial Structure and Function, Rocky Mountain Laboratories, Hamilton, Montana 59840*

John F. Anderson (559), *Connecticut Agricultural Experiment Station, New Haven, Connecticut 06504*

Adam S. Aragon (91), *Department of Biology, University of New Mexico, Albuquerque, New Mexico 87131*

Michael S. Ascher (133), *Department of Medicine, Infectious Diseases Division, University of California, Irvine, California 92717*

Jeanette Ashwood, *Albion, Washington 99102*

William H. Atkinson (411), *Department of Microbiology and Immunology, University of South Alabama College of Medicine, Mobile, Alabama 36688*

Ernest Austin (179), *Department of Pediatrics, Duke University Medical Center, Durham, North Carolina 27710*

Oswald G. Baca (91), *Department of Biology, University of New Mexico, Albuquerque, New Mexico 87131*

J. Howard Barrick (159), *Department of Public Health, State of Tennessee, Nashville, Tennessee 37219*

Jorge L. Benach (149, 603, 611), *New York State Department of Health, SUNY at Stony Brook, Stony Brook, New York 11794*

A. Louis Bourgeois (61, 71, 201), *Department of Microbiology, Naval Medical Research Institute, National Naval Medical Center, Bethesda, Maryland 20014*

Marilyn F. Bozeman, *Bureau of Biologics, Bethesda, Maryland 20014*

David B. Bromely, *Department of Microbiology, West Virginia University Medical Center, Morgantown, West Virginia 26506*

John B. Brooks, (631), *Center for Disease Control, Atlanta, Georgia 30333*

Willy Burgdorfer (139, 255, 281, 559, 585, 595), *Epidemiology Branch, Rocky Mountain Laboratories, Hamilton, Montana 59840*

Barbara G. Cain (347), *Department of Pathology, School of Medicine, University of North Carolina, Chapel Hill, North Carolina 27514*

John L. Cantrell (115), *Laboratory of Microbial Structure and Function, Rocky Mountain Laboratories, Hamilton, Montana 59840*

Elizabeth A. Casper (139, 171, 179, 575), *Epidemiology Branch, Rocky Mountain Laboratories, Hamilton, Montana 59840*

Bobbe Christenson, *School of Public Health, University of Texas, Houston, Texas 77025*

Herald R. Cox (11), *Hamilton, Montana 59840*

Carolyn Crump (159), *Department of General Services, Division of Consolidated Laboratory Services, Commonwealth of Virginia, Richmond, Virginia 23298*

Todd A. Damrow (115), *Laboratory of Microbial Structure and Function, Rocky Mountain Laboratories, Hamilton, Montana 59840*

Gregory A. Dasch (61, 71), *Department of Microbiology, Naval Medical Research Institute, National Naval Medical Center, Bethesda, Maryland 20014*

Jeffrey P. Davis (139), *Department of Pediatrics, Duke University Medical Center, Durham, North Carolina 27710*

David T. Dennis (201), *U. S. Naval Medical Research Unit, Number Two, Jakarta, Indonesia*

Vivian Dickinson (179), *Department of Pediatrics, Duke University Medical Center, Durham, North Carolina 27710*

John P. Donahue (441), *Department of Microbiology, West Virginia University Medical Center, Morgantown, West Virginia 26506*

Harold Dowda, Jr. (159), *South Carolina Department of Health and Environmental Control, Columbia, South Carolina 29201*

Richard J. Duma, *Medical College of Virginia, Virginia Commonwealth University, Richmond, Virginia 23298*

Robert Edelman, *NIAID, MIDP, National Institutes of Health, Bethesda, Maryland 20205*

E. Edlinger, *Virus Diagnostic and Rickettsial Unit, Pasteur Institute, Paris, France*

Bennett L. Elisberg, *Bureau of Biologics, Bethesda, Maryland 20014*

L. Bruce Elliott (159), *Texas Department of Health, Austin, Texas 78756*

Richard W. Emmons, *Viral and Rickettsial Disease Laboratory, California Department of Health Services, Berkeley, California 94704*

Richard C. Y. Fang (201), *Penghu Naval Base Hospital, Pescadores Islands, Taiwan*

Abdulrahman Farhang-Azad (363, 569), *Department of Microbiology, University of Maryland School of Medicine, Baltimore, Maryland 21201*

William F. Firth, *Department of Pathology, University of North Carolina at Chapel Hill, Chapel Hill, North Carolina 27514*

Harvey R. Fischman (569), *Johns Hopkins School of Public Health, Baltimore, Maryland 21205*

Paul Fiset (569), *Department of Microbiology, University of Maryland School of Medicine, Baltimore, Maryland 21201*

James D. Folds, *Department of Bacteriology and Immunology, University of North Carolina School of Medicine, Chapel Hill, North Carolina 27514*

John P. Fox, *Department of Epidemiology and International Health, University of Washington, Seattle, Washington 98195*

Frank R. Gonzales (453, 493), *Department of Microbiology, University of Kansas, Lawrence, Kansas 66045*

James R. Greenwood (133), *Department of Medicine, University of California, Irvine, California 92717*

Gail S. Habicht (149), *Department of Pathology, School of Medicine, SUNY at Stony Brook, Stony Brook, New York 11794*

Ted Hackstadt (267, 431), *Laboratory of Microbial Structure and Function, Rocky Mountain Laboratories, Hamilton, Montana 59840*

Barbara Hanson (503), *Department of Microbiology, University of Maryland School of Medicine, Baltimore, Maryland 21201*

Alyne Harrison (347), *Center for Disease Control, Atlanta, Georgia 30333*

Stanley F. Hayes (281, 585, 595), *Epidemiology Branch, Rocky Mountain Laboratories, Hamilton, Montana 59840*

Karim E. Hechemy (159, 171), *New York State Department of Health, Albany, New York 12201*

Charles G. Helmick (547), *Viral Disease Division, Center for Disease Control, Atlanta, Georgia 30333*

Jane Lea Hicks (171, 179), *North Carolina State Laboratory of Public Health, Raleigh, North Carolina 27611*

James C. Hill, *Development and Applications Branch, NIAID, National Institutes of Health, Bethesda, Maryland 20205*

Jerry R. Hindman (159), *Department of Public Health, State of Tennessee, Nashville, Tennessee 37202*

David Hinrichs, *Washington State University, Pullman, Washington 99163*

Joseph T. Horman (569), *Communicable Disease Division, Maryland Department of Health and Mental Hygiene, Baltimore, Maryland 21201*

Alexander A. Hubert, *Preventive Medicine Activity, Madigan Army Medical Center, Tacoma, Washington 98431*

Robert C. Humphres, *Leprosy Research Unit, U. S. Public Health Service Hospital, San Francisco, California 94122*

Susumu Ito (213, 229), *Department of Anatomy, Harvard Medical School, Boston, Massachusetts 02115*

William L. Jellison (517), *Hamilton, Montana 59840*

Thomas R. Jerrells (191), *Department of Rickettsial Diseases, Walter Reed Army Institute of Research, Walter Reed Army Medical Center, Washington, D. C. 20012*

James W. Johnson, *Aerobiology Division, U. S. Army Medical Research Institute of Infectious Diseases, Fort Detrick, Frederick, Maryland 21701*

William S. Jordan, Jr., *NIAID, National Institutes of Health, Bethesda, Maryland 20205*

J. Mehsen Joseph (159), *Department of Health and Mental Hygiene, State of Maryland, Baltimore, Maryland 21201*

Bernard Kaaserer, *Kitzbühel, Austria*

Theodor Khavkin (335), *333-C Growells Rd., Highland Park, New Jersey 08904*

George Killgore (159), *Kentucky Bureau for Health Services, Commonwealth of Kentucky, Frankfort, Kentucky 40601*

Robert C. Kimbrough III (125), *Good Samaritan Hospital and Medical Center, Portland, Oregon 97210*

Claes-Otto L. Kindmark (103), *Department of Infectious Diseases, University Hospital, Uppsala, Sweden*

Henry N. Kirkman (621), *Department of Pediatrics, University of North Carolina School of Medicine, Chapel Hill, North Carolina 27514*

Karl T. Kleeman (159, 171, 179), *North Carolina State Laboratory of Public Health, Raleigh, North Carolina 27611*

Jerry Kudlac (159), *Oklahoma State Department of Health, Oklahoma City, Oklahoma 73105*

William E. Kuriger (483), *Department of Plant Pathology, Georgia Experiment Station, University of Georgia, Experiment, Georgia 30312*

Jay L. Lancaster, Jr. (595), *Department of Entomology, Division of Agriculture, University of Arkansas, Fayetteville, Arkansas 72701*

Robert S. Lane (575), *Agricultural Experiment Station, Division of Entomology and Parasitology, University of California, Berkeley, California 94720*

Mike N. Laney, *Research Triangle Institute, Research Triangle Park, North Carolina 27709*

James V. Lange (347), *Department of Pathology, University of North Carolina, School of Medicine, Chapel Hill, North Carolina 27514*

Michael S. Loving, *Division of Vector Control, South Carolina Department of Health and Environmental Control, Columbia, South Carolina 29201*

J. Newton MacCormack (171, 179), *Division of Health Services, North Carolina Department of Human Resources, Raleigh, North Carolina 27602*

Louis A. Magnarelli (559), *Connecticut Agricultural Experiment Station, New Haven, Connecticut 06504*

Louis P. Mallavia, *Department of Bacteriology and Public Health, Washington State University, Pullman, Washington 99164*

Nyven J. Marchette, *Department of Tropical Medicine and Medical Microbiology, University of Hawaii at Manoa, Honolulu, Hawaii 96816*

Irene L. Martinez (91), *Department of Biology, University of New Mexico, Albuquerque, New Mexico 87131*

Anthony J. Mavros (255, 585) *Epidemiology Branch, Rocky Mountain Laboratories, Hamilton, Montana 59840*

Thomas F. McCaul (267), *Laboratory of Microbial Structure and Function, Rocky Mountain Laboratories, Hamilton, Montana 59840*

Joseph E. McDade (631), *Center for Disease Control, Atlanta, Georgia 30333*

Edith E. Michaelson (159), *New York State Department of Health, Albany, New York 12201*

Elizabeth T. Miller (327), *Department of Microbiology and Immunology, University of South Alabama College of Medicine, Mobile, Alabama 36688*

James R. Murphy, *Department of Microbiology, University of Maryland School of Medicine, Baltimore, Maryland 21201*

William F. Myers (313), *Department of Microbiology, University of Maryland School of Medicine, Baltimore, Maryland 21201*

Beverly R. Norment *Epidemiology Branch, Rocky Mountain Laboratories, Hamilton, Montana 59840*

Edwin V. Oaks (461), *Department of Microbiology, University of Maryland School of Medicine, Baltimore, Maryland 21201*

James G. Olson (201), *Yale Arbovirus Research Unit, Yale University, New Haven, Connecticut 06510*

Richard A. Ormsbee (125), *Hamilton, Montana 59840*

Joseph V. Osterman (43, 191), *Department of Rickettsial Diseases, Walter Reed Army Institute of Research, Walter Reed Army Medical Center, Washington, D. C. 20012*

Soo P. Ouyang (603), *Department of Applied Mathematics, SUNY at Stony Brook, Stony Brook, New York 11794*

David Paretsky (453, 493), *Department of Microbiology, University of Kansas, Lawrence, Kansas 66045*

Jagdish Patel (159), *Department of Health and Mental Hygiene, State of Maryland, Baltimore, Maryland 21201*

Marius G. Peacock (103, 125, 375), *Epidemiology Branch, Rocky Mountain Laboratories, Hamilton, Montana 59840*

Olivier Péter, *Institute of Zoology, University of Neuchâtel, Neuchâtel, Switzerland*

Paul V. Phibbs, Jr. (421), *MCV Station, Medical College of Virginia, Richmond, Virginia 23298*

Cornelius B. Philip, *California Academy of Sciences, San Francisco, California 94118*

Robert N. Philip (139, 159, 171, 179, 575), *Epidemiology Branch, Rocky Mountain Laboratories, Hamilton, Montana 59840*

Horace Rees, *Environmental and Life Sciences Division, U. S. Army Dugway Proving Ground, Dugway, Utah 84022*

Yasuko Rikihisa (213, 229), *Department of Anatomy, Harvard Medical School, Boston, Massachusetts 02115*

James Rust, *Pan American Health Organization, Washington, D. C. 20037*

Pekka Saikku, *Department of Pathobiology, School of Public Health and Community Medicine, University of Washington, Seattle, Washington 98195*

Sandra J. Sasowski (159), *New York State Department of Health, Albany, New York 12201*

Norman W. Schaad (483), *Department of Plant Pathology, University of Georgia, Georgia Experiment Station, Experiment, Georgia 30312*

John R. Seal (3), *NIAID, National Institutes of Health, Bethesda, Maryland 20205*

Kenneth W. Sell, *NIAID, National Institutes of Health, Bethesda, Maryland 20205*

Daniel J. Sexton (139), *Department of Medicine, Duke University Medical Center, Durham, North Carolina 27710*

David J. Silverman (241), *Department of Microbiology, University of Maryland School of Medicine, Baltimore, Maryland 21201*

Jonathan F. Smith (461), *Department of Microbiology, University of Maryland School of Medicine, Baltimore, Maryland 21201*

Laurel A. Smith (603, 611), *Department of Applied Mathematics, SUNY at Stony Brook, Stony Brook, New York 11794*

D. Sorley (569), *Communicable Disease Division, Maryland Department of Health and Mental Hygiene, Baltimore, Maryland 21201*

Alan J. Spicer (375), *British Military Hospital, Münster, West Germany*

James H. Steele, *Health Science Center at Houston, University of Texas, Houston, Texas 77025*

Herbert G. Stoenner, *Rocky Mountain Laboratories, Hamilton, Montana 59840*

Leo A. Thomas (595), *Epidemiology Branch, Rocky Mountain Laboratories, Hamilton, Montana 59840*

Herbert A. Thompson (441), *Department of Microbiology, West Virginia University Medical Center, Morgantown, West Virginia 26506*

Mary F. Thornton (133), *Department of Medicine, University of California, Irvine California, Public Health Laboratory, Orange County Health Department, Santa Ana, California*

William J. Todd (255), *Epidemiology Branch, Rocky Mountain Laboratories, Hamilton, Montana 59840*

Robert Traub (363, 517), *Department of Microbiology, University of Maryland School of Medicine, Baltimore, Maryland 21201*

Jenifer Turco (81), *Department of Microbiology and Immunology, University of South Alabama College of Medicine, Mobile, Alabama 36688*

Anna D. Waddell (241), *Department of Microbiology, University of Maryland School of Medicine, Baltimore, Maryland 21201*

David H. Walker (347, 621), *Department of Pathology, University of North Carolina School of Medicine, Chapel Hill, North Carolina 27514*

Noel L. Warner (91), *Department of Biology, University of New Mexico, Albuquerque, New Mexico 87131*

Emilio Weiss (387), *Department of Microbiology, Naval Medical Research Institute, National Naval Medical Center, Bethesda, Maryland 20014*

David E. Wells (631), *Center for Disease Control, Atlanta, Georgia 30333*

Dennis J. White (603, 611), *New York State Department of Health, Saranac Lake, New York 12983*

Jack E. Whitescarver, *NIAID, National Institutes of Health, Bethesda, Maryland 20205*

Catherine M. Wilfert (139, 171, 179), *Department of Pediatrics, Duke University Medical Center, Durham, North Carolina 27710*

Jim C. Williams (103, 115, 267, 375, 431, 473), *Laboratory of Microbial Structure and Function, Rocky Mountain Laboratories, Hamilton, Montana 59840*

Herbert H. Winkler (81, 327, 401, 411, 421), *Department of Microbiology and Immunology, University of South Alabama College of Medicine, Mobile, Alabama 36688*

William G. Winkler (547), *Viral Disease Division, Center for Disease Control, Atlanta, Georgia 30333*

Laura Winters, *Pullman, Washington 99163*

Charles L. Wisseman, Jr. (241, 293, 313, 363, 461, 503, 569), *Department of Microbiology, University of Maryland School of Medicine, Baltimore, Maryland 21201*

Peter H. Wittenberg (621), *Department of Pathology, Gaston Memorial Hospital, Gastonia, North Carolina 28052*

Theodore E. Woodward (17), *University of Maryland Hospital, University of Maryland School of Medicine, Baltimore, Maryland 21201*

William E. Woodward, *The University of Texas Medical School, Houston, Texas 77030*

George P. Wray (255), *Department of Molecular, Cellular, and Developmental Biology, University of Colorado, Boulder, Colorado 80309*

Diane Young (159), *Kentucky Bureau for Health Services, Commonwealth of Kentucky, Frankfort, Kentucky 40601*

Robert J. Zahorchak (401), *Department of Microbiology and Immunology, University of South Alabama College of Medicine, Mobile, Alabama 36688*

Michael Zdeb (159), *New York Department of Health, Albany, New York 12201*

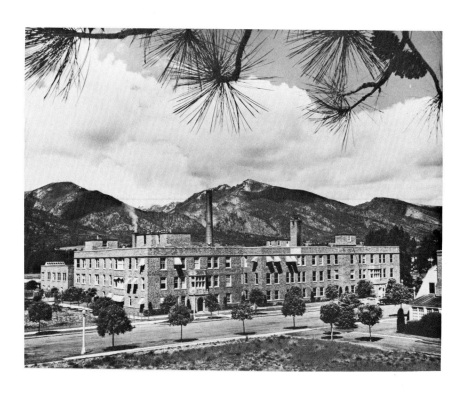

The Rocky Mountain Laboratories in Hamilton, Montana

FOREWORD

Because the initial discovery of the cause of Rocky Mountain spotted fever was made in the Bitterroot Valley, it is indeed fitting that this conference was held at the Rocky Mountain Laboratories, Hamilton, Montana, the "birthplace" of rickettsiology. Nearly 75 years have elapsed since Dr. Howard Ricketts of the University of Chicago demonstrated conclusively that the tick, *Dermacentor andersoni,* was the vector of the spotted fever agent, which was later named *Rickettsia rickettsii* in his honor. Early studies on the problem were supported partially by Montana and various universities, but after 1932, when the Rocky Mountain Laboratory became a field station of the U.S. Public Health Service, all research and control program on spotted fever was supported by the federal government. Many of the highlights of this long period of research on rickettsial diseases are listed in the introductory remarks of Dr. John Seal, Deputy Director, National Institute of Allergy and Infectious Diseases.

The program for this conference is a blend of modern molecular biology and the more traditional investigations on the epidemiology, serology, and immunology of rickettsial diseases and on the ecology of these obligate intracellular parasites. Of 55 papers presented at the conference, 19 dealt with research on the ultrastructure, biochemistry, and metabolism of rickettsiae. Although none dealt specifically with attempts to obtain *in vitro* growth, many of the research efforts were designed to elucidate complex host–parasite subcellular interrelationships that affect their metabolism.

Another major section of the conference was concerned with immunologic aspects of rickettsial diseases, isolation and characterization of antigens, and the development of improved methods of diagnostic serology. Many of the latter studies were done in combination with epidemiologic investigations of spotted fever in eastern states, where the prevalence of the disease has increased remarkably since 1960. Successful in soliciting the participation of the more prominent American rickettsiologists in the program, the organizing committee has assembled an interesting and informative compilation of the latest information on rickettsial diseases.

Herbert G. Stoenner
Asst. Scientific Director, NIAID
Rocky Mountain Laboratories

PREFACE

The Conference on Rickettsiae and Rickettsial Diseases held September 3–5, 1980, at the Rocky Mountain Laboratories in Hamilton, Montana, was organized to assess the state of rickettsial research in the United States where in recent years a steady increase in the number of Rocky Mountain spotted fever cases and revolutionary advances in methodology have rekindled interest in rickettsial research, particularly of Rocky Mountain spotted fever. Ninety-eight scientists from 22 different states and 5 from European countries attended the conference program, which included papers in immunity and immunology, ultrastructure, biology, biochemistry and metabolism, and ecology and epidemiology of rickettsiae and/or rickettsial diseases. Each of these topics was introduced by a lecture providing a general review of the particular subject or of the papers to be presented.

This book is a complete collection of talks, lectures, and research papers given at the conference. Its primary purpose is to provide rickettsiologists, microbiologists, parasitologists, physicians, epidemiologists, health educators and administrators, as well as interested students, a thorough insight into the many challenging aspects of current rickettsial research conducted in the United States. It should also serve as a comprehensive reference source for specialists engaged in rickettsial research and in health and educational activities.

The conference was partly funded by the National Institute of Allergy and Infectious Diseases of the National Institutes of Health. We, therefore, gratefully acknowledge the support and encouragement provided by Dr. Richard Krause, Director, and by Dr. Kenneth Sell, Scientific Director of that Institute. We would also like to express our appreciation to the administrators of the Rocky Mountain Laboratories, particularly Dr. Robert N. Philip, Acting Chief of the Epidemiology Branch, and Mr. Robert W. Steiner,

Chief of the Operations Branch, as well as to all those staff members who assisted with the organization of the conference. Finally, we wish to acknowledge the superb help of Mrs. Helen Donovan in assembling this book.

Willy Burgdorfer
Robert L. Anacker

INTRODUCTION AND GENERAL ADDRESS

THE UNITED STATES PUBLIC HEALTH SERVICE
AND RICKETTSIAL DISEASES,
PAST, PRESENT, FUTURE

John R. Seal

National Institute of Allergy and
Infectious Diseases
National Institutes of Health
Bethesda, Maryland

I. INTRODUCTION

Your co-chairmen, Drs. Burgdorfer and Anacker, kindly in-
vited me to open the conference. I am to welcome you and that
I do. I am glad to be here with you because it has been 5
years since I have visited the Rocky Mountain Laboratory. I
am doubly pleased to be able to attend this conference and to
revisit the laboratory. I also bring you greetings from
Dr. Krause, our Director, who is in China this week.

I was also asked to say a few words about NIAID support
for rickettsial disease research, past, present and future.
For any that might not be familiar with government jargon,
NIAID means the National Institute of Allergy and Infectious
Diseases of the National Institutes of Health.

Before going further, I should say that NIAID is the direct lineal descendant of the one-room laboratory established
by Dr. Joseph Kinyoun in 1887 at the Marine Hospital on Staten
Island, New York, for the study of cholera and other quaran-
tinable diseases. By 1891, that laboratory had been named the
Hygienic Laboratory, moved to Washington, and enlarged. The
Marine Hospital Service became the U.S. Public Health Service
in 1912. Since the histories of the Public Health Service
(PHS) and rickettsial diseases research are inextricably
bound in this century, I must talk about the PHS rather than
NIAID.

3

ISBN 0-12-143150-9

A. The Past

The major Public Health Service involvement has been with Rocky Mountain spotted fever (RMSF), one of the few truly American diseases. It was responsible for the Laboratory where we meet today. I have compiled a listing of significant events between 1902, when this involvement began, to 1980. These events, labeled milestones, were too many to recount here. I have had them copied so you can take them home and review them at your leisure.[1] I cannot vouch for the correctness of every item and hope that anyone that can correct or add to the list will write me. Neither will I pretend that these are as complete as some might desire.

The history divides well into several periods. One, from 1902 to 1910, was a period of intense interest in a newly discovered disease. Brilliant work by two University of Minnesota pathologists, described both the clinical and pathological features of RMSF; the peculiarity of its occurrence on the west side of the Bitterroot Valley; identified the wood tick as the probable vector and the Columbian ground squirrel as the probable infected host. These two, Drs. Wilson and Chowning, had come to the Bitterroot at the request of the Montana State Board of Health. Also at the request of the State, PHS officers came from the Hygienic Laboratory each summer, reporting the Wilson and Chowning findings to Washington, and adding data of their own.

In 1904, one PHS officer, Dr. Charles Stiles, questioned the Wilson and Chowning findings, setting off the controversy that brought Dr. Howard Ricketts from the University of Chicago to the Bitterroot in 1906. Independently and under state auspices, Dr. W. V. King, an entomologist, arrived the same year. There was close collaboration between King's work on the ecology and Ricketts' experimental work. By 1908, Ricketts and King had firmly established the wood tick as the vector, defined the basics of the tick-host system, demonstrated transmission in vertebrates by infected ticks, and described the organism in microscopic studies. This description was confirmed by Wolbach 10 years later who gave Ricketts' name to the organism. Ricketts also suggested that control could be obtained by exterminating the rodent host of ticks and by dipping large animal hosts. In 1909, the Montana Legislature appropriated $6,000 to continue Ricketts' work. The State Treasury had to wait until it accumulated the money and did not release the funds until December. By this time Ricketts had gone to Mexico where he died of typhus a few months later.

---

[1]Available on request.

The second period, 1911 to 1921, was largely marked by further ecological studies and the development of control measures. In 1911, the sending of a PHS officer, Dr. Thomas McClintic, to the Bitterroot to initiate a control program created a bitter controversy because the Board of Health had bypassed Dr. Robert Cooley, a leading entomologist, who had already organized a control program following Ricketts' suggestions. This controversy led to the establishment of the Montana Board of Entomology; its Director, Dr. Cooley, brought Dr. Ralph Parker from Massachusetts and in 1916 placed him in charge of a laboratory to study RMSF. This laboratory was moved to Victor in 1918.

The third period, 1921 to 1948, was centered about development and production of vaccines in response to public and political pressures arising from the death of a prominent Montana legislator from the disease.

Pressure from the U.S. Congress caused the PHS to employ Dr. Parker, move his laboratory to an abandoned schoolhouse in Hamilton, and designate it as a field station of the PHS. Dr. Roscoe Spencer was sent from the Hygienic Laboratory to work with Dr. Parker and develop a vaccine. By 1924, following the lead of a Czechoslovakian report on a typhus vaccine, Spencer had developed from ticks a vaccine that protected guinea pigs. Returning to Hamilton he and Parker further perfected the vaccine and Spencer initiated human trials by taking it himself. Parker and Cooley followed when Spencer survived. Soon vaccine was made available to the public.

By 1927, demands for vaccine far outstripped production. The Montana Board of Entomology obtained a $60,000 appropriation and built a new tick-proof building in Hamilton for vaccine production. This was leased by the PHS. In 1932, following a Congressional Act that changed the Hygienic Laboratory into the National Institute of Health, Drs. Spencer and Cooley engineered the PHS purchase of the building from the State of Montana and funds for its expansion to accommodate the further demand for vaccine from neighboring states. In 1936, Dr. Herald Cox joined the laboratory and converted the production process from infected ticks to the chick embryo. This set the stage for the World War II years when the Laboratory produced a high percentage of the egg-grown RMSF, typhus and yellow fever vaccines needed by the U.S. military. Additional buildings needed for this effort brought the RML to about its present size.

In 1937, RML became a field activity of the Division of Infectious Diseases of the National Institute of Health.

The fourth period was from 1948 to now. In 1948, the Division of Infectious Diseases, National Institute of Health, became the National Microbiological Institute, National Institutes of Health. The RML became an intramural laboratory.

In 1955, the name was further changed to the National Institute of Allergy and Infectious Diseases (NIAID). RML lost its vaccine production mission in 1949 and its research staff was expanded for work on other zoonoses, arthropod-borne viruses, tuberculosis and slow virus diseases. Research on rickettsial diseases was focused on further definition of the ecology and epidemiology, on laboratory diagnosis, and on Q fever vaccine. Most of its work on RMSF in the 1970's has been in the southeastern U.S., there being little or no disease in the West. I need not say more because you will be hearing from those more directly responsible for recent history.

The history prior to 1948 is thus marked by brilliant initial work on a newly discovered disease, followed by nearly 40 years of applied work on control and prevention dictated by public and political pressures. The need for developing control measures for rickettsial diseases, particularly typhus, Q fever, and scrub typhus, also created the Armed Forces Epidemiological Board's Commission on Rickettsial Diseases. The demise of that Commission in 1973 and the later cutback in Army funding at Congressional direction has left the NIAID in the awkward spot of being the principal Government supporter of rickettsial research but not having been given any extra funds to meet this responsibility.

B.   The Present

Grants are initiated by the investigators and with few exceptions awarded strictly on the basis of merit judgments by peers on NIH Study Sections as far as the money will let us go. Contracts are initiated by the Institute and have well-defined, short-range objectives.

The following series of tables will summarize NIAID dollar support to rickettsial diseases research in fiscal year 1979. I have a handout of these data for your convenience. Table 1 reflects the total of investigator-originated applications that were judged sufficiently meritorious by Study Sections to be funded in competition with all other applications.

TABLE 1. NIAID Grants for Rickettsial Diseases
Research, 1979

Walker, David H., University of North Carolina Pathogenesis of Cell Injury	$ 56,815
Waner, Joseph L., Harvard University Spotted Fever in Dogs, Ticks and Man on Cape Cod	2,484
Winkler, Herbert H., University of South Alabama Permeability of Epidemic Typhus Rickettsia	117,350
Total	$176,649

Table 2 summarizes our contract program. It reflects our
recent entry into support of the Army effort to develop a vaccine and to find suitable field conditions for its testing.
Not reflected is the support to a volunteer facility at the
University of Maryland where vaccinated volunteers will be
challenged during the next year. That one trial involving
about 20 volunteers will cost about $100,000.

TABLE 2. NIAID Contracts for Rickettsial Diseases
Research, 1979

Wilfert, Catherine, Duke University Medical Center Epidemiologic Study of RMSF	$102,209
Fischman, Harvey R. Johns Hopkins University Epidemiologic Study of RMSF	484,241
Walker, David, University of North Carolina Rocky Mountain Spotted Fever Vaccine	102,513
U.S. Army, RMSF Vaccine	10,821
Total	$699,784

Table 3 reflects the total of fellowship training applications that have made it through Study Sections. An institu-
tional training application in recent years has had to be in
the top 5 to 10% of priority scores to be funded. None on

rickettsial research have made it. This table does not reflect students receiving training by employment as assistants
on research grants.

TABLE 3. NIAID Training in Rickettsial Diseases
Research, 1979

Turco, Jennifer, University of South Alabama   ca $15,000
Phospholipid and Fatty Acid Composition of
    Rickettsiae

Zahorchak, Robert J., University of South Alabama   15,000
Energy Transduction in Rickettsia prowazekii

| | Total | $30,000 |

Table 4 summarizes the total in extramural and intramural
expenditures. Intramural spending may be overestimated and
might actually be closer to $1 million.

TABLE 4. NIAID Dollar Support to Rickettsial
Diseases Research, 1979

Total, extramural projects		$ 906,433
Intramural projects		1,531,584
	Total	$2,438,017

C. The Future

Despite the extraordinary and partially successful efforts
of our Director to mobilize support for increased budgets for
the NIAID, we still lag behind from the wide-spread belief
that antibiotics had ended the problem of infectious diseases
and failure to get adequate budget increases to more than
offset inflation in past years. Concern for the economy as a
whole has forced sympathetic Congressmen to curtail efforts
to increase appropriations for the NIAID in 1981, and we have
no reason to be overly optimistic about 1982 or beyond. The
bright spot is that last week the House restored funds for

training in 1981 to the 1980 level, there having been no
funds for competing training in the President's budget.

It will do rickettsiologists no good to band together into
an old boys' club, moan for the old days when the money was
easy, and, like the auto industry, demand protection because
you can't compete. There is no validity to the plea of being
an endangered species, because new Wilsons, Chownings,
Ricketts, Cooleys, Parkers, Spencers, or other giants of yore
will arise again should the need demand.

Rickettsial diseases research will have a future in the
ability of a new generation of scientists to ask important
questions, design good experiments, and convince their peers
that the results will be important, not only to rickettsial
diseases in particular but to microbiological research as a
whole. We do not know enough about obligate parasitism and
the ability of a pathogenic organism to live indefinitely in
symbiosis with its human host. We don't know enough about
immunity to such organisms. There are thousands of things
to be done. Few people want to work on pathogenic rickettsiae
because of the dangers involved, but new technologies now
make it possible to circumvent some of the hazards.

You must stay in the mainstreams of science. Results of
your research should be reported at such meetings as the
American Society of Microbiology where you can learn from
others and perhaps excite newcomers to the field. I have no
objection to meetings of the kind held here and at Port
Deposit on a periodic basis; but these should be secondary
outlets for your research, not primary.

Finally, I should say that you have a mentor at the NIAID
who is sympathetic to your interests. Dr. William Jordan,
Director of the Microbiology and Infectious Diseases Extramural Program, has served with the Armed Forces Epidemiological
Board for many years and is a consultant to the Bureau of Biologics. His interest is reflected in our recent contract activities related to an RMSF vaccine.

I am encouraged to see so many new and young faces. This
whole meeting presents a much brighter outlook than was the
case in 1972 when the NIAID convened rickettsiologists in
Atlanta to assess the state of the art and its practitioners.
My estimate is that rickettsial diseases research is on the
way up. This, as my West Virginia mountaineer cousins would
say -- "Pleasures me greatly."

REMINISCENCES

Herald R. Cox, Sc.D. - Retired

When I first came to the Rocky Mountain Laboratory in May
1936, it was distinctly understood that my primary task was
to try to develop a new type of vaccine for Rocky Mountain
spotted fever, to replace the wood-tick vaccine that had been
developed by Drs. Roscoe R. Spencer and Ralph R. Parker, and
which was recognized to be quite hazardous, as well as expensive to prepare. Prior to coming to Hamilton, I had spent 4
years at the Rockefeller Institute for Medical Research in
New York City. During this period, I had acquired considerable experience using chicken embryo tissue cultures in 50 ml
Ehrlenmeyer flasks for the cultivation of such viruses as
Eastern equine encephalomyelitis, Western equine encephalomyelitis, St. Louis encephalitis and both the Indiana and New
Jersey strains of vesicular stomatitis. Thus, at Hamilton,
for the better part of 2 years, I used Ehrlenmeyer flask cultures of tissues derived from chicken embryos and chorio-
allantoic membranes, with a number of different preparations
of suspending nutrient media, in trying to grow rickettsial
organisms, without a bit of worthwhile success. Finally, I
became so depressed with my lack of success, that I offered
my resignation to our director, Dr. Parker, telling him that
perhaps he could find someone else who could succeed in doing
the job. Fortunately, Dr. Parker was an understanding person.
He told me to keep on trying, because he felt that sooner or
later I would get a break, and that he couldn't think of anyone trying any harder than I had to get the job done.
    In a little less than a month, I was able to go back and
tell Dr. Parker that I had found a tissue for growing rickettsiae, in what appeared to be goodly numbers, which, as you
know, was the yolk sac membrane of developing chicken embryos.
This was in the latter half of February 1938. This finding
came about in an experiment in which I was trying to cultivate
Q fever organisms (Coxiella burnetii), which we then knew as
Nine Mile fever. Since I didn't have enough chorio-allantoic

membrane or chicken embryonic tissues to carry out the controlled experiment that I had planned, I fortunately decided
to use yolk sac membrane tissue, which had been removed aseptically, because I was still using Ehrlenmeyer cultures in my
work. You can imagine my surprise and delight when on examining these cultures 5 to 6 days later, I found literally thousands of Q fever rickettsiae in the yolk sac cultures, but no
organisms in the cultures prepared from chorio-allantoic membranes or other chicken embryonic tissues. That night I was
too excited to sleep, and I thought why take the trouble to
prepare tissue cultures, when it would be so much simpler to
inoculate fertile hen's eggs directly into the yolk sac area,
through the air sac end of the egg. So at 4 o'clock in the
morning, I went back to the lab and did that. I may add that
it was just a short distance to the lab, because I then lived
just across the street from the lab, in the house in which
Dr. Jim Williams now lives. Anyway, as you know, that simple
procedure worked and made it possible to cultivate all members
of the rickettsial family of organisms, as well as a number
of other agents also.

Then in the early part of May 1938, Dr. Parker came into
my lab at about 11:00 one morning, and it was obvious that he
was very nervous and ill at ease, because he was chain smoking
cigarettes and coughing more than usual. He said, "Cox, Dr.
Dyer, Director of the Division of Infectious Diseases at the
National Institutes of Health in Bethesda, has just telephoned
me from Missoula. Dr. Dyer stated that he will be down to
Hamilton by about 1:00 or 1:30 this afternoon, and he doesn't
believe what you have written in your April report to the
National Institutes of Health, that you are able to cultivate
rickettsiae in great numbers in the fertile hen's egg." I
said to Dr. Parker, "Well let Dr. Dyer come, and just relax.
We have some good things to show Dr. Dyer in the way of slides
and titration tests in infected guinea pigs, and we are confident in the work that has been done."

I should add that my laboratory associates at that time
were John Bell and Gene Hughes, now both retired, and better
known now as Dr. E. John Bell and Lyndahl E. Hughes.[1]

---

[1]Since this paper was presented, all of us have been
greatly saddened by the untimely, accidental death of Gene
Hughes on Oct. 14, 1980. Both John Bell and Gene Hughes were
most honest, loyal and trusted workers and when I went to
Lederle Laboratories on Dec. 1, 1942, to be in charge of all
research and production activities in the viral and rickettsial field, there was many a time when I fervently wished I
had them with me, to give a helping hand.

Dr. Dyer came into the lab at about 1:30 p.m. It was the
first time we had ever met, and I soon learned that he was
one that came immediately to the point in his speech and did
not stand for any monkey business. The first thing that Dr.
Dyer said to me was, "Cox, I don't believe a damned word in
that recent monthly report of yours, in which you state that
you are able to cultivate rickettsiae in great numbers in fertile hen's eggs, because Dr. Ida Bengtson and I tried for
about 3 years to grow rickettsiae in fertile hen's eggs and
we didn't have a bit of luck." I said, "Dr. Dyer, did you
ever examine the yolk sac membrane tissue in those eggs to
see if any rickettsiae were there?" He said, "No, we didn't."
I said, "Well, that was your mistake, because that is where
you would find the rickettsiae. Now, let's quit arguing and
you sit down and look at these representative slides of spotted fever, epidemic typhus and Nine Mile fever, and then tell
me what you think of them." Well, Dr. Dyer sat down and
looked at slides for about 10-15 minutes. Then he turned
around and said, "Well, I'll be, but you've convinced me.
You surely have done what you stated you did." Then he stood
up and shook my hand, as if to seal the bargain. I can only
say, that from then on, both Dr. Dyer and Dr. Parker were my
firm and steadfast friends for as long as they lived, and I
certainly appreciated their friendship.

Before I left the Rocky Mountain Laboratory to go east to
Lederle Laboratories at Pearl River, N.Y., my associates and
I were using something like 750 to 1,000 fertile hen's eggs
a week, primarily to produce better vaccines, and we felt that
we were doing a pretty good job in using such a number of
eggs. However, when I got to Lederle, I really learned how
things can be in industry. First, I learned that Lederle had
prepared almost $800,000 worth of epidemic typhus vaccine that
wouldn't pass the required government potency test, and thus
had to be discarded. Further, Lederle then had contracts for
12,000 fertile hen's eggs per day for 6 days per week, with
the eggs costing 13 1/2 cents each, yet they had no tested
seed virus system in operation, whereby to consistently manufacture a good vaccine. It took approximately a 2 months'
period to get these troublesome things straightened out. In
the meantime, all the 12,000 eggs per day had to be diverted
into production of fertilizer, because if we had broken the
suppliers' contracts, it would have taken months for us to
get back into production again. After getting the seed virus
system into satisfactory operation, we used the 12,000 eggs
per day for approximately a 3-year period in making epidemic
typhus vaccine.

Then about 10 months after getting typhus vaccine into
production, we were asked by the Armed Forces to manufacture

two badly needed military items, namely, influenza vaccine
and Japanese B encephalitis vaccine. These contracts were accepted by Lederle, and thus we ended up using 46,000 fertile
hen's eggs a day, 12,000 eggs per day for typhus vaccine and
34,000 eggs per day for influenza vaccine. For Japanese B
encephalitis vaccine, we used the brain tissue from 6,000,
12-day-old infected white mice per day. At one time during
this episode, practically every commercial white mouse breeding laboratory in the United States was under contract to fur-
nish their mice to Lederle, and the Navy Medical Research Labs
had to come to us to get help so that they could get enough
mice to work with in some of their research projects.

For the 46,000 eggs per day contracts, Lederle had only
two suppliers. The first was Kerr Chickeries, located at
Flemington, N.J., about 80 miles distant from Lederle, who
supplied us with 19,000 eggs per day, and Pulis Farms, located
at Wyckoff, N.J., about 12 miles distant, who supplied us with
27,000 eggs per day. It may be of interest to note that Mr.
Peter Pulis of Pulis Farms later became president of the bank
in Wyckoff, N.J., which shows how some things work out.

Anyway, it is obvious that we at Lederle got quite a bit
of production experience during those months of the war years,
since it was claimed that Lederle over-all produced about 60
to 70 percent of all the vaccines used by the Allied Armies
during World War II.

I'm glad to report that all production lots of Lederle
typhus vaccine were required to pass potency tests at least
twice as high as were required by the government. Further,
no batches of typhus vaccine or influenza vaccine ever had to
be discarded and declared faulty, once we got the tested seed
virus system into operation. For this achievement, I wish to
give full credit to Timothy Kurotchkin, M.D., a white Russian
refugee from communist Russia, now deceased, who so ably
helped me to get the seed virus systems into operation during
those hectic years. I regret to state that Dr. Kurotchkin's
death came about following an attack of Cape Cod spotted fever, which at the time he believed to be a strain of epidemic
typhus. In addition, we had three other of our personnel to
die from acute laboratory infections during that period. The
first died from scrub typhus or tsutsugamushi disease, the
second from Russian Spring-Summer encephalitis virus and the
third from B virus (Brebner's virus) or simian herpes virus.

In looking back at those earlier days, particularly in
the rickettsial field, it doesn't seem possible that so much
progress has been made, especially in the areas of serological
diagnosis and immunological typing and identification of these
agents. Of course, one of the main stumbling blocks to progress was the fact that there was no easy or practical way to

grow the rickettsial agents in any quantity, until the yolk
sac membrane procedure was found. Following that finding,
Dr. Ida Bengtson of the National Institutes of Health was the
first to develop the complement-fixation test for rickettsial
agents, which has been widely used since then.

   In conclusion, there is now, of course, a whole battery
of more refined and definitive serological tests that have
been developed, such as: direct agglutination tests, microagglutination tests, so-called toxin neutralization tests,
antiglobulin tests, radio-immuno-precipitation (RIP) tests,
direct and indirect fluorescent antibody techniques, micro-
indirect fluorescent antibody techniques, and lastly, but not
necessarily the last, enzyme immuno-assays or enzyme immunosorbent assays (ELISA tests).

RICKETTSIAL DISEASES: CERTAIN UNSETTLED PROBLEMS IN THEIR HISTORICAL PERSPECTIVE

Theodore E. Woodward

Department of Medicine
University of Maryland
School of Medicine and Hospital
Baltimore, Maryland

I. INTRODUCTION

The rickettsial diseases, particularly epidemic typhus fever and Rocky Mountain spotted fever, to a lesser extent, have caused human deaths and suffering for many years. Their serious threat stimulated remarkable medical research and clinical observations which clarified their specific etiology, mode of transmission, pathogenesis, abnormal pathophysiologic changes, clinical manifestations, therapy and means of control.

All rickettsiae have similar morphologic appearances and behavior in arthropods and animals; yet, each specific rickettsial infection has its own distinctive clinical manifestations, host response and specific immunity. There was remarkable progress from 1906 when Ricketts first incriminated the tick and in 1909 when Nicolle showed the louse transmission of typhus until 1948 when the broad spectrum antibiotics were shown to be specifically and therapeutically effective. Yet, these diseases are unconquered, although they are relatively restricted as causes of human illness. Their potential is ever present and the possibility of their return is unlimited should health standards deteriorate to a level which would permit spread by their arthropod vectors, especially by the louse and ticks.

To be discussed are but a few unanswered problems where new information is needed with focus upon their historical perspective.

17

A.   Nature of the Angiitis: Agent Visualization

In 1919, S. Burt Wolbach published his Bible on Rocky
Mountain spotted fever (RMSF) on his thorough postmortem and
experimental studies (1). He studied the agent in primates
and reported the detailed postmortem findings of five cases
of RMSF. In his classic, he described the histologic lesions
and attributed the vasculitis to the parasite: "an acute specific endangiitis chiefly of the peripheral blood vessels."
The endovasculitis which typifies the disease was thoroughly
described and utilizing a modified Giemsa technique, he noted
intracytoplasmic rickettsiae in endothelial and muscle cells.
The character and evolution of the rash, the skin necrosis and
gangrene were attributed to the angiitis. Endothelial cells
were shown attached to intima in swollen arterial lesions with
fragmentation of the elastic lamina and the presence of the
lanceolate formed parasites in large numbers in free and attached endothelial cells and in smooth muscle cells of media.
The parasite was noted in vascular lesions of the skin. Shown
in Figure 1 is a vascular lesion with rickettsia in an endothelial cell.

Wolbach was struck by the similarities of the clinical and
pathological picture in laboratory animals and humans. Now, 60
years later, there is little to add to Wolbach's explanation
except that a toxin is known to promote capillary leakage and
that pathologic abnormalities may result from either immune

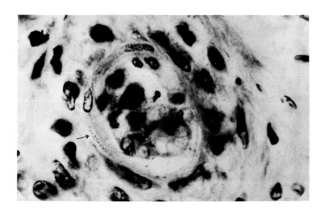

Fig. 1. Rocky Mountain spotted fever. An arteriolar lesion from the scrotal skin of a fatal case showing endothelial
proliferation: intracellular rickettsiae and a perivascular
reaction. [Reference (1)].

complex or cellular immune (hypersensitivity) reactions or
both. Pathologically there is correlation between endothelial
changes with identifiable rickettsiae in the vascular lesions
of the skin and other tissues.

B. Difficulties in Agent Identification

It is not very respectful to question any of Ricketts'
findings, particularly in view of the meticulous care with
which his studies were performed. In his early publication
(January 30, 1909), he described "diplococcoid bodies" and
short bacillary forms with considerable constancy in the blood
of guinea pigs and monkeys infected with RMSF and "no so frequently in the blood of men" (2). Giemsa stain was used exclusively. In his carefully prepared laboratory notes, Ricketts
made drawings of his parasite. Wolbach reported having observed the causative organism in an endothelial cell of a human
case in an ordinary blood film stained with Giemsa. He felt
that the bodies, when present in the circulating blood, were
only within phagocytic cells. On this point of identification
of the parasite, Wolbach compared one of Ricketts' original
preparations with those of his own made from the eggs of infected ticks. He felt "while Ricketts may have encountered the
true parasite of the disease in ticks, he was led hopelessly
astray by the occurrence of bacteria in his infected as well as
noninfected ticks" (1).
Lillie reported the autopsy findings of five cases of RMSF
(3). Although he made no special search for rickettsiae, he
found several clumps of minute basophilic, rod-shaped inclusions in swollen endothelial cells of thrombosed capillaries in
the skin, thyroid, liver and brain. In 1933, Harris showed
rickettsiae in the skin of a patient who contracted RMSF in
Tennessee (4). This 5-year-old girl died in June 1931. In
order to obviate some of the difficulties with Giemsa staining,
he utilized a modified method of Goodpasture's carbol anilin
fuchsin method staining and decolorized four times. The
stained rickettsial bodies which he visualized in endothelial
and muscle cells resembled classic rickettsiae. There was
significant myocarditis in this fatal case (see later discussion).
In 1931, Pinkerton and Maxcy reported the pathologic findings of a case of endemic typhus in Virginia in which rickettsial bodies, visualized in endothelial cells of skin specimens,
were stained by Wolbach's modification of the Giemsa method
(5). The bodies appear morphologically similar to rickettsiae
in endothelial cells. However, Maxcy's patient most likely
died of RMSF (or possibly <u>Rickettsia</u> <u>prowazekii</u> infection related to squirrels). The patient, a farmer, died of his acute

illness in June 1930. Of addiional interest was the histologic
presence of myocarditis in this case (to be discussed later).

C. Demonstration by Immune Fluorescence

It was only logical that the skin biopsy method of confirmation of RMSF be attempted since the illness is characterized by a progressive vasculitis and exanthem. Hence, the causative antigen would be expected to be present in the dermal
lesion.
    In 1976, Rickettsia rickettsii were positively identified
by the immune fluorescence technique in specimens of skin from
patients with RMSF taken as early as the third and as late as
the ninth day of illness (6). Skin specimens examined promptly
or held at -70°C are preferred although formalin-fixed paraffin
sections are adaptable to immune fluorescent methods (7).

D. Mechanism of Vasculitis

Harrell favored an abnormal antigen-antibody reaction (immune complex) to explain certain aspects of the vasculitis late
in illness; he noted that patients with spotted fever treated
with hyperimmune convalescent serum showed more capillary leakage and tissue edema than patients not given serum (8). Cutaneous capillary changes, vascular thrombosis and dermal ecchy-
moses are more prevalent late in the course of RMSF when humoral antibodies could interact with antigen and exaggerate the
vasculitis. Evidence which partially refutes the immune complex concept was derived from a well-studied patient who showed
no abnormalities of complement levels early or later in illness
(9). Successful treatment may have obviated a later, more
severe reaction. Complement interacts in immune complex

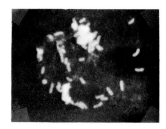

    Fig. 2. Immunofluorescent preparation of Rickettsia rick-
ettsii in a skin section from a macule taken on day 4 of RMSF.
Note coccal and bacillary forms (1000 x). [Reference (6)].

reactions; its role in late vascular abnormalities during RMSF is unclear.

Cell-mediated immunity may be an important mechanism useful for inhibition and eradication of rickettsiae in tissues. Patients convalescent from various rickettsioses exhibit delayed type hypersensitivity reactions to injected rickettsial antigen. Wisseman showed this in patients given the attenuated E strain of R. prowazekii who later developed positive skin tests to antigen injected intradermally 7 to 10 days later when humoral antibodies are present in variable titers (10). Cellular immune changes of the delayed hypersensitivity-type could contribute to the vasculitis.

Evaluation of T lymphocytes, lymphoblast formation and lymphokine production were reported by Ascher at USA Medical Research Institute of Infectious Diseases (11). These reactions are to be extended in volunteer studies now designed to evaluate more effective vaccines. Better clarification of the mechanism of vasculitis in RMSF should follow.

Wolbach's explanation for the vasculitis has come full circle -- vasculitis resulting from rickettsial parasitization of endothelial and muscle cells, toxic capillary action, immune complex and cellular (hypersensitivity) immune reactions, back to direct effects of rickettsiae.

II.   THE BRILL-MAXCY-DYER CONTRIBUTION TO
RECRUDESCENCE AND RAT-FLEA CYCLE OF TYPHUS

A. Brill's Disease

Acting against the advice of associates in 1910, Nathan Brill reported the results of his clinical observations in 221 febrile patients whose illness in New York City reminded him more of typhus than typhoid fever (12). Negative blood cultures and Widal reactions and lack of communicability of the illness led him to call it an illness of unknown cause, which is now correctly referred to as Brill-Zinsser disease or recrudescent typhus fever. Brill, in his classic publications said:

"In as much as these cases have been considered by almost all my colleagues in New York, in the past, as typhoid fever cases, it will be necessary to show the marks of differentiation.

"Clinically, this disease resembles typhus fever more than it does any other disease, and I should have felt that I had offered nothing to our nosology if it had been proved that typhus fever had lost its virulence, that it was constantly present in a community, that it was not communicable, that when it was present, epidemics of it

did not occur, and that it was no longer a grave and
fatal disease. But with typhus fever, as the great
masters of medicine have taught, such a conception
would be unjustifiable. Therefore, I believe this
disease not to be typhus fever.

"I should emphatically deprecate calling the disease 'pseudo typhoid fever' because the affection has
nothing in common with typhoid, paratyphoid, and
typhoid-colon or intermediate group infections. I
prefer to speak of it as an 'acute infectious disease
of unknown origin'."

During the late 19th century and for three decades in the
20th century, clinicians recognized sporadic cases of typhus
fever, often called endemic typhus, in the southeastern states
and in large harbor cities. Occasionally, the illness was er-
roneously referred to as Brill's disease.

The nature of Brill's disease was clarified by Zinsser who
correctly recognized it as a recrudescence of a milder epidemic
typhus infection which had occurred initially years earlier as
a primary illness in European countries where the illness was
endemic (13). It is possible that recurrent infections of the
other rickettsioses occur but such have not been recognized.
Viable rickettsiae remain in the tissues of humans long after
their recovery from the acute illness.

B. Rat-Flea Typhus (Maxcy)

In 1926, Kenneth Maxcy, a wise epidemiologist with a clinical background, observed patients and the environments related
to their illnesses, particularly in Alabama, Georgia, North
Carolina and Virginia. He appraised the geographic settings,
isolated rickettsiae from the blood of patients and noted their
antigenic similarity and differences when compared with R.
prowazekii and R. rickettsii (14). Based on his observations,
Maxcy concluded so perceptively:

"It is suggested as an hypothesis which seems to
afford a more plausible explanation of the mode of
transmission that a reservoir exists other than in
man, and this reservoir is in rodents, probably rats
and mice, from which this disease is occasionally
transmitted to man.

"The epidemiological characteristics afford no
evidence suggesting louse transmission and are
interpreted as being at variance with man to man
transfer by lice. The parasitic intermediaries
which are first suspected are fleas, mites or
possibly ticks."

Several Baltimore physicians played a part in confirmation
of Maxcy's prophecy. In 1930, a patient, Dr. Joseph Lipsky, a
physician-pharmacist, became ill with fever, headache and rash.
He was hospitalized at the Mercy Hospital on September 23,
1930. Dr. Louis A.M. Krause was his physician and Dr. Maurice
C. Pincoffs, Professor of Medicine at Maryland, consulted.
Their initial impression was typhoid fever. Blood cultures and
the Widal reaction were negative while the Proteus OX19 titer
reached 1/320 (15).

Epidemic typhus fever was the discharge diagnosis. On the
day of discharge, Doctor Lipsky's female clerk was hospitalized and placed in the same room with the same illness, as was
the male clerk 3 weeks later.

Appropriate specimens of sera and clinical data were sent
to the National Institutes of Health for confirmation. This
small epidemic led to the trapping of rats in the basement of
Doctor Lipsky's pharmacy at Pennsylvania Avenue and Laurens
Street, just across from Lafayette Market. Dyer and his associates, Rumreich and Badger, were successful in transmitting
the rickettsial agent to guinea pigs from brain suspensions and
from fleas taken from these rodents. They identified the murine reservoir of the rickettsia, incriminated the flea as a
vector fulfilling Maxcy's prophecy (16).

In 1969, I located Doctor Lipsky from a hint given by
Doctor Krause. He was busily practicing medicine in Odenton,
Maryland, near Fort Meade at age 77 and played tennis daily,
when possible. He recalled the large number of rats in the
basement of his store and attributed them to the foodstuffs
stored there by an Italian merchant who operated a stall across
the street. Doctor Lipsky remarked that fleas literally
swarmed through cracks in the floor "like pepper". Then, 40
years after his initial illness, Doctor Lipsky's serum showed
a low titer of complement fixing antibodies to murine typhus
antigen. He was the index case which prompted investigation
and identification of the rodent reservoir and flea vector.

Doctor Dyer confirmed for me, when I spoke to him in
Atlanta a few years later, that the traps were set by Rumreich
in the basement of the pharmacy. Dyer did not come to
Baltimore.

Doctor Lipsky allowed me to give him a 1.0 ml subcutaneous
injection of purified epidemic rickettsial vaccine (Breinl
strain); his lymphocytes and plasma cells demonstrated a phe-
nomenal 40-year memory; in 3 days he showed very high titers
of CF antibodies to R. prowazekii antigen of the 7 S type.
This is a typical antibody-globulin pattern of recall. Doctor
Lipsky died of natural causes at age 81.

Earlier we found about 10 percent rat infestation with murine typhus in the locale of food markets and grain depots in
Baltimore (15).

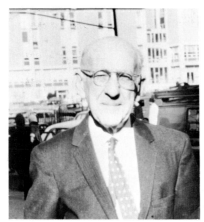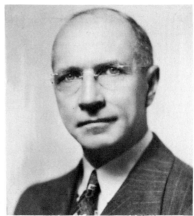

Fig. 3.   Joseph Lipsky, M.D., Odenton, Maryland.   Died
1971.
Fig. 4.   Kenneth F. Maxcy, M.D. (Courtesy of Mrs. Kenneth F.
Maxcy).

Maxcy settled in Baltimore after his departure from
Charlottesville and for may years directed the epidemiological
program at the Johns Hopkins School of Public Health and
Hygiene. He stimulated many young scientists to take their
proper places in academic medicine.
    We need to know why murine typhus rickettsiae are relative-
ly mild for animals, fleas and humans and yet its epidemic
counterpart is just the reverse in its behavior. Can murine
rickettsiae revert to epidemic forms and vice versa by simple
shift in one or two peptides or for similar reasons?

        III.   MYOCARDITIS MAY BE A SIGNIFICANT CONTRIBUTING
               CAUSE OF DEATH IN RICKETTSIAL DISEASES

    Approximately 7 percent of patients with RMSF in the United
States usually die because of a delay in diagnosis and institution of proper specific and supportive care. However, death in
some patients is unavoidable since rickettsiae and the disease
process may attack so rapidly as to outdistance treatment. The
usual cause of death is general organ failure with specific
vascular involvement of brains, lungs, liver, myocardium, ad-
renals and kidneys -- all vital organs. Advanced age, a short

incubation period, rapidity of development of a petechial echymotic rash, and azotemia, with shock, are harbingers of more virulent infections. Wolbach and Lilly stressed the widespread involvement of vascular changes in various organ systems. One of Wolbach's wise admonitions was "don't forget the liver" (17).

A. Histologic Changes in Myocardium

Too little attention is given the myocardium and its possible relationship to the immediate cause of death. Wolbach described histologic changes in the myocardium but did not direct specific attention to their significance (1). Lillie, more direct in his account of five well-studied fatal cases of RMSF, described myocardial changes in two patients: "focal areas of myocardial muscle fiber oxyphilia, hyalinization and karyolysis or karyorrhexis, grading into coagulative necrosis" (2). He noted, "vascular endothelial swelling, proliferation to several layers, and necrosis with or without occlusion by masses of granular oxyphil material -- vessels often surrounded by adventitial cellular infiltrations, comprising chiefly lymphocytes, and, to a lesser extent, plasma cells, macrophages, mast cells and eosinophils." Similar, often dense, focal cellular infiltrations were seen not obviously associated with vessels. Rickettsiae were not identified in the vascular lesions.

Maxcy and Pinkerton reported a fatal case of endemic typhus in 1931 in Charlottesville, Virginia, which, after consideration, was felt to be RMSF (5). In this case, the heart showed numerous lesions -- "many of the precapillaries showed definite intimal proliferation and thrombus formation with perivascular accumulation of macrophages and lymphocytes. The thrombi were comprised chiefly of endothelial cells and platelets but in one instance eight or ten polymorphonuclears were present. A second type of lesion consisted of fusiform collection of cells between spread-apart, but not obviously damaged muscle fibers. These cells included macrophages, endothelial cells, lymphocytes, plasma cells, mast cells and polymorphonuclears, their frequency being in the order mentioned. Lesions in the myocardium were entirely similar to those described by Wolbach, Todd and Palfrey in their European cases of typhus (18). There were clinical clues to the cause of death by either arrhythmia or cardiac failure; details were not given.

Harris' case, a 5-year-old girl, died on about the 12th day of RMSF (4). There were no clinical suggestions of arrhythmia or myocarditis but the description was brief. Postmortem findings showed myocardial edema, many foci in which myocardial cells were necrotic and invasion by polymorphonuclear and large mononuclear leukocytes. "There are a great many foci not definitely associated with either myocardial necrosis or with

thromboses of the blood vessels in which the interstitial tissue is infiltrated by large numbers of plasma cells and large
mononuclear leukocytes and few lymphocytes."

Generally, the myocardium functions well and sustains most
cases of RMSF, epidemic typhus and scrub typhus during their
severe vascular illness. In some patients, death does not
appear to be the result of failure of cerebral, pulmonary,
hepatic or renal systems. Rather, death by arrhythmia or cardiac arrest or pump failure may be the cause.

Of all the rickettsioses the clinical and pathologic manifestations of myocarditis are said to be the greatest in scrub
typhus fever. Levine found little evidence of cardiovascular
abnormalities in scrub typhus patients one to 2 months after
recovery (19). Follow-up studies of scrub typhus patients
failed to reveal significant prevalence of residual damage or
late sequelae (20). Ash and Spitz remarked specifically about
the striking cardiac lesions in scrub typhus of diffuse interstitial myocarditis and a predominance of large basophilic
mononuclear cells (21). They likened the less pronounced myocardial involvement in RMSF to the changes in epidemic typhus.
The older American and European clinical literature referred
particularly to epidemic typhus and RMSF with caution expressed
on use of fluids intravenously because of the potential deleterious effect upon the myocardium. These admonitions were
over-stressed as was the use of digitalis alkaloids.

B. Sudden Death

Although the significance of myocarditis as a contributing
factor to death in RMSF is unclear, there may be a relationship. In his classic paper on sudden death in 1934, Hamman
presented evidence that approximately 8 percent of unanticipated fatalities result from myocardial disorders associated with
myocarditis (22). He pointed out that trivial lesions in the
myocardium may be enough to initiate a fatal rhythm. Keenan
et al. showed that focal disseminated necrosis occurs in the
myocardium of Beagle dogs inoculated with R. rickettsii. Elec-
trocardiographic abnormalities occurred in three dogs (23).

Patients with RMSF have been observed or come to my attention whose fatal outcome is best explained by the clinical effects of an associated myocarditis (24).

C. Case Reports

A 70-year-old man with proven RMSF was first treated with
tetracycline on the 7th day of illness. In spite of appropriate supportive and specific treatment, he became much worse on

the 8th day of illness, the blood pressure fell from 120/80 to 90/60, and pulse became totally irregular (atrial fibrillation) with a radial rate of 120. The electrocardiogram confirmed the arrhythmia and findings indicative of myocardial damage. He died on the 2nd hospital day (9th day of illness). The myocardium showed interstitial edema, mononuclear and plasma cell infiltration and capillary congestion (Fig. 5).

The histologic findings of another patient, a 25-year-old woman who died suddenly and expectedly on the 6th day of RMSF, are shown in Figure 6. The clinical and histologic findings suggest strongly that myocarditis was an immediate contributing cause of her sudden death.

In another patient, a male adult with RMSF, there were similar clinical and histologic findings of myocarditis associated with unanticipated death.

Myocardial involvement during the course of any of the severe rickettsioses must be a relatively rare event. However, to deny its existence is unrealistic and the possibility poses a problem needing solution. Using immunofluorescent techniques we have visualized rickettsiae in the myocardium of fatal cases. These studies should be extended to better identify the specific rickettsial antigen and/or antibody globulin in cardiac tissues. Presently, there are no ready answers although in selected cases, the early use of an anti-arrhythmic medication might be useful. It is doubtful that hyperimmune serum would be beneficial.

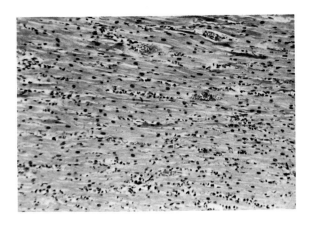

Fig. 5. Rocky Mountain spotted fever. Myocardium showing mononuclear and plasma cell infiltration with interstitial edema in a fatal case.

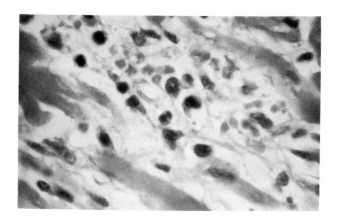

Fig. 6. Rocky Mountain spotted fever. Myocardial changes showing mononuclear infiltration and interstitial edema in a 25-year-old adult. Fatal case with sudden death.

IV. PROTEUS OX19 AS A DEFENSIVE WEAPON; PROTEUS SEROTHERAPY;
     EPIDEMIC TYPHUS ANTIBODIES IN RATS: SQUIRREL TYPHUS

A. Proteus OX19 as a Defense Weapon

Several vignettes are of historical interest to rickettsi-ologists. Hans Zinsser vividly described in "Rats, Lice and History" how lice and typhus influenced the outcome of wars more than bullets or generals (25). Yet, who could have been more ingenious than two Polish physicians, E. S. Lazowsky and S. Matulwicz, who used the Proteus OX19 serologic reaction to influence German military authorities to walk wide of about a dozen Polish villages during World War II (26). They were de-clared "an epidemic area" and its men were freed from oppres-sion, conscription of hard labor elsewhere, incarceration in prison concentration camps or execution. They waged a "private immunological war" by systematically administering Proteus OX19 antigen to persons in these villages during fall and winter months which coincided with the natural seasonal occurrence of typhus. Patients with any suggestion of symptoms of epidemic typhus were selected and given killed suspensions of Proteus OX19 as "protein stimulation therapy" to build up general im-munological resistance!! German health authorities who exa-mined the sera falsely interpreted a positive Weil-Felix reac-tion with a titer of 1/500 or more as evidence of active louse-borne typhus infection. Thus, the artificially induced Weil-

Felix reaction was used as a defensive measure against the savage policies of the German Occupation Government.

Adolph Felix, the co-discoverer of the Weil-Felix reaction in 1916, isolated a strain of "Proteus X" from the urine of patients with typhus in Poland (27). The strain, later designated OX19, was agglutinated by the patient's serum and also by sera of other typhus convalescents. This test became a simple, useful, nonspecific, practical diagnostic reaction for detection of many of the serious rickettsial diseases, such as epidemic and murine typhus and Rocky Mountain spotted fever. Felix maintained that Proteus bacteria and R. prowazekii, which caused epidemic typhus, were genetically related and maintained this concept without relenting.

B.   Trial of Proteus OX19 Immune Serum in Epidemic Typhus

During World War II, I met Felix in London where he was busily engaged in preparing very high titered Proteus OX19 serum in horses by repeated injection of antigen. My clinical work with typhus patients in Morocco provided an ideal setting for testing his therapeutic concept which he eagerly encouraged. Large quantities of serum were made available for evaluation in typhus patients given as early in the clinical course as possible. Four patients were selected in the 4th or 5th days of typhus. After appropriate skin and ocular testing, horse serum was given subcutaneously and intravenously. Although there was no noticeable measurable effect upon the clinical course, including nonabatement of fever or other manifestations, the young medical officer gained considerable more knowledge about how to treat serum sickness!!

C.   Epidemic Typhus Antibodies in Rats in Manila

Another unsolved vignette involves a paradox noted in the sera of rats trapped in Manila, Philippine Islands, during the American re-occupation. Rats (Rattus norvegicus) were trapped, anesthetized, bled and allowed to recover. Those rats whose sera showed CF antibodies to typhus antigens were sacrificed and suspensions of their brains inoculated into guinea pigs yielded murine typhus rickettsiae in several attempts; rat brains were pooled. Of special interest was the unanticipated finding that titers of CF antibody in rat sera were higher for epidemic typhus (Breinl) than murine typhus (Wilmington) antigens (28). This unusual reaction was reconfirmed in Manila and also by Plotz in the Rickettsial Disease Laboratory at the Walter Reed Army Institute of Research. This paradox, higher

antibody titers to epidemic than to murine typhus antigens in
rats, is unexplained. This artifact may relate to the crude
antigens used which caused strong cross-over serologic reactions. It merits further study. Conceivably, there may be a
relation between this reaction and the next vignette involving
squirrels and R. prowazekii infection.

Brigham conducted a thorough serologic study of the Weil-
Felix and complement fixation reactions in wild rats in his
evaluation of the incidence of murine typhus infestation (29).
Most were Norway R. rattus norvegicus rats; a few were R.
rattus rattus. Proteus OX19 agglutinins and CF antibodies
indicative of murine typhus infection were present. Unfortu-
nately, the CF antigen was not described; it is presumed that
the test employed the R. mooseri (Wilmington) strain since this
was the standard antigen used.

              D. Epidemic Typhus as a Natural Infection
                    in the United States

In February 1980, the clinical data of a youth, aged 12,
was discussed during a short tour as Visiting Professor at the
Princeton, New Jersey, Hospital (Rutgers Medical School affili-
ate). Dr. Alexander Ackley presented the data of the boy who
became ill in early December 1979 after a visit to West
Virginia with fever, rash, lethargy, headache, sullenness for
a few days and general malaise. The boy spent the Thanksgiving
holiday in West Virginia, played in wooded areas, and it is
probable that he handled the carcasses of deer or squirrels.
The rash consisted of macules 1-2 mm in diameter which
blanched; later it became petechial and was prevalent on the
trunk. It became morbilliform and "blotchy". It abated in
about 5 days after hospitalization and he recovered fully after
a total acute illness of about 7 days. Treatment consisted of
penicillin, chloramphenicol and tetracycline.

Dr. McDade, Center for Disease Control, confirmed for
Doctor Ackley that the serum indicated a recent epidemic typhus
infection. McDade reported the findings of eight such patients
with serologic evidence of epidemic typhus in the United States
acquired possibly from squirrels and their ectoparasites (30).

The prevalence of R. prowazekii infections in humans and
squirrels in the United States (31) raises several important
questions including the validity of the man-louse-man reservoir
and transmission solely by the human body louse. Could there
have been an antigenic shift, such as from R. typhi to R.
prowazekii in squirrels and their ectoparasites which has resulted in a milder human type of epidemic typhus? Zinsser and
many others struggled with this possibility. On this important
point, Zinsser held that murine and European typhus rickettsiae

were distinct varieties of agents, distinguishable by biologic
methods each of which could occur endemically and epidemically
(13). Working in Boston and Mexico with his associate,
Castaneda, he showed the louse capable of epidemic transmission
of murine rickettsiae and that such strains passed through the
cycle man-louse-man were temporarily, not permanently, modified
in the direction of European type characteristics. His studies
of Brill's disease convinced him that secondary cases of epidemic typhus could result from louse infestation and transmission from recrudescent cases; yet, he did not believe that
latent human infections were the only source of origin or
reservoir of classical European disease (13,32). Influenza
viruses characteristically shift their characters and lepto-
spira are suspected of such antigenic variation. The Manila
rat sera raise the possibility of an antigenic shift as does
the clinical mildness of human-squirrel associated epidemic
typhus; ordinarily, murine typhus is mild and louse-borne typhus is clinically severe.

V. IMMUNE SERUM, PARA-AMINOBENZOIC ACID AND SPECIFIC ANTIBIOTIC THERAPY OF RICKETTSIOSES

A. Immune Therapy; Limitations

Attempts to ameliorate the manifestations of the rickettsial diseases soon followed the discovery of protective substances, "antibodies", present in the serum of convalescent
animals or humans. Ricketts and Gomez produced a serum with
neutralizing value only in guinea pigs; the antibody titer was
not increased by a second injection of serum (33). Later, guinea pig passage rickettsiae produced high neutralizing serum
titers in horses (34,35). Horse serum was concentrated by methods similar to those used to concentrate diphtheria antitoxin
which increased the neutralizing value. Therapeutic efficacy
in humans was not attempted. In 1923, Noguchi reported that
guinea pigs were protected against rickettsial challenge if
given rabbit immune serum during the incubation period (36).
Therapeutic value was claimed if the challenge infectious doses
were greatly reduced. In 1933, Parker reported the therapeutic
benefit of goat immune serum stimulated by tick virus. Later,
he reported his inability to confirm the results.

Topping rejuvenated interest in immune serum therapy. Initially, he reported the results in guinea pigs and monkeys infected with R. rickettsii treated with crude immune rabbit serum (39). He concentrated and purified the antibody similar to
methods used for anti-pneumococcus antibody. As a sequel to
this work, Kurotchin et al., using highly infectious yolk sac

material, prepared immune rabbit serum with a high neutralizing
titer which contained much higher concentrations of antibody
protein (40). Topping followed these preliminary studies with
use of hyperimmune rabbit serum for treatment of laboratory
animals and patients with RMSF during the summers of 1941 and
1942 (41). Results were inconclusive particularly when serum
was given after the first week of illness. Serum was regarded
as effective in reducing fatality if administered on or before
the 3rd day of rash. No attempt was made at case selection or
use of controls. Seventy-one patients were treated with serum
by various physicians throughout the United States. Although
detailed relevant clinical data were not given, there was no
evidence that serum shortened the febrile period significantly.
Fatality was said to have been reduced in serum treated cases.
In epidemic typhus fever, the therapeutic efficacy of serum
treatment was not clear-cut and rickettsemia persisted up to
72 hrs after administration of immune serum (42).

B.   Therapy with Para-aminobenzoic Acid and
              Methylene Blue

     Specific chemotherapy for the rickettsioses began with
methylene blue and para-aminobenzoic acid which showed anti-
rickettsial properties when evaluated in animals (43-45). Each
drug was thought to act through its ability to produce a chemical environment unfavorable for growth of rickettsiae (46-48).
Rickettsiae are obligate intracellular organisms which multiply
rapidly in slowly metabolizing or dying cells, first noted when
abundant yields were observed in the dying chick embryo. The
reverse occurred when rickettsial growth was impeded in rapidly
metabolizing cells such as in mice fed methylene or toluidine
blue or when infected hens' eggs were incubated at temperatures
higher than the usual 37°C.
     Methylene blue is a catalyst which alters the respiration
of tissues; PABA is known to increase the oxygen consumption
of cells. Inhibitory effect was thought to be by direct action
on the enzymes concerned with the metabolism of rickettsiae or
by modifying metabolism of entoderma cells sufficient to alter
the equilibrium between rickettsiae and host cells.
     Para-aminobenzoic acid significantly benefited patients
with classical louse-borne typhus (49), Rocky Mountain spotted
fever (50,51) and scrub typhus fever (52). Very large doses
were required given every 2 hrs in order to achieve satisfactory sustained blood levels of about 10 mg/100 ml. It was
noted that treatment with PABA early in illness led to a delay
in emergence of proteus agglutinins and CF antibodies. Although the general results were favorable, PABA was limited in
its use because of troublesome nausea, vomiting and diarrhea.

Methylene blue was of no practical use for treatment of scrub typhus patients and larger doses cause methemoglobinemia.

Shown in Figure 7 are the clinical data of a patient with Rocky Mountain spotted fever treated successfully with PABA. Rickettsemia ceased after several days of treatment; the duration of fever and progression of the rash were abated. In one series of 40 patients treated, there were no fatalities.

C. Antibiotic Treatment

The advent of specific and dramatically effective antibiotic therapy for the rickettsioses was in 1948. Displayed in Figures 8, 9, and 10 are the first specifically treated cases of scrub, Rocky Mountain spotted and murine typhus fevers (53-56).

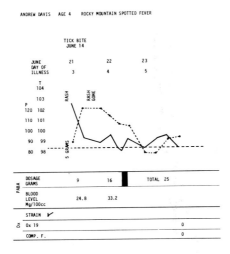

Fig. 7. Rocky Mountain spotted fever. Four-year-old patient treated successfully with para-aminobenzoic acid initiated on 3rd day of illness. Rapid defervescence and abatement of rash. Total dose of 25.0 grams. Reference: (49).

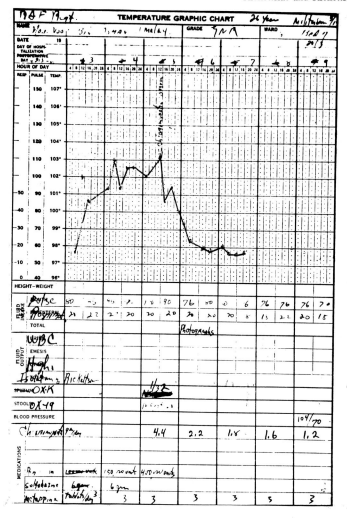

Fig. 8. Scrub typhus fever. Initial patient treated with chloramphenicol in Kuala Lumpur, Malaya, 1948. Note rapid defervescence. [Reference: (53)].

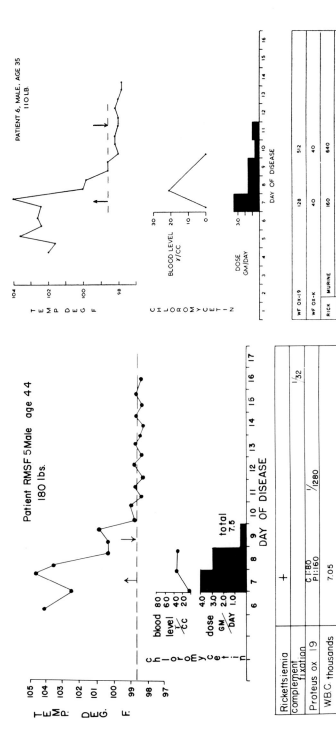

Fig. 9. RMSF. Treatment of 44-year-old adult with chloramphenicol. Note Proteus OX19, 1/1280; CF 1/32. [Reference: (54)].

Fig. 10. Murine typhus fever. Prompt response in 35-year-old man treated with chloramphenicol. Weil-Felix and CF reactions positive. [Reference: (55)].

In each figure are given the dosage regimens, rapidity of defervescence, abatement of clinical manifestations and pertinent laboratory values. The initial cases of louse-borne typhus fever were treated with chloromycetin by Payne in Bolivia, which showed similar responses (57).

VI.   RICKETTSIAL VACCINES: A UNIQUE VIABLE
FLEA-FECES (BLANC) VACCINE

A.   Early Inactivated Vaccines

The first inactivated vaccines for rickettsial infections were made from infected tick tissues by Spencer and Parker (35-38). Favorable results were reported. When tested much later in volunteers in a controlled vaccine trial, there was little, if any, protective value (58).

The Weigl vaccine was difficult to produce since lice were inoculated intrarectally (a louse enema) with viable R. prowazekii (59). Rickettsiae multiply in intestinal cells and lice were fed on the skin of convalescent patients twice daily for a week or more. The louse intestine was harvested, the rickettsiae inactivated with formalin; the resultant vaccine contained many rickettsiae. One hundred louse intestines represented one vaccine dose. Later, Castaneda produced an inactivated typhus vaccine by forcing mice to inhale droplets of rickettsial-laden emulsions; on being placed in a cold room, rickettsial pneumonitis developed (60). Lungs were harvested, the rickettsiae inactivated with formalin and an effective rickettsial-laden vaccine was produced. Giroud extended this method to include rabbits, dogs, sheep and even considered camels in his search for a larger vaccine factory. When such animals, including mice, sneezed virulent rickettsiae into the room, they often infected the inoculator and others. Herald Cox's adaptation of the Goodpasture egg embryo technique simplified the method of vaccine production which, along with ether extraction and freeze-thawing of infected chorioallantoic membranes, led to an effective vaccine particularly when care was taken to produce a product with high titers of antigen (61).

B.   Viable Murine Typhus Vaccine (Blanc)

A vaccine for typhus more unique than Weigl's was developed by Georges Blanc and Marcel Baltazard of the Institut Pasteur, Casablanca. I observed this technique first as a young medical officer soon after arrival in North Africa in 1942. Guinea

pigs infected with R. mooseri (typhi) were placed in deep por-
celain lined sawdust pits, each of which contained 30 to 40
thousand starved fleas; the infected animal soon died of ex-
sanguination. Several additional infected guinea pigs were
placed into the tubs until the fleas were well infected. To
collect the rickettsial-laden flea feces, healthy cotton rats
were placed into the pit. In only a few hours, they died of
blood loss and then appeared brown in color because of a coat
of flea feces. In such tubs, fleas could feed on many rats.
The dead animal was removed and technicians, without any real
protection, picked the brownish rat hair, rubbed it over a fine
mesh which permitted the flea feces to drop into a glass petri
dish. Such heaps of flea feces were then measured in milligram
amounts and sealed in glass ampoules. These ampoules were then
crated along with a diluent of saline water with a small amount
of ox bile. These cartons were dispatched throughout Morocco
and Algeria to various district health stations. Huge numbers
of Muslim citizens, who came for a regular sugar ration, were
then injected with the vaccine which was reconstituted just
before inoculation, i.e., dried flea feces placed in a small
amount of ox bile/saline diluent. This so-called "attenuated"
vaccine produced an unknown number of cases of murine typhus
fever said to be milder than usual because of the attenuating
effect of the ox bile. Incidentally, Zinsser always argued
with Blanc during international meetings that rickettsiae were
not made less virulent in this manner. It was known from prior
studies in animals and observations in humans that murine typhus fever provided resistance to the more virulent epidemic
louse-borne typhus fever.
     Careful studies of the Blanc vaccine were conducted in vol-
unteers with pre- and post-vaccine antibody studies and clinical evaluation of vaccinees. In two separate series, it appeared that approximately 10 percent of the vaccinees developed
murine typhus fever suggesting that they were the benefactors
of most of the particles of flea feces from a particular vial
of dried material. One vial of dried flea feces was said to
contain enough antigen for 100 doses. Another interesting
finding was the development of fever in other vaccine recipients who were not clinically ill and who did not develop Proteus OX19 or CF antibodies to rickettsial antigens. Indeed, I
learned that the simple taking of oral temperature in a large
number of persons will show a small percentage of elevations
without an obvious cause!
     A later study of this vaccine in volunteers showed that
protection to epidemic typhus occurred only when the flea-feces
in the vaccine was viable and caused a mild murine typhus infection with serologic conversion after vaccination. Most vaccinees received no antigen and developed no immunity.

REFERENCES

1. Wolbach, S. R., J. Med. Res. XLI, 1 (1919).
2. Ricketts, H. T., JAMA LII, 379 (1909).
3. Lillie, R. D., Pub. Health Rep. 46, 2840 (1931).
4. Harris, P. N., Am. J. Path. 9, 71 (1933).
5. Pinkerton, H., and Maxcy, K. F., Am. J. Path. 7, 95 (1931).
6. Woodward, T. E. Pedersen, C. E., Jr., Oster, C. N.,
    Bagley, L. R., Romberger, J., and Snyder, M. J., J. Infect.
    Dis. 134, 297 (1976).
7. Walker, D. H., and Cain, B. G., J. Infect. Dis. 137, 206
    (1978).
8. Harrell, G. T., Medicine 28, 333 (1949).
9. Fine, D., Mosher, D., Yamada, T., Burke, D., and Kenyon,
    R., Arch. Int. Med. 138, 735 (1978).
10. Wisseman, C. L., Jr., Batawi, Y., Wood, W. H., Jr., and
    Noriega, A. R., J. Immunol. 98, 194 (1967).
11. Oster, C. N., Burke, D. S., Kenyon, R. H., Ascher, M. S.,
    Harber, P., and Pedersen, C. E., Jr., New Engl. J. Med.
    297, 859 (1977).
12. Brill, N. E., Am. J. Med. Sci. 139, 484 (1910).
13. Zinsser, H., Am. J. Hyg. 25, 430 (1937).
14. Maxcy, K. F., Pub. Health Rep. 44, 1735 (1929).
15. Woodward, T. E., J. Infect. Dis. 127, 583 (1973).
16. Dyer, R. E., Rumreich, A., and Badger, L. F., Pub. Health
    Rep. 46, 334 (1931).
17. Wolbach, S. B., in "Rickettsial Diseases of Man". Publica-
    tion of the American Association for the Advancement of
    Science, Boston (1948).
18. Wolbach, S. B., Todd, J. L., and Palfrey, F. W. "The
    Etiology and Pathology of Typhus," Harvard University
    Press, Cambridge (1922).
19. Levine, H. D., War Med. 7, 76 (1945).
20. Elsom, K. A., Beebe, G. W., Sayen, J. J., Scheie, H. G.,
    Gammon, G. D., and Wood, F. C., Ann. Int. Med. 55, 784
    (1961).
21. Ash, J. E., and Spitz, S., in "Pathology of Tropical Dis-
    eases," Chapter 4, W. B. Saunders Co., Philadelphia (1945).
22. Hamman, L., Johns Hopkins Med. Bull. 53, 387 (1934).
23. Keenan, K. P., Buhles, W. C., Jr., Huxsoll, D. L.,
    Williams, R. G., and Hildebrandt, P. H. Am. J. Vet. Res.
    38, 851 (1977).
24. Woodward, T. E., Togo, Y., Lee, Y. C., and Hornick, R. B.,
    Arch. Int. Med. 120, 270 (1967).
25. Zinsser, H., "Rats, Lice and History", The Atlantic
    Monthly Press (Little, Brown and Company), Boston (1935).
26. Lazowski, E. S., and Matulewicz, S., ASH News 43, 300
    (1977).

27. Weil, E., and Felix, A., Wien. Klin. Wschr. 29, 33 (1916).
28. Woodward, T. E., Philip, C. B., and Loranger, G. L., J. Infect. Dis. 78, 167 (1946).
29. Brigham, G. D., and Bengtson, I. A., Pub. Health Rep. 60, 29 (1945).
30. McDade, J. E., Shepard, C. C., Redus, M. A., Newhouse, V. F., and Smith, J. D., Am. J. Trop. Med. Hyg. 29, 277 (1980).
31. Sonenshine, D. E., Bozeman, F. M., Williams, M. S., Masiello, S. A., Chadwick, D. P., Stocks, N. I., Lauer, D. M., and Elisberg, B. L., J. Trop. Med. Hyg. 27, 339 (1978).
32. Zinsser, H., and Castaneda, M. R., New Engl. J. Med. 209, 815 (1933).
33. Ricketts, H. T., and Gomez, L., J. Infect. Dis. 5, 221 (1908).
34. Heinemann, P. G., and Moore, J. J., JAMA 57, 198 (1911).
35. Heinemann, P. G., and Moore, J. J., J. Infect. Dis. 10, 294 (1912).
36. Noguchi, H., J. Exp. Med. 37, 383 (1923).
37. Parker, R. R., J. Infect. Dis. 57, 78 (1935).
38. Spencer, R. R., and Parker, R. R., Pub. Health Rep. 40, 2159 (1925).
39. Topping, N. H., Pub. Health Rep. 55, 41 (1940).
40. Kurotchkin, T. J., Van der Scheer, J., and Wyckoff, R.W.G., Proc. Soc. Exp. Biol. Med. 45, 323 (1940).
41. Topping, N. H., Pub. Health Rep. 58, 757 (1943).
42. Plotz, H., Bennett, B. L., and Tabet, F., Proc. Soc. Exp. Biol. Med. 63, 176 (1946).
43. Snyder, J. C., Maier, J., and Anderson, C. R., Report to the Division of Medical Sciences, National Research Council, December 26 (1942).
44. Hamilton, H. L., Proc. Soc. Exp. Biol. Med. 59, 220 (1945).
45. Peterson, O. L., Proc. Soc. Exp. Biol. Med. 55, 155 (1944).
46. Greiff, D., Pinkerton, H., and Moragues, V., J. Exp. Med. 80, 561 (1944).
47. Greiff, D., and Pinkerton, H., J. Exp. Med. 82, 193 (1945).
48. Greiff, D., in "The Rickettsial Diseases of Man," Symposium, American Association for the Advancement of Science, (1948).
49. Yeomans, A., Snyder, J. C., Murray, E. E., Zarafonetis, C.J.D., and Ecke, R. S., JAMA 126, 349 (1944).
50. Rose, H. M., Duane, R. B., and Fischel, E. E., JAMA 129, 1160 (1945).
51. Woodward, T. E., and Raby, W. T., South. Med. J. 41, 997 (1948).
52. Tierney, N. A., JAMA 131, 280 (1946).

53. Smadel, J. E., Woodward, T. E., Ley, H. L., Jr., and
     Lewthwaite, R., *J. Clin. Invest.* 28, 1196 (1949).
54. Pincoffs, M. C., Guy, E. G., Lister, L. M., Woodward,
     T. E., and Smadel, J. E., *Ann. Int. Med.* 29, 656 (1948).
55. Ley, H. L., Jr., Woodward, T. E., and Smadel, J. E., *JAMA*
     143, 217 (1950).
56. Woodward, T. E., *Ann. Int. Med.* 31, 53 (1949).
57. Payne, E. H., Sharp, E. A., and Knauolt, J. A., *Trans.
     Roy. Soc. Trop. Med. Hyg.* 42, 163 (1948).
58. DuPont, H. L., Hornick, R. B., Dawkins, A. T., Heiner,
     G. G., Fabricant, I. B., Wisseman, C. L., Jr., and
     Woodward, T. E., *J. Infect. Dis.* 128, 340 (1973).
59. Weigl, R., *Bull. Intern. Acad. Polonaise Sci. Lettres
     (Cl. Med.)*, July, 25 (1930).
60. Castaneda, M. R., *Am. J. Path.* 15, 467 (1939).
61. Cox, H. R., *Science* 94, 399 (1941).

IMMUNITY AND IMMUNOLOGY

IMMUNITY AND IMMUNOLOGY OF RICKETTSIAL DISEASES

Joseph V. Osterman

Department of Rickettsial Diseases
Walter Reed Army Institute of Research
Washington, DC

Recent investigations in the immune response to rickett-sial infections have been highlighted by the emerging recog-nition of the role of cellular immune events in modulating disease. The production of humoral antibody specific for rickettsiae has been recognized and employed for diagnostic purposes for many years, but only recently have we been chal-lenged to understand the mechanism of protection mediated through the interaction of lymphocytes and macrophages. Rec-ognition of the role of these cells in resistance to rickett-sial infection has also caused us to seek in vitro correlates of cellular immunocompetency which accurately reflect the immune status of the host.

An early study on the immunology of scrub typhus had shown that infection of mice with any strain of R. tsutsugamushi conferred on the survivors protection against subsequent challenge not only with the homologous strain, but also with heterologous strains of the scrub typhus group (1). The un-derlying mechanism for this group specific protection was not immediately apparent, because antibody neutralization studies indicated substantial differences among strains (2). Shirai et al. postulated that a cellular immune mechanism might be operative and began studies using inbred BALB/c mice. These animals were found to be susceptible to lethal infection with the Karp strain, but relatively resistant to the Gilliam strain which could be used to establish nonlethal immunizing infections. The employment of inbred mice was important, be-cause it allowed transfer of potentially immunocompetent cells between animals without subsequent immunological rejection.

Using the Gilliam-Karp system, Shirai and co-workers were able to assess the cellular contribution to host protection by

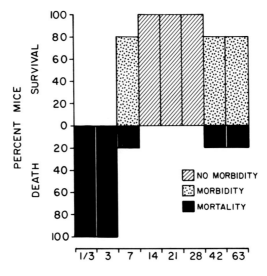

Fig. 1. Survival of BALB/c mice after receipt of immune
spleen cells followed by challenge infection with R. tsutsugamushi, strain Karp (1,000 MLD$_{50}$). All mice serving as
spleen cell donors were immunized with Gilliam (100 MID$_{50}$).
On the days indicated, one spleen equivalent was transferred
to each recipient mouse, which was challenged 8 h later with
Karp. Sample size for each challenge infection was five mice.

cell transfer experiments (3). Mice were immunized with 1 x
10^2 50% mouse infectious doses (MID$_{50}$) of the Gilliam strain,
and at various days after inoculation five mice were sacrificed, their spleens removed aseptically, and a suspension of
single cells was prepared. One spleen equivalent, or approximately 1 x 10^8 leukocytes in 0.2 ml, was given to each recipient. The animals were challenged 8 hours later with 1 x 10^3
50% mouse lethal doses (MLD$_{50}$) of the Karp strain. The results (Fig. 1) indicated that spleen cells from animals immunized 3 days previously with Gilliam conferred no protection
against the Karp challenge. When spleen cells were transferred 7 days postimmunization, 80% of the challenged mice
became ill but survived, and complete protection against illness as well as death was observed when cells were transferred
14 to 28 days after Gilliam immunization. The protective
capacity of immune spleen cells was somewhat lower on days 42
and 63 when the experiment was terminated.

TABLE 1. Effect of Specific Cytotoxic Antilymphocyte Serum on Mouse Survival and Cellular Proliferation

Treatment of spleen cells	Mouse survival (sample size/ survivors [%])	ConA stimulation (counts/min x 10^3/ control [%])	LPS stimulation (counts/min x 10^3/ control [%])
Control[a]	5/100	78/100	19/100
Untreated[b]	10/70	57/73	12/63
Anti-theta serum + complement	10/20	8/10	8/42
Anti-immunoglobulin + complement	10/100	82/105	4/20

[a]Spleen cells were transferred immediately after harvest.
[b]Spleen cells were untreated with either antiserum but incubated under similar temperature conditions and transferred in parallel with treated cells.

Subsequent studies indicated that the cells necessary for transfer of protection were nonadherent to a tissue-culture plastic surface, and were more than 95% lymphocytes by morphologic criteria. The number of nonadherent lymphoid cells necessary to achieve protection was determined with spleens harvested from mice infected 21 days previously with Gilliam. Complete protection from a 1×10^3 MLD_{50} Karp challenge was achieved with 3×10^7 cells. The identity of the lymphocyte subpopulation responsible for protection was determined by treating aliquots of these cells with either anti-theta or anti-immunoglobulin serum and complement. The results (Table 1) indicated that anti-theta serum abrogated most of the protective effect of immune splenic lymphocytes and the ability of such cells to respond to concanavalin A. Anti-immunoglobulin serum had no effect on the protective ability of immune spleen lymphocytes but reduced lipopolysaccharide (LPS)-stimulated proliferation. These data strongly implied that the protective cell was a thymus-derived lymphocyte or T-cell.

Concomitant histopathological studies on the intraperitoneal infection of BALB/c mice with Karp indicated that most pathological alterations were confined to the peritoneal cavity (4). It was concluded, on microscopic and morphologic data, that the survival of an animal following intraperitoneal infection with scrub typhus rickettsiae depended on its ability to concentrate a sufficiently vigorous immune response in the peritoneal cavity. The morphologic data also suggested that the evolution of rickettsiacidal macrophages was important in suppressing infection. The photomicrograph in Figure 2 suggests intimate contact between lymphocytes and macrophages in the peritoneal cavity of an infected mouse.

Shirai's initial cell transfer studies had all employed immune spleen lymphocytes injected into the peritoneal cavity of recipient mice, followed by an intraperitoneal challenge with Karp. However, the histopathological studies suggested that lymphocytes in the peritoneal exudate could also play an important role in the cellular defense mechanism against rickettsial infection. To examine the role of various lymphoid cell populations in host protection, Catanzaro et al. immunized mice with 1×10^2 MLD_{50} of strain Gilliam, then at various days after infection, harvested spleens or peritoneal exudate cells (5). Recipient mice were inoculated intraperitoneally with cell suspensions containing 3×10^7 lymphocytes, and were challenged 8 hours later with 1×10^3 MLD_{50} Karp.

Protection afforded by transfer of splenic lymphocytes was quite similar to that observed previously (Fig. 3). Not until 7 days after Gilliam immunization were splenic lymphocytes able to transfer partial (80%) protection against challenge with strain Karp. Complete protection was achieved with

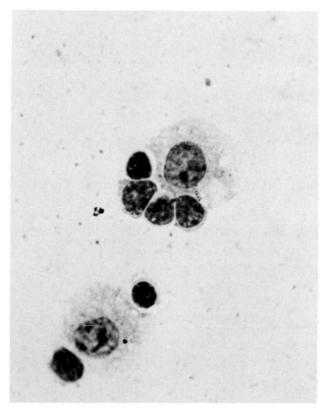

Fig. 2. Peritoneal scraping prepared 3 days after Karp
infection. Early in the infectious period with either Karp or
Gilliam, intimate contact between lymphocytes and macrophages
was observed but was not seen at later times. (Giemsa,
x1,000)

splenic lymphocytes transferred 14 to 28 days after immunization. The protective capacity of immune splenic lymphocytes
was slightly less on days 35 and 42, when experiments were
terminated. The protection afforded by peritoneal exudate
lymphocytes differed from that seen with splenic lymphocytes.
Partial protection was achieved with peritoneal exudate lymphocytes as early as 3 days after immunization and complete
protection was observed following transfer of lymphocytes on
day 7. In addition, the protective capacity of peritoneal
exudate lymphocytes persisted until termination of the experiment, and did not show the decline exhibited by splenic lymphocytes 35 and 42 days postimmunization. It is also interesting
to note that the protection afforded by transfer of immune

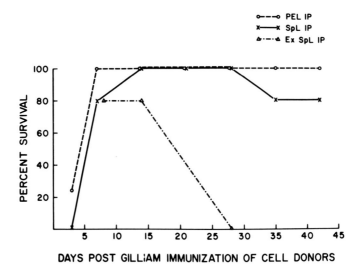

Fig. 3. Comparison of the protective effects of Gilliam immune peritoneal exudate lymphocytes (o) and splenic lymphocytes (x) transferred intraperitoneally before Karp challenge of recipients. In some experiments, immune splenic lymphocytes were harvested from donors bearing a mineral oil-induced peritoneal exudate (Δ). Ordinate indicates percent survival of recipients.

splenic lymphocytes could be reduced by inducing a sterile peritoneal exudate in these animals with mineral oil. It was clear from these studies that peritoneal exudate lymphocytes were more efficient immune cells than splenic lymphocytes, and it seemed that the peritoneal exudate lymphocyte was the mediator of cellular protection against intraperitoneal infection with scrub typhus rickettsiae. It was also interesting to find that splenic lymphocytes capable of suppressing rickettsial infection were mobile. Induction of a sterile exudate may have mobilized protective cells into the exudate itself, or alternatively a phenomenon of negative lymphoid trapping may have excluded immunocompetent lymphocytes from the spleen.
    Since peritoneal exudate lymphocytes were potent mediators of protection against rickettsial infection, it was important to examine their effect on the interaction of rickettsiae with resident peritoneal macrophages. Nacy and Osterman showed that macrophages from normal BALB/c mice cultured in vitro supported the unrestrained growth of scrub typhus rickettsiae (6). After 5 days incubation of infected macrophages, the entire cytoplasm was often filled with organisms, as shown in

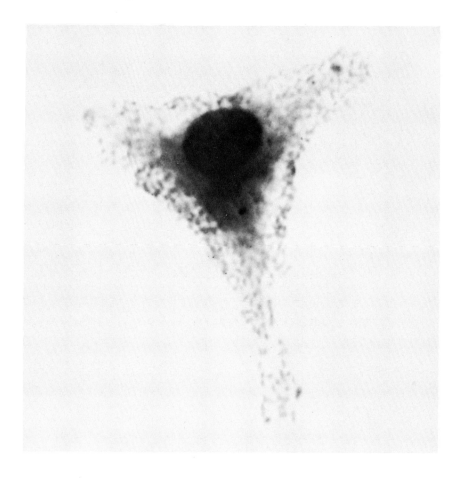

Fig. 4. Rickettsial growth in peritoneal macrophages 5
days after in vitro infection with R. tsutsugamushi strain
Gilliam.

Figure 4. If a spleen cell supernatant containing lymphokines
were applied to normal macrophage monolayers for 4 hours prior
to inoculation with rickettsiae, a substantial diminution in
infection was noted. As seen in Figure 5, rickettsial replication was slowed, and the percentage of infected macrophages
was reduced. When peritoneal macrophages were harvested from
immune animals and infected, a similar interaction occurred
and the percentage of infect-macrophages was very low. However, lymphokine activation of macrophages was not the only
mechanism by which effector cells could kill rickettsiae. If
scrub typhus organisms were mixed with antiserum prior to exposure to macrophages from a normal animal, the uptake of

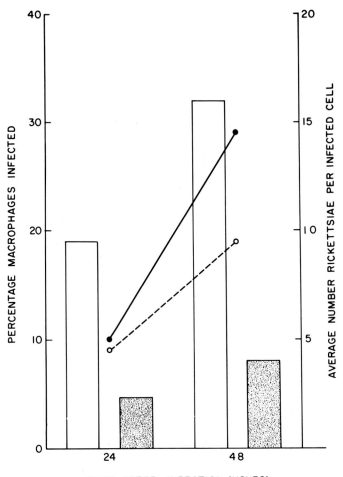

Fig. 5. Rickettsial growth in normal and activated macrophages. Open bars indicate the percentage of infected macrophages in cultures pretreated with spleen cell supernatants
without lymphokine activity; solid bars indicate the percentage of infected macrophages in cultures pretreated with lym-
phokine-containing culture supernatants. Symbols: ●, rickettsial replication in normal macrophage cultures; o, rickettsial replication in lymphokine-activated macrophage cultures.

rickettsiae was slightly enhanced, and the intracellular destruction of organisms was augmented. There also seemed to be
some enhancing effect of antibody on the intracellular killing
of rickettsiae in lymphokine-activated macrophages, but this

TABLE 2. Response of Inbred Mouse Strains to R. tsutsugamushi Gilliam

Inbred strain	MID50 (log10)	MLD50 (log10)	Resistance index (log10)	H-2 haplotype	Response pattern
A/HeJ	8.7	8.5	0.2	a	Susceptible
A/J	7.8	6.0	1.8	a	Selectively resistant
AKR/J	8.0	3.9	4.1	k	Resistant
BALB/cDub	7.4	<3.0	>4.4	d	Resistant
BALB/cJ	7.0	<3.0	>4.0	d	Resistant
C3H/HeDub	9.5	9.0	0.5	k	Susceptible
C3H/HeJ	8.3	8.3	0	k	Susceptible
C3H/HeN	8.7	8.5	0.2	k	Susceptible
C3H/St	8.5	8.5	0	k	Susceptible
C57BL/6J	7.5	<3.0	>4.5	b	Resistant
C57L/J	8.8	<3.0	>5.8	b	Resistant
CBA/J	7.7	7.7	0	k	Susceptible
DBA/1J	8.4	8.4	0	q	Susceptible
DBA/2J	8.0	8.0	0	d	Susceptible
SJL/J	8.2	8.2	0	s	Susceptible
SWR/J	7.5	<3.0	>4.5	q	Resistant

was difficult to quantify, because of the inherent rickettsiacidal capacity of the macrophages.

As these studies in mice began to describe the mechanism
of immunity to experimental scrub typhus infection, another
major line of investigation was beginning to provide alternative data on the pathogenesis of disease and the effect of
immune factors in modulating the severity of infection. Studies by Groves et al. focused on the genetic background of
mice, and the role of genetic factors in resistance to rickettsial infection. An initial survey study of inbred strains
of mice infected with strain Gilliam or strain Karp showed
that Karp was uniformly lethal for over 30 inbred strains, inbred hybrids and outbred stocks of mice (7). The Gilliam
strain, however, showed selective virulence for certain inbred
strains of mice. The data in Table 2 indicate that A/HeJ, the
C3H strains, CBA/J, the DBA strains, and SJL/J mice were all
susceptible to Gilliam infection, with a lethal dose being
less than 10 organisms. When susceptible C3H/HeDub animals
were mated with resistant BALB/cDub mice, it was found that
resistance was dominant. Study of F_1, F_2 and parental back-
cross generations indicated that resistance was controlled by
a single gene or closely linked cluster of genes that were
autosomal and not linked to coat color. The resistance of
BALB/cDub mice to strain Gilliam was not due to an inability
of host cells to support rickettsial growth, since both C3H/
HeDub and BALB/cDub embryo cell cultures supported similar
growth of rickettsiae. C3H/HeDub mice, although susceptible
to intraperitoneal Gilliam infection, were capable of mounting
an immune response to Gilliam antigens. Subcutaneous infection with this strain of rickettsiae was not lethal and did
protect animals against subsequent intraperitoneal challenge
with either the Gilliam or Karp strains of R. tsutsugamushi.

These genetic studies were continued, and recombinant inbred mice were employed to map the gene locus conferring resistance to Gilliam infection (8). Recombinant inbred mouse
strains are derived by inbreeding randomly chosen pairs of
mice from the F_2 generation of the cross between two dissimilar progenitor strains. These studies employed the two recombinant inbred strains shown in Table 3. B x D strains were
derived from the cross of C57BL/6J (resistant) with DBA/2J
(susceptible) and B x H strains were a cross of C57BL/6J
(resistant) with C3H/HeJ (susceptible). All mice were challenged intraperitoneally with 1×10^3 MLD$_{50}$ of Gilliam. The
Ric gene, the gene locus controlling resistance to lethal
Gilliam infection in mice, of C57BL/6J was found in 13 of 25
B x D strains and 4 of 13 B x H strains, for a ratio of 17
resistant to 21 susceptible strains. This is in close agreement with the 1:1 ratio expected under the hypothesis that

TABLE 3. Inheritance of Chromosome 5 Markers Pgm-1, Ric, rd, and Gus in the B x D, B x H, and RI strains[a]

B x D

Locus	1	2	5	6	8	9	11	12	13	14	15	16	18	19	20	21	22	23	24	25	27	28	29	30	31
Pgm-1	B	D	D	B	B	B	B	B	B	B	B	B	D	B	D	D	D	D	D	B	B	B	D	B	D
(x)						x				x				x								x	x		x
Ric	B	D	D	B	B	B	D	D	D	D	D	D	D	D	D	D	D	D	D	D	D	B	B	D	B

B x H

Locus	2	3	4	5	6	7	8	9	10	11	12	14	19
Pgm-1	H	H	H	B	B	B	H	H	H	B	B	H	H
(x)				x	x								
Ric	H	H	H	H	B	H	H	H	H	B	B	H	H
rd	H	H	H	H	B	H	H	H	H	B	B	H	H
(x)	x					x	x		x				
Gus	B	H	H	H	B	B	H	H	H	B	B	B	H

[a] The letters B, D, and H are used as generic symbols for alleles inherited from strains C57BL/6J, DBA/2J, and C3H/HeJ, respectively. An x is used to indicate regions of recombination. The B x D-31 strain arose in the course of propagating the neurologic mutation, vibrator (vb).

resistance is controlled by a single autosomal locus. The
patterns of inheritance of the <u>Ric</u> locus in the recombinant
inbred strains were compared with the patterns available for
other loci which had been previously typed. Ten of 25 B x D
strains demonstrated recombination between <u>Ric</u> and <u>Pgm-1</u>
(phosphoglucomutase-1 locus), the only chromosome 5 marker
available in these strains. Of the 13 B x H strains, 2 exhibited recombination between <u>Ric</u> and <u>Pgm-1</u>, 4 between <u>Ric</u>
and <u>Gus</u> (glucuronidase locus), but there were no recombinants
between <u>Ric</u> and <u>rd</u> (retinal degeneration locus). These data
strongly suggest that the <u>Ric</u> gene locus is closely linked to
the retinal degeneration locus on chromosome 5.

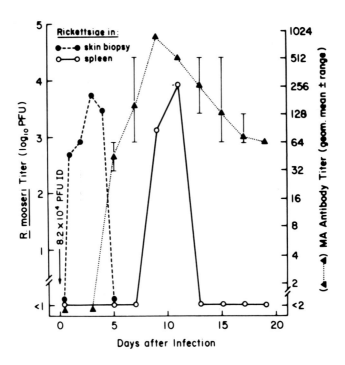

Fig. 6. Dynamics of infection in skin at sites of inoculation, infection in spleen, and serum antibody response after
i.d. inoculation of 8.2 x 10^4 PFU of R. mooseri into each of
three sites on the back. Symbols: (o) PFU per biopsy of inoculation site; (o) PFU per spleen; and (Δ) reciprocal of
microagglutination antibody titer. At each interval, tissues
from 3 guinea pigs were pooled for rickettsial determinations,
and 3 individual serum samples were employed for serology.

Other investigators have been pursuing immunological studies which suggest that cell-mediated immunity may also be
important in resistance to typhus group organisms. Murphy et
al. have published a recent series of papers dealing with the
immune response of inbred guinea pigs to infection with R.
typhi (R. mooseri). A model system was established in which
guinea pigs were infected with approximately 1×10^3 plaque-
forming units (PFU) of rickettsiae by the intradermal (i.d.)
route. The proliferation and spread of organisms was quantified, as was the humoral antibody response (9). The data in
Figure 6 combined with other results, indicated that rickettsiae were recovered first from the site of inoculation, then
from the draining lymph nodes, and subsequently from deep organs. Systemic infection occurred at about the time serum
antibody was detected. It was concluded that the dynamics of
infection involved a sequential evolution and resolution of
infection in the skin prior to the onset of systemic infection, and that the systemic infection progressed in the face
of rising antibody titers. A role for cell-mediated immunity
was suspected, but no delayed-type hypersensitivity to typhus
antigens could be demonstrated.

Histological examination of the dermal lesions revealed
an early acute inflammation which progressed to a predominantly monocyte/macrophage inflammation and subsequently condensed
into lymphocyte-containing granulomatous foci (10). Rickettsial proliferation declined markedly with the appearance of
granulomatous foci. Immune guinea pigs, when given a similar
challenge, displayed an accelerated response to infection.
The inflammatory response was of a greater magnitude, and the
evolution of the response from acute inflammation to the formation of granulomatous lesions was accelerated in comparison
to nonimmune animals.

Further studies by these authors demonstrated that immune
spleen cells could adoptively transfer immunity to R. typhi
(11). Fig. 7 indicates that recipient guinea pigs inoculated
with 2×10^9 viable spleen cells from R. typhi-immune guinea
pigs showed substantial protection against the development of
dermal lesions. This capacity to transfer protection against
challenge was seen in donor animals by day 10 and persisted at
least through day 21 after primary infection. However, immune
serum recovered from donors on the same days, and transferred
in a 10 ml volume to recipients, was not able to restrain the
local proliferation of rickettsiae. In fact, recipients developed slightly larger dermal lesions after challenge than
did untreated normal guinea pigs. Titration of immune spleen
cells indicated that adoptive immunization was possible with
either 2×10^9 or 2×10^8 cells, but that 2×10^7 or fewer
cells were incapable of suppressing the dermal lesion.

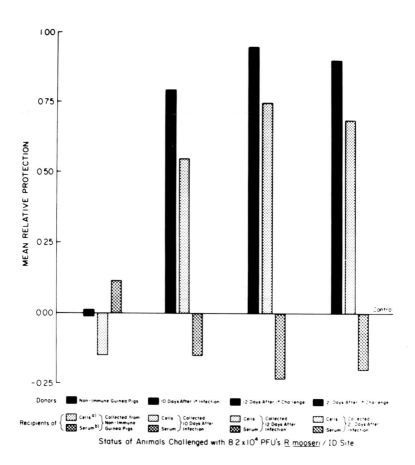

Fig. 7. Demonstration that immune splenic cells adoptively immunize naive recipients against i.d. R. mooseri challenge.
The immune status of donor animals was determined before R.
mooseri infection and at days 10, 12, and 21 after infection
by i.d. challenge. Sera or splenic cells collected at similar
intervals were delivered to recipients, 10 ml of serum or 2 x
10^9 cells; 6 h later, recipients, donors, and normal animals
were challenged with R. mooseri, 8.2 x 10^4 PFU, inoculated
into each of 3 i.d. sites. The development of lesions on
experimental animals was compared with controls inoculated
with the same inoculum.

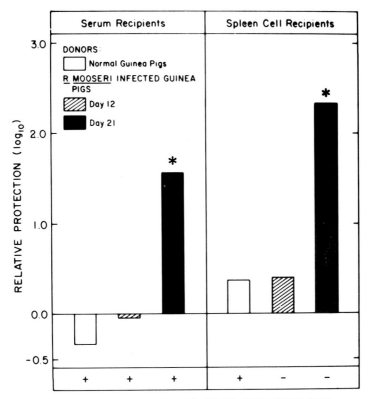

LESION DEVELOPMENT AT I.D. CHALLENGE SITE

Fig. 8. Demonstration that recipients of immune serum or
immune splenic cells are protected from systemic R. mooseri
infection. Sera or splenic cells were collected from the indicated donors and transferred to recipients as described in
the text. Subsequently, recipient and normal animals were
challenged with R. mooseri by i.d. inoculation on the back,
and 11 days later the animals were sacrificed and the numbers
of rickettsiae in their kidneys were determined. The histo-
grams show the difference between the $\log_{10}$ geometric mean
numbers of rickettsiae recovered from normal control and
treated animals. Asterisks denote groups of recipient animals
from which no rickettsiae were recovered. The sites of i.d.
challenges were observed daily through day 5 after challenge.
The groups of recipient animals which developed lesions of
approximately the same magnitude as those of nonimmune controls are denoted by a plus sign, whereas groups of animals
which did not develop large lesions are signified by a minus
sign.

The capacity /f immune spleen cells and immune serum to
protect against systemic infection was then examined (12).
Recipient guinea pigs were inoculated with either 10 ml of
immune serum or 2 x 10^9 viable spleen cells and challenged
with approximately 8 x 10^4 PFU of R. typhi. Recipients of
serum were given a second 5 ml inoculation of the same serum
6 days after challenge. At 11 days after challenge, animals
were sacrificed and the number of viable rickettsiae in the
kidneys was determined. Figure 8 shows that both serum and
cells collected 21 days after donor infection provided recipients with protection from systemic R. typhi infection. Recipients of either serum or cells were devoid of detectable
rickettsiae in the kidneys, whereas untreated animals had a
rickettsial burden of approximately 1 x 10^4 organisms/kidney.
The serum recipients, although protected against systemic infection, did develop large lesions at the site of intradermal
challenge, while cell recipients were protected against both
dermal lesions and systemic infection. When animals receiving
immune serum or spleen cells were examined at later periods
in the infection (day 15 or 21) it was found that the rickettsial burden in the kidneys was identical to that of infected
nonimmune guinea pigs. The authors concluded that inoculation
of immune serum or immune spleen cells delayed the onset of
systemic infection, but did not prevent it.

REFERENCES

1. Blake, F. G., Maxcy, K. F., Sadusk, J. F., Jr., Kohls,
   G. M., and Bell, E. J., Am. J. Hyg. 41, 243 (1945).
2. Bennett, B. L., Smadel, J. E., and Gauld, R. L., J.
   Immunol. 62, 453 (1949).
3. Shirai, A., Catanzaro, P. J., Phillips, S. M., and
   Osterman, J. V., Infect. Immun. 14, 39 (1976).
4. Catanzaro, P. J., Shirai, A., Hildebrandt, P. K., and
   Osterman, J. V., Infect. Immun. 13, 861 (1976).
5. Catanzaro, P. J., Shirai, A., Agniel, L. D., Jr., and
   Osterman, J. V., Infect. Immun. 18, 118 (1977).
6. Nacy, C. A., and Osterman, J. V., Infect. Immun. 26, 744
   (1979).
7. Groves, M. G., and Osterman, J. V., Infect. Immun. 19,
   583 (1978).
8. Groves, M. G., Rosenstreich, D. L., Taylor, B. A., and
   Osterman, J. V., J. Immunol. 125, 1395 (1980).
9. Murphy, J. R., Wisseman, C. L., Jr., and Fiset, P.,
   Infect. Immun. 21, 417 (1978).

10. Murphy, J. R., Wisseman, C. L., Jr., and Fiset, P., Infect. Immun. 22, 810 (1978).
11. Murphy, J. R., Wisseman, C. L., Jr., and Fiset, P., Infect. Immun. 24, 387 (1979).
12. Murphy, J. R., Wisseman, C. L., Jr., and Fiset, P., Infect. Immun. 27, 730 (1980).

ANTIGENS OF THE TYPHUS GROUP OF RICKETTSIAE: IMPORTANCE OF THE SPECIES-SPECIFIC SURFACE PROTEIN ANTIGENS IN ELICITING IMMUNITY[1]

Gregory A. Dasch
A. Louis Bourgeois

Naval Medical Research Institute
Bethesda, Maryland

I. INTRODUCTION

The Cox-type, ether-extracted, killed epidemic typhus vaccine developed during World War II is effective but does not
meet present standards for bacterial vaccines in that it contains large amounts of yolk sac and effective immunizing doses
elicit strong local and systemic reactions, probably due to
their high endotoxin content (1). The current guinea pig potency test for typhus vaccines is an imprecise measure of potency based on antibody titer and the immediate toxicity of
rickettsiae in high dosages (2, 3). Since recent studies
suggest that cellular immunity is more important than humoral
immunity in defense against rickettsial infections, the value
of the current potency test is questionable (4).
   Our laboratory has been developing an improved combined
vaccine against murine and epidemic typhus over the past five
years. A combined vaccine was chosen because of the current
similar global incidence of the two diseases, the great antigenic and chemical similarity of R. typhi and R. prowazekii,
and the apparent effectiveness of earlier combined vaccines of
British (5) and Mexican workers (6). The Renografin density

---

[1] Supported by the Naval Medical Research and Development
Command, Department of the Navy, Research Task Nos.
MR0410501.0030 and M0095PN002.5060.

gradient centrifugation technique permitted the isolation of
viable rickettsiae that were free of contaminating yolk sac
materials (7). In this paper and the next (8), we describe
the preparation and characterization of subunit vaccines from
Renografin purified R. typhi and R. prowazekii.
  Earlier pioneering studies on typhus vaccines provided
initial insight into the nature of essential antigens that
might be suitable for a subunit vaccine (Table 1). These
studies suggested that the R. prowazekii antigen which was
essential for the protective efficacy of the vaccine was heat-
labile and species-specific. Vaccines treated at $60^{o}C$ were
not protective, although they readily elicited the formation
of group-reactive antibodies and were themselves group-reactive antigens (9-11). We have identified and purified major,
heat-labile, species-specific, protein antigens (SPAs) from
soluble extracts of R. typhi and R. prowazekii (12). We recently developed a simple procedure for their selective extraction from the rickettsial cell surface (13). In this report, some characteristics of the SPA extracts of R. typhi, R.
prowazekii, and R. canada are compared. The endotoxin content
and importance of the SPAs of R. typhi and R. prowazekii in
humoral and cellular immunity to typhus rickettsiae are also
examined. The protective efficacy of the SPA of R. typhi in
a guinea pig protection model is described in the following
paper (8).

TABLE 1. Response of Guinea Pigs to Inoculation with Soluble
            Antigen Fractions of R. prowazekii

Antigen treatment	Mouse toxin neutralization titer against:		Protection against fever after challenge by:		Refer- ence
	R. prow- azekii	R. typhi	R. prow- azekii	R. typhi	
None	181	-[a]	-	-	10
60°C 45 min	24	-	-	-	
None	128	32	Complete	None	9
60°C 4 min	4	4	None	None	
None	320	-	Complete	-	11
60°C 60 min	0	-	Partial	-	
100°C 100 min	0	-	None	-	

[a]Not done.

II. METHODS

Antigens were prepared from Renografin density gradient
purified R. typhi Wilmington or R. prowazekii Breinl or Madrid
E (7, 14). For the enzyme-linked immunosorbent assay (ELISA),
total rickettsial extracts were prepared by French pressure
cell disruption (15). DE52 purified SPAs (12) and the supernatant fraction of the French pressure cell extract were used
in human lymphocyte transformation assays (16). Antigens obtained with a selective Tris extraction and sonication procedure (13) were used in all other experiments. Briefly, cells
were extracted twice in 10 mM Tris HCl, pH 7.6 for 20 min at
45°C; SPAs were in the supernatant fraction of the pooled Tris
extracts obtained by centrifugation at 200,000 x g for 2 hr.
Sonic extracts of the Tris-extracted, SPA-depleted cells were
separated similarly into supernatant and membrane fractions.

Polyacrylamide gel electrophoresis (PAGE) of native proteins was done on 7.5% acrylamide disc gels or 3 mm preparative
slab gels with a BioRad Laboratories Model 220 adapter kit
(17). Discontinuous sodium dodecyl sulfate (SDS) PAGE was done
on 1.5 mm, 9% acrylamide slabs with the Model 220 cell (18).

Ouchterlony double diffusion assays in 1% agarose in phosphate buffered saline were incubated for 48 hr at 20°C and
employed the same hyperimmune rabbit antisera used previously
in rocket and crossed immunoelectrophoresis (RIE, CrIE) (12).

The Limulus amoebocyte lysate gelation assay for endotoxin
(19) was standardized with Reference Endotoxin Lot EC4 from
the Bureau of Biologics, Food and Drug Administration.

The mouse spleen cell mitogenicity assay and whole guinea
pig blood transformation assay were modified slightly from
published procedures (20, 21) and were similar to the human
lymphocyte transformation assay (16). Normal NMRI mouse
spleen cells (2.5×10^{6} cells/ml) were incubated in complete
RPMI (16) containing 5% heat-inactivated fetal bovine serum
with added antigen or mitogen (4 replicate wells) for three
days. Whole guinea pig blood, diluted 1:10 in complete RPMI
containing heparin, was incubated with antigen or controls (6
replicate wells) for 6 days. ^{3}H-thymidine (1 μCi/well) was
added 18 hr prior to harvesting the cells with a multiple
automated sample harvester (MASH) (22, 16). Guinea pig cells
were washed on the MASH sequentially with 3% acetic acid,
water, and methanol prior to liquid scintillation counting.
Transformation responses were calculated as stimulation indi-
ces--the ratio of the mean disintegrations per min (dpm) of
stimulated cultures to the mean dpm of unstimulated cultures.
An index greater than 3 was significant ($P < 0.01$).

III.   RESULTS

Although the antisera used reacted against rickettsial
group antigens (23), the SPAs of R. typhi, R. prowazekii,
and R. canada gave single specific immunoprecipitates by
Ouchterlony double diffusion analysis (Fig. 1).   Only the
R. prowazekii SPA had heterologous cross-reactivity with the
R. typhi antiserum.   Similar results were obtained by RIE,
and a slight cross-reaction of R. typhi SPA with R. prowazekii antiserum was also detected by ELISA (not shown).   The
Tris extracts of the 3 species migrated by Davis PAGE as one
major and 1-3 minor bands with SPA activity (not shown).   For
both R. typhi and R. prowazekii the whole extract and the two
most rapidly migrating SPA bands (major band I, minor band II)
purified by preparative PAGE had similar SDS-PAGE patterns
(Fig. 2, R. typhi band II poorly shown).   Bands II were shown
to be dimers of bands I by sucrose gradient centrifugation
(not shown).   In contrast, although the purified minor doublet
fraction I and slower major band II of R. canada SPA consisted
of different polypeptides by SDS-PAGE, they were not distinguished on sucrose gradients.   R. canada fraction I polypeptides appeared to arise from band II by proteolysis.   In conclusion, Tris extracts of each typhus rickettsia contained
immunologically similar, molecular variants of SPA but were
nearly free of non-SPA polypeptides.
     By the Limulus amoebocyte lysate gelation assay, endotoxin
levels in the Tris-extracted SPAs of R. typhi and R. prowazekii were reduced by 10^3 compared to fractions obtained from
Tris-extracted cells (Table 2).   Similarly, the SPAs lacked

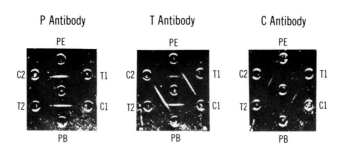

Fig. 1.   Immunodiffusion analysis of Tris-extracted SPAs
of typhus rickettsiae.   Outer wells: 2-10 µg of SPA protein;
center wells: 5 µl of undiluted rabbit anti-rickettsial
antiserum.   R. prowazekii Breinl (PB) or Madrid E (PE), R.
typhi (T), R. canada (C).

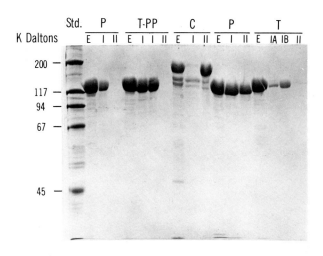

Fig. 2.   SDS-PAGE analysis of Tris-extracted SPAs (E) and preparative PAGE purified SPA bands I and II. Abbreviations as in Fig. 1 except SPA from plaque purified R. typhi (T-PP).

the potent mitogenic effect for mouse lymphocytes of other rickettsial fractions, which, as with other Gram-negative bacteria, is probably due to the presence of endotoxin.

TABLE 2.   Endotoxin Content and Mitogenicity for Mouse Spleen Cells of Antigen Fractions of Typhus Rickettsiae

Antigen fraction	µg endotoxin/ mg rickettsial protein[a]	Mitogen response[b]
Rickettsia typhi		
Specific antigen	0.02	1.3 ± 0.1
Sonicate supernatant	4.0	10.8 ± 0.4
Sonicate pellet	40.0	12.1 ± 0.2
Rickettsia prowazekii		
Specific antigen	0.03	1.3 ± 0.1
Sonicate supernatant	70.0	8.6 ± 0.5
Sonicate pellet	20.0	11.9 ± 0.5

[a]Limulus amoebocyte lysate gelation assay.
[b]Mean stimulation index + S. E. of spleen cells of unimmunized mice at 3 days of culture with 25 µg rickettsial antigen per well (0.2 ml).

The importance of SPAs in humoral and cellular immunity to typhus rickettsiae was examined in infected guinea pigs and humans. Although ELISA titers of sera of infected guinea pigs were species-specific and of comparable magnitude with either the total rickettsial extracts or SPAs, anti-SPA titers were somewhat more species-specific (not shown). With lymphocytes of control animals, occasional non-specific mitogenic effects were obtained with membrane fractions but not with SPAs (Table 3). Specific anti-rickettsial transformation responses were detected with either fraction in infected guinea pigs. However, responses to SPA-deficient membranes were not species-specific and were lower than the species-specific anti-SPA responses (Table 3).

Every human serum in which we have detected anti-typhus antibodies by ELISA with total rickettsial antigens also had significant anti-SPA titers (not shown). The ELISA and cellular immune status of one control and four typhus exposed individuals are shown in Table 4. Although ELISA titers were present in all exposed cases, in only two could the titer (> 500) be considered diagnostic of previous typhus infection (15); however all had significant cellular responses against both antigens. Anti-SPA cellular responses were lower but more specific for the infecting agent, when known, than those against total supernatant extracts. The occupationally exposed individual probably had a subclinical Madrid E infection and had the anticipated specific anti-R. prowazekii SPA response.

TABLE 3.   Whole Blood Lymphocyte Transformation Response of Guinea Pigs Following Infection with Rickettsiae

| Intradermal infection | Mean stimulation index[a] | | | |
| | Sonicate pellet | | Specific antigen | |
	Rt Ag[b]	Rp Ag[b]	Rt Ag	Rp Ag
Sham control	1.4	3.7	1.4	2.2
$10^{6.4}$ PFU of R. typhi	7.9	7.6	12.0	2.7
$10^{6.2}$ PFU of R. prowazekii	7.2	7.1	1.2	25.0

[a]Blood collected at 12 days post infection and incubated with 2 μg/well of each antigen (0.2 ml per well).

[b]Rt Ag = R. typhi antigen; Rp Ag = R. prowazekii antigen.

TABLE 4. Lymphocyte Transformation, Response in Humans to Fractions of Typhus Group Rickettsiae

Exposure to rickettsiae	Years since last exposure	ELISA IgG titer[a]		Mean stimulation index[b]			
				Total supernatant antigen		Specific antigen	
		R. typhi	R. prow-azekii	R. typhi	R. prow.	R. typhi	R. prow.
None	0	100	100	1.5	1.9	1.3	1.1
R. typhi infection (1961)	0	3500	600	22.7	19.6	14.7	8.0
R. prowazekii vaccine (1969); R. typhi infection (1974)	3	1700	2200	17.6	11.4	8.2	2.3
R. prowazekii infection (1946)	33	200	410	4.8	8.1	2.1	5.0
Occupational: to both	0	270	170	10.8	9.9	5.7	10.6

[a] Total French pressure cell extract antigens, titer is serum dilution giving an absorbance 0.2 units above no serum controls at 60 min with a goat anti-human IgG-alkaline phosphatase conjugate.

[b] 0.5 µg antigen per well tested (0.2 ml/well), results at 5 days of culture.

IV. DISCUSSION

The SPAs of R. typhi and R. prowazekii have many properties which make them attractive as possible subunit vaccines:
First, the SPAs of these rickettsiae can be obtained simply in excellent purity and yields (10-15 mg protein per 100
mg of rickettsiae) (13). Similar SPA fractions have also been
obtained from R. canada, as shown here, and from R. akari
(Dasch et al., manuscript in preparation). Other spotted fever group rickettsiae with the major 120,000 Dalton polypeptide (24) probably also contain similar SPAs. It will be of
interest whether all SPAs are important in eliciting their
respective anti-rickettsial immunities, and whether these
proteins may have arisen from a common ancestral protein.
Second, the SPAs of R. typhi and R. prowazekii are very
large polypeptides which associate into forms that may reflect
their native organization on the surface of the rickettsiae.
Since immunogenicity generally increases with molecular weight
and even small forms of the SPAs, probably derived by proteolysis, retain most of their immunological reactivity (12),
the SPAs may be very potent immunogens.
Third, endotoxin levels in the SPAs of R. typhi and R.
prowazekii were suitably low for use as bacterial vaccines, as
expected from their freedom from contaminating outer membrane
proteins (13). Although it is not known whether all rickettsial toxic reactions are due to the endotoxin, the absence of
significant local reactions in guinea pigs immunized with the
SPA of R. typhi supports this view (8).
Fourth, because the antigen and chemical contents of the
SPAs may be readily determined by several assays (12, 13),
production of uniform SPA vaccine lots may be easier than with
Cox-type vaccines. Similarly, less cumbersome and more meaningful vaccine potency assays than the current guinea pig test
may also be possible with the SPA subunit vaccines.
Finally, the SPAs are avidly recognized by both the humoral and cellular arms of the immune system of guinea pigs and
man. This is important in two respects. First, the SPAs are
excellent antigens for the in vitro detection of rickettsial
infections and immune status following vaccination. In particular, their lack of non-specific mitogenicity in lymphocyte
transformation assays makes them more satisfactory than other
rickettsial antigens for use with animals or human individuals
who are responsive to endotoxin. Furthermore, infections with
R. typhi or R. prowazekii are more readily distinguished with
the SPAs than with other rickettsial extracts which contain
significant amounts of typhus group antigens. Second, we detected potent CMI responses to the SPAs in all four human

typhus exposures, even in an individual 33 years after his infection with R. prowazekii. It is impossible to assess the relative protective importance of individual antigens solely from the magnitudes of the humoral and CMI responses to them, but the strong anti-SPA responses measured here are fully consistent with the conclusions drawn from earlier studies about the essential role of the SPAs in protective immunity (Table 1).

Of course, the real value of the SPAs in eliciting immunity in man and animals against the typhus rickettsiae can only be determined by direct in vivo evaluation of their immunogenicity and protective efficacy. Results that directly confirm the efficacy of the SPA of R. typhi in eliciting immunity in a guinea pig intradermal challenge model are provided in the following paper (8).

V. SUMMARY

Early studies which suggested that the species-specific protein antigens (SPAs) of typhus rickettsiae are essential for the protective efficacy of typhus vaccines are reviewed. A simple method for the isolation of SPAs from R. typhi, R. prowazekii, and R. canada is described. The SPAs of each species exist in several molecular forms, each with very similar immunological properties. SPA fractions of R. typhi and R. prowazekii did not have significant endotoxin content by two assays. Guinea pigs and man previously infected with R. typhi or R. prowazekii have significant levels of humoral and cellular immunity against the SPAs of these rickettsiae, as measured respectively by enzyme-linked immunosorbent assay and lymphocyte transformation. These findings suggest that the SPAs of R. typhi and R. prowazekii are excellent materials for evaluation as possible highly immunogenic, non-toxic, subunit vaccines against murine and epidemic typhus.

ACKNOWLEDGMENTS

We gratefully acknowledge the devoted and expert technical assistance of J. R. Samms, M. Klingseis, W. G. Sewell, and B. L. Ward in this investigation. We also thank Emilio Weiss for his encouragement and assistance with the manuscript.

REFERENCES

1. Mason, R. A., Wenzel, R. P., Seligmann, E. B. Jr., and
    Ginn, R. K., J. Biol. Stand. 4, 217 (1976).
2. Mason, R. A., Seligmann, E. B. Jr., and Ginn, R. K.,
    J. Biol. Stand. 4, 209 (1976).
3. Barker, L. F., and Patt, J. K., Am. J. Epidemiol. 86,
    500 (1967).
4. Murphy, J. R., Wisseman, C. L. Jr., and Fiset, P.,
    Infect. Immun. 27, 730 (1980).
5. Davis, W. A., Ann. Int. Med. 34, 448 (1951).
6. Castaneda, M. R., J. Immunol. 58, 283 (1948).
7. Weiss, E., Coolbaugh, J. C., and Williams, J. C.,
    Appl. Microbiol. 30, 456 (1975).
8. Bourgeois, A. L., and Dasch, G. A., in "Rickettsiae
    and Rickettsial Diseases," (W. Burgdorfer and R. L.
    Anacker, eds.), p. 71. Academic Press, New York (1981).
9. Shepard, C. C., in "Studies of Typhus Fever," p. 93.
    National Institutes of Health Bull. No. 183 (1945).
10. Craigie, J., Watson, D. W., Clark, E. M., and Malcomson,
    M. E., Can. J. Res. E24, 84 (1946).
11. Golinevitch, H. M., and Voronova, Z. A., J. Hyg.
    Epidemiol. Microbiol. Immunol. 12, 413 (1966).
12. Dasch, G. A., Samms, J. R., and Williams, J. C., Infect.
    Immun. 31, 276 (1981).
13. Dasch, G. A. Manuscript submitted for publication (1981).
14. Dasch, G. A., and Weiss, E., Infect. Immun. 15, 280
    (1977).
15. Halle, S., and Dasch, G. A., J. Clin. Microbiol. 12, 343
    (1980).
16. Bourgeois, A. L., Dasch, G. A., and Strong, D. M.,
    Infect. Immun. 27, 483 (1980).
17. Davis, B. J., Ann. N. Y. Acad. Sci. 121, 404 (1964).
18. Laemmli, U. K., Nature (London) 227, 680 (1970).
19. Jorgensen, J. H., and Smith, R. F., Appl. Microbiol. 26,
    43 (1973).
20. Strong, D. M., Ahmed, A. A., Thurman, G. B., and Sell,
    K. W., J. Immunol. Meth. 2, 279 (1972).
21. Kenyon, R. H., Ascher, M. S., Kishimoto, R. A., and
    Pedersen, C. E. Jr., Infect. Immun. 18, 840 (1977).
22. Hartzman, R. J., Bach, M. L., Bach, F. H., Thurman,
    G. B., and Sell, K. W., Cell. Immunol. 4, 182 (1972).
23. Halle, S., Dasch, G. A., and Weiss, E., J. Clin.
    Microbiol. 6, 101 (1977).
24. Pedersen, C. E. Jr., and Walters, V. D., Life Sci.
    22, 583 (1978).

THE SPECIES-SPECIFIC SURFACE PROTEIN ANTIGEN
OF RICKETTSIA TYPHI: IMMUNOGENICITY
AND PROTECTIVE EFFICACY IN GUINEA PIGS[1]

A. Louis Bourgeois
Gregory A. Dasch

Naval Medical Research Institute
Bethesda, Maryland

I. INTRODUCTION

As discussed in the previous paper (1) the species-specific protein antigens (SPAs) of Rickettsia typhi and Rickettsia prowazekii have several characteristics which make them ideal candidates for use as subunit typhus vaccines. Therefore, we examined the immunogenicity and vaccine potential of the SPA of R. typhi in guinea pigs. Humoral and cell-mediated immune (CMI) responses following SPA immunization were monitored by ELISA (2) and whole blood lymphocyte transformation (1), respectively. Protective efficacy was evaluated in the guinea pig intradermal (ID) challenge model of Castaneda (3) as modified recently by Murphy, Wisseman, and Fiset (4, 5). Protection in this model is based on an animal's ability to suppress cutaneous lesion formation at ID challenge sites and to prevent the systemic spread of rickettsiae.

The federal typhus vaccine guinea pig potency test (6) is an indirect and imprecise measure of vaccine efficacy (1). Nevertheless, sera from SPA immunized guinea pigs were assayed for toxin-neutralizing antibodies (7) against R. typhi to determine whether such antibodies were elicited by SPA immunization and, if they were, what SPA dosage would be needed to approximate the titer required in the federal potency test.

[1]Supported by the Naval Medical Research and Development Command, Department of the Navy, Research Task Nos. MR0410501.0030 and M0095PN002.5060.

II. METHODS

The total French pressure cell extract antigens, Tris-extracted SPAs and sonic extract membranes of R. typhi and R. prowazekii were prepared as previously described (1). The SPA and 0.1% formalin treated membrane fraction of R. typhi were dialyzed for 18 h at 4°C against 500-1000 volumes of Dulbecco's phosphate buffered saline (PBS) before use as an immunogen or in lymphocyte transformation assays.

The immunogenicity and protective efficacy of the SPA of R. typhi were examined in male Hartley strain guinea pigs pur-chased from the Walter Reed Army Institute of Research, Wash-ington, D.C. Following primary and booster immunization, anti-rickettsial humoral and CMI responses were monitored in vitro by ELISA and whole blood lymphocyte transformation, respectively. The ELISA was modified slightly from that of Halle and Dasch (2). Total antigens, SPAs and membrane fractions of R. typhi and R. prowazekii were used as antigens at a coating concentration of 3.2 µg/ml. All sera were screened at a fixed 1:100 dilution, and plates were read directly in a Titertek Multiskan ELISA reader (Flow Labs.) at 405 nm. Wells with off scale readings were diluted and re-read. The whole blood lymphocyte transformation assay was performed as described (1).

The intradermal (ID) challenge model of Murphy et al. (4, 5) was used to assess cutaneous and systemic immunity in guinea pigs following immunization. Animals were challenged ID with R. typhi (bovine plasma albumin-purified seed; step 2, ref. 8) and local skin reactions were observed for 10 days post-challenge (4). The number of rickettsiae in the blood, spleen, and kidneys of animals at 12 days post-challenge was determined by plaque assay on irradiated L-cell monolayers used at 5 days post-irradiation (9). Blood and tissue speci-mens from individual animals were diluted in sucrose-phos-phate-glutamate solution (10) supplemented with 1% Renografin and 5 mM $MgCl_2$ (11) for inoculation. Following inoculation, flasks were rocked for 75 min at room temperature and centri-fuged at 600 x g for 10 min (12). After centrifugation, flasks were overlayed and incubated for 12 days at 32°C in a 5% CO_2 humidified atmosphere. Flasks received a second over-lay on day 6 and were stained as described (13).

The toxin-neutralizing antibody titers of pooled guinea pig sera were determined in NMRI mice as described (7), ex-cept that the total volume injected was 0.25 ml to reduce the number of non-specific deaths.

III. RESULTS

Anti-SPA antibody is readily detected in the sera of man
and animals following infection with R. typhi (1, 14). To
determine whether the SPA is also immunogenic in the absence
of other rickettsial antigens or infection, groups of guinea
pigs were immunized subcutaneously with 50, 5, 0.5, or 0.05 µg
SPA, or sham immunized with PBS. Antibody responses for the
5 groups were measured by ELISA using the total rickettsial
antigen extract of R. typhi (Fig. 1). Animals immunized with
50 and 5 µg of SPA exhibited strong antibody responses which
persisted for at least 70 days, but immunization with lower
SPA doses failed to elicit a significant response. On day
62 post-primary immunization, all animal groups including
the initial controls received a booster immunization with
2 µg of SPA (Fig. 1), a dose that elicited antibody levels
in control animals that were only slightly lower than those
achieved by 5 µg of SPA (Fig. 1). All of the previously
immunized animals had marked rises in antibody levels. However, the kinetics of their responses were quite different
from those of the 2 µg primary group (Fig. 1). The accelerated response at 7 days post booster immunization of animals
initially receiving 0.5 and 0.05 µg SPA indicated that they

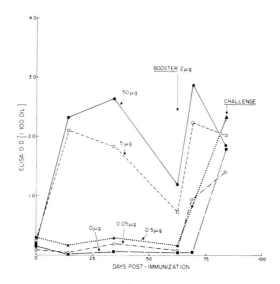

Fig. 1. Mean antibody response of guinea pigs against the
total antigen extract of R. typhi following primary and
booster immunization with the SPA of R. typhi.

had been sensitized by these small amounts of antigen.

To confirm that the antibody responses elicited by the SPA were directed against the specific antigen, the SPAs of R. typhi and R. prowazekii also were used in the ELISA (Table 1). The antibody response after either primary or booster immunization was highly specific. Similar specificity was also obtained when total rickettsial extracts or extracted membranes of these organisms were employed in the ELISA. However, ELISA optical densities were generally lower with the membrane antigens (data not shown), possibly because of the relatively low SPA content of these fractions.

Because CMI plays an important role in anti-typhus immunity (4, 5), the ability of the SPA to elicit CMI was next examined in vitro with a whole blood lymphocyte transformation assay (Table 2). At 34 days post-immunization, only guinea pigs receiving 50 or 5 µg of SPA had significant stimulation indices against the SPA. In contrast, all guinea pigs boosted with 2 µg of SPA exhibited excellent transformation responses at 7 days post-immunization, even though a primary 2 µg dose alone was insufficient to elicit a significant cellular response (Table 2). As was found for the humoral response to the SPA (Fig. 1), single 0.5 and 0.05 µg doses of this antigen were sufficient to sensitize these animals for accelerated cellular responses. Stimulation

TABLE 1. Specificity of the Guinea Pig Antibody Response Following Immunization with the SPA of R. typhi

Primary immunization dose	ELISA O.D.[c] (1:100 dil.)			
	14 days P.I.		69 days P.I.[a]	
	RT SPA	RP SPA	RT SPA	RP SPA
None (3, 2)[b]	0.10	0.19	0.19	0.13
0.05 µg (3, 2)	0.16	0.18	1.61	0.61
0.50 µg (3, 1)	0.44	0.30	0.55	0.35
5.00 µg (3, 3)	1.73	0.43	2.87	1.41
50.00 µg (2, 2)	2.76	0.67	3.48	1.57

[a] 7 days after SPA booster immunization (2 µg) of all groups including the unimmunized control.

[b] (No. animals in primary immunization group, No. animals in groups receiving booster immunization).

[c] Optical density.

TABLE 2. Whole Blood Lymphocyte Transformation Response of
Individual Guinea Pigs to the SPA of R. typhi

Primary immunization dose	Mean stimulation index $\pm$ S.E.[a]	
	34 days P.I.	69 days P.I.[b]
	2.5 µg SPA	1 µg SPA
None	1.7 + 0.2 1.0 + 0.1	1.0 + 0.2 1.0 + 0.2
0.05 µg	1.0 + 0.1 1.2 + 0.2	6.0 + 0.6 Not done
0.50 µg	1.0 + 0.1 2.0 + 0.3	4.0 + 0.5 Not done
5.00 µg	5.0 + 0.6 6.0 + 0.6 Not done	9.0 + 0.9 6.0 + 0.7 20.0 + 3.0
50.00 µg	1.0 + 0.1 3.0 + 0.4	18.0 + 2.0 11.0 + 1.0

[a] Stimulation indices > 3 are significant at the 0.01 level
and are considered indicative of CMI to R. typhi.

[b] 7 days post 2 µg booster immunization in all groups.

indices were somewhat lower when the extracted (SPA-poor)
membrane fraction was substituted for the SPA (data not
shown).

The ability of guinea pigs to suppress local and systemic
rickettsial infection 21 days after booster immunization was
determined by challenging animals ID in the back with both
10^7 (high dose) and 10^5 (low dose) PFU of R. typhi (4). At
high (not shown) and low dose (Fig. 2) challenge sites, the
time course and severity of lesion development due to rickettsial growth was significantly modified in immunized animals.
Due to the toxicity of the higher dose, differences in lesion
size were more obvious with the lower dose. The degree of
lesion suppression, particularly its magnitude and persistence, correlated very strongly to the amount of the initial
SPA immunization (Fig. 2). Lesion suppression with 2 µg alone
was similar to that in the 5 + 2 µg regimen group (data not
shown).

SPA immunization of guinea pigs also enhanced their ability to reduce or prevent the systemic spread of rickettsiae
from ID sites to the peripheral blood and deep tissues

(Table 3). SPA immunized animals exhibited insignificant
levels of rickettsiae in their blood. Although the spleens

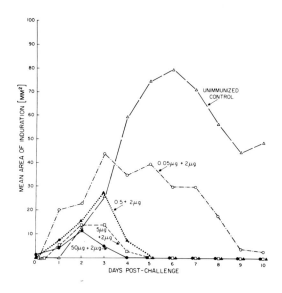

Fig. 2. Cutaneous lesion development in guinea pigs
following ID challenge with 10^5 PFU of R. typhi.

TABLE 3. Rickettsial Plaque-Forming Units (PFU) in Guinea Pig
Tissues Following Immunization
with the SPA of R. typhi and Challenge[a]

Total immunization regimen	Mean PFU per gram of tissue		
	Whole blood	Spleen	Kidney
None	1,700	13,000	63,000
2 μg	< 10	Not done	5,800
0.05 μg + 2 μg	40	Not done	2,500
0.50 μg + 2 μg	< 10	Not done	1,400
5.00 μg + 2 μg	< 10	300	< 50
50.00 μg + 2 μg	< 10	< 50	< 50

[a] PFUs assayed at 12 days after intradermal challenge with
$10^{7.5}$ PFU of R. typhi 21 days post 2 μg SPA immunization in
all groups.

TABLE 4. Toxin-Neutralizing Antibody Titers of Guinea Pig Sera
Following Immunization with the SPA of R. typhi

Primary immunization dose	Reciprocal dilution	
	34 days P.I.	83 days P.I.[a]
None	< 8	10
0.05 μg	< 8	< 8
0.50 μg	< 8	9
5.00 μg	8	27
50.00 μg	8	37
5.00 μg (IFA)[b]	Not done	115
Infected control[c]	41	Not done

[a] 21 days post 2 μg booster immunization in all groups.

[b] Primary immunization (5 μg) given in incomplete Freund's adjuvant.

[c] Intradermal infection with 10^5 PFU of R. typhi.

and kidneys of these animals also had substantially reduced
levels of rickettsiae, the reduction was complete in the
kidney only with the 5 + 2 and 50 + 2 μg SPA regimens
(Table 3).

Although the toxin-neutralizing antibody titers were
only of borderline significance following primary immunization, very significant titers were obtained following
booster SPA immunization, especially following primary SPA
immunization in incomplete Freund's adjuvant (Table 4).   It
was of interest that the toxin-neutralizing titers stimulated
by the 50 + 2 and 5 + 2 μg SPA immunization regimens were
comparable to the minimum titer of 1:32 specified for release
of a vaccine lot for human use in the federal guinea pig
typhus vaccine potency test (6).

IV. DISCUSSION

Characteristics of SPAs which make them highly attractive
vaccine candidates were discussed in the preceding paper (1).
This paper establishes that the SPA of R. typhi is highly
immunogenic and stimulates significant levels of protective
immunity in a guinea pig infection model.   Protective immun-

ity in guinea pigs following SPA immunization correlated
closely with the ability of animals to mount a strong anti-
SPA lymphocyte transformation response. This apparent relationship between protection and anti-rickettsial CMI was
not unexpected since Murphy et al. (4, 5) previously have
shown that anti-typhus immunity is cell-mediated and possibly
independent of antibody. In these and in subsequent experiments, primary immunization with intermediate SPA doses
(2-5 µg) elicited only weak transformation responses (Table
2) and variable levels of local (not shown) and systemic
immunity (Table 3) which failed to persist for 60 days. In
contrast, after booster immunization, animals exhibited
highly significant transformation responses (Table 2) and
protective immunity (Fig. 2 and Table 3) that persisted and
were comparable to those seen in guinea pigs following infection (not shown). A 2-dose regimen appears necessary to
obtain protection equivalent to naturally acquired immunity.
We do not know whether primary immunization with higher SPA
doses (> 5 µg) would be as effective as the 2-dose regime.

The strong CMI elicited by immunization with the purified
SPA was surprising since even killed whole cell bacterial vaccines may require an adjuvant to elicit detectable levels of
CMI. Kenyon and co-workers (15) observed that guinea pigs
receiving multiple injections of killed R. rickettsii vaccine
failed to exhibit significant lymphocyte transformation unless an adjuvant was used. Although they suggested that infection with R. rickettsii might be required to elicit a
cellular immune response, this is clearly not the case for
the typhus rickettsiae. Purified bacterial proteins are
often poor immunogens. For example, N. meningitidis outer
membrane proteins are poor immunogens without added capsular
polysaccharide (16). Similarly, phase I polysaccharide antigen of Coxiella burnetii acts as an adjuvant for phase II
antigen (17). It is possible that endogenous adjuvants may
be potentiating the response to the SPA. The Tris-extracted
SPAs contain RNA fragments (14), that, by analogy with ribosomal vaccines (18), may act as an adjuvant. Alternatively
the protein itself may have unusual properties which confer
strong immunogenicity on it. Very large proteins like the
SPAs (1) are generally effective immunogens (19). Since the
SPA is a surface antigen, one may speculate that this protein
plays a role in rickettsiae-host cell interactions. Extracted SPA may bind to host cell surfaces (macrophages or endothelial cells) thereby facilitating its ability to stimulate anti-rickettsial immunity.

The federal guinea pig typhus vaccine potency assay is
cumbersome, imprecise, and possibly not relevant to a
vaccine's efficacy (1). The results detailed here suggest

several alternative methods. Immunization with SPA elicits
protective immunity and a toxin–neutralizing antibody response in guinea pigs (Table 4). Assays which measure anti-
SPA antibody or CMI in vaccinated test animals may be more
accurate and meaningful predictors of immunity than is the
current test. However, the guinea pig ID challenge model
may be even better since in vivo efficacy is measured.

   In conclusion, the SPA of R. typhi is an effective protective immunogen. Studies to be reported elsewhere have
also demonstrated the efficacy of a combined murine–epidemic
typhus SPA vaccine in guinea pigs. Consequently, combined
murine–epidemic SPA vaccines are being prepared for evaluation of their efficacy in human volunteers.

V. SUMMARY

   The immunogenicity and protective efficacy of the SPA of
R. typhi were examined in guinea pigs. Primary immunization
with 50 and 5 µg of protein elicited strong species–specific
anti–rickettsial antibody responses, and weak, but significant
lymphocyte transformation reactions. Immunization with lower
SPA doses (0.5 and 0.05 µg) did not trigger primary antibody or cellular responses, but were sufficiently immunogenic
to sensitize animals for both humoral and cell–mediated
immunity. Following booster immunization all animals exhibited accelerated antibody and lymphoproliferative responses.
Intradermal challenge experiments indicated that two SPA immu-
nizations dramatically modified the course of cutaneous lesion
development and prevented the dissemination of R. typhi from
the skin into the deep tissues. Booster immunization with
SPA also stimulated the production of sufficient toxin neutralizing antibodies to meet the federal potency requirement
for typhus vaccine. By all criteria examined, the SPA of
R. typhi is a highly protective subunit vaccine for murine
typhus.

ACKNOWLEDGMENTS

   We thank Richard Grays for the preparation of tissue culture materials and Byron L. Ward and Walter G. Sewell for
their excellent technical assistance. We also thank Emilio
Weiss for his encouragement and assistance with this manuscript.

REFERENCES

1. Dasch, G. A., and Bourgeois, A. L., in "Rickettsiae and Rickettsial Diseases," (W. Burgdorfer and R. L. Anacker, eds.), p. 61. Academic Press, New York (1981).
2. Halle, S., and Dasch, G. A., J. Clin. Microbiol. 12, 343 (1980).
3. Castaneda, M. R., J. Exp. Med. 64, 701 (1936).
4. Murphy, J. R., Wisseman, C. L., Jr., and Fiset, P., Infect. Immun. 22, 810 (1978).
5. Murphy, J. R., Wisseman, C. L., Jr., and Fiset, P., Infect. Immun. 27, 730 (1980).
6. "Minimum Requirements: Typhus Vaccine." DHEW, PHS, NIH, Bethesda, Maryland, 6th revision, 22 July (1954).
7. Henderson, R. G., and Topping, N. H., Nat. Inst. Health Bull. 183, 41 (1945).
8. Weiss, E., Coolbaugh, J. C., and Williams, J. C., Appl. Microbiol. 30, 456 (1975).
9. Oaks, S. C., Jr., Osterman, J. V., and Hetrick, F. M., J. Clin. Microbiol. 6, 76 (1977).
10. Bovarnick, M. R., Miller, J. C., and Synder, J. C., J. Bacteriol. 59, 509 (1950).
11. Bourgeois, A. L., and Dasch, G. A., Abstr. Am. Soc. Microbiol. D7 (1980).
12. Ormsbee, R., Peacock, M., Gerloff, R., Tallent, G., and Wike, D., Infect. Immun. 19, 239 (1978).
13. Woodman, D. R., Weiss, E., Dasch, G. A., and Bozeman, F. M., Infect. Immun. 16, 853 (1977).
14. Dasch, G. A., Manuscript submitted for publication (1981).
15. Kenyon, R. H., Ascher, M. S., Kishimoto, R. A., and Pedersen, C. E., Infect. Immun. 18, 840 (1977).
16. Zollinger, W. D., Mandrell, R. E., Griffiss, J. M., Altieri, P., and Berman, S., J. Clin. Invest. 63, 836 (1979).
17. Fiset, P., and Ormsbee, R. A., Zbl. Bakt. (Orig.) 206, 321 (1968).
18. Collins, F. M., Bacteriol. Rev. 38, 371 (1974).
19. Borek, F., in "Immunogenicity," (F. Borek, ed.), p. 45. American Elsevier Publishing Co., New York (1972).

INTERACTION OF RICKETTSIA PROWAZEKI AND MACROPHAGE-LIKE CELL LINES[1]

Jenifer Turco[2]
Herbert H. Winkler

Department of Microbiology
University of South Alabama
College of Medicine
Mobile, Alabama

I. INTRODUCTION

Bacteria of the genus Rickettsia are obligate intracellular parasites which grow in the cytoplasm (and sometimes in the nucleus) of their host cells. Such intracellular organisms might be expected to have developed some mechanism(s) for avoiding destruction in phagocytic cells. The interactions of certain Rickettsia species and macrophages in particular have been partially characterized in several studies.

The recent work of Nacy and Osterman (1) described the growth of R. tsutsugamushi in resident mouse peritoneal macrophages. Destruction of many of the organisms within the macrophages resulted if the rickettsiae were treated with immune serum before they were allowed to infect the cells. Other experiments indicated that activated macrophages were important in host defense against R. tsutsugamushi (1,2).

The growth of both R. typhi and the virulent Breinl strain of R. prowazeki in human monocyte-derived macrophages was reported by Gambrill and Wisseman (3). Destruction of the organisms within the cells resulted if the rickettsiae

[1]Supported by NIH grant AI 15035 and U.S. Army Medical Research and Development Contract C-9018.
[2]Supported by a National Science Foundation postdoctoral fellowship.

were treated with immune serum before infection of the cells
(4,5). Whereas the virulent Breinl strain of R. prowazeki
grew in human macrophages, the avirulent E strain did not
grow in most human macrophages (3). This observation
suggested that the difference in virulence between the E and
Breinl strains somehow involved their interaction with
macrophages.

Determination of the basis for the difference in
virulence between the E and Breinl strains would be
facilitated by development of a convenient, reproducible
experimental system in which the E and Breinl strains could
be differentiated. Continuous macrophage-like cell lines are
now available which exhibit many properties characteristic
of macrophages (6, 7, 8, 9). The interaction of Rickettsia
species and macrophage-like cell lines had not previously
been investigated; hence we determined the fate of avirulent
and virulent strains of R. prowazeki in several
macrophage-like cell lines. Our results are presented
briefly in this report. A complete manuscript detailing our
experiments has been submitted for publication.

II. METHODS

A. Cell Lines

The mouse macrophage-like cell lines P388D1 and PU5 were
kindly provided by Dr. Janet Oliver. The mouse
macrophage-like cell lines RAW264.7 and J774.1 were sent to
us by the Cell Distribution Center at the Salk Institute.
The human macrophage-like cell line U937-1 was the gift of
Dr. Hillel S. Koren. We purchased L929 mouse fibroblasts
from Flow Laboratories.

Mouse macrophage-like cell lines were grown in
Dulbecco's Modified Eagle Medium supplemented with calf
serum, fetal calf serum, or a combination of fetal calf
serum and horse serum. U937-1 cells were grown in fetal calf
serum-supplemented RPMI 1640 medium. L929 cells were grown
in calf serum-supplemented Eagle's Minimal Essential Medium.
All cells were grown at 34^0 C in a humidified CO_2 incubator.

B. Rickettsiae

The Madrid E and Breinl strains of Rickettsia prowazeki
were purified from infected yolk sacs as described
previously (10). The final rickettsial suspensions in the

sucrose phosphate glutamate solution of Bovarnick et al.
(11) were aliquoted and stored at -70°C. The numbers of
viable rickettsiae/ml in these suspensions were determined
by the antibody hemolysis method (12).

C. Infection of Cells

Cell division was inhibited by X-irradiation of the
cells before infection with rickettsiae. Cells which grew
attached to the substratum (RAW264.7, J774.1, and L929) were
seeded in chamber slides 36 to 48 hours prior to infection.
Nonadherent (U937-1) or partially adherent cells (PU5 and
P388D1) were infected in suspension.

Immediately before infection, cells were washed in
Hank's balanced salt solution supplemented with 0.1% gelatin
and 4.9 mM glutamate. Rickettsiae diluted in the same
solution were then added to the cells at various
multiplicities of infection. After incubation with
rickettsiae for 1 hr at 34°C, the cells were washed and
fresh medium was added. Chamber slides or suspension
cultures were then incubated at 34°C for up to 48 hours. At
various times after infection, slides were stained by a
modified Giménez technique, as outlined by Wisseman et al.
(13). Collection of data involved counting the number of
rickettsiae in each of 100 cells for each duplicate of each
experimental treatment. Cells which contained more than 100
rickettsiae were assigned a value of 100 rickettsiae.

D. Antiserum

Antiserum was obtained from rabbits immunized with the E
strain of Rickettsia prowazeki (14), and was heated at 56°C
for 1 hour before use.

III. RESULTS

A. Growth of the Madrid E and Breinl Strains of
Rickettsia prowazeki in L929 Cells
or Macrophage-Like Cell Lines

The E and Breinl strains displayed similar patterns of
growth in the mouse fibroblast line L929. In these cells,
the average number of E strain rickettsiae per cell
increased about 35 fold and the average number of Breinl

strain rickettsiae per cell increased about 38 fold from 0
to 48 hours after infection. With either rickettsial strain
the percentage of L929 cells infected remained stable or
increased slightly during the same period of time.

In contrast, the interactions of the E and Breinl
strains of Rickettsia prowazeki with mouse macrophage-like
cell lines were strikingly different. On one hand, the
Breinl strain grew well in all of these cell lines. From 0
to 48 hours after infection, the average number of Breinl
strain rickettsiae per cell increased from 13 to 28 fold in
the various cell lines. The percentage of cells infected
with Breinl strain rickettsiae remained stable or increased
during this 48 hour period. On the other hand, the E strain
grew poorly or failed to grow in these mouse macrophage-like
cell lines. In RAW264.7 cells, there was a 2 fold increase
in the average number of E strain rickettsiae per cell from
0 to 48 hours after infection. In the remaining three cell
lines, the average number of E strain rickettsiae per cell
at 48 hours after infection was less than or about the same
as that observed immediately after infection. In RAW264.7,
J774.1, and P388D1 cells, the percentage of cells infected
with E strain rickettsiae decreased dramatically between 0
and 48 hours after infection. In these three cell lines, the
percentages of cells infected at 48 hours ranged from as
high as one-third to as low as one-tenth of the percentages
of cells infected at 0 hours post infection. Thus, for
example, in RAW264.7 cells, E strain rickettsiae were
cleared from most of the cells by 48 hours post infection,
but persisted and multiplied in some of the remaining
infected cells.

Whereas the growth of the E strain was dramatically
suppressed in comparison with that of the Breinl strain in
all four mouse macrophage-like cell lines, the difference in
the proliferation of the E and Breinl strains in the human
macrophage-like line U937-1 was much less striking. There
was a 16 fold increase in the average number of Breinl
strain rickettsiae per cell and a 6 fold increase in the
average number of E strain rickettsiae per cell from 0 to 48
hours post infection.

        B. Infection of L-929 Cells or Macrophage-Like Cell Lines
            with Antiserum-Treated, Normal Rabbit Serum-Treated,
                        or Untreated Rickettsiae
          and Subsequent Fate of the Rickettsiae in These Cells

    Incubation of L929 cells with untreated Breinl strain
rickettsiae or with Breinl strain rickettsiae plus 10%

normal rabbit serum resulted in comparable initial
infections. Both the percentages of cells infected and the
average numbers of rickettsiae per cell were similar with
normal rabbit serum-treated and untreated rickettsiae.
Normal rabbit serum-treated rickettsiae also grew as well as
untreated rickettsiae in L929 cells. Suspensions of E or
Breinl strain rickettsiae plus 10% rabbit antirickettsial
antiserum were very poorly infectious for L929 cells.
However, those antiserum-treated rickettsiae which did
infect L929 cells multiplied as well as did untreated
rickettsiae.

The results in the mouse macrophage-like cell lines are
in striking contrast to the results in the L929 fibroblasts.
In the macrophage-like cell line RAW264.7, untreated and
normal rabbit serum-treated Breinl strain rickettsiae caused
similar initial infections and multiplied comparably.
However, suspensions of E or Breinl strain rickettsiae plus
10% rabbit antirickettsial antiserum caused a comparable or
slightly enhanced initial infection of the cells. Moreover,
the majority of the antiserum-treated E or Breinl strain
rickettsiae were cleared from the cells by 48 hours post
infection. A small proportion of cells, though, did show
rickettsial growth.

Inclusion of 10% rabbit antiserum with the rickettsiae
enhanced the initial infection of J774.1 and PU5 cells and
had no effect on the initial infection of U937-1 cells. Most
of the treated rickettsiae (Breinl strain) were cleared from
J774.1 and PU5 cells, but U937-1 cells were somewhat less
effective at disposing of antiserum-treated rickettsiae than
were the mouse macrophage-like cell lines. Thus antiserum
treatment of the rickettsiae inhibited the infection of L929
cells but did not inhibit the infection of macrophage-like
cell lines by these organisms. In addition, such treatment
had no effect on the growth of the rickettsiae in L929 cells
but led to clearance of most of the organisms from the mouse
macrophage-like cell lines.

IV. DISCUSSION

The four mouse macrophage-like cell lines tested in this
study clearly distinguished the avirulent E and virulent
Breinl strains of R. prowazeki. In each of these cell lines
the growth of the E strain was suppressed in comparison with
that of the Breinl strain. Both strains of R. prowazeki,
however, grew similarly in the mouse fibroblast line L929.
Wisseman and Waddell (15) had likewise reported that these

two strains of R. prowazeki grew similarly in chicken embryo
cells.

Comparison of our results in mouse macrophage-like cell
lines with those of Gambrill and Wisseman (3), who described
the interaction of the E and Breinl strains with human
monocyte-derived macrophages, is interesting. The two
studies are similar in that the growth of E strain
rickettsiae was inhibited in comparison with the growth of
Breinl strain rickettsiae in both macrophage-like cell lines
and human monocyte-derived macrophages. In addition, both
the human macrophages and some of the macrophage-like cell
lines showed heterogeneity in their interaction with the E
strain: most of the cells cleared the E strain rickettsiae
but a small fraction of the cells supported growth of these
organisms. On the other hand, the percentage of human
macrophages infected with Breinl strain rickettsiae
decreased with time(but not to as great an extent as did the
percentage of human macrophages infected with E strain
rickettsiae) (3), whereas the percentage of cells infected
with Breinl strain rickettsiae remained stable or increased
with time in all macrophage-like cell lines. Perhaps human
macrophages, unlike the macrophage-like cell lines we
tested, have a limited capacity for eliminating the Breinl
strain of R. prowazeki. Interestingly, we found that growth
of the E strain was less dramatically inhibited in human
U937-1 cells than in the mouse macrophage-like cell lines.

Treatment of the rickettsiae with antiserum
differentially affected their ability to infect L929 cells
or macrophage-like cell lines. Rickettsial infection of L929
cells was suppressed after antiserum treatment. A likely
explanation for this suppression is that coating of the
rickettsiae with antibody prevented the rickettsiae from
inducing their phagocytosis by the L929 cells (16). Our
results with L929 cells differ from those reported in
chicken embryo cells where the initial rickettsial infection
was not decreased after treatment of R. prowazeki with human
immune serum (17). In our experiments with macrophage-like
cell lines, which bear receptors for the Fc portion of
immunoglobulin (9,18), the initial rickettsial infection was
unaffected or enhanced by treatment of the rickettsiae with
antiserum.

Treatment of the rickettsiae with antiserum also
differentially affected their ability to grow in L929 cells
or in macrophage-like cell lines. Antiserum-treated
rickettsiae grew as well as untreated rickettsiae in L929
cells. This result is similar to that of Wisseman et al.
(17), who reported that the growth of rickettsiae treated
with human immune serum was not inhibited in chicken embryo

cells. In sharp contrast to the situation in L929 cells, the
majority of the antiserum-treated rickettsiae were destroyed
in the mouse macrophage-like cell lines.

Whether killing of the E strain of R prowazeki in
macrophage-like cell lines occurs in the phagosomes or in
the cytoplasm is unknown. The electron microscopic studies
of Meyer and Wisseman demonstrated the escape of the Breinl
strain of R. prowazeki from the phagosomes of human
macrophages (W.A. Meyer III and C.L. Wisseman, Abstr. Annu.
Meet. Am. Soc. Microbiol. 1980, D10, p.39). Their studies
also depicted the destruction of dead rickettsiae and immune
human serum-treated rickettsiae within the phagosomes of
human macrophages. It is tempting therefore to speculate
that the E strain is destroyed in the phagosomes. On the
other hand, killing of the E strain may occur in the
cytoplasm. Nacy and Meltzer (2) suggested that the
macrophage cytoplasm was the site of killing of R.
tsutsugamushi in their experiments with mouse macrophages
treated with lymphokines after rickettsial infection.

Our experiments indicate that the avirulent E and
virulent Breinl strains of R. prowazeki are clearly
distinguished by the four mouse macrophage-like cell lines
we tested. Resident or elicited mouse peritoneal
macrophages, in contrast, do not distinguish the E and
Breinl strains but destroy them both (Winkler and Daugherty,
in preparation). Therefore, although mouse macrophage-like
cell lines share many properties with mouse peritoneal
macrophages, they must also differ from mouse peritoneal
macrophages in some important respect(s). The mouse
macrophage-like cell lines should be a very useful model
system for further investigation of the difference in
virulence between the E and Breinl strains of R. prowazeki.

V. SUMMARY

1. The avirulent E and virulent Breinl strains of
Rickettsia prowazeki grew comparably in the mouse fibroblast
line L929.
2. In four mouse macrophage-like cell lines, the growth of
the E strain was markedly inhibited in comparison with that
of the Breinl strain.
3. Treatment of the Breinl or E strains of R. prowazeki
with rabbit antirickettsial antiserum led to a marked
suppression in the initial infection of L929 cells but did
not affect the growth of the rickettsiae in these cells.
4. Antiserum treatment of Breinl or E strain rickettsiae

had no effect on or increased the initial infection of
macrophage-like cell lines. However, most of the
antiserum-treated rickettsiae (Breinl or E strain) were
cleared from the mouse macrophage-like cell lines.
5. Inhibition of the growth of the E strain and disposal of
antiserum-treated rickettsiae were less efficient in the
human macrophage-like cell line U937-1 than in the mouse
macrophage-like cell lines.

ACKNOWLEDGMENTS

We thank Drs. Koren and Oliver for the gift of
macrophage-like cell lines.

REFERENCES

1. Nacy, C.A., and Osterman, J.V., Infect. Immun. 26,
   744(1979).
2. Nacy, C.A., and Meltzer, M.S., J. Immunol. 123,
   2544(1979).
3. Gambrill, M.R., and Wisseman, C.L., Jr., Infect. Immun.
   8, 519(1973).
4. Beaman, L., and Wisseman, C.L., Jr., Infect. Immun. 14,
   1071(1976).
5. Gambrill, M.R. and Wisseman, C.L., Jr., Infect. Immun.
   8, 631(1973).
6. Defendi, V., in "Immunobiology of the Macrophage" (D.S.
   Nelson, ed.), p. 275. Academic Press, New York, (1976).
7. Koren, H.S., Anderson, S.J., and Larrick, J.W., Nature
   279, 328(1979).
8. Morahan, P.S., J. Reticuloendothel. Soc. 27, 223(1980).
9. Ralph, P., Nakoinz, I., Broxmeyer, H.E., and Schrader,
   S., Natl Cancer Inst. Monogr. 48, 303(1978).
10. Winkler, H.H., Infect. Immun. 9, 119(1974).
11. Bovarnick, M.R., Miller, J.C., and Snyder, J.C., J.
    Bacteriol. 59, 509(1950).
12. Walker, T.S., and Winkler, H.H., J. Clin. Microbiol. 9,
    645(1979).
13. Wisseman, C.L., Jr., Waddell, A.D., and Walsh, W.T., J.
    Infect. Dis. 130, 564(1974).
14. Winkler, H.H., Infect. Immun. 17, 607(1977).
15. Wisseman, C.L., Jr., and Waddell, A.D., Infect. Immun.
    11, 1391(1975).
16. Walker, T.S., and Winkler, H.H., Infect. Immun. 22,

200(1978).
17. Wisseman, C.L., Jr., Waddell, A.D., and Walsh, W.T., Infect. Immun. 9, 571(1974).
18. Larrick, J.W., Fischer, D.G., Anderson, S.J., and Koren, H.S., J. Immunol. 125, 6(1980).

INTERACTION OF <u>COXIELLA BURNETII</u> WITH MACROPHAGE-LIKE TUMOR CELL LINES

O.G. Baca
A.S. Aragon
E.T. Akporiaye
I.L. Martinez
N.L. Warner[1]

Department of Biology and the School of Medicine
Departments of Pathology and Medicine[1]
The University of New Mexico
Albuquerque, New Mexico

I. INTRODUCTION

There are several facultative and obligate intracellular parasites that are not destroyed by phagocytes but, instead, proliferate within them. The properties of these microorganisms and the mechanisms involved in avoiding intracellular killing, are, for the most part, unknown. In the case of the diverse group of obligate intracellular prokaryotic parasites classified as the rickettsiae, virtually nothing is known about how they avoid destruction within macrophages and polymorphonuclear leukocytes. Studies have shown that several rickettsial species, including <u>Coxiella burnetii</u>, multiply within normal macrophages (1, 2, 3, 4, 5, 6, 7). In the case of <u>C. burnetii</u> both the naturally occurring phase I organism and the phase II variant that appears after serial passage in embryonated eggs (8) grow within the phagocytes. One of the long-range goals of our research is to determine the mechanism(s) that accounts

for the intracellular survival of C. burnetii; this includes
the identification of its properties (i.e. surface
components) that allow proliferation. We are currently
examining the interaction, including the entry and fate, of
Coxiella with a series of macrophage-like tumor cell lines:
PU-5-IR, J774, P388D1, WEHI-3, and WEHI-274. These cell
lines exhibit varying capacities to interiorize particles and
possess various properties characteristic of macrophages (9,
10).

In this report, evidence is presented that shows that
phase I C. burnetii can proliferate and establish a
persistent infection in some of the above cell lines and not
in others. The kinetics of uptake of the rickettsiae by the
cell lines are presented.

II. MATERIALS AND METHODS

A. C. burnetii: Propagation, Radiolabeling, and Purification

Phase I Coxiella burnetii, Nine Mile strain, was used in
these studies. The rickettsiae were obtained from Dr. R. A.
Ormsbee, Rocky Mountain Laboratory, U.S. Public Health
Service, Hamilton, MT. The organisms were plaque-purified by
Ormsbee and Peacock (11) in primary chick embryo cells. For
these studies, the rickettsiae were propagated in mouse
fibroblast L cells (L-929) maintained in suspension culture
(12). Infected cells were disrupted in a Ten Broeck
homogenizer and the released rickettsiae purified by
differential centrifugation. Three cycles of low speed-high
speed centrifugation (800 x g and 10,000 x g) resulted in
rickettsiae essentially free of host material. Further
purification was obtained by passage through 30% - 60%
continuous sucrose gradients (13). The purified organisms
were suspended in Dulbecco's Balanced Salt Solution and
stored at -70°C until required. Rickettsial concentrations
were determined by the methods of Silberman and Fiset (14).

Radioactively labeled rickettsiae were obtained by
exposure of infected L cells to [^{32}P]-orthophosphoric acid
(1.0 mCi/50 ml culture) for 3 to 4 days. Purification of the
radiolabeled rickettsiae was performed as described above.
The specific radioactivity was such that circa 0.6 Coxiella
associated per macrophage could be detected.

B. Macrophage Tumor Cell Lines

All tumor cell lines used in these studies were from established tissue culture cell lines maintained in appropriate media conditions with 5-10% fetal calf serum also containing non-essential amino acids for the PU-5 line. The cultures were passaged every 3 to 4 days as their cell densities approached 10^6/ml. The monocyte macrophage cell lines (including original reference) used were: J774 (15), P388D1 (16), PU-5-IR (17), WEHI-3 (18), and WEHI-274 (19). All of these lines were derived from the BALB/c mouse, except P388D1, which originated from the DBA/2 mouse strain. The cultures were maintained in suspension culture in plastic Petri dishes at 37^0C in a 4% CO_2 atmosphere. Cell viabilities were determined by the dye (erythrosin B or trypan blue) exclusion technique.

C. Experimental Procedures

All the macrophage cell lines were exposed to C. burnetii and examined periodically for the presence or absence of cell-associated rickettsiae. Bright-field microscopy of Giménez-stained cells (20) and transmission electron microscopy were employed. All the lines were washed and resuspended to appropriate concentrations in complete antibiotic-free growth medium and exposed to multiplicities of infection (MOI) of 5, 50, and 500 rickettsiae. The macrophage cell concentrations, at the time of exposure, were 2×10^4 cells/ml, except P388D1 which was 4×10^4/ml. The cells were kept at 37^0C in a 4% CO_2 atmosphere and passaged every three days at which time samples were removed and examined for the presence of cell-associated rickettsiae. At least 200 Giménez-stained cells from each sample were examined.

The uptake of radiolabeled rickettsiae by all the cell lines was followed over a 3 hour time period. Macrophages (10^6/ml) and rickettsiae (MOI of 500) were mixed in 50 ml screw-capped Erlenmeyer flasks and incubated at 37^0C in a shaking incubator at 100 rpm. Periodically aliquots were removed and subjected to centrifugation at 160 x g at 4^0C for 5 min. The pelleted macrophages and associated rickettsiae were washed with HBSS four times (optimum number of washes) to remove unassociated rickettsiae. The washed rickettsiae-macrophage pellets were placed in liquid scintillation fluid and the radioactivity determined in a liquid scintillation spectrometer. From the specific radioactivity, the number of C. burnetii per macrophage was determined.

Phase I radiolabeled <u>Coxiella</u> were exposed to antisera
containing antibodies to both phase I and II rickettsiae or
normal rabbit sera for 30 min at 37°C. After such treatment,
the organisms were exposed to J774, WEHI-3, and WEHI-274 and
their uptake by the macrophages monitored over a 3 h period.
Late rabbit antiserum containing phase I and phase II
antibodies was prepared according to the procedure of Fiset
(21).

III.   RESULTS

A.   Fate of <u>C. burnetii</u>

The fate of phase I <u>C. burnetii</u> after exposure to the
various macrophage cell lines was followed over a period of
weeks to months. Fig. 1 shows that initially all of the
lines were associated with one or more rickettsiae with some
of the lines containing a higher percentage of infected cells
than others. By the third day post-infection, the J774 and
P388D1 populations contained the highest percentage of cells
that were associated with rickettsiae. By the tenth day, the
majority (75%-85%) of the J774 and P388D1 cells were
infected; within 13 and 25 days, 100% of the P388D1 and J774
cells, respectively, contained rickettsiae. Electron
microscopy of thin sections of infected J774 (Fig. 2) and
P388D1 (not shown) cells revealed the presence of numerous
rickettsiae within vacuoles. Many of the cells contained
over a thousand parasites. Both of these lines became and
remained persistently infected. This, of course, implies a
dividing, viable population. Fig. 1 is an electron
micrograph of cells that had been persistently infected for
155 days. The viability of the infected J774 and P388D1
populations, as determined by dye exclusion, was relatively
high. During this experiment, the P388D1 and J774 cells were
approximately 90% viable. The results described were from
macrophages exposed to 500 rickettsiae per cell. At other
MOI's (5 and 50) the results were the same, although, there
was a proportional delay in the attainment of 100% infection.
In other experiments, persistently infected populations of
P388D1 and J774 have been maintained for 200 and over 100
days, respectively.
Fig. 1 shows that the other cell lines (WEHI-3, WEHI-274,
PU-5-IR) were associated with the highest number of
rickettsiae by the sixth day post-infection but thereafter
the number of parasites declined and eventually disappeared.
By the 13th day, none of the WEHI-3 or WEHI-274 cells

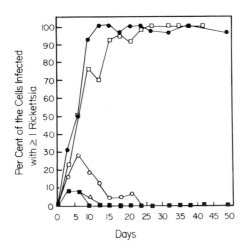

Fig. 1.   Fate of phase I C. burnetii in macrophage-like cell lines J774 (□), P388D1 (●), PU-5-IR (○), WEHI-3 (△), and WEHI-274 (■).   Infectivities were determined as described in "Methods" section.

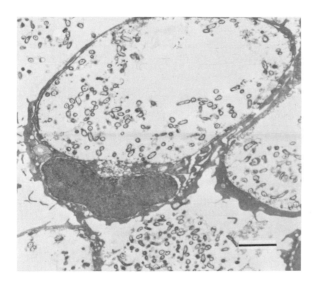

Fig. 2.   Phase I C. burnetii-infected J774 cell at 155 days post-infection.   Marker represents 5 μm.

appeared to contain rickettsiae. After the 23rd day, no
rickettsiae were observed in the PU-5-IR population. At
other MOI's (5 and 50) similar results were obtained with
these three cell lines.

The disappearance of the parasites from the PU-5-IR,
WEHI-3, and WEHI-274 populations indicated that either the
parasites were interiorized and destroyed or, although they
may have attached to the outer surface, they never entered
into the cells and were subsequently diluted out upon
subsequent passages. In the case of the PU-5-IR cells,
electron microscopy clearly showed that, at least by the 6th
day, rickettsiae had entered some of the cells and, possibly,
proliferated within vacuoles. Very few cells (possibly 1 in
100) contained rickettsiae. Other micrographs showed what
appeared to be rickettsiae within vacuoles undergoing
destruction. Electron and bright-field microscopy of stained
PU-5-IR macrophages at 3 to 4 weeks post-infection showed no
evidence of intracellular or extracellular rickettsiae.
Similar EM studies are currently being performed with WEHI-3
and WEHI-274 cells.

The results obtained with the PU-5-IR cells were repeated
in 8 independent experiments. In two recent experiments,
however, we have found that at a MOI of 500 they became
infected. At this time we do not know the reason for the
sudden ability of this cell line to permit rickettsial
multiplication whereas before it caused its disappearance.
We are currently examining various possibilities that may
account for this change. After one year of experimentation,
consistent results have been obtained with the other cell
lines.

B. Uptake of Phase I ^{32}P-Coxiella

The kinetics of uptake of radiolabeled phase I C.
burnetii by all the cell lines was determined. After 3 h
incubation, the J774 macrophages were associated with the
largest number of parasites (Fig. 3); the P388D1 and PU-5-IR
cells associated with approximately one-third the number of
rickettsiae as did the J774 cells. WEHI-3 and WEHI-274
picked up about one-ninth the number of Coxiella as did J774
(Fig. 3). With the exception of PU-5-IR, the uptake of
Coxiella by the five cell lines reflects their differential
ability to ingest latex microspheres in which the order of
activity is PU-5-IR > J774 > P388D1 > WEHI-3 > WEHI-274 (10).
Exposure of the cell lines to the phase I rickettsiae at 0°C
for 5 min also showed the same order of rickettsial
association (Fig. 4). Since endocytosis is an energy-
requiring process that is inhibited by low temperature (22),

the associated rickettsiae are probably attached to the
macrophage surface and not interiorized.

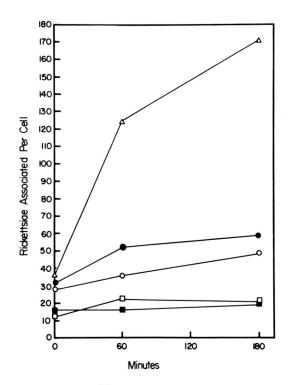

Fig. 3.   Uptake of ^{32}P-labeled C. burnetii by
macrophage-like cell lines J774 ($\triangle$), P388D1 ($\bullet$), PU-5-IR
($\bigcirc$), WEHI-274 ($\square$), and WEHI-3 ($\blacksquare$). The experimental
protocol is described in the "Methods" section.

C.   Effect of Antibody on the Uptake of Phase I Coxiella

     The effect of antibody on rickettsial uptake by J774 (a
highly phagocytic line), WEHI-3 (a moderately phagocytic
line) and WEHI-274 (a poorly phagocytic line) was examined.
Preincubation of the ^{32}P-rickettsiae with serum containing
antibodies versus phase I Coxiella, followed by mixing with
the cell lines, resulted in a 6-fold increase in the number
of rickettsiae that became associated with the J774 cells
during a 3 h incubation period (data not shown). The other
two lines showed no significant increase in rickettsial

uptake with antibody treatment although both are reported to
contain Fc receptor (9, 10).

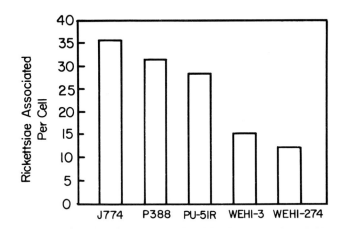

Fig. 4. Association of C. burnetii with various
macrophage-like cell lines after incubation for 5 min at 0°C.
Radiolabeled rickettsiae and macrophages were held separately
at 0°C and then mixed and kept at 0°C for 5 min after which
duplicate aliquots were removed and prepared for
radioactivity determination as described in the "Methods".

IV.   DISCUSSION

    Several in vitro studies have shown that phase I and
phase II C. burnetii enter and proliferate within monocytes
and macrophages and eventually destroy the phagocytes (1, 3,
4, 5, 6). These in vitro studies may reflect the in vivo
state in humans and experimental animals in which Q fever
occasionally results in a chronic persistent infection (23,
24). With both types of infection (in vivo and in vitro) the
interactions between parasite and host that account for
persistent infection are totally unknown. The types of cells
that may sequester the rickettsiae during the latent state
have not been identified. Although there is no evidence,
phagocytic cells such as macrophages might be the cells in
which the parasite establishes a latent infection. Because
the cells of the monocytic series play a key role in the
control of infectious agents, it is important to attain an

understanding of the mechanisms involved in the control of
such agents. Such knowledge would also provide insight into
the conditions leading to persistent infection. The in vitro
system that we have chosen to study, may provide clues to
such mechanisms since in some of the cell lines phase I C.
burnetii proliferates while in others it does not (Fig. 1).
In these studies we have demonstrated that phase I C.
burnetii is capable of entering and establishing a
persistent infection of highly phagocytic cell lines. Not
only did phase I C. burnetii cause a persistent infection of
the most phagocytically active cells, but it also appeared to
enter (Fig. 3) and attach (Fig. 4) more readily to them.
That the most active lines became infected while the others
did not may be due simply to the ingestion of larger numbers
of parasites exceeding the phagocyte's capacity to kill. At
this time we do not know whether or not the rickettsia even
enters into the WEHI-3 and WEHI-274 cells.

Along with C. burnetii, and possibly other intracellular
parasites, these lines may serve as excellent in vitro model
systems for exploring the mechanisms that account for the
survival of the parasite. That the phase I Q fever agent
does not establish infection of some of the cell lines
examined is very interesting since their use may also provide
a model for examining the mechanisms involved in the
avoidance of infections and, possibly, intracellular
destruction. Recently we have found that phase II C.
burnetii enters and multiplies in all five cell lines used in
this investigation (manuscript in preparation). This is an
extremely interesting finding because it strongly suggests
that surface differences between the two phases may account
for their differential fate. It therefore becomes important
to identify such surface component(s) that may ultimately be
responsible for obviating or promoting intracellular
destruction.

V. SUMMARY

We have examined the interaction, including the entry
and fate, of phase I Coxiella burnetii with several
macrophage-like tumor cell lines of murine origin which
previous workers have found to exhibit a range of phagocytic
capabilities. The parasite proliferated and established a
persistent infection of two of the cell lines (J774, P388D1)
and not of two others (WEHI-3, WEHI-274). In some
experiments C. burnetii entered and proliferated within
PU-5-IR cells while in other experiments it did not. In
those experiments where it did not proliferate within the

PU-5-IR cells, the parasite had entered but eventually
disappeared. Whether or not the parasite even enters into
the WEHI-3 and WEHI-274 cells is not known at this time. The
kinetics of uptake of ^{32}P-labeled rickettsiae was examined.
The effect of antibody on uptake was also examined. Since
the parasite proliferates in some of the cell lines and not
in others, we now have a model system that should greatly aid
in elucidating the interactions between parasite and
phagocyte that result in either rickettsial survival or,
possibly, destruction.

ACKNOWLEDGMENTS

    The technical assistance of Eva Berry, Maria Robles, and
Pam Valverde is gratefully acknowledged.
    This study was supported by grants from the National
Science Foundation (PCM 77-01559, PCM 8010633) and the Public
Health Service, Division of Research Resources, Minority
Biomedical Support Program, National Institutes of Health
(RR-08139-04).

REFERENCES

1. Downs, C. M., Zentralbl. Bakt. Parasit. Inf. Hyg. I
    (Orig.) 206, 329 (1968).
2. Gambrill, M.R., and Wisseman, C. L., Jr., Infect. Immun.
    8, 631 (1973).
3. Hinrichs, D. J., and Jerrells, T. J., J. Immunol. 117,
    996 (1976).
4. Kishimoto, R. A., Veltri, B. J., Canonico, P. G.,
    Shirey, F. G., and Walker, J.S., Infect. Immun. 14,
    1087 (1976).
5. Kishimoto, R. A., Veltri, B. J., Shirey, F. G.,
    Canonico, P. G., and Walker, J.S., Infect. Immun. 15,
    601 (1977).
6. Kishimoto, R. A., and Walker, J. S., Infect. Immun. 14,
    416 (1976).

7. Nacy, C. A., and Osterman, J. V., _Infect. Immun._ 26, 744 (1979).

8. Stoker, M. G. P., and Fiset, P., _Can. J. Microbiol._ 2, 310 (1956).

9. Morahan, P. S., _J. Reticuloendothel. Soc._ 27, 223 (1980).

10. Warner, N. L., Burchiel, S. W., Walker, E. B., Richey, J. B., Leary, J. F., and McGlaughlin, S., _in_ "Immunobiology and immunotherapy of cancer" (W. Terry and Y. Yamamura, ed.), p. 243. Elsevier-North Holland, New York, (1979).

11. Ormsbee, R. A., and Peacock, M. G., _Tissue Culture Assoc. Manual._ 2, 475 (1976).

12. Burton, P. R., Stueckemann, J., Welsh, R. M., and Paretsky, D., _Infect. Immun._ 21, 556 (1978).

13. Thompson, H. A., Baca, O. G., and Paretsky, D., _Biochem. J._ 125, 365 (1971).

14. Silberman, R., and Fiset, P., _J. Bact._ 95, 259 (1968).

15. Ralph, P., Prichard, J., and Cohn, ·M., _J. Immunol._ 114, 898 (1975).

16. Koren, H. S., Handwerger, B. S., and Wunderlich, J. R., _J. Immunol._ 114, 894 (1975).

17. Ralph, P., Moore, M. A. S., and Nilsson, K., _J. Exp. Med._ 143, 1528 (1976).

18. Warner, N. L., Moore, M. A. S., and Metcalf, D., _J. Natl. Cancer Inst._ 43, 963 (1969)

19. Walker, E., Richey, J. B., and Warner, N. L., _Fed. Proc._ 38, 1418 (1979).

20. Giménez, D. F., _Stain Technol._ 39, 135 (1964).

21. Fiset, P., _in_ "Techniques in experimental virology" (R. J. C. Harris, ed.), p. 225-255. Academic Press, London, (1964).

22. Stossel, T. P., _Sem. Hematol._ 12, 83 (1975).

23. Marmion, B. P., _J. Hyg. Epidem._, Praha 6, 79 (1962).

24. Syrucek, L., Sobeslavsky, O., and Gutvirth, I., _J. Hyg. Epidem._, Praha 2, 29 (1958).

DETECTION OF COXIELLA BURNETII SOLUBLE ANTIGENS
BY IMMUNOELECTROPHORESIS: DEMONSTRATION
OF ANTIGEN IN THE SERA OF GUINEA PIGS
DURING EXPERIMENTAL Q FEVER

Jim C. Williams
Marius G. Peacock

Laboratory of Microbial Structure and Function
Rocky Mountain Laboratories
Hamilton, Montana

Claes-Otto L. Kindmark

Department of Infectious Diseases
University Hospital
Uppsala, Sweden

I.   INTRODUCTION

Coxiella burnetii is primarily a parasite of phagocytic
cells where the microbe carries out its developmental cycle
in the phagolysosome (1-7). The host cell becomes filled
with organisms and eventual lysis of the cell establishes a
new round of infection. Since C. burnetii occupies the phagolysosomal niche, lysis of host cells results in the release
of lysosomal contents, C. burnetii and, perhaps, soluble
antigens and fragments of the parasite. Recently, in this
laboratory ultrastructural analysis of C. burnetii in phagocytic cells and of highly purified organisms (8) indicated
that endospore formation was characteristic of a large cell
variant (LCV) and that the outer membrane and other components
were easily released from the LCV, thus suggesting that C.
burnetii cells, endospores and subcellular fragments might
also be released during the infection cycle. Other investigators have shown that C. burnetii contains polysaccharides that

exhibit some characteristics of other Gram-negative bacterial
endotoxins and lipopolysaccharides (LPS) (9). We recently
observed that C. burnetii cells, upon exposure to anti-C.
burnetii serum, have a fibrillar network of antigen-antibody
(Ag-Ab) on their surfaces (McCaul and Williams, unpublished
observations) similar to that observed for other rickettsial
organisms (10). Release of lysosomal enzymes, C. burnetii
whole cells, endospores and shedding of outer membrane components as well as soluble antigens during the infectious
process might lead to circulating complexes of Ag-Ab or some
other serum components.

Circulating Ag-Ab complexes (immune complexes, IC) have
been detected in several bacterial diseases (11). These IC
have been implicated in the immunopathology of viral and
bacterial infections (11) and schistosomiasis (12). In particular, pneumococcal polysaccharide is present in the circu-
latory system and other body fluids of some patients with
pneumococcal infection, and this antigen can be detected by
immunoelectrophoretic techniques (13). The purpose of our
study was to examine sera of experimentally infected guinea
pigs for the presence of circulating antigens. We report
that a soluble antigen is present in sera of infected guinea
pigs. The soluble antigen is apparently circulating as an IC
which seems to correlate with the anti-complementary activity
of the sera. Further, a phenol soluble antigen of C. burnetii
was observed to form a line of identity with the circulating
antigen.

II. MATERIALS AND METHODS

A. Preparation of C. burnetii Seed Stocks and Antisera

C. burnetii (Phase I, Ohio strain CBOI) were propagated
in SPF type 5, antibiotic-free, fertile hen egg yolk sacs
(H and N Hatchery, Redmond, Wash.) and purified as previously
described (14). Viable rickettsial seed stocks were prepared
from the purified organisms in a diluent of 50% BHI in phosphate-buffered saline (pH 7.35) at 5.2 mg rickettsiae per ml
or 19.8 X 10^{10} organisms per ml.

Hyperimmune sera directed against rickettsial antigens
were prepared in guinea pigs by injecting killed whole cells
of CBOI followed by infection or a second injection with the
same strain. Q174 antiserum was prepared as follows: i) on
day zero, animals were injected subcutaneously with graded
doses of killed whole cells (CBOI) ranging from 10 to 100 µg
per animal; ii) two weeks later an identical second injection

was made; iii) after two more weeks, 30 days after the first
injection, the animals were challenged with 1.4 X 10^{10} PFU
per guinea pig; and iv) surviving animals were exsanguinated
on day 57 of the experiment. This sera was employed as the
developing sera in the immunoelectrophoretic techniques.

Antisera to be tested for the presence of soluble antigen
was obtained from infected guinea pigs (Table 1). Viable CBOI
were used to infect guinea pigs (Hartley strain) via intraperitoneal (i.p.) injections (see Table 1).

B. Immunoelectrophoresis (IEP)

Sodium barbital buffer (0.05 M, pH 8.2) was routinely
employed in all of the electrophoretic procedures.

Agarose was prepared at a concentration of 0.75% (wt/vol)
in the sodium barbital buffer. Litex agarose for gel electrophoresis type number HSA was obtained from Accurate Chemical
and Scientific Corp., Hicksville, N.Y.

Electrophoresis of the antigen or treated antiserum was
carried out at 4°C employing an LKB2117 Multiphor (LKB Instruments Inc., Rockville, Md.) equipped with a refrigerated circulating bath (RTE-8, Neslab Inst, Portsmouth, N.H.). A
voltage gradient of 5 V/cm was applied across the gel slab
(Electrophoresis Power Supply, Model 494, ISCO Inst., Lincoln,
Neb.) at the initiation of electrophoresis. Electrophoresis
was carried out under constant voltage for 1.5 hr. After
electrophoresis, the agarose was removed from the pre-cut
trough, and the respective antigen or antiserum was placed in
the trough. Diffusion was carried out at room temperature or
4°C for 48 hr or 7 days, respectively. Gel slabs were washed
in 1% saline containing 0.2% sodium azide for 48 hr with four
changes of diluent. Gel slabs were photographed, pressed to
dryness and stained in an aqueous solution of 0.5 g of
Coomassie brilliant blue per liter containing 7.5% acetic acid
and 25% isopropyl alcohol for 1 hr. These stained gel slabs
were destained, in the above solution without Coomassie
brilliant blue, and photographed again so that a direct comparison of immune precipitate could be made before and after
the above procedures.

C. Treatment of Serum

Normal and anti-C. burnetii sera used in these studies
were treated with iodide salts. Dissolution of IC was performed as described by Avrameas and Ternynck (15) by adding
potassium iodide crystals (reagent grade, Fisher Scientific

TABLE 1. Serological Response of Q171 Sera Collected from Experimentally Infected Guinea Pigs

Postinfection[a]	Serologic activity[b]						
	Microagglutination		Complement fixation			Immunofluorescence	
(day)	Ph II	Ph I	Ph II	AC[c]	Ph I	Ph II	Ph I
11	1024	2	128	2	2	1024	<8
43	1024	64	1024	16	128	4096	512
56	1024	64	2048	16	128	8192	4096
81	256	64	256	8	256	8192	$\geq$32,768
95	2048	64	2048	2	1024	2048	$\geq$32,768

[a]Fifty-five male guinea pigs weighing 400 to 500 g were infected i.p. with 2×10^5 PFU of CBOI on day zero. The animals were bled on day 11, 43, 56, 81 and 95 post-infection, and the sera from each bleeding were pooled. Animals were challenged with 7×10^9 PFU i.p. on day 47.

[b]Microagglutination (20), complement fixation (18) and microimmunofluorescence (21) titers were determined on pooled sera from each bleeding. Microimmunofluorescence titer represents the 7S globulin.

[c]AC = anticomplementary activity employing 5 units of complement.

Co.) directly to the serum so that a final concentration of
3.5 M was obtained. The solution was incubated at 56°C for
30 min. The treated serum was used immediately as described
for IEP. Serum from normal guinea pigs as well as guinea pigs
that had been vaccinated against Q fever were treated with
iodide salt and used as controls.

D. Extraction of Soluble Antigen from C. burnetii

Phenol soluble antigens (PSA) of CBOI was prepared from
chloroform-methanol extracted cells (16) according to the
Westphal procedure (17). The PSA preparation showed a positive serologic reaction against standard guinea pig anti-C.
burnetii serum by the CF test (18). The lowest concentration
of PSA that reacted with standard hyperimmune serum was
0.5 µg per ml at a serum dilution of 1:64. In the CF block
titration (18) the PSA preparation reacted as a pure Phase I
antigen.

E. Hemolytic Assay

Lysis of sheep red blood cells (SRBC) by the sera employed
in these studies was tested. SRBC were collected in Alsever's
solution (19) and stored at 4°C for 24 hr. SRBC were washed
three times in PBS (pH 6.5), and the packed cell pellet was
resuspended as a 2.5% suspension in PBS. One ml of 2.5% SRBC
was added to 1 ml of the respective antiserum. Incubation was
carried out for 30 min at 37°C. Hemolytic activity was scored
according to degree of hemolysis by visual analysis.

III. RESULTS

A. Serologic Reactivity of the Anti-C. burnetii Sera

Serological analysis of Q171 sera suggested that a temporal development of antibodies to Phase I and II antigens (20)
was evolving (Table 1). However, an atypical antibody response to Phase I antigen was unfolding. The MA test indicated that the anti-Phase I titer was not increased after day
43, yet the anti-Phase II titer continued to increase although
there was a drop in titer on day 81. The CF test showed an
increasing titer to the Phase II antigen with a decrease in
titer on day 81 which paralleled the drop in MA titer, whereas
the Phase I titer continued to increase. However, anticomplementary (AC) activity was associated with the temporal sequence

of antibody response. The AC activity employing 5 units of
complement showed an increase on day 43, and this titer was
unchanged at day 56, but a declining AC activity was observed
on days 81 and 95. An analysis of the 7S globulin response
by the IF test during this time sequence showed a temporal
development of anti-Phase II antibody and a continuous increase
in the anti-Phase I response. The activity of the sera on
day 81 and 95 was >32,768.

Although the above-described response was quite similar
to vaccination of guinea pigs with WC (unpublished observation), there was a remarkable departure in that the MA titer
continued to increase and the AC activity was not observed
during the temporal development of antibodies during vaccination. We reasoned that an IC in the serum might account for
the AC activity (11).

Serological reactivity of the developing anti-C. burnetii
Q174 sera indicated that high titers to Phase I and Phase II
antigens were obtained. The MA and CF tests showed titers for
Phase I and II of 4096 and 2048 and 2048 and 1024, respectively. However, AC activity was not detected in the Q174 sera.

B. Hemolytic Test of Complement Activity

Normal guinea pig serum which has not been heat inactivated at 56°C for 30 min will lyse SRBC (18). Therefore, we
tested the Q171, Q174 and normal sera for their ability to
lyse SRBC. The results were scored as - for no lysis and 5+
for complete lysis. The hemolytic activity was 5+, 2+ and -
with normal guinea pig, Q174 and all of the sera from the
Q171 series, respectively. Although normal and Q174 sera
retained hemolytic activity, serum obtained from infected
animals did not lyse SRBC. Therefore, IC formation during Q
fever infections in guinea pigs effectively depletes the serum
of complement.

C. Dissolution of Immune Complex with Potassium Iodide

We preferred antigen-specific methods (11) for the detection of IC formation. Thus, the methods described by Avrameas
and Ternynck (15) and Coonrod and Leach (22) were employed to
detect antigen in the serum of experimentally infected guinea
pigs.

The series of Q171 sera were treated with or without KI
at 56°C for 30 min and used immediately in IEP (Fig. 1). An
immunoprecipitate was observed with serum that had been treated

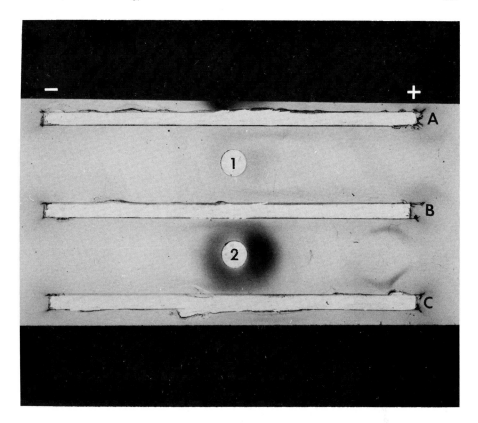

Fig. 1. Immunoelectrophoresis of Q171 serum collected on day 43 postinfection containing <u>Coxiella</u> <u>burnetii</u> soluble antigens. The center wells contained the following materials: (1) Q171 sera heated at 56°C for 30 min without KI; (2) Q171 sera heated at 56°C for 30 min with 3.5M KI. The troughs (A, B and C) contained Q174 serum. The precipitin arcs (arrows) indicate the migration of the antigen in Q171 sera. Precipitin arcs were observed in sera collected on 11, 43, 56, 81 and 95 days postinfection of guinea pigs with <u>C. burnetii</u> (data not shown). Normal and Q174 guinea pig sera did not show a precipitin band (data not shown).

with KI, thus demonstrating the requirement for KI treatment to dissolve the IC.

All of the Q171 sera contained an apparent soluble antigen, whereas normal serum showed no immunoprecipitates (data not shown). Control experiments were performed employing

KI-treated Q174 developing antisera and electrophoresed sera.
Q174 sera did not show a corresponding precipitin arc.

D. Demonstration of Soluble Antigen in the Series of Q171 Sera

   A modified technique of IEP (23) was used to facilitate
the identification of specific precipitin arcs. The major
antigen involved in the IC could be demonstrated by employing
PSA (see Materials and Methods) suspended at 5 mg/ml of
saline, Q171 and Q174 sera as follows (Fig. 2): Treated Q171
serum was electrophoresed, the PSA was placed in the upper
trough (A) and the developing Q174 serum was placed in the
lower trough (B). The plate was then placed in a moist chamber at 4°C for one week. At the position of the electrophoretic migration of the antigen in the Q171 serum sample,
a reaction of identity occurred, thus bending and fusing with
the corresponding component in the PSA preparation. A dense
precipitin arc was produced as a result of the interaction of
the soluble antigen with the precipitin arc of the Q171 serum
containing soluble antigen. The arc was displaced with a con-
vex orientation toward the Q174 serum containing trough (Fig.
2, arrow).

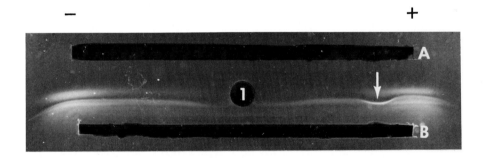

   Fig. 2. Modified immunoelectrophoresis of Q171 serum
collected on day 43 postinfection containing Coxiella burnetii
soluble antigens. The center well contained 20 μl of Q171
serum treated with 3.5M KI for 30 min at 56°C. The troughs
contained the following materials: (A) soluble antigen and
(B) Q174 serum. (arrow) This line of precipitation is observed to bend and fuse with one of the six precipitin bands,
thus identifying the soluble antigen present in the Q171 serum
which was electrophoretically separated. At least six precipitin lines were observed in this PSA preparation.

IV. DISCUSSION

Inhalation of C. burnetii appears to be the common mode of infection, thus the target organ is the lung. Experimental infection of the lung (24) shows that only those organisms which escape a fatal interaction with resident (fixed) alveolar macrophages have a chance of becoming established in the lung and, perhaps, disseminated systemically. Since C. burnetii multiplies within the phagolysosomal space of phagocytic cells (1), this microbe has a clear advantage in a non-immune host. After the infection has been established, the microbe is apparently circulated throughout the host, thus facilitating infection of fixed phagocytes (i.e., Kupffer cells) and mobile monocytes (25). Indeed, in the guinea pig (26), monkey (27), and human (28), there appears to be an underlying mechanism of systemically spreading the microbe throughout host tissues. Q fever infections in monkeys closely resemble the infection in humans (29). Guinea pigs infected by aerosols of C. burnetii were shown to develop interstitial pneumonia, lung lesions, granulomas of the liver and spleen, lymphoreticular myocarditis and epicarditis (26). Furthermore, the humoral and cellular immune responses have been shown to be of critical importance during Q fever infection (29-31).

In our studies guinea pigs were infected by i.p. injections of 10^5 PFU per animal. Circulating antigens of C. burnetii were demonstrated by day 11, our earliest time point, postinfection. The appearance of the antigen paralleled the AC activity of the pooled sera and the inability of sera to lyse SRBC. The soluble antigen was apparently circulating as an IC with antibody and complement or some other serum component. The IC was very stable as evidenced by resistance to dissociation by heating at 56°C for 30 min, but heating in the presence of 3.5M iodide released the antigen from the IC. The circulating soluble antigen was shown to form a line of identity with a phenol extracted soluble component. The nature of this component is unknown at this time; however, the phenol extract contained at least six soluble antigens. We hope to purify the antigen(s) involved in the IC so that the chemical composition and localization on the microbe can be described. More important, the development of monoclonal antibody (32, 33) to the soluble antigen will be sought so that specific antibodies can be employed as diagnostic reagents.

Our demonstration of soluble antigen in the serum of experimentally infected guinea pigs suggests that it should be possible to demonstrate C. burnetii antigen in the serum of patients during acute and, perhaps, chronic Q fever infections.

V.   SUMMARY

Coxiella burnetii releases a soluble component which
forms a circulating immune complex (IC) in the sera of experimentally infected guinea pigs. The appearance of a soluble
antigen in the sera paralleled the anti-complementary activity
and the inability of sera to lyse sheep red blood cells. The
IC was very stable as evidenced by resistance to dissociation
by heating at 56°C for 30 min, but heating in the presence of
3.5M iodide released an antigen from the IC. The circulating
soluble antigen was shown to form a line of identity with a
phenol-extracted soluble component by employing a modified
immunoelectrophoretic technique. Establishment of the sensitivity and specificity of the method for the detection of
circulating antigen may lead to a rapid diagnostic test in
human acute and chronic infections.

ACKNOWLEDGMENTS

We are indebted to John Coe for many helpful discussions.
The expert secretarial assistance of S. Smaus is gratefully
acknowledged.

REFERENCES

1.   Hackstadt, T., and Williams, J. C., Proc. Natl. Acad.
     Sci. U.S.A. (in press).
2.   Victor, J., Raymond, R., Valliant, J., Wagner, J. C., and
     Pollack, A. D., J. Exp. Med. 95, 61 (1952).
3.   Wisseman, C. L. Jr., Fiset, P., and Ormsbee, R. A., J.
     Immunol. 99, 669 (1967).
4.   Downs, C. M., Zentralbl. Bakteriol. (Orig. A) 206, 329
     (1967).
5.   Kazar, J., Skultetyona, E., and Brezina, R., Acta Virol.
     19, 428 (1975).
6.   Hinrichs, D. J., and Jerrells, T. R., J. Immunol. 117,
     996 (1976).
7.   Kishimoto, R. A., and Walker, J. S., Infect. Immun. 14,
     416 (1976).
8.   McCaul, T. F., and Williams, J. C., J. Bact. (in press).
9.   Baca, O. G., and Paretsky, D., Infect. Immun. 9, 939
     (1974).
10. Silverman, D. J., Wisseman, C. L. Jr., Waddell, A. D.,
     and Jones, M., Infect. Immun. 22, 233 (1978).

11. Zubler, R. H., and Lambert, P. H., Prog. Allergy 24, 1 (1978).
12. Phillips, S. M., and Colley, D. G., Prog. Allergy 24, 49 (1978).
13. Coonrod, J. D., and Drennan, D. P., Ann. Inter. Med. 84, 254 (1976).
14. Williams, J. C., Peacock, M. G., and McCaul, T. F., Infect. Immun. (in press).
15. Avrameas, S., and Ternynck, T., Biochem. J. 102, 37c (1967).
16. Cantrell, J. L., and Williams, J. C., Infect. Immun. (in press).
17. Westphal, O., and Jann, K., in "Methods in Carbohydrate Chemistry" (R. L. Whistler, ed.), Vol 5, p. 83. Academic Press, New York (1965).
18. Palmer, D. F., and Casey, H. L., Public Health Monograph, No. 74 (PHS Publ. No. 1228) (1969).
19. Alsever, J. B., and Ainslie, R. B., N.Y. State J. Med. 41, 126 (1941).
20. Fiset, P., and Ormsbee, R. A., Zentralbl. Bakteriol. (Orig. A) 206, 321 (1968).
21. Philip, R. N., Casper, E. A., Burgdorfer, W., Gerloff, R. K., Hughes, L. E., and Bell, E. J., J. Immunol. 121, 1961 (1978).
22. Coonrod, J. D., and Leach, R. P., J. Clin. Microbiol. 8, 257 (1978).
23. Osserman, E. F., J. Immunol. 84, 93 (1960).
24. Truitt, G. L., and Mackaness, G. B., Am. Rev. Resp. Dis. 104, 829 (1971).
25. North, R. J., J. Exp. Med. 132, 521 (1970).
26. Kishimoto, R. A., and Burger, G. T., Infect. Immun. 16, 518 (1977).
27. Gonder, J. C., Kishimoto, R. A., Kastello, M. D., Pedersen, C. E., and Larson, E. W., J. Infect. Dis. 139, 191 (1979).
28. Turck, W. P. G., Howitt, G., Turnberg, L. A., Fox, H., Longson, M., Matthews, M. B., and Gupta, R. D., Quarterly J. Med. 178, 193 (1976).
29. Heggers, J. P., Mallavia, L. P., and Hinrichs, D. J., Can. J. Microbiol. 20, 657 (1974).
30. Kishimoto, R. A., Johnson, J. W., Kenyon, R. H., Ascher, M. S., Larson, E. W., and Pedersen, C. E. Jr., Infect. Immun. 19, 194 (1978).
31. Jerrells, T. R., Mallavia, L. P., and Hinrichs, D. J., Infect. Immun. 11, 280 (1975).
32. Kohler, G., and Milstein, C., Nature 256, 495 (1975).
33. Kohler, G., and Milstein, C., Eur J. Immunol. 6, 511 (1976).

MODIFICATION OF IMMUNE COMPETENCE
IN MICE BY Q FEVER VACCINE

Todd A. Damrow[1]

Department of Microbiology
University of Montana
Missoula, Montana

John L. Cantrell
Jim C. Williams

Laboratory of Microbial Structure and Function
Rocky Mountain Laboratories
Hamilton, Montana

I.   INTRODUCTION

Despite the prophylactic efficacy of the Q fever whole
cell vaccine (1-5), adverse physiologic effects consisting of
local skin reaction, fever, anorexia and malaise in vaccinated
individuals were noted by Smadel et al. (1). Other workers
since then have described various other severe local reactions
(2, 5, 6), and occasional systemic reactions (7). The vaccine
has been shown to be pyrogenic for both man and animals (1, 7).
Recently, Cantrell and Williams reported on the toxic activity
of a whole cell vaccine, and showed that formaldehyde killed
Coxiella burnetii whole cells are capable of inducing severe
splenomegaly, hepatomegaly and liver necrosis in C57BL/10 mice
(8). These undesirable effects have been defined largely in
terms of gross pathological changes. In light of increasing
awareness of naturally-occurring biological immunosuppressive

---

[1] Recipient of a USPHS, COSTEP training grant for scientist.

RICKETTSIAE AND RICKETTSIAL DISEASES

115

factors and their relationship to disease (9), we became
interested in studying the effect of this vaccine on the
immunologic functions of the C57BL/10 mouse.

Humoral and cellular immune responses were evaluated in
C57BL/10 mice using both in vivo and in vitro techniques.
Our results show that in addition to splenomegaly, hepatomegaly, liver necrosis and increased blastogenic activity,
administration of Q fever whole cell vaccine to mice resulted
in marked and chronic suppression of the normal proliferative
response of host spleen cells to various phytomitogens. In
contrast, the antibody-producing capacity in vaccinated mice
remained intact. Moreover, killed C. burnetii whole cells
were found to confer upon recipient mice, a nonspecific
resistance to heterologous bacterial challenge.

II. MATERIALS AND METHODS

A. Animals and Antigens

C57BL/10 male mice were obtained from the specific
pathogen-free production colony maintained at NIH Rocky Mountain Laboratories, Hamilton, MT. The mice were 9 to 12 weeks
of age and weighed 18 to 22 g. Outbred Swiss-Webster 10-week-
old male mice that weighed 20 to 25 g were obtained from the
above source.

C. burnetii (Ohio strain, Phase I) were cultivated and
purified as described by Williams et al. (10). Purified
organisms were inactivated with 1% formaldehyde solution for
24 hr at 25°C and dialyzed against sterile, de-mineralized
and distilled water at 4°C and then lyophilized. The inactivated status of this preparation was verified by egg inoculation according to the safety test for Q fever vaccine
devised by Berman et al. (11). Whole cells of inactivated
C. burnetii (1 mg = 3.78 X 10^{10} organisms) were administered
to mice intraperitoneally in 0.5 ml volumes of phosphate-
buffered saline (PBS, pH 7.2). Mice injected with 0.5 ml PBS
served as controls.

B. Immunological and Cytotoxicity Assays

All in vitro studies of immunologic activity were performed with leucocytes obtained from the spleen of animals as
described by Cantrell and Wheat (12). Suspensions of cells
were adjusted to a concentration of 2 X 10^6 cells per ml in
Eagle's minimal essential medium (MEM) (12). Leucocyte

viability, as determined by trypan blue exclusion, was always greater than 95%. Measurements of blastogenic activity (i.e., ^{3}H-TdR incorporation during the first 24 hr of cultivation of splenic leucocytes) were made according to the procedure of Cantrell and Wheat (12).

Sera of mice were evaluated for Phase I and Phase II $\underline{C}$. $\underline{burnetii}$ agglutinins by the microagglutination assay (MA) of Fiset et al. (13).

Lymphocyte transformation (LT) assays were conducted using the microculture system described by Strong et al. (14). The following mitogens were employed in this study: concanavalin A (Con A; P-L Biochemicals, Inc., Milwaukee, WI), phytohemagglutinin-P (PHA; Difco, Detroit, MI) and pokeweed mitogen (PWM; Grand Island Biological Co., Grand Island, NY). Con A, PHA and PWM were added to cell cultures at a final concentration of 1, 10 and 30 μg per well, respectively. These concentrations of mitogens were previously determined to result in maximal stimulation (data not shown). $\underline{C}$. $\underline{burnetii}$ whole cells (WC), when tested for mitogenic activity, were added to cell cultures to a final concentration of 5 μg per ml. Controls consisted of cultures to which only 20 μl of MEM was added. Cell cultures (4 X 10^5 cells per well) were incubated for 96 hr at 37°C in a humidified atmosphere of 5% CO_2 in air with a terminal 24 hr pulse of 1.0 μCi of ^{3}H-TdR (2 Ci per mmol). Samples were harvested and counted as described above (12). All determinations were conducted on a pooled suspension of cells from 3 to 5 mice. Results are presented as the arithmetic mean stimulation index (SI) and range of 4 replicate samples. SI was calculated as the ratio of counts per minute in stimulated cultures divided by the counts per minute in non-stimulated cultures.

The ^{51}Cr-release assay introduced by Goodman (15) was used to determine cell damage by WC. Results are expressed as the arithmetic mean counts per minute of 4 replicate cultures.

C. Susceptibility of C57BL/10 Mice to Listeriosis

A culture of $\underline{Listeria}$ $\underline{monocytogenes}$ (ATCC #15313) was maintained on brain-heart infusion agar (Difco, Detroit, MI) slants at 4°C. Prior to use, these organisms were passed repeatedly in mice to ensure full virulence of the strain. Susceptibility of mice to a challenge infection was measured in terms of survival after injection with serial 10-fold dilutions of challenge organisms into separate groups of mice. Experimental and control groups of 6 mice each were injected i.p. with 0.5 ml of each dilution of $\underline{L}$. $\underline{monocytogenes}$. One hundred μg of WC was injected i.p. into groups of test mice

2 weeks prior to challenge. Deaths among challenged mice
were recorded daily for 14 days. LD_{50} values were calculated
according to the method of Reed and Muench (16).

III. RESULTS

A. Biological Responses of C57BL/10 Mice
to Killed C. burnetii Whole Cells

Administration in vivo of WC to mice resulted in enhanced
in vitro blastogenic activity of splenic leucocytes. Increases in the blastogenic index (BI) were dose and time dependent in WC-injected mice (Fig. 1). The blastogenic response
of spleen cells peaked at 14 days postinjection. At this
time, cells from mice injected with 100 μg or more of WC,
displayed a rate of blastogenesis which was approximately 20
times greater than that of cells from control mice. Significantly elevated levels of blastogenic activity were still
demonstrable on day 35. An interesting, additional finding
was the presence of rickettsiae, detected by fluorescent antibody technique (17), in spleen impression mounts, prepared
from mice injected 5 weeks previously with 100 μg of WC.

B. Immunological and Cytotoxic Responsiveness of C57BL/10
Splenic Leucocytes

The administration in vivo of WC to mice resulted in a
marked inhibition of the in vitro mitogenic response of spleen
cells to Con A, PHA and PWM (Fig. 2). i) Hyporesponsiveness
to Con A was first detected on day 3 after treatment of mice
with 100 μg of WC and on day 7 after treatment with 10 μg of
WC (Fig. 2A). Maximal levels of inhibition were observed on
day 14 when 100 μg of WC was administered and on day 21 when
10 μg of WC was given and persisted through the duration of
the experimental period. The degree and time of onset of
suppression were related to the amount of WC administered. ii)
Hyporesponsiveness to PHA mitogenesis (Fig. 2B) indicated that
similar levels of inhibition resulted following injection of
mice with either 10 or 100 μg of WC. Suppression was initially
detected on day 3, whereas maximal levels of inhibition were
observed from day 14 to day 35. iii) Hyporesponsiveness to
PWM response was not as consistent when compared to that of
Con A and PHA (Fig. 2C). Reduction of the responsiveness of
spleen cells to PWM was observed on day 3. Maximal hyporesponsiveness was noted on day 14 postinjection of mice with

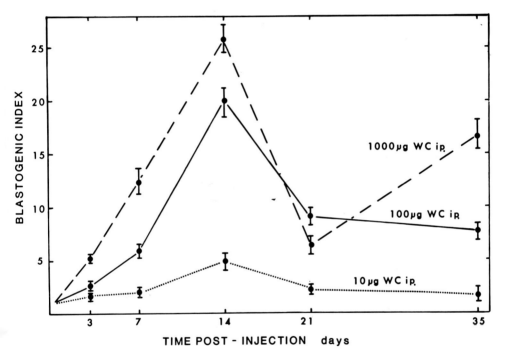

Fig. 1. Comparison of blastogenic activity in suspensions of splenic leucocytes from C57BL/10 mice injected with graded doses of killed C. burnetii whole cells. Mice were injected i.p. with 10 µg (•••••), 100 µg (-----) and 1000 µg (- - -) of killed C. burnetii whole cells. Data points represent the arithmetic mean of quadruplicate counts conducted on a pooled suspension of cells from 3 to 5 mice; bars = range. Background activity for the unsensitized and unstimulated control mice averaged 647 CPM.

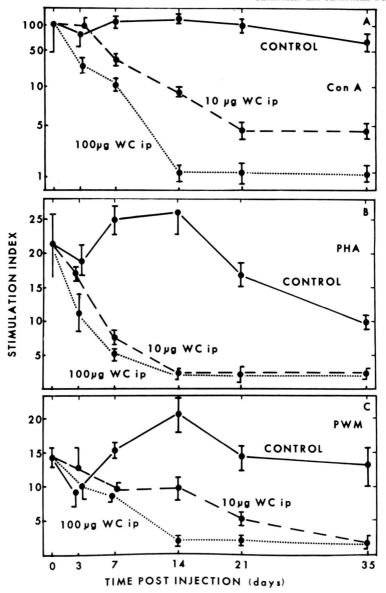

Fig. 2. Mitogenic response of C57BL/10 splenic leucocytes to Con A (A), PHA (B) and PWM (C) at various times postinjection of C. burnetii WC into mice. Mice were injected i.p. with 0.5 ml PBS (——), 10 μg WC (- - -) and 100 μg WC (·····). Data points represent the arithmetic mean of quadruplicate counts conducted on a pooled suspension of cells from 3 to 5 mice; bars = range. Background activity for the control groups, 10 μg and 100 μg groups were 222, 866 and 930 CPM, respectively.

100 µg of WC. This period of time was extended to 21 days when 10 µg of WC was administered. With either dose, however, similar levels of inhibition were eventually attained by day 35.

To determine if the mitogen hyporesponsiveness may be the result of a direct adverse action of WC on the integrity of the leucocyte membrane, the effect of WC on the release of ^{51}Cr from labeled C57BL/10 spleen cells was investigated. The presence of WC in normal and previously sensitized splenic leucocyte cultures had no effect on the rate at which ^{51}Cr was released from labeled cells (data not shown). Moreover, trypan blue dye exclusion viability determinations revealed that WC had no adverse effect on cell viability (data not shown).

When WC were presented in vitro to cultures of normal splenic leucocytes, a mitogenic response was observed. ^{3}H–TdR incorporation was stimulated 2.6 ± 0.4-fold as compared to unstimulated cultures. These findings indicate that WC were not toxic for sensitized or normal splenic leucocyte cultures.

C. Susceptibility of C. burnetii Treated Mice to Listeriosis

Immunocompetence of mice previously sensitized with WC was tested by challenging these mice with L. monocytogenes. Swiss–Webster mice were injected i.p. with 100 µg of WC. After a period of 2 weeks, groups of mice were inoculated with serial 10-fold dilutions of viable L. monocytogenes. Likewise, groups of PBS-treated mice were also inoculated. The LD_{50} value of L. monocytogenes was 1.9×10^2 colony forming units (CFU) in the control mice, whereas WC-treated mice exhibited an LD_{50} of 5.6×10^6 CFU. Thus, WC-treated mice were approximately 30,000 times more resistant to infection with L. monocytogenes as compared to PBS-treated controls.

IV. DISCUSSION

Disease-related immunosuppression has been reported during infection with members of various classes of infectious agents including viruses (18-21), bacteria (22), fungi (23), protozoa (24) and rickettsiae (25, 26). Our studies demonstrate that nonviable C. burnetii whole cells are also capable of suppressing host immune responsiveness. The administration of inactivated C. burnetii whole cells to C57BL/10 mice, genetically unresponsive to endotoxin (27), resulted in a severe depression of the in vitro lymphocyte transformation (LT) response to various mitogens. The chronic nature of the immunosuppressive

response to C. burnetii whole cells is uncommon among other
agents. We have not ruled out the possibility that the C57BL/
10 mouse may be genetically predisposed to immunosuppression
by inactivated C. burnetii whole cells.

The suppression of immune responsiveness reported to occur
during infection with various other organisms in other animal
models is, in most cases, transient. Even among other
rickettsiae, C. burnetii may be unique with respect to the
duration of the immunosuppressive response. Oster et al. (25)
observed that suppression of LT in guinea pigs infected with
Rickettsia rickettsii subsided by day 17; R. sibirica and R.
conorii caused suppression of LT only through day 7. Kishimoto
and Gonder (26) reported that the mitogen responsiveness of
lymphocytes from guinea pigs and monkeys was suppressed only
between 14 and 28 days after infection with C. burnetii. In
addition, they reported that suppression of LT occurs only
following an active infection and not merely antigenic exposure; no suppression of LT was detected in animals vaccinated
with killed Q fever vaccine.

The mechanism of immune suppression is not known at this
time. However, several observations can be made from our data
which show that the condition results from a subtle or indirect action of C. burnetii whole cells. The lack of effect
of WC on the release of ^{51}Cr from host leucocytes and the
finding that exposure to killed whole cells does not reduce
cell viability, as determined by trypan blue dye exclusion,
suggest that the hyporesponsive state is not the result of a
lethal interaction directly between C. burnetii and the host
target cell.

Killed C. burnetii cells have been shown by others to be
readily phagocytized by macrophages (28). Because macrophages
play a vital role in the regulation of numerous immune responses (29, 30), it is possible that the suppression demonstrated following vaccination of mice against Q fever results
from modulation by macrophages. Indeed, macrophage-mediated
immunosuppression has already been demonstrated in numerous
infectious diseases (31, 32). In this study, nonspecific
immunity implicated in the response of mice to WC in that
vaccinated mice were found to be approximately 30,000 times
more resistant than nonvaccinated mice to the lethal effects
of L. monocytogenes challenge. This finding is consistent
with other studies reporting nonspecific activation of macrophages by killed C. burnetii (33). Activated macrophages have
been shown to markedly influence mitogen-induced LT (34, 35).
Additional studies are necessary to define the cellular basis
of the immunosuppressive response which we have described.

V. SUMMARY

Various immunological parameters were investigated in C57BL/10 mice following i.p. administration of formalin-inactivated <u>Coxiella burnetii</u> whole cells (WC). Spleen cells explanted from mice pretreated with <u>C</u>. <u>burnetii</u> WC displayed a 20-fold increase in blastogenic activity as determined by increased ^{3}H-TdR uptake. Pretreatment of mice with WC, however, suppressed the normal mitogenic response of spleen cells to Con A, PHA and PWM. Suppression of the mitogenic response by WC was time and dose dependent. However, mice pretreated with WC demonstrated heightened resistance to infection with <u>Listeria monocytogenes</u>. Thus, nonviable <u>C</u>. <u>burnetii</u> whole cells are capable of suppressing host immune responsiveness to lymphocyte transformation by various mitogens while promoting a nonspecific resistance to heterologous challenge. The nature of the cellular and subcellular components responsible for the noted biological effects are currently under investigation.

ACKNOWLEDGMENT

The expert secretarial assistance of S. Smaus is gratefully acknowledged.

REFERENCES

1. Smadel, J. E., Snyder, M. J., and Robbins, F. C., <u>Am. J. Hyg.</u> <u>47</u>, 71 (1948).
2. Luoto, L., Bell, J. F., Casey, M., and Lackman, D. B., <u>Am. J. Hyg.</u> <u>78</u>, 1 (1963).
3. Kishimoto, R. A., Johnson, J. W., Kenyon, R. H., Ascher, M. S., Larson, E. W., and Pederson, C. E. Jr., <u>Infect. Immun.</u> <u>19</u>, 194 (1978).
4. Behymer, D. E., Biberstein, E. L., Rieman, H. P., Franti, C. E., Sawyer, M., Ruppanner, R., and Crenshaw, G. L., <u>Am. J. Vet. Res.</u> <u>37</u>, 631 (1976).
5. Meiklejohn, G., and Lennette, E. H., <u>Am. J. Hyg.</u> <u>52</u>, 54 (1950).
6. Stoker, M. G. P., <u>Brit. Med. J.</u> <u>1</u>, 425 (1957).
7. Anacker, R. L., Lackman, D. B., Pickens, E. G., and Ribi, E., <u>J. Immunol.</u> <u>89</u>, 145 (1962).
8. Cantrell, J. L., and Williams, J. C., <u>Infect. Immun.</u> (in press).

9. Neubauer, R. H. (ed.) CRC Press (1979).
10. Williams, J. C., Peacock, M. G., and McCaul, T. F.,
    Infect. Immun. (in press).
11. Berman, S., Cole, G., Lowenthal, J. P., and Gochenour,
    R. B., J. Bact. 79, 747 (1960).
12. Cantrell, J. L., and Wheat, R. W., Cancer Res. 39,
    3554 (1979).
13. Fiset, P, Ormsbee, R. A., Silberman, R., Peacock, M.,
    and Spielman, S. H., Acta Virol. 13, 60 (1969).
14. Strong, D. M., Ahmed, A. A., Thurman, G. B., and Sell,
    K. W., J. Immumol. Methods 2, 279 (1973).
15. Goodman, H. S., Nature (London) 190, 269 (1961).
16. Reed, L. J., and Muench, H., Am. J. Hyg. 27, 493 (1938).
17. Peacock, M. W., Burgdorfer, W., and Ormsbee, R. A.,
    Infect. Immun. 3, 355 (1971).
18. Kantzler, G. B., Lauteria, S. F., Cusumano, C. L.,
    Lee, J. D., Ganguly, R., and Waldman, R. H., Infect.
    Immun. 10, 996 (1974).
19. Ganguly, R., Cusumano, C. L., and Waldman, R. H.,
    Infect. Immun. 13, 464 (1976).
20. Fireman, P., Friday, G., and Kumate, J., Pediatrics
    43, 264 (1969).
21. Ten Napel, C. H. H., and The, T. H., J. Infect. Dis.
    141, 716 (1980).
22. Schwab, J. H., Bact. Rev. 39, 121 (1975).
23. Stobo, J. D., Paul, S., VanScoy, R. E., and Hermans,
    P. E., J. Clin. Invest. 57, 319 (1976).
24. Cunningham, D. S., Grogl, M., and Kuhn, R. E., Infect.
    Immun. 30, 496 (1980).
25. Oster, C. N., Kenyon, R. H., and Pederson, C. E. Jr.,
    Infect. Immun. 22, 411 (1978).
26. Kishimoto, R. A., and Gonder, J. C., Can. J. Microbiol.
    25, 949 (1979).
27. McAdam, K. P. W. J., and Ryan, J. L., J. Immunol. 120,
    249 (1978).
28. Kazar, J., Skultetyova, E., and Brezina, R., Acta
    Virol. 19, 426 (1975).
29. Pierce, C. W., Kapp, J. A., Wood, D. D., and Benacerraf,
    B., J. Immunol. 112, 1181 (1974).
30. Murahata, R. I., Cantrell, J. C., Lichtenstein, A.,
    and Zighelboim, J., Int. J. Immunopharmac. 2, 47 (1980).
31. Wellhausen, S. R., and Mansfield, J. M., Cell. Immunol.
    54, 414 (1980).
32. Rinaldo, C. R. Jr., Carney, W. P., Richter, B. S., Black,
    P. H., and Hirsch, M. S., J. Infect. Dis. 141, 488 (1980).
33. Kelley, M. T., Cell. Immunol. 28, 198 (1977).
34. Keller, R., Cell. Immunol. 17, 542 (1975).
35. Nelson, D. A., Nature (London) 246, 306 (1973).

Q FEVER ENDOCARDITIS: A THREE AND ONE-HALF YEAR FOLLOW-UP

Robert C. Kimbrough, III

Good Samaritan Hospital
and Medical Center
Portland, Oregon

Richard A. Ormsbee
Marius G. Peacock

Rocky Mountain Laboratories
Hamilton, Montana

I.   INTRODUCTION

In September of 1979 we presented a case of Q fever endo-carditis (1). The diagnosis was made by serology and recovery of the organism from the patient's aortic valve obtained at the time of valve replacement. At the time of publication we felt that this was the first case so documented from the United States. Since then, four other cases have been referred to the Rocky Mountain Laboratories. One of the four has had the organism recovered from valvular tissue. We present this case to further expand upon the clinical history, to report further serologic data, and to present serologic data of the patient's family and cattle.

A.   Case History

The patient is a 58-year-old white male maintenance supervisor of a creosoting plant in Portland, Oregon. He is now 4 years past aortic valve replacement and 2½ years from last antibiotic therapy. Since 1961 he has raised cattle and sheep as a hobby. His daughter helped with this hobby, his wife did

not. The patient aided in numerous deliveries in both small
herds. In the lambing season of 1971 he had a 3-week, self-
limited illness of fever, chills, sweating, chest pain and
weight loss. In November of 1975 and again in February of
1976 he assisted in cattle births; the last calf was stillborn
with a foul smelling placenta.

In January 1976 he first noted night sweats and easy fatig-
ability. In February 1976 he complained of weight loss, loss
of libido, and joint pain in the knees. In March 1976 he had
a sudden onset of left-sided headache, intermittent right
visual field loss, and facial paresthesia. He was eventually
referred to the Neurological Surgery Service of Good Samaritan
Hospital & Medical Center in May 1976. Initial physical examination was negative except for elevated temperature. Initial laboratory data revealed an elevated erythrocyte sedimen-
tation rate, mildly increased liver function tests, hema-
turia, and abnormal cerebrospinal fluid. Computed tomography,
EEG and brain scan were normal. Cerebral angiography showed a
blocked left internal carotid artery.

Repeat physical examination revealed a systolic heart murmur and a recent splinter hemorrhage on the left index finger.
A presumptive diagnosis of endocarditis and meningitis was
made, and after appropriate blood cultures were done, the patient was started on methicillin, penicillin and chloramphenicol. He became asymptomatic in 72 hrs. One week later a dia-
stolic murmur of aortic regurgitation was heard.

Two weeks later, because of thrombocytopenia, the patient
sustained intestinal bleeding. Chloramphenicol was discontin-
ued, but other antibiotics were continued. Four weeks after
admission the first serologic results were returned: all were
negative except for a complement-fixation (CF) test for Q
fever which was reported at 1:256 without phase specification.
Tetracycline treatment was started and later changed to doxycycline for better gastrointestinal acceptance. The state
laboratory reported a CF titer for Q fever of 1:4096 without
phase specification. A presumptive diagnosis of Q fever endocarditis was entertained, and because of a report from Britain
(2) the patient was discharged in mid-June on doxycycline 100
mg every 12 hrs and double strength sulfatrimethoprim, one
tablet, every 12 hrs.

He returned in August 1978 with angina and congestive heart
failure. Cardiac catheterization revealed poor function of the
left ventricle and a damaged aortic valve. He underwent aortic
valve replacement and a coronary artery bypass on August 20,
1976. He was discharged on August 26, 1976 on the same regimen
mentioned above. The sulfatrimethoprim was stopped in November
1976 because of gastrointestinal problems. Rifampin, 600 mg
daily, was added to the doxycycline in January 1977. Rifampin

was discovered to be more potent than tetracycline by a factor
of at least 100 in plaque inhibition tests (unpublished findings of one of the authors, RAO, of plaque inhibition by rifampin incorporated in the nutrient agar overlay of monolayers of
primary chick embryo cells previously inoculated with Coxiella
burnetii). In March 1977 the patient suffered a subendocardial
myocardial infarction. Anticoagulation was difficult because
of the rifampin. In April 1978 he sustained another gastrointestinal bleed and all antibiotics were stopped. In July
1978 angina again led to a cardiac catheterization which revealed mild mitral valve function, improved left ventricular
function, and the bypass graft was opened.

He was re-examined at 6-month to 1-year intervals. He continued to have mild fatigue, mild headache, and some palpita-
tions following exertion. He had no fever, weight loss,
sweats, and had good vision. A recent electrocardiogram showed
only left ventricular hypertrophy. All laboratory tests were
normal.

Results of serologic testing of his family and cattle herd
are presented below. Prior to the onset of his cardiovascular
symptoms the patient sold or slaughtered all of his sheep. His
cattle herd has changed in composition markedly since 1971 due
to sales and slaughter.

II.   MATERIALS AND METHODS

Parts of the aortic valve were processed for light microscopy. Another part of the valve was frozen in liquid nitrogen and shipped to the Rocky Mountain Laboratories. This was
quickly thawed in a small volume of sodium chloride, warmed
gently under the water tap and ground in a high speed micro-
blender. Portions of the suspension were stained by the
Giménez method or by antiserum tagged with fluorescein isothiocyanate for microscopic observation, or used in immediate
isolation attempts (3).

A.   Isolation of C. burnetii

Portions of the valve suspension, thawed but held at 0°C
until used, were inoculated intraperitoneally into 300 to 400 g
guinea pigs, embryonated chicken eggs via the yolk sac, and
primary cultures of chick embryo cells. Guinea pigs that responded with fever (rectal temperatures of $\geq 40°C$) were sacrificed 5 days after inoculation while they were still febrile;
and spleen, liver, and kidney suspensions were inoculated into guinea pigs, embryonated eggs, and primary chick embryo

cultures. Yolk sac suspensions from inoculated eggs and inoculated primay chick embryo cultures were similarly subpassaged.

B.   Serologic Studies

The following three purified antigens (4) were used at the
concentration of 200 mcg/ml in indirect microimmunofluorescence (micro-IF) tests: a) C. burnetii, Nine Mile strain,
phase I, 306 guinea pig (GP) passages, cloned from primary
chick embryo cell culture plaques, six passages in chick embryos (EP); b) C. burnetii, Nine Mile strain, phase II, 306 GP,
4 EP, 1 GP, 3 EP, cloned from primary chick embryo cell culture
plaques and extracted with trichloracetic acid to remove any
trace of phase I antigen (5) and render the antigen reactive
only to phase II antibodies (6), c) a natural phase II antigen
prepared from a cloned Nine Mile, 94 EP. Titrations of phase I
antibody were performed by microagglutination (MA), indirect
micro-IF, and CF with both a) and an antigen made from the isolate from the patient. MA titrations of phase II antibodies
were performed with b). The CF and micro-IF titrations of phase
II antibodies were performed with c). Rabbit antisera against
human IgG and IgM were rendered completely specific to the respective heavy chain components of IgG and IgM (7), tagged with
fluorescein isothiocyanate (8), and used in the indirect micro-
IF tests (9).

III.   RESULTS

A.   Isolation

The tricuspid aortic valve was calcified and displayed partially fused commissures. It was quite difficult to cut. The
right coronary cusp was perforated and much of the superior aspect of the valve was covered with fine, granular, amber vege-
tations that extended slightly onto the ventricular septum.
Bacterial, mycobacterial, and fungal studies of the valve were
all negative. Microscopic examination of the tissue suspension
in Giménez-stained preparations showed micro-organisms with the
size, shape, and tinctorial properties of C. burnetii. Valve
tissue fragments stained with fluorescein isothiocyanate-tagged
guinea pig antisera against C. burnetii and examined microscopically by ultraviolet light contained hundreds of fluorescent
particles with the size and shape of C. burnetii.
Inoculated guinea pigs, that had responded with fever, produced specific antibodies against C. burnetii. Subpassage of
suspensions of tissues from these animals into embryonated eggs

produced abundant growth of C. burnetii identified by direct
MA reactions with standard guinea pig antisera. Inoculation of
aortic valve material into embryonated eggs also resulted in
abundant growth of C. burnetii by the second egg passage. Inoculation of valve suspension into primary chick embryo cell
cultures, followed by subpassage into embryonated eggs, also
produced growth of a microorganism indistinguishable from C.
burnetii. Attempts to isolate C. burnetii from blood taken
the day before valve replacement were unsuccessful.

B. Serology

Titrations of serum antibodies are summarized in the following tables. Table 1 is a chronological summary of CF and
MA tests. Table 2 is a chronologic summary of the micro-IF
test data. These data indicate the high levels of specific
phase I antibodies which are almost entirely IgG.

TABLE 1. Phase I and Phase II Antibody Levels

Date		Complement Fixation II	I	Microagglutination II	I
5/7/76	(0)[a]	64	512	1024	1024
8/19/76	(15)	128	1024	2048	2048
11/10/76	(27)	64	2048	2048	1024
1/18/77	(36)	128	1024	2048	512
3/9/77	(44)	64	512	1024	256
6/14/77	(58)	64	2048	512	256
10/5/77	(74)	128	32	256	64
3/30/78	(99)	128	32	128	32
7/11/78	(109)	128	32	256	64
12/5/78	(130)	128	32	128	64
6/3/80	(208)	256	128	256	32

[a]Number of weeks.

TABLE 2.   Phase I and Phase II Antibody Levels

Date		IgG II	IgG I	IgM II	IgM I
5/7/76	(0)[a]	2048	16384	8	512
8/19/76	(15)	1024	128000	<8	512
11/10/76	(27)	2048	65536	<8	256
1/18/77	(36)	65536	262273	<16	<16
3/9/77	(44)	4096	>262273	<16	16
6/14/77	(58)	256	32768	32	512
10//5/77	(74)	256	16384	32	1024
3/30/78	(99)	512	32768	64	1024
7/11/78	(109)	16384	32768	128	512
12/5/78	(130)	>16384	16384	1024	1024
6/3/80	(208)	4096	256	128	16

[a]Number of weeks.

Table 3 is the CF data on the serum of the wife and daughter. The wife had no detectable antibodies, and she did not help with the management of the herds. The daughter had low levels of phase I and phase II antibodies; she did help with the management of the herd.

TABLE 3.   Phase I and Phase II Antibody Levels
of Wife and Daughter

	Complement Fixation II	Complement Fixation I
Wife	<1:8	<1:8
Daughter	1:32	1:8

Table 4 is a summary of the CF and MA data from the cattle remaining in the patient's possession at the time of his valve replacement. These data indicate that only one of these cattle (#5) had any significant antibody to C. burnetii.

TABLE 4. Phase I and Phase II Antibody Levels
of Patient's Cattle

Cattle	Complement Fixation		Microagglutination	
	II	I	II	I
#1	<1:8	<1:8	1:4	<1:2
#2	<1:8	<1:8	1:8	<1:2
#3	<1:8	<1:8	1:8	<1:2
#4	<1:8	<1:8	1:8	<1:2
#5	<1:8	<1:8	1:32	<1:2

IV. DISCUSSION

Rickettsial endocarditis typically occurs 3 to 20 years after Q fever, most often in men exposed to the body fluids or dust associated with infected sheep or cattle (10,11). Usually it occurs on previously damaged heart valves. Until recently, survival time from onset of illness seldom had exceeded 3 years. Valve replacement as an aid in eradicating the rickettsial infection was still unproved (10).

Turck and associates (10) observed little antibody change in the first year, but a gradual lowering of antibody levels after 3-5 years of therapy. Our findings are similar for the period that this patient has been observed (Tables 1 and 2). The increase of titers by indirect micro-IF tests in late 1978 are unexplained. In this case, high levels of IgG antibody against C. burnetii and low levels of IgM antibody were found (Table 2) even though the overall IgM levels were in the normal range.

No ready explanation presents itself for the changes in micro-IF titers observed in 1978 after cessation of antibiotic treatment. They may have been the result of a) persistent infection of the left carotid artery, b) valve ring abscess, or c) residual foci of C. burnetii in the reticuloendothelial portion of the liver so small as to be undetected by liver function tests. It should be noted that the apparent titer changes revealed by micro-IF were not mirrored in either CF or MA titers.

We believe that one should use specific phase I antigen, for unequivocal serologic diagnosis of rickettsial endocarditis. With this antigen, any of the three tests which we have used will differentiate between the high phase I antibody responses characteristic of rickettsial endocarditis and the low phase I antibody responses seen in primary Q fever. Phase II antigen alone or a mixture of phase I and phase II antigen may give results that are impossible to interpret.

V. SUMMARY

Q fever endocarditis should be considered in the diagnosis of disease in patients who have been in contact with sheep or cattle or their products and who show features of culture-negative endocarditis. Serologic testing should be done with phase specific antigens, especially phase I. Family and others who have had contact with the patient's cattle herds should also be tested.

REFERENCES

1. Kimbrough, R. C., Ormsbee, R. A., Peacock, M., Rogers, W. R., Bennetts, R. W., Raaf, J., Krause, A., and Gardner, C., Ann. Int. Med. 91, 400 (1979).
2. Freeman, R., and Hodson, M. E., Br. Med. J. 1, 419 (1972).
3. Giménez, D. F., Stain Technol. 39, 135 (1964).
4. Ormsbee, R., Peacock, M., Philip, R., Casper, E., Plorde, J., Gabre-Kidan, T., and Wright, L., Am. J. Epidemiol. 105, 261 (1977).
5. Anacker, R. L., Lackman, D. B., Pickens, E. G., and Ribi, E., J. Immunol. 89, 145 (1962).
6. Fiset, P., Ormsbee, R. A., Silberman, R., Peacock, M., and Spielman, S. H., Acta Virol. 13, 60 (1969).
7. Fahey, J. L., and McKelvey, E. M., J. Immunol. 94, 84 (1965).
8. Peacock, M., Burgdorfer, W., and Ormsbee, R. A., Infect. Immunol. 3, 355 (1971).
9. Philip, R. N., Casper, E. A., Ormsbee, R. A., Peacock, M. G., and Burgdorfer, W., J. Clin. Microbiol. 3, 51 (1976).
10. Turck, W.P.G., Howitt, G., Turnberg, L. A., Fox, H., Longson, M., Matthews, M. B., and Das Gupta, R., Quarterly J. Med. 45, 193 (1976).
11. Wilson, H. G., Neilson, G. H., Galea, E. G., Stafford, G., and O'Brien, M. F., Circulation 53, 680 (1976).

A RAPID IMMUNOFLUORESCENT PROCEDURE FOR SERODIAGNOSIS OF Q FEVER

Michael S. Ascher
James R. Greenwood
Mary F. Thornton

Department of Medicine
University of California, Irvine
Irvine, California
and
Public Health Laboratory
Orange County Health Department
Santa Ana, California

I. INTRODUCTION

Recent developments in technology have made it possible to accurately quantitate the results of fluorescent antibody procedures and eliminate much of the subjective component of such assays. These techniques have been successfully implemented on a commercial basis in the assay of antibody to rubella and anti-nuclear antibody(1,2), and additional antigenic systems are forthcoming from the manufacturer(3). The acronym for this procedure is FIAX. We have adapted this assay to the study of antibody in Q fever.

II. METHODS

In this procedure the carrier slide is replaced by a plastic "dipstick" coated on two sides with special paper. The assay instrument is a quantitative fluorometer specifically designed for this purpose. In these studies we have used as antigens two U.S. Army investigational Q Fever vaccines, one in Phase I and one in Phase II. The technical

details involve placing 25 ul of antigen suspension on one
side of the stick and allowing it to air dry. The stick is
then passed through tubes containing serum and conjugate along
with intervening washes for a total assay time of one hour.
The stick is then placed in the fluorometer chamber and each
side is measured. The results appear in digital form on the
instrument. The specific fluorescence of the sample (FSU) is
defined as the result in arbitrary units of the antigen side
less the result of the control side.

III. RESULTS

Table 1 shows the results of this assay applied to serum
obtained from guinea pigs three weeks after immunization with
12 ug Phase I vaccine in Freund's complete adjuvant. Results
are presented for four serial dilutions of serum. Under these
conditions, we note a marked difference between immune serum
and control serum. These results were obtained after minimal
manipulation of variables to obtain optimal concentrations of
reagents.

TABLE 1. FIAX Immunofluorescence Assay of Guinea Pig
Serum Antibodies to Phase I Q Fever Antigen

Immunization	Serum Dilution (reciprocal)			
	160	320	640	1280
None	2.4[a]	3.2	0.7	1.0
Phase I vaccine (12µg) + FCA	113.0	97.0	72.0	58.0

[a]FSU

A major question in the development of an immunologic
assay for Q fever is the sensitivity of the test. Table 2
shows the antibody response of guinea pigs three weeks after
immunization with varying amounts of phase I vaccine. The
procedure detects a response in animals which received only 60
ng of antigen in the form of a skin test and shows a graded
dose response from that form of immunization up to the
Freund's complete adjuvant group. The data also illustrate

the effect of varying the concentration of antigen on the sticks.

TABLE 2. Effect of Varying Doses of Immunizing Vaccine
on Immunofluorescence of Guinea Pig Sera
with Phase I Q Fever Antigen

Vaccine (µg)	Adjuvant	Antigen dilution (reciprocal)		
		32	16	8
None	None	8.9[a]	8.6	15.9
0.06	None	14.5	21.5	37.4
12.0	None	28.7	46.3	94.3
12.0	FCA	50.9	69.8	129.9

[a]FSU

In Table 3 we present the relationship between standard phase II complement fixation results and those obtained with the FIAX assay applied to human samples. The sera were obtained in the course of a biosurveillance program surrounding a recent outbreak of Q fever in a research laboratory.

TABLE 3. Immunofluorescence Assay of Human Serum Antibody
to Phase I and II Q Fever Antigens

Phase II CF Value	Phase II Antigen		Phase I Antigen	
	N	Mean FSU (SD)	N	Mean FSU (SD)
<8	68	26.9 (15.8)	34	0.1 (4.8)
8	11	41.1 (21.1)	11	3.0 (2.9)
16-32	12	76.1 (18.7)	5	11.5 (7.2)
≥64	6	74.3 (19.7)	−	Not Done

The CF results are arbitrarily divided into four groups and the following observations can be made. One, all of the sera with clear positive results on CF, i.e. a titer of 1:16 or greater have FIAX values of 50 or more. Two, the sera with borderline CF titers of 8 center on the value of about 50 units. Three, sera negative by CF have a few results overlapping the positive range. In these few high grade reactors, we postulate that this assay is more sensitive than CF(4). One problem with these data is that the fluorescent values of the nonimmune human sera are considerably higher than those seen with sera from nonimmune guinea pigs. This noise in the assay has been reduced in other antigenic systems by the use of a tissue culture control antigen on the reverse surface of the stick and experiments of that type attempting to characterize this nonspecific background are in progress. Nevertheless, the overall performance of this assay to date suggests that it would serve as an excellent rapid screening procedure in the serodiagnosis of Q fever. In simple terms, any FIAX value of less than 50 can be assumed to be negative by CF and only those greater than 50 would be subjected to more cumbersome CF testing.

Finally, we tested this assay in man with phase I vaccine as antigen in addition to the phase II antigen. Table 3 demonstrates a similar degree of separation between CF positives and negatives but at a much lower level of response. We consider it significant that phase I reactivity can be detected in these individuals and this finding will be pursued in recipients of the new phase I vaccine.

IV.   SUMMARY

We have used a new simplified FIAX immunofluorescent procedure to demonstrate antibody to C. burnetii in guinea pigs and man. The test is extremely sensitive and correlates very well with standard Phase II CF serology. The widespread dissemination of FIAX instruments to clinical laboratories should make it possible for more facilities to perform their own screening tests for Q fever and may relieve the burden placed on reference laboratories by biosurveillance of sheep research programs.

ACKNOWLEDGMENTS

Supported by the US Army Medical Research and Development
Command under Contract DAMD17-80-C-0154

REFERENCES

1. Brody, J.P., Binkley, J.H., and Harding, S.A., J. Clin.
    Microbiol. 10, 708 (1979).
2. Ross, G.L., Barland, P., and Grayzel, A.I., J. Rheum. 5,
    373 (1978).
3. Walls, K.W., and Barnhart, E.R., J. Clin. Microbiol. 7,
    234 (1978).
4. Kazar, J., Brezina, R., Kovacova, E., and Urvölgyi, J.,
    Acta Virol. 17, 512 (1973).

SEROLOGIC COMPARISON OF R. RICKETTSII ISOLATED
FROM PATIENTS IN NORTH CAROLINA TO R. RICKETTSII
ISOLATED FROM PATIENTS IN MONTANA

Jeffrey P. Davis[1,2]
Catherine M. Wilfert

Department of Pediatrics
Duke University Medical Center
Durham, North Carolina

Daniel J. Sexton[3]

Department of Medicine
Duke University Medical Center
Durham, North Carolina

Willy Burgdorfer
Elizabeth A. Casper
Robert N. Philip

Epidemiology Branch
Rocky Mountain Laboratories
Hamilton, Montana

[1]Supported in part by a Bristol Fellowship in Infectious
Diseases from Bristol Laboratories and in part by NIH grant
1-F32-AI-05582-01A1.
[2]Present address: Bureau of Prevention, Division of
Health, Madison, Wisconsin.
[3]Present address: Internal Medicine-Infectious Diseases,
Oklahoma City Clinic, Oklahoma City, Oklahoma.

I.   INTRODUCTION

Variations in ultrastructure, pathogenicity and immunogenicity have been recognized among spotted fever group (SFG)
rickettsiae isolated from various species of ticks in
different regions of the United States (1-4).   Similar
comparisons of immunogenicity and pathogenicity among
rickettsial isolates from humans are few (5-6).   We studied
six isolates of R. rickettsii from patients with Rocky
Mountain spotted fever (RMSF) from North Carolina and compared
their serologic reactivity with that of five isolates from
patients with RMSF from Montana and the Sheila Smith strain
of R. rickettsii which has been widely used in vaccine and
laboratory investigations.   In addition, the serologic
responses of the patients were studied.   The results of these
studies are reported here.   Also noted are two instances
in which R. rickettsii was isolated from patients after
specific antirickettsial therapy had been instituted.

II.   MATERIALS AND METHODS

North Carolina isolates of R. rickettsii were obtained
from 4 patients hospitalized at Duke University Medical Center
and from 2 patients at Cabarrus County Hospital in 1975.
Blood specimens were obtained soon after admission to the
hospital.   Specimens were collected prior to the institution
of either tetracycline or chloramphenicol in all but 2
patients.   Approximately 15 ml. of whole blood was promptly
frozen at -70°C and kept frozen until the clots could be
inoculated into meadow voles, Microtus pennsylvanicus.   Serum
samples were collected from the same patients before, during
and after the institution of antirickettsial therapy.
    Montana isolates of R. rickettsii were made from five
patients evaluated between 1970-1975.   The Sheila Smith strain
originated in Missoula, Montana and was isolated in 1946 from
a patient with RMSF (7).

A.   Rickettsial Isolation and Antigens

Approximately one-half of the blood clot from each patient
was triturated with an equal volume of cold brain heart
infusion broth (Difco) and 0.25 ml of suspension was injected
intraperitoneally into each of two male and two female meadow
voles.   The subsequent processing of the voles and the

inoculation of chicken embryo yolk sacs is described in
earlier studies (4,8).

Rickettsiae were cultured in chicken-embryo yolk sacs
according to the method of Bell and Pickens (7). Dilutions of
rickettsiae in inocula were adjusted to give optimal embryo
death patterns. Eggs were incubated at 35°C for an additional
48-72 hours after embryo death to obtain maximal yields of
rickettsiae. Rickettsiae from the third to fifth passage in
chick embryos were used to prepare crude yolk sac preparations
of stock antigen by methods previously described (6). Three
to 5% yolk sac suspensions of viable rickettsiae were made and
stored at -65°C. Part of the stock antigen was used to
prepare antiserum and part (stored in 0.2 ml amounts) was used
as test antigen.

B. Rickettsial Strains

All strains were tested for group-reactive antigens
by direct immunofluorescence by using serial two-fold
dilutions of fluorescein-labeled guinea pig or rabbit antisera
prepared against the "R" and Sawtooth-strains of R. rickettsii
and the Breinl strain of R. prowazekii. All patient strains
reacted only to spotted fever group conjugates.

C. Antisera

Antisera were prepared in random-bred, weanling Swiss
mice from the Rocky Mountain Laboratory colony using stock
antigens and employing methods and materials previously
described (6).

D. R. rickettsii Serology

The microimmunofluorescent (micro-IF) test was used to
test patient sera. The materials and procedure on micro-IF
tests was a modification of that of Wang(9) detailed
elsewhere (10,11).

E. Cross Micro-IF Test

Cross-testing of each of the low (third to fifth) egg
passage test antigens against mouse antisera was
completed using methods previously described by Philip
et al, (6). The test antigen made from the Sheila Smith
Strain was a preparation from the eleventh egg passage.
Yolk sac suspensions of other SFG rickettsiae including R.
parkeri, R. sibirica, R. conorii, and R. prowazekii and the

respective mouse antisera for each of these strains were
included for comparison.

III.   RESULTS

Five of the six North Carolina patients and four of the
five Montana patients (Table 1) had typical signs and symptoms
of RMSF and had demonstrable serologic conversion (Table 2).
Two patients had atypical disease. North Carolina patient
SIM became abruptly ill with fever, headache, and faint rash.
Oral tetracycline therapy was instituted within 2-3 hours of
the onset of her illness. Approximately 12 hours after the
onset of her illness she was completely well. R. rickettsii
was isolated from her blood but no serologic evidence of
rickettsial infection could be demonstrated 60 days after
onset of illness (Table 2).

Montana patient SWA had atypical disease notable for
the absence of rash until six hours before death on the sixth
day of illness. Rickettsiae were recovered from clotted blood
obtained on the second day and stored at refrigerator
temperatures for one week.

Patient HUD had received chloramphenicol therapy during
the 4 days prior to the drawing of the blood sample from
which the isolate was made. Patient MCD had G-6-PD deficiency.
Appropriate antibiotic therapy was not initiated until late
in the course of his illness. He developed severe vasculitis,
acral gangrene eventually requiring amputation of several
fingers and one leg, and renal failure requiring dialysis.

Cross micro-IF testing of low egg passage preparations
of rickettsiae with mouse antisera demonstrated that the
North Carolina strains were not detectably different from the
Montana strains (Table 3). Low egg passage preparations of
each of these were indistinguishable from the Sheila Smith
strain of R. rickettsii. In contrast, distinct differences
were evident in patterns of cross-reaction between isolates
from RMSF patients and four other species of rickettsiae.

IV.   DISCUSSION

We were unable to demonstrate serologic differences
among strains of R. rickettsii isolated from humans.
Rickettsiae obtained from these six North Carolina patients
were not detectably different from Montana strains of
rickettsiae used in this study, and all isolates were

indistinguishable from the Sheila Smith strain used in
serologic and vaccine studies. The similarities among human
isolates is in contrast to the wide range of antigenic
and pathogenic characteristics noted in spotted fever group
rickettsiae isolated from ticks (12-14). This suggests that
only certain spotted fever group rickettsiae in nature have
pathogenic potential for humans. Our study is by no means
definitive. The findings of a lack of serologic differences
among strains noted in this study need to be confirmed by
further investigation, particularly that which could relate
the cross micro-IF results to the specificity of cell-mediated
immunity assays, vaccination-challenge experiments, and
virulence tests in animal models.

Table 1. Age, location and timing of rickettsial culture in six patients
          from North Carolina and in five patients from Montana with Rocky
          Mountain spotted fever.

Patient	Age (yrs.)	Geographic Location	Rickettsial Isolation (day of illness sample obtained)
HUD	6	Durham, NC	11 *
SIM	4	Durham, NC	12 hrs.**
MCD	29	Broadway, NC	11
WHI	24	Durham, NC	6
GRA	2	Concord, NC	2
MOR	2	Kannapolis, NC	2
SIN	5	Hamilton, MT	4
HAN	25	Hamilton, MT	0
WAC	6	Darby, MT	2
SWA	30	Missoula, MT	2 ***
NOR	12	Missoula, MT	3

  * received chloramphenicol for four days immediately preceding
    sampling

 ** received two doses of tetracycline during the nine hours
    immediately preceding sampling

*** fatal case: isolation obtained from clotted blood obtained on the
    second day of illness and stored for one week unfrozen at refrigerator
    temperatures.

Table 2. Antibody status of six patients from North Carolina and five
          patients from Montana with Rocky Mountain spotted fever
          as determined by microimmunofluorescence (micro-IF) tests.

| Patient | Day of Illness | Date Serum Obtained | Micro-IF Antibody Titers | | |
			All Immuno-globulins	IgM	IgG
HUD	10	4-14-75	–	0	–
	11	4-15-75	32	0	–
	60	6-12-75	4096	tr.	4096
SIM	1	4-17-75	0	0	0
	60	6-18-75	0	0	0
MCD	11	6-9-75	512	64	512
	16	6-14-75	2048	128	2048
	21	6-19-75	1024	256	1024
WHI	6	4-22-75	0	0	0
	8	4-24-75	0	0	0
	23	5-9-75	4096	4096	–
GRA	2	5-17-75	0	0	0
	14	5-29-75	2048	512	32
MOR	2	5-12-75	0	0	0
	17	5-27-75	256	128	16
SIN	4	7-17-70	0	0	–
	25	8-7-70	8192	8192	–
HAN	0	6-2-73	0	0	–
	40	7-12-73	64	64	–
	137	10-17-73	8192	0	–
WAC	2	5-6-74	0	0	–
	24	5-28-74	256	256	–
	51	6-24-74	16	0	–
SWA*	6	8-6-75	tr.	tr.	0
NOR	3	8-15-75	0	0	0
	21	9-5-75	256	128	16

* fatal case: antibiotic therapy initiated a few hours before death.

Table 3. Cross microimmunofluorescence tests of mouse antisera against rickettsial isolates from Montana and North Carolina cases of Rocky Mountain spotted fever.

RICKETTSIAE	SOURCE	PATIENT	S. SMITH	SIN	HAN	WAC	SWA	NOR	WIS	MOR	WHI	HUD	GRA	MCD	R. PARKERI	R. SIBIRICA	R. CONORII	R. PROWAZEKII
ISOLATES FROM RMSF CASES	MONT.	S. SMITH	512	512	512	512	512	512	512	512	512	512	512	512	128	64	32	0
		SIN	512	512	1024	1024	1024	512	512	512	512	512	512	512	128	64	32	0
		HAN	512	512	512	512	512	512	512	512	512	256	512	256	64	64	32	0
		WAC	1024	1024	1024	1024	1024	1024	1024	1024	1024	1024	1024	1024	128	128	32	0
		SWA	1024	512	512	512	512	512	512	512	512	512	512	512	64	64	32	0
		NOR	512	512	512	512	512	512	512	512	512	512	512	512	64	32	16	0
	N.C.	SIM	2048	1024	1024	1024	1024	1024	1024	1024	1024	2048	1024	1024	128	128	32	0
		MOR	1024	512	512	1024	1024	1024	1024	1024	512	1024	1024	1024	64	64	32	0
		WHI	1024	1024	1024	1024	1024	1024	1024	512	1024	1024	1024	1024	64	64	32	0
		HUD	1024	1024	1024	1024	1024	512	512	512	1024	1024	1024	1024	64	64	32	0
		GRA	1024	1024	1024	1024	1024	1024	1024	1024	1024	1024	1024	1024	64	64	32	0
		MCD	1024	1024	1024	1024	1024	512	1024	1024	1024	1024	1024	1024	64	64	32	0
OTHER SPECIES		R. PARKERI	64	32	64	64	64	32	32	32	32	32	32	32	512	128	64	0
		R. SIBIRICA	128	128	128	128	256	128	128	128	128	256	128	128	512	2048	128	0
		R. CONORII	16	16	32	32	32	16	16	16	16	16	16	16	64	64	2048	0
		R. PROWAZEKII	0	0	0	0	0	0	0	0	0	0	0	0	0	0	0	1024

ANTIGENS*

* 5% crude yolk sac preparations containing viable rickettsiae from the fourth or fifth passge in chick embryo.

The isolation of R. rickettsii from a patient receiving
chloramphenicol has been previously reported (15).   Patient
SIM is notable since a strain of R. rickettsii virulent for
laboratory animals was isolated from her blood after two doses
of tetracycline.   Her illness was treated promptly after onset
and a subsequent antirickettsial antibody response was
completely absent 60 days after illness onset.   Early antimicrobial therapy of patients with RMSF has been known to
blunt the subsequent antirickettsial antibody titer (16-18)
but proof that early therapy can completely abolish the
subsequent antibody response can only be documented if
R. rickettsii is actually isolated from blood.   Early
antirickettsial therapy may explain why some typical cases
of RMSF are not able to be serologically confirmed.

ACKNOWLEDGMENTS

We wish to thank Linda Holzbauer for manuscript preparation.

REFERENCES

1.   Bell, E.J., Kohls, G.M., Stoenner, H.G., and Lackman,
     D.B. J. Immunol. 90, 770 (1963).
2.   Price, W.H. Science. 118, 49 (1953).
3.   Ormsbee, R., Peacock, M., Gerloff, R., Tallent, G.,
     and Wike, D. Infect. Immun. 19, 239 (1978).
4.   Burgdorfer, W., Sexton, D.J., Gerloff, R.K., Anacker,
     R.L., Philip, R.N., and Thomas, L.A. Infect.
     Immun. 12, 205 (1975).
5.   Bell, E.J., and Stoenner, H.G. J. Immunol.
     84, 171 (1960).
6.   Philip, R.N., Casper, E.A., Burgdorfer, W., Gerloff,
     R.K., Hughes, L.E., and Bell, E.J. J. Immunol. 121, 1961
     (1978).
7.   Bell, E.J., and Pickens, E.G. J. Immunol. 70,
     461 (1953).
8.   Magnarelli, L.A., Anderson, J.F., and Burgdorfer, W.
     Am. J. Epidemiol. 110, 148 (1979).
9.   Wang, S-P. In "Trachoma and related disorders caused
     by chlamydial agents" (Nichols, R.L., ed), p. 273.
     Excerpta Medica, Amsterdam, (1971).
10. Philip, R.N., Casper, E.A., Ormsbee, R.A., Peacock, M.G.,
     and Burgdorfer, W. J. Clin. Micro. 3, 51 (1976).

11. Philip, R.N., and Casper, E.A. In "Proceedings
     of the 2nd International Symposium on Rickettsiae and
     rickettsial diseases" (Kazar, J., Ormsbee, R.A., and
     Tarasevich, I.N., eds), p.307. VEDA, Bratislava,
     (1978).
12. Robertson, R.G., and Wisseman, C.L., Jr. Am. J.
     Epidemiol. 97, 55 (1973).
13. Goldwasser, R.A., Steiman, Y., Klingberg, W., Swartz,
     T.A., and Klingberg, M.A. Scand. J. Infec. Dis.
     6, 53 (1974).
14. Philip, R.N., and Casper, E.A. Am. J. Trop. Med. Hyg.
     (in press).
15. Meaderis, D.N. N. Engl. J. Med. 298, 1071 (1978).
16. Schubert, J.H. Public Health Lab. 10, 38 (1952).
17. Lackman, D.B., and Gerloff, R.K. Public Health
     Lab. 11, 97 (1953).
18. Philip, R.N., Casper, E.A., MacCormack, J.N., Sexton,
     D.J., Thomas, L.A., Anacker, R.L., Burgdorfer, W., and
     Vick, S. Am. J. Epidemiol. 105, 56 (1977).

LYMPHOCYTE TRANSFORMATION USING THREE STRAINS OF SPOTTED FEVER GROUP RICKETTSIAE[1]

Jorge L. Benach

State of New York Department of Health and
Department of Pathology
School of Medicine,
State University of New York at Stony Brook
Stony Brook, New York

Gail S. Habicht

Department of Pathology
School of Medicine
State University of New York at Stony Brook
Stony Brook, New York

I. INTRODUCTION

Rocky Mountain spotted fever (RMSF) has been endemic in Long Island, New York, for over 50 years (1-3). Increases in RMSF incidence during the early part of the last decade (4) prompted local investigations into the epizootiology of this disease. The hemolymph test (5) provided a simple method for determining the presence of rickettsiae in ticks. Since 1976, a majority of the spotted fever-group rickettsiae present in hemolymph-positive ticks from Long Island and from other RMSF endemic areas in the eastern states have been identified as Rickettsia montana (3,6) by isolation procedures (3,6,7). The specific microimmunofluorescence (micro-IF) test for rickettsial antibodies (8) allowed testing of human sera for antibodies specific for purified rickettsial species and strains.

---

[1]Supported in part by Grant No. 1746 of the New York State Health Research Council.

RICKETTSIAE AND RICKETTSIAL DISEASES

149

Monotypic antibody titers to R. rickettsii are seldom found in
human cases on Long Island; serological reactivity to R. montana is generally lower than to R. rickettsii. Agent 369-C,
although never isolated from Long Island ticks, can be identified morphologically from tick hemolymph preparations. The
serological reactivity of RMSF cases to this agent has frequently been equal and sometimes greater than to R. rickettsii
by micro-IF (9). Previous studies have shown considerable
heterogeneity among the spotted fever-group rickettsiae by a
variety of methods (10-12).

Because of discrepancies between our epidemiological and
serological data we chose to use the lymphoproliferative assay
to determine whether the cellular immune response to three
strains of the spotted fever group was more discriminatory than
available serologic techniques. The lymphocyte transformation
(LT) assay has been used to determine stimulation of lymphocytes by various species of rickettsiae since 1971 (13-17).
In all these studies, the LT assays have shown sensitivity as
well as long-term antigen recognition.

II. MATERIALS AND METHODS

Volunteers: nine volunteers were selected as lymphocyte
donors for this project. Table 1 presents histories of the
volunteers. Three separate LT assays were done and numbered
1-3. Sex and age matched controls were secured for assays 2
and 3.

Lymphocyte transformation assay: blood for the assays was
collected in sterile heparinized vacuum tubes and diluted 1:2
with RPMI-1640 medium supplemented with L-glutamine and antibiotics (culture medium). Mononuclear cells were harvested by
density gradient centrifugation (Ficoll), washed twice and resuspended in culture medium. The assays were performed in
flat-bottomed microculture plates. Each well received 1×10^5
cells in culture medium containing heat inactivated human serum
from an AB positive donor so that the final well concentration
was 10%. Plates were incubated at 37°C in 5% CO_2 until harvest. Cultures were pulsed with 10 μl containing 1 μCi of 3H-thymidine 20 to 24 hrs prior to harvest. LT assay 1 was harvested at 72, 96 and 120 hours and LT assays 2 and 3 were harvested at 72 and 96 hrs with a multiple sample automatic harvester. Samples were counted in a liquid scintillation counter. LT results are expressed as mean disintegrations per min
(DPM) ± standard error of the mean of quintuplicate cultures.
Stimulation indices (SI) were calculated as mean DPMs/mean
DPMs of unstimulated control culture containing serum alone.
Statistical analyses were done by Student's test.

TABLE 1. Histories of Lymphocyte Donors

	Age	Sex	Remarks
LT Assay No. 1			
Case 1A	52	F	RMSF in previous year
Case 1B	48	F	RMSF in previous year
Control 1V	34	M	Lederle RMSF vaccine series in 1976 and booster in 1977
Control 1A	38	F	No known exposure to rickettsiae; tick bites in California.
LT Assay No. 2			
Case 2	32	M	RMSF with onset 12 days before blood collection
Control 2A	32	M	No known exposure to rickettsiae or ticks
LT Assay No. 3			
Case 3	23	M	RMSF with onset 18 days before blood collection
Control 3A	23	M	No known exposure to rickettsiae or ticks
Control 3B	23	M	No known illness due to rickettsiae; this volunteer performed hemolymph test on ticks during 1979 and 1980.

Mitogens and antigens: two mitogens, Concanavalin A (Con A), and Pokeweed (PWM) were used in LT assay 1. Phytohemagglutinin P (PHA) and Escherichia coli lipopolysaccharide 0111-B4 (LPS) were added to LT assays 2 and 3. All mitogens were used at a final concentration of 0.01 mg/ml. The antigens used were 1) high salt method purified (18) R. rickettsii, R strain, SF200; 2) renografin density gradient purified (19) R. montana, M/5-6 strain; and 3) renografin density gradient purified 369-C, Dermacentor variabilis agent, Sheephead 130 strain. All rickettsial strains were grown in Vero cells, inactivated with 0.5% formalin, kept at 4°C, washed prior to culture, and used at final concentrations of 1 μg/ml and 10 μg/ml per culture well. Concentrations of stock solutions of rickettsial antigens were determined by dry weight analysis.

Lymphocyte subpopulations, serology, and additional tests: T lymphocyte ratios were determined by sheep red blood cell rosetting (25); B lymphocytes were enumerated by polyvalent anti-Ig and anti-IgD immunofluorescence microscopy (20).

Serology on all donors was by the micro-IF test (21) using
rickettsial antigens of the same origin as those used for the
LT assays. Complete blood counts (CBC) and serum chemistries
were done on all specimens.

III. RESULTS

All controls were well at the time of the LT assays. Complete blood counts including differentials for all volunteers
were within normal limits. Serum chemistries for all volunteers were also within normal limits except for Case 3 who had
elevated levels of lactic dehydrogenase, and serum glutamic-
oxalic transaminase. Ratios of lymphocyte subpopulations for
all volunteers were within the normal limits for our laboratory
(T-lymphocytes: 65-85% by sheep red blood cell rosetting; B-
lymphocytes: 6-13% by polyvalent Ig and 3-8% for IgD).
All controls including the vaccinated control were non-
reactive at 1:16 by micro-IF to rickettsial antigens. Differential serologies one year apart are provided for Cases 1A and
1B (Table 2). Responses to nonspecific mitogens were greatest
at 120 hrs in LT assay 1 (Con A, PWM), and at 96 hrs in LT
assays 2 and 3 (PHA, Con A, PWM). LPS failed to induce blast
transformation in any case in which it was tested (LT assays 2
and 3).
The proliferative responses of rickettsial antigens at
1 µg/ml at 96 hrs are shown in Table 3. Cases 1A and 1B showed
peak responses to R. rickettsii in the culture harvested at 96
hrs with lower responses to R. montana and to 369-C. Case 2
responded strongly to R. rickettsii antigen at both 72 and 96
hrs; significant stimulation was also obtained using 369-C and
R. montana. Case 3, who experienced a severe illness, exhibited a large proliferative response to R. rickettsii at 96 hrs
but not at 72 hrs; weaker but significant proliferation occurred with the other two strains at 96 hrs. The vaccinated
Control IV mounted significant responses to R. rickettsii of
decreasing magnitude from 72 to 120 hrs. Control 1A was stimulated by R. rickettsii at 96 and 120 hrs. Control 3B showed
significant stimulation at 96 hrs to all three antigens in this
order: 369-C, R. montana, R. rickettsii. This individual,
although never clinically ill, spent the springs and summers of
1979 and 1980 performing hemolymph tests on Long Island ticks.
Overall, responses to 10 µg/ml rickettsial antigens were lower
but paralleled those obtained with 1 µg/ml for both cases and
controls.

TABLE 2. Antibody Titers to Three Strains of Spotted Fever-Group Rickettsiae.

	Ig			IgM			IgG		
	R.r	R.m	369-C	R.r	R.m	369-C	R.r	R.m	369-C
Case 1A 1979[a]	1:2048	1:1024	1:1024	1:2048	1:512	1:512	1:128	1:64	1:512
1980[b]	1:256	1:64	1:128	1:32	tr	tr	1:128	1:64	1:128
Case 1B 1979[a]	1:32768	1:2048	1:8192	1:8192	1:128	1:4096	1:8192	1:2048	1:8192
1980[b]	1:2048	1:512	1:2048	1:512	tr	1:512	1:2048	1:512	1:2048
Case 2 1980[b]	1:64	1:32	1:64	1:16	nr	nr	1:64	1:32	1:32
Case 3 1980[b]	1:32768	1:8192	1:16384	1:2048	1:512	1:1024	1:8192	1:2048	1:8192

[a] Antibody titers from serum taken during convalescent period in 1979. [b] Antibody titers from serum taken on the same day of the LT assays. R.r; Rickettsia rickettsii, R.m; Rickettsia montana,. tr; trace, nr; non-reactive.

TABLE 3. Mean DPMs ± Standard Error of the Mean and Stimulation Indices of Lymphocyte Responses to Three Strains of Spotted Fever-Group Rickettsiae, 1 μg/ml

	R. rickettsii			R. montana			Agent 369-Z		
	72	96	120	72	96	120	72	96	120
Case 1A	3660±194 (2.23)[a]	16540±1908 (6.27)[a]	14620±1786 (5.25)[a]	2960±144 (1.80)	12360±1533 (5.28)[a]	5420±327 (2.33)[a]	3450±289 (2.10)	8060±1124 (3.44)[a]	4980±609 (2.14)[a]
Case 1B	2700±219 (7.50)[a]	5360±693 (12.76)	3000±403 (3.94)[a]	1800±194 (5.00)[a]	4320±383 (10.29)	2060±325 (2.71)[a]	1460±144 (4.05)[a]	1650±118 (3.93)[a]	1680±378 (2.21)[a]
Cont. 1V	11280±5646 (9.25)[a]	14240±1106 (5.98)[a]	14920±3410 (5.45)[a]	920±70 (0.75)	2160±293 (0.90)	2640±559 (0.96)	920±100 (0.75)	2200±134 (0.92)	2160±279 (0.78)
Cont. 1A	1760±238 (1.66)	6250±1513 (6.79)[a]	7480±946 (12.35)[a]	1800±336 (1.69)	1400±148 (1.52)	1780±339 (3.17)	640±31 (0.60)	1400±170 (1.52)	840±70 (1.39)
Case 2	46140±7010 (15.27)[a]	62940±6415 (19.19)[a]	nd	4260±94 (1.41)	6640±384 (2.10)[a]	nd	7440±589 (2.46)[a]	11660±1024 (3.68)[a]	nd
Cont. 2	6300±572 (1.73)	9480±510 (2.70)[a]	nd	3300±171 (0.90)	4150±420 (1.18)	nd	3380±196 (0.92)	4325±496 (1.23)	nd
Case 3	1040±126 (1.86)	27060±1450 (72.16)[a]	nd	1180±77 (2.11)	2700±322 (7.20)[a]	nd	350 (0.62)	2380±100 (6.35)[a]	nd
Cont. 3A	1040±167 (0.96)	700±130 (0.47)	nd	920±202 (0.85)	440±141 (0.29)	nd	900±83 (0.83)	640±161 (0.43)	nd
Cont. 3B	460±44 (1.21)	860±161 (2.69)[a]	nd	400±54 (1.05)	1080±306 (3.38)[a]	nd	560±141 (1.47)	1720±260 (5.38)[a]	nd

[a] Significant stimulation, (p<0.05); nd, not done.

IV. DISCUSSION

Cellular immune responses are essential to the host defense against rickettsial diseases. In this study, both antigen specific cellular responses and general adequacy of the cellular immune response were evaluated in RMSF cases and controls. All volunteers had lymphocyte subpopulation ratios within our normal laboratory limits, and all mounted strongly significant proliferative responses to the mitogens.

We have shown that lymphoproliferative responses can be produced in vitro with very low concentrations of specific rickettsial antigens as shown by greater stimulation produced by 1 µg/ml than did 10 µg/ml. In other studies involving LT assays to R. rickettsii antigens, the concentrations found optimal were slightly higher (13) and much higher (17). One study using R. typhi showed stimulation at a range of concentrations (1-400 µg/ml) but optimal at 10 µg/ml (14). Coxiella burnetii antigens were stimulatory in a range of 200-400 µg/ml (16). R. rickettsii produced the greatest proliferative responses in all the cases reported here. Responses were strongest in Cases 2 and 3 which had RMSF (Cases 1A and 1B); the responses to R. rickettsii had declined to a greater extent than those to R. montana and 369-C so that after one year the LT assay revealed a greater cross reactivity among these antigens. Peak cellular immune responses in a patient with clinical Q fever occurred 10 days after onset with high stimulation indices persisting over a long period of time (16).

Lymphoproliferative responses to rickettsial antigens in controls were lower than in cases. However, Control 1A showed a strong response to R. rickettsii increasing in magnitude from 72 to 120 hrs. Since the response to R. rickettsii in this control did not peak at 96 hrs as in the others in the same assay, it could represent nonspecific stimulation; however, previous subclinical exposure cannot be ruled out for this or any of the other controls. It is possible that some of these responses may be due to nonspecific factors. However, yolk sac derived (15) and duck embryo grown rickettsiae (17) have been previously used for LT assays without apparent stimulation due to possible contaminants. The use of renografin purified whole cell preparations of R. montana and 369-C, and high salt purified R. rickettsii should have reduced the amount of contaminants (14). It is unlikely that the lymphoproliferative responses to rickettsial preparations were due to a nonspecific mitogenic effect. A nonspecific mitogen would be expected to stimulate Control as well as Case lymphocytes. Nonspecific stimulation by a rickettsial lipopolysaccharide is also unlikely since we failed to obtain a response to E. coli LPS in LT assays 2 and 3 at concentrations of 0.01 mg/ml. This is in agreement with studies which have shown that LPS is non-mitogenic for human peripheral blood lymphocytes (22,23). Yet, a more recent study has shown that bacterial LPS can produce a response on or after 7 days of culture and that the response occurs over a broad range of LPS concentrations including 1 μg/ml (21). Crossreactivity between rickettsial antibodies and Proteus OX-19 bacterial LPS is believed to be the basis for the Weil-Felix reaction which can detect both typhus and spotted fever-group antibodies (24). Since LPS of rickettsiae of the typhus group has been isolated and its biological activity assessed (25), we may assume that a similar LPS component exists in the rickettsiae of the spotted fever group. Yet, since a human lymphocyte response to LPS is produced on or after 7 days of culture (21), the lymphoproliferation produced by low concentrations of antigen as in our RMSF cases obtained after 96 hrs of culture can be considered more antigen specific.

Our studies show that both lymphoproliferative and antibody forming responses in RMSF cases were directed preferentially against antigens found on R. rickettsii and thus this organism can be considered to have been the infecting agent. Decreased proliferation upon stimulation with R. montana parallels the serological results. We feel that the criteria for separating R. rickettsii from R montana used in previous studies are justified (10-12). That the antibody responses to 369-C were high while the lymphoproliferative responses were low probably reflects the fact that the B and T lymphocytes were responding to different antigenic determinants on these complex organisms. 369-C has not been studied in great detail and the antigenic determinants shared with other rickettsiae have not been identified.

V. SUMMARY

Four RMSF cases (two current and two from the previous year) and five well controls (one vaccinated to RMSF 4 years earlier) donated blood for lymphocyte transformation assays in which three strains of spotted fever-group rickettsiae (R. rickettsii, R. montana, and 369-C) were used. Normal proliferative responses to mitogens (PHA, Con A, and PWM) were obtained for all donors; no stimulation due to E. coli was obtained in the five volunteers tested. T and B lymphocyte ratios as well as complete blood counts were within normal limits for all donors. The greatest lymphoproliferative response to rickettsial antigens was obtained by stimulation with R. rickettsii (1 μg/ml). All of the RMSF cases were stimulated to a lesser degree by R. montana, and least by 369-C. Responses to rickettsial antigens at 10 μg/ml paralleled the results

obtained at 1 μg/ml but were quantitatively lower. Slight responses to the antigens were obtained in the controls.

ACKNOWLEDGMENTS

We gratefully acknowledge Dr. Robert Philip for providing
the antigens and performing the serology. We wish to thank
Mr. David Dubocq, Mr. Jim Coleman, Mr. Anthony Viscardi and
Mr. Edward Irwin for their technical help. Finally, we wish
to thank all of the volunteers for donating the large amounts
of blood needed for this work.

REFERENCES

1. Miller, J. K., Ann. Int. Med. 33, 1398 (1950).
2. Vianna, N. J., and Hinman, A. R., Am. J. Med. 51, 725
    (1971).
3. Benach, J. L., White, D. J., Burgdorfer, W., Keelan, T. R.,
    Guirgis, S., and Altieri, R. H., Am. J. Epidemiol. 106,
    380 (1977).
4. Hattwick, M.A.W., O'Brien, R. J., and Hanson, B. F., Ann.
    Intern. Med. 84, 732 (1976).
5. Burgdorfer, W., Am. J. Trop. Med. Hyg. 19, 1010 (1970).
6. Bell, E. J., Kohls, G. M., Stoenner, H. G., and Lackman,
    D. B., J. Immunol. 90, 770 (1963).
7. Linnemann, C. C., Jr., Schaeffer, A. E., Burgdorfer, W.,
    Hutchinson, L., and Philip, R. N., Am. J. Epidemiol. 111,
    31 (1980).
8. Philip, R. N., Casper, E. A., Ormsbee, R. A., Peacock,
    M. G., and Burgdorfer, W., J. Clin. Microbiol. 3, 51
    (1976).
9. Benach, J. L., unpublished information, 1978.
10. Philip, R. N., Casper, E. A., Burgdorfer, W., Gerloff,
    R. K., Hughes, L. E., and Bell, E. J., J. Immunol. 121,
    1961 (1978).
11. Anacker, R. L., McCaul, T. F., Burgdorfer, W., and
    Gerloff, R. K., Infect. Immun. 27, 468 (1980).
12. Lackman, D. B., Bell, E. J., Stoenner, H. G., and Pickens,
    E. G., Health Lab. Sci. 2, 135 (1965).
13. Ascher, M. S., Oster, C. N., Harber, P. I., Kenyon, R. H.,
    and Pedersen, C. E., J. Infect. Dis. 138, 217 (1978).
14. Bourgeois, A. L., Dasch, G. A., and Strong, D. M., Infect.
    Immun. 27, 483 (1980).
15. Coonrod, J. D., and Shepard, C. C., J. Immunol. 106, 209
    (1971).

16. Jerrels, T. R., Mallavia, L. P., and Hinrichs, D. J.,
     Infect. Immun. 11, 280 (1975).
17. Oster, C. N., Burke, D. S., Kenyon, R. H., Ascher, M. S.,
     Harber, P., and Pedersen, C. E., N. Engl. J. Med. 297,
     859 (1977).
18. Ormsbee, R. A., J. Immunol. 88, 100 (1962).
19. Weiss, E., Coolbaugh, J. C., and Williams, J. C., Appl.
     Microbiol. 30, 456 (1975).
20. Winchester, R. J., and Ross, G., in "Manual of Clinical
     Immunology" (N. R. Rose and H. Friedman, eds.), p. 64.
     American Society for Microbiology, Washington, D.C. (1976).
21. Miller, R. A., Gartner, S., and Kaplan, H. S., J. Immunol.
     121, 2160 (1978).
22. Peavy, D. L., Adler, W. H., and Smith, R. T., J. Immunol.
     105, 1453 (1970).
23. Ringden, O., Scand. J. Immunol. 5, 891 (1976).
24. Bendich, A., and Chargaff, E., J. Biol. Chem. 166, 283
     (1946).
25. Schramek, S., Brezina, R., and Kazar, J., Acta Virol. 21,
     439 (1977).

ROCKY MOUNTAIN SPOTTED FEVER: FIRST-YEAR
EVALUATION OF A LATEX AGGLUTINATION TEST
FOR ANTIBODIES TO <u>RICKETTSIA</u> <u>RICKETTSII</u>

Karim E. Hechemy[1]
Sandra J. Sasowski
Edith E. Michaelson
Michael Zdeb

New York State Department of Health
Albany, New York

Robert L. Anacker
Robert N. Philip

Epidemiology Branch
Rocky Mountain Laboratories
Hamilton, Montana

Karl T. Kleeman

N.C. State Laboratory of Public Health
Raleigh, North Carolina

Carolyn Crump

Department of General Services
Division of Consolidated Laboratory Services
Commonwealth of Virginia
Richmond, Virginia

───────────────────────

[1]Supported by New York State Health Research Council
awards No. 9-032 and No. 1507.

159

Jerry Kudlac

Oklahoma State Department of Health
Oklahoma City, Oklahoma

J. Mehsen Joseph
Jagdish Patel

Department of Health and Mental Hygiene
State of Maryland
Baltimore, Maryland

Harold Dowda, Jr.

South Carolina Department of Health
and Environmental Control
Columbia, South Carolina

George Killgore
Diane Young

Kentucky Bureau for Health Services
Commonwealth of Kentucky
Frankfort, Kentucky

J. Howard Barrick
Jerry R. Hindman

Department of Public Health
State of Tennessee
Nashville, Tennessee

L. Bruce Elliott

Texas Department of Health
Austin, Texas

Richard H. Altieri

Nassau County Department of Health
Hempstead, New York

I. INTRODUCTION

This is a preliminary report on the first year of a two-year collaborative evaluation of a new latex test for detection of antibodies to Rickettsia rickettsii. The test, developed in the New York State (Albany) laboratory (1), was designed to be specific, sensitive, simple, easy to perform, and capable of reducing workload by 80%.

The evaluation was done in the Albany laboratory in collaboration with the nine other health departments.

II. METHODS

A. Sera and Tests

Specimens submitted to each collaborating laboratory for Rocky Mountain spotted fever (RMSF) testing during the 1979 RMSF season were included in this study.

Each laboratory tested the specimens submitted to it by its current technique. All except two laboratories used the complement fixation (CF) test; the Albany and Texas laboratories used the microimmunofluorescence (micro-IF) test (2). The laboratories then forwarded a portion of each specimen to the Albany laboratory for testing by latex-R. rickettsii and micro-IF. These results were sent to the collaborating laboratory, which added its own test results and clinical information if available. The complete results were then sent to Albany for compilation and statistical analysis.

A total of 3,868 sera from 2,656 patients were tested by latex-R. rickettsii and micro-IF. Of these, CF results were available for 2,655 sera from 1,732 patients.

B. Test Procedures

In this evaluation, sera to be tested by latex-R. rickettsii were diluted at 1:16 and inactivated at 56 C for 30 min; the test was then performed as previously described (1). Micro-IF and CF were also performed as described (2-3).

During the course of this evaluation we developed an improved method of preparing the latex-R. rickettsii reagent. This method (patent application pending) superseded the procedure described earlier (1).

To determine stability, five reactive sera were
initially titrated with five batches of latex-R. rickettsii
reagent at the time of reagent preparation and then retested
after 5 to 17 months for a total of 50 trials.

C.   Threshold Values of Reactivity

The threshold values of reactivity for all three tests
have previously been determined (1-3). One titer below
threshold value was considered to be weakly reactive. However, for the purposes of this report, all titers below
diagnostic level have been grouped together as nonreactive.

III.   RESULTS

A.   Sensitivity

The latex-R. rickettsii test was in agreement for 382 of
407 patients whose sera had diagnostic titers by micro-IF
using a polyvalent conjugate (micro-IF/Ig) (Table 1). This
indicates a sensitivity of 93.86%.

Of these 382 patients sera from 314 had IgG and IgM response to R. rickettsii; 32 had IgG only; and 29 had IgM
only. This was determined using micro-IF/IgM and -IgG conjugates (1). For 7 patients whose sera were insufficient for
further study, only micro-IF/Ig results were determined.

TABLE 1.   Comparison of Latex-R. rickettsii with
           Micro-IF Results

| Latex-R. rickettsii results | Micro-IF results | | No. of patients |
	Reactive	Nonreactive	
Reactive	382	24	406
Nonreactive	25	2225	2250
No. of patients	407	2249	2656

The sera from 25 patients who did not have latex-R. rickettsii diagnostic titers were divided into six categories (Table 2). Of the 25 patients 11 were clinically diagnosed as recent RMSF cases. Of these 11, 4 had both an IgM and IgG response to RMSF; 6 had IgG response only; and 1 could not be determined because the serum was insufficient. One of the 6 patients with IgG response, on serotyping, had a micro-IF titer against Rickettsia rhipicephali of 16,384 and against R. rickettsii of 1,024.

Five patients had had a clinically diagnosed RMSF infection with onset more than 1 year earlier. These sera did not show IgM to R. rickettsii.

Four patients were laboratory-confirmed typhus cases. The micro-IF titers against Rickettsia typhi antigen were fourfold higher than those for R. rickettsii. These results were substantiated by latex-R. typhi tests (4).

Three patients had nonrickettsial infections: two cases of Q fever and one of tularemia. Of the two remaining patients, one was a clinically unconfirmed case of RMSF (micro-IF/Ig titer, 128; micro-IF/IgM, 8). For the other no clinical information was available (micro-IF/Ig, 128; micro-IF/IgM, 8).

B. Accuracy

The accuracy of the new test was determined as described (4) with reactive single sera or second specimens of pairs or with first specimens of pairs if there was a decrease in titer. Of the 382 sera 83 were ties. Of the 299 nonties 163 had a higher ratio by the latex test and 136 by micro-IF.

TABLE 2. Latex False Negatives (Relative to Micro-IF)

Clinically diagnosed RMSF	
Recent infection	11
Onset $\geq$ 1 year	5
Typhus infection	4
Infection other than rickettsial	3
Clinically unconfirmed to RMSF	1
Clinical information not available	1
Total	25

These nontie values did not fall in the critical region
(<133,>166).   Thus the accuracy of latex-R. rickettsii was
not statistically different from that of micro-IF.

C.   Time Course of Reactivity

The frequency of early detectable reaction for latex-R.
rickettsii was determined (1) and was similar to that for
micro-IF.   Of 266 first specimens 218 were ties.   For the 48
nonties latex-R. rickettsii showed a reaction earlier in 17
and micro-IF in 31 cases.   Since these nontie values did not
fall in the critical region (<17,>31), the frequency of early
detection for latex-R. rickettsii was not statistically different from that of micro-IF.

D. Specificity

The latex-R. rickettsii test was in agreement for 2,225
patients of the 2,249 whose sera had nondiagnostic titers by
micro-IF.   This indicates a specificity of 98.93%.   Eighty-
one patients whose sera were nonreactive by both tests were
diagnosed as having other pathologic conditions (Table 3).
The 24 remaining patients with sera reactive by latex-R.
rickettsii only were divided into three categories.   One
patient was diagnosed by the attending physician as having
moderately severe RMSF, which responded to tetracycline
therapy; 7 were diagnosed as typhus cases; for the remaining
16 no clinical information was available.

TABLE 3.   Diagnoses for 81 Patients with Sera
           Nonreactive by Latex-R. rickettsii
           and Micro-IF

Leptospirosis	1	Influenza	1
Typhus	4	Herpes	15
Q fever	2	Coccidiomycosis	1
Chlamydia	2	Mycoplasma	11
Measles	19	Cytomegalovirus	9
Rubella	7	Adenovirus	4
Varicella	1	Viral encephalitis	2
Mumps	1	Respiratory syncytial virus	1

For the 7 typhus patients micro-IF titers against R. typhi were fourfold higher than those against R. rickettsii. These results were substantiated by latex-R. typhi tests.

Of the 16 patients with clinical information unavailable 7 had single specimens with latex-R. rickettsii titers of 64. Of the 9 patients with paired sera 5 had a $\geq$ 4-fold rise in titer from 8 to $\geq$ 64; 2 had a twofold drop in titer from 32 to 8; and 2 had standing titers of 64. All specimens had IgM titers of 8, except 2 for which results were equivocal.

E. Complement Fixation Test

Sera from 1,353 of 1,732 patients had nondiagnostic titers by latex-R. rickettsii, micro-IF, and CF. The remaining 379 patients had diagnostic titers by one or more tests, 211 by all three (Table 4).

Sera from 105 patients had diagnostic titers by latex-R. rickettsii and micro-IF only. Clinical information available for 53 patients indicates 17 confirmed, 2 probable, and 34 possible cases (for criteria see ref. 1). There was a fourfold change in micro-IF titer for 44 of these cases; the remaining 62 had either a twofold change or none.

Three patients had diagnostic titers by latex-R. rickettsii only. One of these was diagnosed as having typhus. The other two were false positives; the first specimens of these pairs were either anticomplementary or not done, and the second specimens had CF titers of 8.

Eleven patients had diagnostic titers by micro-IF and CF only. Six of these patients had clinically diagnosed recent RMSF infections; four of these had had RMSF onset within 1 year; and one was clinically unconfirmed (CF titer, 8; micro-IF/Ig, 128; micro-IF/IgM, 8).

Sera from 10 patients with clinically unconfirmed cases had diagnostic titers by latex-R. rickettsii only. They are part of the 29 micro-IF/Ig-nonreactive sera (Section III. A).

Five patients had sera with diagnostic titers by micro-IF alone; four of these had recent infections, and one had had RMSF onset within 1 year.

Thirty-four patients had diagnostic titers by CF alone: 28 had minimal titers of 8; 4 had titers of 16; and 2 had titers of 32 and 128 respectively (onset within 1 year).

TABLE 4. Number of Patients Serologically Reactive for RMSF by One or More Tests

Serologically reactive by test(s)*

Collaborating laboratory code no.	Latex Micro-IF CF	Latex Micro-IF		Latex CF	Micro-IF CF	Latex		Micro-IF		CF
		a	b			a	b	a	b	
001	83	61	12	0	5	6	1	4	2	4
002	36	10	14	1	3	3	1	0		10
003	42	7	2	1	2	0		1		15
004	6	8	10	0	0	0		0	2	3
005	25	6		0	0	0		0		0
006	10	7		1	0	0		0		0
007	6	5	3	0	1	1		0		2
008	3	1		0	0	0		0		0
009	0	0	14	0	0	0	3	0		0
010	0	0	11	0	0	0	6	0	5	0
No. of patients	211	105	66	3	11	10	11	5	9	34

* a = CF negative. b = CF not available or anticomplementary.

F. Predictive Value

The predictive value of the latex-R. rickettsii test, relative to micro-IF was 94.10% for a positive result and 98.93% for a negative result. The overall efficiency of the test was 98.16%. The correlation statistic kappa (1) was used to demonstrate agreement between micro-IF and latex-R. rickettsii: K = 0.929 (p <0.0001).

G. Stability

In 42 of 50 trials the variation in titers of the latex-R. rickettsii reagent batches agreed within a twofold dilution. The remaining 8 trials agreed within a fourfold dilution, of which 7 showed an increase in titer. These results indicate that the latex-R. rickettsii reagent has not lost appreciable reactivity over a 17-month period to date.

IV. DISCUSSION

In this evaluation we used all sera submitted for RMSF testing, regardless of reactivity. The values obtained using such specimens are a more valid indicator of the diagnostic potential of a new test than values obtained using a group of samples with preselected ratios of reactivity, as is customarily used during the development of a test.

The latex-R. rickettsii test appears to be sensitive for detection of active infection but does not appear to detect old RMSF infections. Therefore the test is inappropriate for epidemiologic studies. In active infections the latex-R. rickettsii reagent particles appear to aggregate specifically with anti-R. rickettsii IgG and IgM or with either one alone.

In early infection, when micro-IF/IgM titers are high, latex-R. rickettsii titers are also elevated. However, in late convalescence, when the IgM titer drops, latex titers were below the threshold values of reactivity.

Sera from 32 patients who had micro-IF/IgG response only had high titers by latex-R. rickettsii. Thus the test reactivity is not linked solely to the presence of anti-R. rickettsii IgM. It would be of interest (i) to study the composition of anti-R. rickettsii IgG subclasses in active and old RMSF infections to determine their effect on latex reactivity and (ii) to determine the relative accuracy (titer/threshold value) of the latex test with sera containing various ratios of anti-R. rickettsii IgG and -IgM or either one alone.

Of the 11 clinically diagnosed patients with recent infections not detected by latex-R. rickettsii, approximately half did not have a micro-IF/IgM response. Ormsbee et al. (5) have proposed that the failure of the micro-agglutination system with certain sera may be due to the presence of incomplete antibody. In addition serum factors may inhibit the specific aggregation of the particles; these factors may be characteristic of these sera or may be present in larger amounts than normal. In sera with anti-R. rickettsii IgG response only, the IgG subclass composition may be such that the aggregation of specific particles does not occur.

The latex-R. rickettsii test appears to have high specificity. Among the sera submitted were 81 from patients with pathologic conditions other than RMSF. Latex-R. rickettsii and micro-IF were nonreactive with these specimens.

As regards cross-reactivity with other rickettsiae, both tests using R. rickettsii antigen seem to vary in their reactivity with sera from typhus patients.

Best results with the latex test were obtained when the sera were clear, contained no particles, and were not lipemic. Heating the dilute sera (1:16) at 56 C for 30 min greatly decreased the number of latex false-reactive sera.

Sixteen specimens from patients with clinically unconfirmed cases had latex-R. rickettsii titers of 64. At this minimum threshold value the probability of these patients having RMSF is 50% (1). However, the specimens may have contained factors, e.g. lipid, which might cause nonspecific aggregation of particles (6).

Since CF has been considered the test of choice for laboratory confirmation of RMSF and is used by most collaborating laboratories, we compared the CF results to those of latex-R. rickettsii and micro-IF. The comparison confirmed previous findings (5,7,8) that CF is relatively insensitive. Latex-R. rickettsii and micro-IF tests detected antibodies sooner than CF, as shown previously (1).

V.   CONCLUSION

The results of this first year evaluation concur with the findings obtained during the development of the test. A total of 2,656 specimens were tested by latex-R. rickettsii and micro-IF. The latex test had an overall efficiency of 98.16% relative to the reference micro-IF.

REFERENCES

1. Hechemy, K. E., Anacker, R. L., Philip, R. N., Kleeman,
    K. T., MacCormack, J. N., Sasowski, S. J., and Michaelson,
    E. E., J. Clin. Microbiol. 12, 144 (1980).
2. Philip, R. N., Casper, E. A., Ormsbee, R. A., Peacock,
    M. G., and Burgdorfer, W., J. Clin. Microbiol. 3, 51
    (1976).
3. US Dept. Health, Education and Welfare, PHS, Diagnostic
    Complement Fixation Method (LBCF), CDC Laboratory Train-
    ing Manual, Atlanta, GA (1962).
4. Hechemy, K. E., Osterman, J. V., Eisemann, C. S., Elliott,
    L. B., and Sasowski, S. J., J. Clin. Microbiol. 13, in
    press (1981).
5. Ormsbee, R., Peacock, M., Philip, R., Casper, E., Plorde,
    J., Gabre-Kidan, T., and Wright, L., Amer. J. Epid. 105,
    261 (1977).
6. Hechemy, K. E., Stevens, R. W., and Gaafar, H. A., Appl.
    Microbiol. 28, 306 (1974).
7. Hechemy, K. E., N. Eng. J. Med. 300, 859 (1979).
8. Philip, R. N., Casper, E. A., MacCormack, J. N., Sexton,
    D. J., Thomas, L. A., Anacker, R. L., Burgdorfer, W.,
    and Vick, S., Amer. J. Epid. 105, 56 (1977).

EARLY DETECTION OF ANTIBODY TO RICKETTSIA
RICKETTSII: A COMPARISON OF FOUR SEROLOGICAL
METHODS: INDIRECT HEMAGGLUTINATION, INDIRECT
FLUORESCENT ANTIBODY, LATEX AGGLUTINATION,
AND COMPLEMENT FIXATION

K. T. Kleeman
J. L. Hicks

N.C. State Laboratory of Public Health
Raleigh, North Carolina

R. L. Anacker
R. N. Philip
E. A. Casper

Epidemiology Branch
Rocky Mountain Laboratories
Hamilton, Montana

K. E. Hechemy

Division of Laboratory and Research
N.Y. State Department of Health
Albany, New York

C. M. Wilfert

Duke University Medical School
Durham, North Carolina

J. N. MacCormack
N.C. Division of Health Services
Raleigh, North Carolina

I. INTRODUCTION

Rocky Mountain Spotted Fever (RMSF) is a severe, potentially fatal disease caused by infection with Rickettsia
rickettsii. Laboratory confirmation of R. rickettsii
infection may be accomplished by the demonstration of a
specific antibody response in the patient. Several methods
are currently being used to detect antibodies to R. rickettsii. These include the indirect hemagglutination test (IHA),
the indirect fluorescent antibody test (IFA), the latex-R.
rickettsii test (LA), and the complement fixation test (CF).
The purpose of this study was to analyze data derived from
the testing of sera from serologically confirmed cases of
RMSF to determine which procedure would permit the earliest
detection of an antibody titer rise to R. rickettsii.

II. METHODS

A. Sera

Routinely submitted paired sera from North Carolina with
four-fold or greater antibody titer rises to R. rickettsii
by one or more of the four methods used in the study were
selected for data analysis. Sera were stored frozen (-20°C)
until tested or shipped to Montana and/or New York for testing. Sera were shipped at ambient temperature with 0.1%
sodium azide added as a preservative.

TABLE 1. Number of Paired Sera with Four-fold or Greater
Titer Rises by Test Procedure

No. Tested/ Result	Number of sera giving result by test			
	IHA	IFA	LA	CF
Number of paired sera tested	91	60	91	63
≥ Four-fold titer rise	89 (97.8%)	57 (95.0%)	83 (91.2%)	24 (38.1%)
Stationary titer	2 (2.2%)	3 (5.0%)	5 (5.5%)	4 (6.3%)
Negative	0	0	3 (3.3%)	35 (55.5%)

B.   Indirect Hemagglutination Test

The IHA test was performed as previously described (1)
using fresh erythrocytes coated with erythrocyte-sensitizing
substance (ESS). The North Carolina State Laboratory of
Public Health used sheep erythrocytes and the NIAID Rocky
Mountain Laboratories used human type O erythrocytes. The
ESS was prepared at the Rocky Mountain Laboratory in Hamilton,
Montana by sodium hydroxide digestion of purified R. rickettsii, strain R (1). All sera were preabsorbed with normal
sheep erythrocytes when sheep erythrocytes were used in the
test system.

C.   Indirect Fluorescent Antibody Test

The IFA test was performed using the previously described
microimmunofluorescence procedure (Micro-IF-Ig) and reagents
(2).

D.   Latex R. rickettsii Test

The LA test was performed using latex particles coated
with ESS (1) as recently described (3).

E.   Complement Fixation Test

The CF test was performed using the Laboratory Branch
Complement Fixation (LBCF) method (4). Spotted fever group
yolk sac antigen prepared from R. rickettsii, Sheila Smith
strain, obtained from the Center for Disease Control, was
used in the CF test.

III.   RESULTS

Paired sera were tested for each patient included in this
study. All ninety-three paired sera selected for analysis
showed a four-fold or greater titer rise by one or more of
the serologic methods used in the study. The North Carolina
State Laboratory of Public Health performed the IHA test (81
pairs), the LA test (40 pairs), and the CF test (63 pairs).
The NIAID Rocky Mountain Laboratories performed the IHA test
(10 pairs) and the IFA test (19 pairs). The New York State
Department of Health performed the LA test (51 pairs) and the
IFA test (41 pairs). Table 1 shows the number of paired sera
with four-fold or greater titer rises by each test procedure.

TABLE 2.   Percent Positive First Sera by Test Method

Test Method	Total paired sera tested[a]	Total 1st sera titer $\geq$1:16	% Positive first sera
IHA	91[b]	34	37.4
IFA	60[b]	15	25.0
LA	91[b]	18	19.8
CF	63[b]	2	3.2

[a]All paired sera showed a four-fold or greater titer rise
by at least one method.

[b]Of the 93 paired sera used for data analysis, IHA and LA
results were available on 91 pairs, IFA test results were
available on 60 pairs and CF results were available on 63
pairs.

For those fifty-two serum pairs upon which all four tests
were performed, 17 (32.6%) were positive by all four tests,
27 (51.9%) were positive by three tests, 6 (11.5%) were
positive by two tests, and 2 (3.8%) were positive by only one
test procedure.

Based on the onset dates provided on the submission forms,
the first or acute sera were collected as early as the day of
onset of clinical symptoms and as late as twelve days after
onset. However, most acute sera were collected within three
days of onset.

The most sensitive procedure for the early detection of
antibody to R. rickettsii might be expected to be the one
that gives a positive result more frequently when the first
or acute serum of each pair is tested. The results of IHA,
IFA, LA and CF tests of first or acute sera can be seen in
Table 2. A threshold titer of $\geq$ 1:16 was used to indicate
the presence of antibody.

As can be seen in Table 2, the IHA test was able to
detect antibody in 37.4% of first or acute sera. The IFA and
LA methods detected antibody in 25.0% and 19.8% of first sera
respectively. This might indicate the IHA test is somewhat
more sensitive for the early detection of specific antibody
to R. rickettsii. The least sensitive method was the CF
test by which only 3.2% of the first or acute sera gave a
specific antibody titer of $\geq$ 1:16.

A more detailed analysis was performed by comparing
antibody levels during the period of 0 to 24 days after onset
of illness as detected by each of the four methods studied.

TABLE 3. Median Antibody Titers for Each
Test Method by Days after Onset

Days after onset[a]	Median reciprocal antibody titer			
	IHA[b]	IFA[b]	LA[b]	CF[b]
0 - 3	< 8	< 16	< 16	< 8
4 - 6	16	< 16	< 16	< 8
7 - 9	$\geq$ 1024	32	16	< 8
10 - 12	$\geq$ 1024	256	128	< 8
13 - 15	$\geq$ 1024	$\geq$ 512[c]	512	32[c]
16 - 18	$\geq$ 1024	$\geq$ 512	256	< 8
19 - 21	$\geq$ 1024	$\geq$ 512	128	8
22 - 24	$\geq$ 1024	$\geq$ 512	128	64[c]

[a]Based on unconfirmed submission data.
[b]Initial testing dilution was 1:8 for IHA and CF. Initial dilution was 1:16 for IFA and LA.
[c]Median based on three or fewer sera.

This analysis was performed by determining the median antibody titer for each of eight 3-day intervals. The results can be seen in Table 3.

Based on this analysis, by testing an acute serum collected on the day of onset paired with a second serum collected as early as a week after onset, one might expect to demonstrate a four-fold or greater antibody titer rise using the IHA test. The IFA and LA tests may take a few days longer to show a significant titer rise. The CF test may take 2-3 weeks to demonstrate an antibody response.

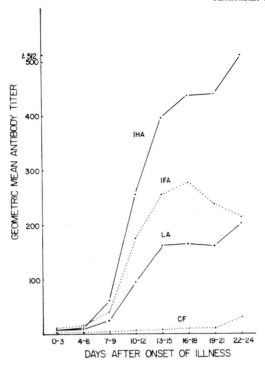

Fig. 1. Geometric mean R. rickettsii antibody titers by serological methods according to day after onset of RMSF.

Finally, the geometric mean antibody titer was calculated for each three day time interval for each test method. A moving average was then plotted as seen in Figure 1. The moving average was computed using the titers for the depicted three day interval plus the titers for the three day intervals immediately preceding and following that interval.

As seen in this analysis, the IHA antibody titer to R. rickettsii appears to rise slightly earlier in the course of RMSF.

IV.   DISCUSSION

In this study, the IHA test was shown to detect antibody to R. rickettsii in a higher percentage of first or acute sera from serologically confirmed cases of RMSF. In their study, Hechemy, et al. (3), found that for the first specimen of reactive pairs, a detectable reaction was obtained

significantly more often in the latex-R. rickettsii test
than in the CF test, but less often than in the IHA test.

Although we do not have a significant number of measurements at all time intervals observed in this study,
some trends related to the early detection of a R. rickettsii
antibody response in RMSF seem clear. In cases of RMSF, a
four-fold or greater antibody titer rise to R. rickettsii
may be detected with an acute serum collected within 3 days
of onset of illness and a second serum collected as early as
one week after onset using the IHA test. A four-fold or
greater titer rise by the IFA and LA methods may not be
detected as early as by the IHA test, but a significant
antibody response may be demonstrated by 7-12 days after
onset. The CF test is less sensitive than all other tests
and a significant antibody response may not be detected
until 2-3 weeks after onset. Similar results were reported
by Philip, et al. (5). In that study, it was shown that
antibody titers to R. rickettsii were first evident five to
six days after onset of symptoms with the more sensitive
tests (IHA and IFA). The CF test was less sensitive.
Moreover, only one-half of patients judged to have RMSF by
the more sensitive tests were positive by the CF test.

V.   SUMMARY

The purpose of this study was to analyze data derived
from the testing of sera from serologically confirmed cases
of RMSF to determine which procedure (IHA, IFA, LA or CF)
would permit the earliest detection of a specific antibody
response to R. rickettsii. Based on this analysis, by
testing an acute serum collected within 3 days of onset of
illness, paired with a second serum collected as early as
a week after onset, one might expect to demonstrate a four-
fold or greater antibody titer rise using the IHA test. A
four-fold or greater titer rise by the IFA or LA methods was
not detected as early as the IHA test in this study, but a
significant antibody response was demonstrated by 7-12
days after onset. The CF test appears to be less sensitive
than all other tests studied and a significant antibody
response may not be detected until two to three weeks
after onset.

REFERENCES

1. Anacker, R.L., Philip, R.N., Thomas, L.A., and Casper,
    E.A., J. Clin. Microbiol. 10, 677 (1979).
2. Philip, R.N., Casper, E.A., Ormsbee, R.A., Peacock, M.G.,
    and Burgdorfer, W., J. Clin. Microbiol. 3, 51 (1976).
3. Hechemy, K.E., Anacker, R.L., Philip, R.N., Kleeman, K.T.,
    MacCormack, J.N., Sasowski, S.J., and Michaelson, E.E.,
    J. Clin. Microbiol. 12, 144 (1980).
4. Center for Disease Control (1974). Standard Diagnostic
    Complement Fixation Method and Adaptation to Micro Test.
5. Philip, R.N., Casper, E.A., MacCormack, J.N., Sexton,
    D.J., Thomas, L.A., Anacker, R.L., Burgdorfer, W. and
    Vick, S., Am. J. Epidemiol. 105, 56 (1977).

THE INCIDENCE OF ROCKY MOUNTAIN SPOTTED FEVER AS
DESCRIBED BY PROSPECTIVE EPIDEMIOLOGIC SURVEILLANCE
AND THE ASSESSMENT OF PERSISTENCE OF ANTIBODIES TO
R. RICKETTSII BY INDIRECT HEMAGGLUTINATION AND
MICROIMMUNOFLUORESCENCE TESTS

Catherine M. Wilfert[1]
Ernest Austin
Vivian Dickinson

Departments of Pediatrics and Microbiology
Duke University Medical Center
Durham, North Carolina

Karl Kleeman
Jane Lea Hicks
J. Newton MacCormack

N.C. State Laboratory of Public Health
Raleigh, North Carolina

Robert L. Anacker
Elizabeth A. Casper
Robert N. Philip

Rocky Mountain Laboratories
Hamilton, Montana

[1]Supported by NIH contract No. NO1 A1-92621.

I. INTRODUCTION

Rocky Mountain spotted fever (RMSF) is endemic in the
Southeastern United States. North Carolina has reported more
cases of the disease than any other state for 1970 through
1979, and again leads the nation in 1980. All estimates of
incidence of RMSF have depended upon the recognition and subsequent reporting of clinically identifiable illness. Not all
cases are reported, and not all reported cases are serologically confirmed.

An epidemiologic study has been undertaken in Cabarrus and
Rowan Counties in North Carolina to better define several aspects of the epidemiology of RMSF. The annualized reported
case rates were 8.5 per 100,000 and 12.2 per 100,000 in
Cabarrus and Rowan Counties, respectively, for the period 1968-
1977. These rates are the two highest reported rates for all
100 North Carolina counties for this 10-year period. There
appears to be a substantially increased risk for the population
in these counties when these estimates are compared to the reported estimate of 0.5 cases per 100,000 of population in the
U.S. and of 1.66 per 100,000 population in the South Atlantic
states (1).

This is a preliminary summary of the epidemiologic study.
During the first year, an attempt was made to define whether
reported disease accurately reflects serologically confirmed
disease. The second aspect of the study examines the persistence of antibodies and sensitivity and specificity of currently employed antibody assays to detect previous infection.
Thirdly, a prevalence study attempts to define the occurrence
of antibody positivity in the general population of this endemic area.

II. MATERIALS AND METHODS

During the first of 3 years of study, case reporting by
the usual means was compared with that of cases identified by
2 field epidemiologists. Epidemiologists (E.A. and V.D.) living in study counties, organized surveillance through the
County Health Departments, the 2 hospitals, and physicians providing primary care. The epidemiologists are notified when a
physician decides to initiate specific antimicrobial therapy
for RMSF. During the first year, physicians did not expect the
study to replace routine reporting of cases to the State Health
Department. Surveillance was initiated in July 1979 with
retrospective case finding from April 1979. Cases were reported through September of 1979.

   Review of medical records in Rowan and Cabarrus Hospitals
of all cases reported to the North Carolina State Health Departments during the last 20 years, and of cases known to local
physicians and Duke University Medical Center consultants,
identified patients with prior diagnoses of RMSF. Sera were
obtained from thirty of these persons during the fall/winter
1979-80.
   The indirect hemagglutination test (IHA) test was performed
using fresh sheep erythrocytes coated with erythrocyte-sensitizing substance (2). All sera were absorbed with sheep erythrocytes prior to testing.
   The indirect fluorescent antibody test (IFA) test was the
previously described microimmunofluorescence (MIF) procedure
at the Rocky Mountain Laboratories (3).
   The antibody prevalence survey was based on several assumptions: 1) that infection may be followed by life-long persistence of detectable antibody; 2) actual incidence of RMSF may
be greater than reported incidence of disease; 3) immigration
of residents from hypo-endemic RMSF areas and emigration of
residents have not significantly affected the prevalence of
seropositivity in the current populations of these counties;
4) a proportion of the population acquires RMSF each year, so
that past rickettsial infection would be cumulative, and testing sera of older residents would increase the likelihood of
detecting past infection; 5) if persons were not known to have
had RMSF they would be less likely to have received antimicrobial therapy with its possible effects on the persistence of
antibody.
   During the winter and spring of 1979-80, sera were obtained
from 181 persons, residing ≥ 40 years in either county. Most
study participants were healthy volunteer blood donors. The
person's age, duration of residence in the county, and past
history of RMSF, or vaccination against RMSF were obtained at
entry into the study. Sera were tested for antibodies by IHA
and MIF tests.

                    III.   RESULTS

        A.   Surveillance and Routine Reporting

   Seventy-eight persons with suspected RMSF were identified
between April and September 1979. Serologically confirmed
cases were defined as those who had $>$4-fold rise in R. rickettsii antibody titers (IHA or MIF), or R. rickettsii IgM antibodies detected by MIF. Individuals with "stationary" titers
were those who had detectable antibodies at constant titer in
at least 2 sera, the second of which was obtained at least

3 weeks after recognition of illness. Those patients who had appropriately timed sera, who lacked demonstrable antibody, are referred to as serologically disconfirmed cases. Incomplete serology indicates either that no serum, or only an acute phase serum, was obtained. Table 1 summarizes the investigation of the 78 suspect cases. Twenty persons had serologically confirmed RMSF. Three of these had stationary titers with an elevated MIF-IgM titer. Two additional patients were identified by the postmortem finding of R. rickettsii in tissues, bringing the total of confirmed cases of RMSF to 22 for the 1979 season. Serological testing revealed 14 individuals who had antibodies of constant titer, indicating that they may have had R. rickettsii infection. Additionally, there were 29 individuals whose illness was not RMSF based on the absence of R. rickettsii antibody. Table 1 also presents data for "routinely reported" cases. Forty cases were reported through the usual channels, but only 10 of these had serologically confirmed RMSF. All reported cases were detected independently by the surveillance system and, in fact, serological evaluation of these persons was largely accomplished through the epidemiologic study. Routine reporting did not detect 12 confirmed cases of RMSF. Thus, the total 40 cases reported for the two counties was nearly twice the number confirmed in the epidemiologic study. Additionally, 24 individuals reported as having RMSF did not have confirmatory serological evidence of infection.

TABLE 1. Routinely Reported RMSF Compared to Epidemiological Surveillance Rowan/Cabarrus Counties, 1979

Total number of routinely reported cases		40
Serological assessment		34
Serologically confirmed	10	
Stationary titer (IHA or MIF)	7	
Serologically disconfirmed	17	
Incomplete serological assessment		6
Epidemiological surveillance		78
Serological assessment		65[a]
Confirmed cases	22[a]	
Stationary titer (IHA or MIF)	14	
Serologically disconfirmed	29	
Incomplete serology	13	

[a]Two cases confirmed by detection of R. rickettsii in tissues.

TABLE 2.   Clinical Diagnosis of RMSF Without Serological
Confirmation at Time of Acute Illness

Patient	Yr. of disease	Date serum obtained	Reciprocal of dilution		
			CF	IHA	IgG-MIF[a]
1	1940	11/14/79	8	64	128
2	1942	11/14/79	<8	<8	128
3	1951	11/15/79	<8	<8	NR
4	1962	10/25/79	<8	128	trace
5	1975	12/5/79	<8	16	64

[a] to R. rickettsii.

B.   Persistence of Antibody After Infection in the Past

Thirty persons who had RMSF in previous years were located.
A serum sample was obtained from each during fall/winter of
1979-80.   Five patients were identified who had been hospitalized with clinically diagnosed disease.   These patients did not
have serological confirmation at the time of their acute illness (Table 2).

Three patients had detectable antibodies by IHA and by
MIF determination.   Two patients with illnesses in 1940 and
1942 could not have received specific antimicrobial therapy.

The 3 patients in Table 3 had clinically diagnosed RMSF
and at least one elevated R. rickettsii antibody titer at the
time of their illness.   These 3 patients had detectable antibodies by the IHA test and one had antibodies detected by MIF.

TABLE 3.   Clinical Diagnosis of RMSF with Temporally
Related Single Elevated R. rickettsii Antibody Titer

Patient	Yr. of disease	Date serum obtained	Reciprocal of dilution		
			CF	IHA	IgG-MIF[a]
1	1962	6/62	64		
		10/30/79	<8	8	NR
2	1974	5/9/74	<8	4096	512
		1/16/80	<8	16	NR
3	1977	4/27/77	<8		
		?/77	16		
		1/7/80	8	8	128

[a] to R. rickettsii.

TABLE 4. Clinical Diagnosis and Documented
4-fold Antibody Rise at Time of Acute Illness

Year of illness	Number of patients	IHA pos. ≥ 8	MIF pos. ≥ 16
1975-77	11	11	8
1969-74	10	9	5
1964	1	1	1
Total	22	21	14

Twenty-two patients had 4-fold rise in antibody titer (CF,
MIF, or IHA) during illness. Table 4 summarizes the antibody
determinations on follow-up sera. Fourteen had antibody detected by both IHA and MIF tests. The IHA assay with R. rickettsii antigen detected antibody in 21 of 22 persons who had
serologically documented infection in the past. Three persons
had IHA titers of 8, and 7 had titers of 16. Eight persons did
not have antibody by MIF. Seven MIF-negative sera had IHA
titers ranging from 16 to 64.

C. Prevalence Study

Serological evaluation of 181 sera was completed from persons resident in either county for greater than 40 years. Sera
were screened at 1:8 dilution, and all positive sera were titered to endpoint (Table 5). One hundred persons were sero-
negative by both IHA and MIF tests. Fifteen persons who had a
positive IHA titer also had a positive MIF level to one or more
of the rickettsial antigens. Forty-three persons had a positive IHA determination but a negative MIF determination. Fourteen persons had a negative IHA assay but a positive MIF assay.

TABLE 5. Evaluation for R. rickettsii Antibodies
in Sera from 181 Persons Resident in Cabarrus or
Rowan Counties 40 or More Years

County	IHA neg MIF neg	IHA pos MIF pos	IHA pos MIF neg	IHA neg MIF pos	MIF pos	MIF neg
Rowan	76	8	30	10	3	6
Cabarrus	24	7	13	4		9[a]
	100	15	43	14		

[a]IHA not done.
IHA positive ≥ 8; MIF ≥ 8.

TABLE 6.   IHA Antibody Titers of Persons Resident in
Cabarrus or Rowan Counties 40 or More Years

Number of persons	IHA titer
22	8
10	16
14	32
10	64
2	128

Nine sera were examined only by MIF test. Three of these were
positive. IHA titers on the seropositive individuals are
depicted in Table 6. The single largest group (22 individuals)
had titers of 8. Two persons had titers of 128 and 10 persons
had titers of 64.

These sera were tested by MIF with antigens representing
various serotypes of the spotted fever and typhus groups.
There were 4 persons with detectable antibodies by MIF who
might be regarded as having serological evidence of past R.
rickettsii infection. Table 7 shows antibody patterns of
persons whose MIF titers to R. rickettsii were equal to or
greater than antibody levels to other spotted fever group or
typhus group organisms. Cross-reactivity among the spotted
fever-group antigens is apparent. One person had antibody detected by IHA. None had received vaccine or were known to have
had RMSF.

TABLE 7.   Serological Evidence (MIF) of R. rickettsii
Infection in Persons Resident in County 40 or More Years

Case	IHA titer	MIF rick	akar	cono	rhip	mont	369C	typh	cana
1		16					tr		
2		16	8	16	16	16	16		
3	QNS	16	8						
4	32	64	32	32	32	32	32		16

rick = R. rickettsii, akar = R. akari, cono = R. conorii,
rhip = R. rhipicephali, mont = R. montana, prow = R. prowazekii,
typh = R. typhi, cana = R. canada.
(Blank spaces denote no detectable titers at 1:8).

Eleven individuals had serological evidence of infection with other members of the spotted fever group of rickettsiae. Seven people had maximum titers to 369C and two to R. montana.

Finally, 19 persons had serological evidence of infection with the typhus group of organisms. Maximum serological responses occurred to R. prowazekii in most persons. Only one person knew he had received typhus vaccine. Two of them denied military service, foreign travel, or receiving typhus vaccine, but were in the military and traveled outside the United States. Two could not be reached for additional information concerning their vaccine status.

IV. DISCUSSION

Current incidence and prevalence data are dependent upon voluntary reporting of suspected RMSF. It has generally been assumed that human R. rickettsii infection usually results in clinical disease. Seasonality of RMSF and its geographic localization influence reporting of suspected cases. Illnesses with fever and/or rash become suspect during the spring and summer. Our comparison of routinely reported cases with those identified by epidemiologic surveillance also recognizes only clinically suspect illness. Our information suggests either that clinically recognized RMSF is reported in endemic areas more often than it actually occurs, or not all patients with RMSF respond with antibody detectable by two of our most sensitive serodiagnostic procedures. Whereas 40 cases of disease were reported through the routine reporting system, only 10 of these patients could be serologically confirmed as having RMSF. Thus, routine reporting of cases reported 3 times as many cases as could be serologically documented. In contrast, our epidemiologic surveillance resulted in the investigation of 78 patients. Two of these were fatal cases which were not reported and a total of 20 patients had serological confirmation of RMSF. The additional 12 documented cases detected by the surveillance raises the seasonal total of 22 patients for these counties. The reported number of cases is therefore almost twice that which could be documented. At the time this study was initiated, it was anticipated that there would be substantial underreporting of illness. We expected to find more overt, serologically proven cases of disease than were reported. Although cases were missed by routine reporting, it appears that there may be overreporting of disease in endemic areas.

We have performed antibody determinations on sera obtained from patients who had R. rickettsii infection in the past. It was important to document persistence of antibodies in proven

cases of disease before undertaking a prevalence survey. The
2 patients who had disease before antimicrobial therapy was
available had relatively high titers of antibody 38 years after
disease. Whereas most patients with previously diagnosed RMSF
had detectable antibodies by either MIF or IHA, the specificity
of low titers is questionable by the determinations. Some patients were positive only by IHA test and not by MIF. Antibodies were detectable in titers as low as 8 or 16 in 10 of 21
persons. It is impossible to totally disregard these titers,
as these patients have had previously confirmed disease. IHA
determinations were reproducible, and 14 of 22 patients had
antibody detectable both by IHA and MIF.

The prevalence study of spotted fever antibodies was conducted in Rowan and Cabarrus Counties, and the initial serological evaluations were accomplished on 181 sera obtained from
healthy persons who had resided in one of these counties for
more than 40 years. A total of 75 persons were seropositive
by either IHA and/or MIF (Table 5). Fifteen were positive by
both tests. Four individuals (Table 7) had serological evidence by microimmunofluorescence suggesting that R. rickettsii
infection was the best explanation for their seropositivity.
Cross-reactivity in the spotted fever group is apparent. None
of these 4 people had received vaccine or were known to have
had RMSF. Thus, the serological determinations performed to
date in the prevalence study suggest that a minimum of 4 individuals, or a maximum of 75 individuals could have encountered
and responded to rickettsial antigens at an undetermined time.
This provides a means of estimating the occurrence of disease
from 55 to 1035 per 100,000 of the population per year for
county residents. Even the minimal estimate suggests that
asymptomatic or unrecognized infection is occurring.

There were 11 individuals with serological evidence of infection with other members of the spotted fever group of rickettsiae. Seven people had their maximum response to 369C and
2 to R. montana. It is of interest that tick drag studies done
in North Carolina have yielded isolates of these rickettsial
organisms (4). At present, there is no clinical evidence to
indicate that human infection with these organisms occurs.
Further study is required to evaluate the significance of these
observations.

V.   SUMMARY

During the 1979-80 epidemiologic year, routine reporting
of RMSF in two high risk counties described three cases for
each one that was subsequently serologically proven. Routine

reporting also failed to identify one-half of clinically evident, serologically confirmed cases. IHA detected antibody in 21 of 22 persons with serologically proven RMSF in the past. MIF detected R. rickettsii antibody in 14 of the 22 persons. IHA antibody titers were detectable in 58 of 172 persons residing for 40 years or more in an endemic area. Twenty-six of these had titers of 32 or greater. Only 32 of 181 persons had positive MIF titers to one or more rickettsial antigens. Fifteen persons had antibody detected by both assays. The lower antibody titers may not be specific indicators of past infection with R. rickettsii if low levels of reactivity are generated by some nonrickettsial stimulants or infection with other rickettsiae.

Eleven of 181 persons had serological evidence suggesting infection with other members of the spotted fever group, predominantly 369C. Eighteen of 181 persons had evidence of prior experience with R. prowazekii.

Thus, the antibodies detected by IHA seem to be a sensitive, but possibly nonspecific indicator of past infection with R. rickettsii. There is serological evidence to substantiate the concept that asymptomatic or unrecognized cases of R. rickettsii infection are occurring in endemic areas. There is similar evidence to suggest that infection with 369C and possibly R. prowazekii are also occurring. Additional work is planned to complete the laboratory evaluation of the prevalence study, looking for detectable titers in younger persons who have been resident in endemic areas for shorter periods of time and taking a comparative look at the antibody status of persons residing in a county where R. rickettsii infection is recognized infrequently.

ACKNOWLEDGMENTS

The authors wish to thank Mr. Klimas and Mr. Hawley of the Cabarrus and Rowan County Health Departments for their enthusiastic support. The physicians of these counties have made these studies possible by their willing collaboration and the Rowan, Cabarrus, and V.A. Hospital (Salisbury) Laboratories' personnel have provided essential help with the collection and storage of specimens.

REFERENCES

1. D'Angelo, L. J., Winkler, W. G., and Bregman, D. J., J. Infect. Dis. 138: 273 (1978).
2. Anacker, R. L., Philip, R. N., Thomas, L. A., and Casper, E. A., J. Clin. Microbiol. 10, 677 (1979).
3. Philip, R. N., Casper, E. A., Ormsbee, R. A., Peacock, M. G., and Burgdorfer, W., J. Clin. Microbiol. 3, 51 (1976).
4. Burgdorfer, W. and authors. Unpublished observation.

INFLAMMATORY RESPONSE OF SUSCEPTIBLE AND RESISTANT CONGENIC C3H MICE TO INFECTION WITH R. TSUTSUGAMUSHI STRAIN GILLIAM

Thomas R. Jerrells
Joseph V. Osterman

Department of Rickettsial Diseases
Walter Reed Army Institute of Research
Washington, DC

I. INTRODUCTION

Previous work from this laboratory has established that susceptibility of inbred mice to lethal rickettsial infection is controlled by factors inherent to the rickettsiae as well as factors determined by the genetic background of the host (1). At least in terms of resistance to lethal infection with the Gilliam strain of R. tsutsugamushi, the host factors are under the control of a single, autosomal, dominant gene designated Ric (2).

In a recent study we established a model system employing congenic strains of C3H mice which were shown to differ at the Ric gene (Jerrells, T. R. and Osterman, J. V., submitted for publication, 1980). In this study we also demonstrated that susceptible C3H/HeDub mice responded to infection with a vigorous inflammatory response consisting of macrophages (MØ), lymphocytes and polymorphonuclear leukocytes (PMN), whereas the response of the resistant mice (C3H/RV) followed similar kinetics but was of a lesser magnitude and essentially mononuclear in character. We demonstrated that indomethacin, an anti-inflammatory drug which inhibits prostaglandin synthesis, prolonged the survival of susceptible animals. We interpreted these data to suggest that in the susceptible animals the inflammatory response was providing cells capable of replicating rickettsiae and/or were inappropriate or nonfunctional in terms of cell-mediated immune (CMI) effector mechanisms.

In the present study we addressed the latter possibility
by examining the cellular composition of the mononuclear cells
responding to infection in terms of lymphocyte surface markers
as well as functional activity of inflammatory MØ. It was
found that the susceptible C3H/HeDub mice responded to Gilliam
infection with an influx of lymphocytes which are predominantly thymus-derived lymphocytes (T-lymphocytes), and which occur
in greater numbers than seen in C3H/RV mice. It was further
found that the MØ component of the inflammatory response in
C3H/HeDub mice was also greater than seen in C3H/RV animals
and, based on the criteria used, was as activated as the C3H/
RV MØ population. Finally, administration of killed C. parvum
to C3H/RV in a regimen previously shown to lower resistance to
Listeria monocytogenes (3) resulted in an apparent decrease in
resistance to rickettsial challenge.

II. MATERIALS AND METHODS

A. Animals

Female C3H/HeDub mice were purchased from Flow Laboratories (Dublin, VA). C3H/RV mice were obtained initially as a
breeding pair from Dr. Robert Jacoby, Yale University School
of Medicine, New Haven, CT, and subsequently reared by Flow
Laboratories under contract to the Walter Reed Army Institute
of Research. All mice were used at 6-8 weeks of age and
weighed 18-22 g. In individual experiments mice were age and
sex matched.

B. Rickettsiae

Gilliam (165th egg passage) and Karp (52nd egg passage)
strains of R. tsutsugamushi were plaque purified in L-929
cells as previously described (4) and propagated in embryonated chicken eggs. Infected yolk sac suspensions were prepared
and stored as previously described (5). Quantification of
rickettsiae was accomplished by intraperitoneal inoculation of
C3H/HeDub mice and calculation of the 50% mouse lethal dose
(MLD_{50}) by the Spearman and Karber procedure (6).

C. Infection

Mice were infected by intraperitoneal (ip) injection of
0.2 ml of infected yolk sac suspension diluted in cold brain-
heart infusion broth to contain 1000 MLD_{50} of rickettsiae.

D. Estimation of Inflammatory Response

At various intervals following infection, animals were
sacrificed by CO_2 asphyxiation, and cells were obtained by
washing the peritoneal cavity twice with 5 ml of Hank's balanced salt solution (HBSS) supplemented with 50 µg/ml of gentamycin and 10 units of heparin/ml. Peritoneal cells obtained from the two washings were pooled, centrifuged at 500 x
g for 10 min at 4°C, and washed once with HBSS. Cytocentri-
fuge preparations (Cytospin, Shandon Elliot, Sewickley, PA)
were Giemsa-stained, and differential cell counts were performed. A total of 200 cells were counted in each sample.

E. Lymphocyte Subpopulation Quantitation

The proportion of T-lymphocytes was determined using a
fluorescein labeled rabbit anti-mouse brain serum (RAMB;
Litton Bionetics Inc., Kensington, MD). The proportion of
lymphocytes with surface immunoglobulin (B-lymphocytes) was
determined using fluorescein labeled goat anti-mouse IgG with
heavy and light chain specificity (Cappel Laboratories Inc.,
Cochranville, PA).

F. Macrophage Functional Activity

Activation of MØ as a result of infection was assayed using tumor cell cytolysis and phagocytosis of ^{51}Cr-labeled
sheep erythrocyte-anti-sheep erythrocyte (EA) complexes. The
cytolysis assay was a modification of the procedure of Ruco
and Meltzer (7). Briefly, inflammatory MØ were adjusted to
8.0 x 10^5 and 1.6 x 10^6 MØ/ml in RPMI 1640 supplemented with
1 % glutamine, 25 mM N-2-hydroxyethylpiperazine-N'-2-ethanesul-
fonic acid (HEPES) buffer, 50 µg/ml gentamycin, and 10% fetal
bovine serum all obtained from MA Bioproducts, Walkersville,
MD. The cells were added in 0.5-ml aliquots to 24 well tissue
culture plates (Costar, Boston, MA) and incubated 60 min at
37°C in a humidified 5% CO_2 atmosphere to allow attachment of
adherent cells. After incubation, nonadherent cells were removed by washing each well 3-4 times with warm RPMI 1640.

The resulting adherent cells were predominantly MØ (>95%) based on latex phagocytosis and uptake of neutral red. The TU-5 tumor target cells were prelabeled with tritiated thymidine (^{3}H-TdR) by incubating nonconfluent monolayers overnight in complete RPMI 1640 media containing 20 µCi ^{3}H-TdR (S.A. 6.7 Ci/mMole; New England Nuclear, Boston, MA). To each well 0.5 ml of TU-5 cells at 8 x 10^4 cells/ml were added. This resulted in effector to tumor target cell (E:T) ratios of 10:1 and 20:1.

The MØ-tumor cell cultures were incubated a further 48 hr at 37°C in a humidified 5% CO_2 atmosphere. Release of ^{3}H-TdR was determined by scintillation counting (Packard Prias Tri-Carb). Total incorporated radioactivity was determined after SDS lysis of target cells. Percent cytolysis was calculated by dividing the CPM released in experimental cultures by the total incorporated (SDS released) CPM.

The phagocytic capacity of macrophages was determined by uptake of ^{51}Cr-labeled EA complexes sensitized with IgG anti-sheep erythrocyte serum (Cappel Laboratories, Cochranville, PA) as described by Boraschi and Meltzer (8). Briefly, sheep erythrocytes were washed 3 times in phosphate buffered saline (PBS) and adjusted to 1 x 10^9/ml in PBS. An equal volume of antiserum diluted to the first subagglutinating concentration in PBS and 10 µCi of ^{51}Cr (New England Nuclear, Boston, MA) were added. This mixture was incubated at 37°C for 60 min, and following incubation, ^{51}Cr-labeled EA complexes were washed 3-4 times and resuspended at 1 x 10^9/ml in PBS. To MØ monolayers at 8 x 10^5/well in 24 well tissue culture plates, isolated as described, 0.2 ml of EA suspension were added. The cultures were incubated at 37°C in a humidified 5% CO_2 atmosphere for 60 min after addition of EA. Each well was washed 3 times to remove free EA followed by treatment with 0.84% ammonium chloride solution to lyse any unphagocytized EA. The MØ monolayers were washed a further 3 times to remove the ammonium chloride and finally lysed with a 0.5% solution of SDS. The CPM were determined using a gamma counter (Packard Prias Auto-Gamma).

G.   Treatment of Mice with Formalin-Killed
Corynebacterium parvum

C. parvum lot number CA771/A (Burroughs Wellcome, Research Triangle Park, NC) was adjusted to 7 mg/ml in PBS, and C3H/RV mice were injected with 0.1 ml either ip or intravenously (iv) 24 hr prior to ip infection with 1000 MLD$_{50}$ of R. tsutsugamushi, strain Gilliam.

III. RESULTS

A. Inflammatory Response

The inflammatory cell influx (Table 1) at 5 and 7 days postinfection was significantly greater in C3H/HeDub than in C3H/RV mice. These data also indicate the number of MØ and lymphocytes was of a greater magnitude in C3H/HeDub animals. The most obvious difference noted between sensitive (C3H/HeDub) and resistant (C3H/RV) animals was the presence of a PMN response in C3H/HeDub animals.

To further characterize the influx as to immunocompetent cells responding to the infection, cells recovered at various points during the inflammatory response were evaluated for the presence of T- and B-lymphocytes. The proportion of cells staining with RAMB (Fig. 1) increased in number from day 5 through day 10 postinfection in the C3H/HeDub animals. In contrast, only a slight peak of T-lymphocyte influx was noted at day 7 in C3H/RV mice. The B-lymphocyte response to Gilliam infection was roughly the same in both groups reaching a maximum level at day 7 postinfection.

TABLE 1. Inflammatory Response of C3H/HeDub and C3H/RV Mice to R. tsutsugamushi Strain Gilliam

Mouse Strain	Day[a]	Total Leukocytes	MØ	Lymph	PMN
C3H/HeDub	0	2.6 ± 0.8[b]	1.2 ± 0.2	1.4 ± 0.3	0
	5	15.1 ± 3.1	4.7 ± 0.1	5.5 ± 0.1	$5.0 + 0.8$
	7	19.6 ± 4.2	11.0 ± 1.0	7.8 ± 2.6	0.9 ± 0.6
C3H/RV	0	3.6 ± 1.6	1.7 ± 0.4	1.9 ± 0.1	0.01 ± 0.01
	5	4.7 ± 0.9	1.7 ± 0.5	2.9 ± 1.3	0.2 ± 0.1
	7	8.0 ± 3.3	3.7 ± 1.8	3.8 ± 1.1	0.5 ± 0.4

[a]Days after ip infection with 1000 MLD$_{50}$ R. tsutsugamushi strain Gilliam.
[b]Mean ± standard deviation of 6 mice x 10^6.

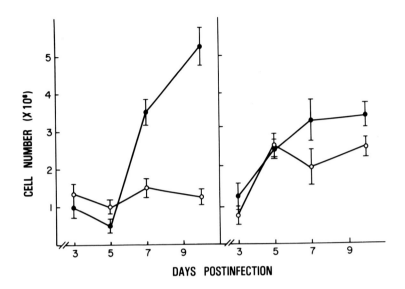

Fig. 1. Left Panel: Influx of lymphocytes staining with rabbit anti-mouse brain serum during progressive infection. Right Panel: Influx of lymphocytes staining with anti-immuno-globulin. ●—● C3H/HeDub o—o C3H/RV.

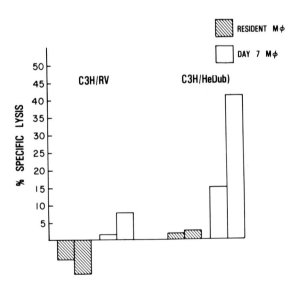

Fig. 2. Cytolytic activity of resident and inflammatory macrophages obtained from C3H/RV and C3H/HeDub mice at E:T ratios of 10:1 and 20:1.

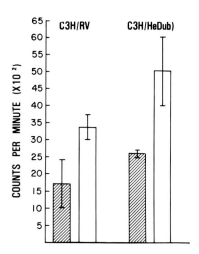

Fig. 3.   Phagocytosis of erythrocyte antibody complexes by resident (▨) and inflammatory (□) macrophages obtained from C3H/RV and C3H/HeDub mice.

B.   Macrophage Functional Activity

Approximately equal numbers of MØ recovered prior to infection (resident MØ), or 7 days postinfection from C3H/HeDub
and C3H/RV mice, were employed in a tumor cell cytolysis assay
and an assay of phagocytic function. Data obtained from the
cytolysis assay are presented in Figure 2. It is evident that
more activity was obtained using C3H/HeDub MØ as effector
cells. A similar pattern was evident when phagocytosis of
^{51}Cr EA was used as the criterion of MØ activity (Fig. 3). In
both groups the MØ recovered 7 days postinfection were more
active than resident MØ, and C3H/HeDub inflammatory MØ were
significantly more active (p $\leq$ 0.05 using Student's t test)
than the C3H/RV MØ. No significant difference in resident
peritoneal MØ activity was detected using these two assays.

C.   Effect of Formalin-Killed C. parvum
on C3H/RV Resistance

It was found that administration of killed C. parvum ip
24 hr prior to rickettsial infection rendered C3H/RV mice susceptible to Gilliam infection (Table 2). The C3H/RV mice injected ip with C. parvum died 16 and 19 days postinfection.
In contrast, the C3H/RV mice injected iv with an equal dose of
C. parvum followed 24 hr later by an ip infection with rickettsiae survived throughout the duration of the experiment.

TABLE 2.   Effect of Killed C. parvum on Resistance
of C3H/RV Mice to R. tsutsugamushi, Strain Gilliam[a]

Mouse strain	Treatment	% Mortality[b]
C3H/He	Saline	100
C3H/RV	Saline	0
C3H/RV	C. parvum iv[c]	0
C3H/RV	C. parvum ip[c]	60

[a]Mice challenged with 1000 MLD_{50} Gilliam ip 24 hr postinjection with C. parvum.
[b]C3H/HeDub control mice died at day 10 postinfection.
Other groups represent cumulative data after 30 days. Mice
receiving killed C. parvum ip died between days 16 and 19
postinfection.
[c]700 μg of C. parvum in PBS injected either iv or ip.

IV.   DISCUSSION

Previous work from this laboratory (Jerrells, T. R. and
Osterman, J. V., submitted for publication, 1980), demonstrated that animals which are susceptible to lethal infections
with the Gilliam strain of R. tsutsugamushi produce an inflammatory response containing what would seem to be the appropriate effector cells previously shown to be important in rickettsial immunity (9-11). We have extended the observation in
this report and show that C3H/HeDub mice respond to Gilliam
infection with an increasing influx of T-lymphocytes which is
of a significantly greater magnitude than the influx noted in
C3H/RV mice. The B-lymphocyte response was of equal magnitude
in both strains of mice. As before, the major difference
noted was the magnitude of response; the kinetics were similar.
    Data presented in Figures 2 and 3 show that MØ which
traffic to the site of infection are apparently more activated
in C3H/HeDub than in C3H/RV animals when assessed by tumoricidal and phagocytic activity. These criteria are often utilized to evaluate MØ activation, and a correlation between
tumoricidal activity and rickettsiacidal activity has previously been suggested (10).

In addition, a recent study of Gilliam infection of BALB/c
and C3H/HeDub mice (Nacy and Meltzer, in press, 1980) has
also demonstrated a correlation between tumoricidal and rickettsiacidal activities.

The ability of formalin-killed C. parvum to modulate the
immune response was recently demonstrated to increase the lethality of L. monocytogenes infection in mice (3). We have
shown a similar trend in Gilliam infected C3H/RV mice administered these inactivated organisms. The mechanism(s) of
action of C. parvum are not clearly defined, but may involve
induction of suppressor cells and/or alteration of effector
function.

The results of this study suggest that the C3H/RV mouse
possesses the necessary cellular components in the peritoneal
cavity, which nonspecifically prevent rickettsial replication.
This effective rickettsiacidal activity limits the ensuing inflammatory response. In C3H/HeDub mice the proposed anti-
rickettsial component may be missing or nonfunctional, allowing early, unrestrained rickettsial replication with an accom-
panying inflammatory cascade.

REFERENCES

1. Groves, M. G., and Osterman, J. V., Infect. Immun. 19,
    583 (1978).
2. Groves, M. G., Rosenstreich, D. L., Taylor, B. A., and
    Osterman, J. V., J. Immunol. 125, 1395 (1980).
3. Wing, E. J., and Kresefsky-Friedman, D. Y., J. Infect.
    Dis. 141, 203 (1980).
4. Oaks, S. C., Jr., Osterman, J. V., and Hetrick, F. M.,
    J. Clin. Microbiol. 6, 76 (1977).
5. Ewing, E. P., Takeuchi, A., Shirai, A., and Osterman,
    J. V., Infect. Immun. 19, 1068 (1978).
6. Finney, D. J., "Statistical Methods in Biological Assay",
    2nd ed. Charles Griffin, London (1971).
7. Ruco, L. P., and Meltzer, M. S., J. Immunol. 119, 889
    (1977).
8. Borachi, D., and Meltzer, M. S., J. Immunol. 122, 1592
    (1979).
9. Catanzaro, P. J., Shirai, A., Hildebrandt, P. K., and
    Osterman, J. V., Infect. Immun. 13, 861 (1976).
10. Nacy, C. A., and Osterman, J. V., Infect. Immun. 26, 744
    (1979).
11. Shirai, A., Catanzaro, P. J., Phillips, S. M., and
    Osterman, J. V., Infect. Immun. 14, 39 (1976).

RISK OF RELAPSE ASSOCIATED WITH DOXYCYCLINE THERAPY FOR SCRUB TYPHUS[1]

James G. Olson[2]
A. Louis Bourgeois[3]

U.S. Naval Medical Research Unit
Number Two, Taipei, Taiwan

Richard C.Y. Fang[4]

Penghu Naval Base Hospital
Pescadores Islands, Taiwan

David T. Dennis[5]

U.S. Naval Medical Research Unit
Number Two, Jakarta, Indonesia

[1]This study was supported through funds provided by the Naval Medical Research and Development Command, Navy Department, for work unit MR 000.01.01-2064.
[2]Present address: Yale Arbovirus Research Unit, Yale University, New Haven, Connecticut.
[3]U.S. Naval Medical Research Institute, Bethesda, Maryland.
[4]Veterans General Hospital, Taipei, Taiwan.
[5]WHO Center for Research and Training in Tropical Diseases, Kuala Lumpur, Malaysia.
The opinions and assertions contained herein are those of the authors and are not to be construed as official or as reflecting the views of the Navy Department.

I.   INTRODUCTION

Chloramphenicol (Chloromycetin) or oxytetracycline (Terra-mycin) are the drugs presently recommended for treatment of patients with scrub typhus (1). These antibiotics are usually given in 250 mg doses every 6 hrs for 5 to 7 days. Since both drugs are rickettsiostatic, relapses can occur following ini-tial treatment unless follow-up antibiotics are administered (2-4).

Scrub typhus outbreaks have occurred in nonimmune military populations whose occupational exposures increased their risk of infection with Rickettsia tsutsugamushi (5,6). Under field conditions, simpler methods of treatment of shorter duration would provide great advantage to medical and paramedical per-sonnel responsible for treatment.

Doxycycline (Vibramycin), a lipophylic congener of oxyte-tracycline, is rapidly and completely absorbed from the gut and maintains high levels in the blood for several days fol-lowing administration (7). It is a candidate antibiotic for single dose therapy for scrub typhus. Single doses of doxy-cycline are effective in the treatment of epidemic louse-borne typhus (8) and are effective in the treatment of scrub typhus in rural populations of Malaysia (9). The present study com-pares the effectiveness of single and weekly-spaced doses of doxycycline with multiple doses of oxytetracycline in a double blind, randomized trial conducted in a population of scrub typhus patients who were exposed in the Pescadores Islands of Taiwan.

II.   MATERIALS AND METHODS

The study population was comprised of 68 Chinese military personnel from Taiwan who were stationed in the Pescadores Islands in 1976, were admitted to the Penghu Naval Base Hospi-tal with suspected scrub typhus and whose illnesses were con-firmed by laboratory means. Subjects were all males, mostly young army recruits who had not previously been exposed to R. tsutsugamushi infections. The epidemiology of scrub typhus in the Pescadores Islands has been discussed elsewhere (10,11).

Patients were acutely ill when they were admitted to the hospital. Most were in early stages of their disease (mean days between onset and treatment was 5.4 days). Oral tempera-tures were 38C or greater in 66 of 68 patients, all had eschars and two-thirds had typical scrub typhus rashes. Patients were examined by a physician before treatment and then twice daily while they remained in the hospital for 3 weeks. The diagnosis of scrub typhus was confirmed by recovering rickettsiae (12) from venous blood collected before antibiotic therapy was begun or by demonstrating a 4-fold increase in antibody from the acute to the convalescent phase of illness by the indirect immunofluorescence method of Bozeman and Elisberg (13) as modified by Bourgeois et al. (10).

Patients were randomly allocated to one of three treatment regimens as follows: doxycycline, 200 mg in a single dose on day 1 of treatment, followed by placebo (DXY I, 22 patients); doxycycline, 200 mg in a single dose on day 1, followed by placebo and a second 200 mg dose of doxycycline on day 7 (DXY II, 23 patients); oxytetracycline, 500 mg every 6 hrs for 7 days (OXY, 23 patients). Drug and placebo were manufactured in such a way and administered every 6 hrs for 7 days so that neither patient nor physician knew to which regimen a given patient was assigned. Randomization was forced in 3 groups and stratified by age to ensure that the groups were of a comparable age distribution.

Cure was defined as a prompt relief of symptoms and a return to normal health using trial treatment only; persons with recrudescent but self-limited fevers (1 or more measurements of 37.6 C on 2 or more consecutive days) were included in this group. Recurrence of fever and other symptoms severe enough to require treatment was classified as a relapse. Two patients vomited shortly after drug administration, had a continuation of symptoms and were considered primary treatment failures. Those patients who experienced relapses and who vomited their drug were retreated with oxytetracycline 500 mg given orally at 6-hr intervals for 7 days.

III.   RESULTS

Table 1 shows the categories of patient response. Two persons who received doxycycline vomited their first drug dose. These patients were excluded from further analysis but were treated with oxytetracycline and promptly cured. All other patients initially responded to antibiotic therapy satisfactorily. Mean times from treatment to return to normal temperature were the same for each group. In general, signs and symptoms disappeared quickly. Most patients were up and about on the third day of study and could have returned to their units for convalescence on day 5-7 following treatment. There were no instances of pneumonitis, encephalitis, heart failure or bleeding. Symptoms persisted for about equal periods in the 3 treatment groups.

TABLE 1. Frequency of Response among Scrub Typhus Patients by Treatment Group

Treatment group	Primary treatment failure	Relapse	Initial Cure with recurrence of fever	Uncomplicated cure	Total
Doxycycline, single dose (200mg)	0	2 (9)[a]	6 (27)	14 (64)	22
Doxycycline, 200mg on day 1 of study, and 200mg on day 7 of study	2 (9)	1 (5)[b]	5 (24)[b]	15 (71)[b]	23[b]
Oxytetracycline, 2g daily on days 1-7 of study	0	1 (4)	2 (9)	20 (87)	23
All Subjects	2 (3)	4 (6)[b]	13 (20)[b]	49 (74)[b]	68

[a] numbers enclosed in parentheses are percentages.

[b] primary treatment failures were excluded from the total before frequencies were calculated.

Four patients, 2 in Group DXY I, 1 in Group DXY II and 1 in
Group OXY, were treated for recurrent illness (Table 2). These
were considered relapses. Patient 171 (Group DXY II) developed
a return of fever greater than 39 C on day 5 and 6. He was
treated with oxytetracycline beginning on day 6 and was promptly cured. Patient 190 (Group DXY I) responded well to treatment and was afebrile on day 3. Fever returned on day 10 and
rickettsiae were isolated from a blood specimen collected on
day 11. Oxytetracycline was given on days 17 through 24 with
slow subsidence of temperature to a range of 37-37.6 C. Subsequent intermittent low-grade fever persisted for several
weeks. This was thought to be associated with a urinary tract
infection but a diagnosis was not clearly established. Patient
139 (Group DXY I) was also enigmatic. He was afebrile within
40 hrs of receiving the first drug dose, but experienced a relapse of fever and mild symptoms during the second week. He
responded slowly and only partially to retreatment with oxytetracycline. Further returns of fever in subsequent weeks,
during which the patient appeared otherwise well, did not seem
to be affected by two courses of oxytetracycline and one course
of doxycycline. Repeated blood cultures for rickettsiae were
negative as were results of standard investigations for fevers
of unknown origin. The patient was discharged on the 20th week
and was well when examined 3 months later. Patient 151 (Group
OXY) experienced temperature elevations on days 7, 9, and 12
which remitted spontaneously; fever returned on days 18 and 19
which was successfully retreated with a second course of oxytetracycline.

All 4 patients who were thought to have had relapses received initial treatment within 4 days after onset of illness
(Table 3). Excluding the 2 patients who vomited their initial
dose of drug, 62 of 66 (94%) were cured following the protocol
treatment alone (Table 4), experiencing rapid initial disappearance of symptoms, usually within 3-5 days. Thirteen
(20%) patients experienced elevations of temperature to 37.6 C
or greater on 2 or more days during the second and third week
of treatment (Table 1). These self-limiting fevers may have
represented mild recurrences of rickettsial illness. Temperature elevations of this sort occurred in 6 patients in Group
DXY I, 5 patients in Group DXY II and 2 patients in Group OXY.
Although these fevers were generally mild and of short duration, sometimes only a single spike of fever on 2 days, they
occasionally reached 39 C and in three instances persisted for
more than 2 days before spontaneous remission. Associated
symptoms were minor or absent and patients were often unaware
of fever and denied feeling of ill health. Rashes and eschars
were not exacerbated. The frequency of uncomplicated cure was
higher in Group OXY than in Groups DXY I and DXY II (Table 5).
The difference approached statistical significance (p=0.0666).

TABLE 2. Frequency of Relapse among Scrub Typhus Patients
by Treatment Group

Treatment group	No. relapses (%) No. treated	
Doxycycline, single dose (200 mg)	2/22	(9)
Doxycycline, 200 mg on day 1 of study and 200 mg on day 7 of study	1/21[a]	(5)
Oxytetracycline, 2g daily on days 1-7 of study	1/23	(4)

[a]Primary treatment failures excluded.

Hypothesis: Frequency of relapse among those treated with doxycycline was greater than among those treated with oxytetracycline. Not statistically significant, P=0.89 by Fisher's exact test.

TABLE 3. Frequency of Relapse among Patients by Duration after Onset when Treatment Was Begun

Days after onset of symptoms	No. relapses (%) No. treated[a]	
less than 5	4/30	(13)
5 or more	0/36	

[a]Primary treatment failures excluded.

Hypothesis: Frequency of relapse among patients treated early in their illnesses was greater than among those treated later in illness. Statistically significant difference, P=0.038 by Fisher's exact test.

TABLE 4. Frequency of Subjects Cured without Retreatment
          by Treatment Group

Treatment group	No. requiring no further treatment No. treated	(%)
Doxycycline, single dose (200 mg)	20/22	(91)
Doxycycline, 200 mg on day 1 of study and 200 mg on day 7 of study	20/21[a]	(95)
Oxytetracycline, 2g daily on days 1-7 of study	22/23	(96)

[a]Primary treatment failure excluded.

Hypothesis: Oxytetracycline resulted in a higher frequency of
cures which did not require further treatment. Not statistically
significant, P=0.829 by Fisher's exact test.

TABLE 5. Frequency of Uncomplicated Cure by Treatment Group

Treatment group	No. with uncomplicated cure No. treated	(%)
Doxycycline single dose (200 mg)	14/22	(64)
Doxycycline, 200 mg on day 1 of study and 200 mg on day 7 of study	15/21[a]	(71)
Oxytetracycline, 2g daily on days 1-7 of study	20/23	(87)

[a]Primary treatment failure excluded.

Hypothesis: Oxytetracycline resulted in a higher frequency of
uncomplicated cure than doxycycline. Nearly statistically
significant P=0.0666 by Fisher's exact test.

IV. DISCUSSSION

Scrub typhus affected thousands of military personnel who were exposed in the Far East and southwest Pacific during World War II (5). The case fatality ratio observed before specific antibiotic therapy was available ranged from 1% to 30% and full convalescence often took 2 or more months (5,6). Scrub typhus was one of the first rickettsial infections found treatable with chloramphenicol and tetracycline (14). Chloramphenicol and tetracycline have been the drugs of choice for treating scrub typhus and their use has reduced mortality and morbidity. Because antibiotics of choice are rickettsiostatic, host immunity is important in achieving cure (15). Persons who were treated early in the course of their disease were likely to experience relapse unless follow-up doses of antibiotics were administered during convalescence (3,16). Relapses of this sort were common among U.S. military personnel treated in the Vietnam conflict whether or not they received follow-up anti-biotics (16). A recent study (9) has shown that single doses of doxycycline can be highly effective for treatment of scrub typhus patients in Malaysia.

In contrast to a study conducted in Malaysia (9), our study a) followed patients in hospital for 3 full weeks instead of one week, b) included 30 patients whose onsets had occurred less than 5 days before treatment was commenced, c) was a double-blind trial, and d) dealt with patients who were drawn from a population from outside the endemic area who had not had lifelong exposure to R. tsutsugamushi infection.

To what degree these differences may account for the con-trasting findings of the two trials is not known. Only one of the 4 patients who experienced relapse in our study would have been identified if we had discharged the patients after 7 days. The follow-up procedure used in the Malaysian trial required an outpatient visit on days 10 and 14 and would probably have identified 3 of 4 relapses in our trial.

The Malaysian study (9) included at least one patient with duration of illness as short as 4 days, but the mean duration of illness of Malaysian patients at time of treatment was 10.6 days compared to 5.4 days in our series. The low incidence of eschar and rash and the fact that scrub typhus is a common cause of febrile illness in Malaysia (9) leads us to speculate that patients in the Malaysian trial may have had previous infections with one or more strains of R. tsutsugamushi. This may have caused the Malaysian patients to be less ill and incu-bate disease longer before the sought treatment.

Our results agree closely with the major finding of Brown et al. (9), in that doxycycline in single doses was highly effective in treating persons acutely ill with scrub typhus.

Doxycycline administered in one or 2 doses cured 40 of 43
(Table 4) patients who retained their medication. The two
patients who vomited their initial dose of doxycycline exem-
plify a concern for single dose therapy. The patient who vomits
his initial dose of standard tetracycline or chloramphenicol
treatment receives another dose 6 hrs later. The patient on a
single dose regimen is without the benefit of additional antibiotic.

    It is extremely important to note that some of the patients
treated in early stages of acute illness (less than 5 days
after onset) experienced relapse of symptoms regardless of
whether they received doxycycline or tetracycline. In our
series, 4 of 30 (13%) persons beginning treatments less than 5
days after onset experienced relapses. Further, 13 of 66 (20%)
patients experienced minor returns of fever which did not require retreatment with antibiotics.

    In conclusion, we recommend doxycycline therapy for scrub
typhus under difficult field conditions where medical support
is limited and drug compliance uncertain. The treatment of
acutely ill patients early in their disease involves significant risk of relapse and must include appropriate follow-up
procedures to identify and retreat patients who experience
return of symptoms.

                         V.   SUMMARY

    During 1976 a scrub typhus treatment trial was conducted
in the Pescadores Islands of Taiwan. Sixty-eight Chinese
military patients with scrub typhus confirmed by recovering R.
tsutsugamushi from acute phase blood or by demonstrating a
diagnostic rise in indirect immunofluorescent antibody from the
acute to the convalescent phase were treated with one of three
different treatment regimens. Twenty-two patients received a
single dose of 200 mg doxycycline by mouth, 23 patients received a single dose of 200 mg doxycycline by mouth on study
day 1 and 7, and 23 patients received oxytetracycline by mouth
500 mg every 6 hours for 7 days. Most patients experienced
rapid cures; there were, however, two primary treatment failures with doxycycline (both of which were due to vomiting of
the initial dose). Four patients had relapse of symptoms severe enough to require retreatment, and 3 of these had received
doxycycline. In addition, 13 patients (doxycycline 11; oxytetracycline 2) had returns of fevers of 37.6C or greater on 2
or more days which resolved without antibiotic intervention but
might be considered recrudescences of rickettsial illness. The
frequency of illness which necessitated retreatment among
patients who received antibiotic therapy less than 5 days after

onset of symptoms was 4 of 30 (13%) and among patients whose
therapy commenced after 5 or more days post-onset was 0 of 36.
These data documented the heightened risk of relapse in scrub
typhus when antibiotic therapy is commenced before 5 days of
illness. Further, the data document the occurrence of relapse
and recrudescence of self-limited fevers in patients treated
with doxycycline.

REFERENCES

1. Crozier, D., in "Current Therapy. Latest Approved Methods
    of Treatment for the Practicing Physicians" (H. F. Conn,
    ed.), p. 86. E. B. Saunders, Philadelphia, (1977).
2. Smadel, J. E., Woodward, T. E., Ley, H. L., Jr., and
    Lewthwaite, R., J. Clin. Invest. 28, 1196 (1949).
3. Bailey, C. A., Ley, H. L., Jr., Diercks, F. H., Lewthwaite,
    R., and Smadel, J. E., Antibiot. Chemother. 1, 16 (1951).
4. Prezyna, A. P., Teh-Ling, C., Tsu-Lin, W., Dougherty, W.J.,
    and Bond, H. B., Am. J. Trop. Med. Hyg. 3, 608 (1954).
5. Zarafonetis, C.J.D., and Baker, M. D., in "Internal Medi-
    cine in World War II. Vol. II. Infectious Diseases", p.
    111. Office of the Surgeon General, Department of the
    Army, Washington, D.C. (1963).
6. Sayen, J. J., Pond, H. S., Forrester, J. S., and Wood,
    F. C., Baltimore Medicine 25, 155 (1946).
7. Barza, M., and Shiefe, R. T., Am. J. Hosp. Pharm. 34, 48
    (1977).
8. Perine, P. L., Krause, D. W., Awoke, S., and McDade,
    J. E., Lancet II, 742 (1974).
9. Brown, G. W., Saunders, J. P., Singh, S., Huxsoll, D. L.,
    and Shirai, A., Trans. Roy. Soc. Trop. Med. Hyg. 72, 412
    (1978).
10. Bourgeois, A. L., Olson, J. G., Ho, C. M., Fang, R.C.Y.,
    and Van Peenen, P.F.D., Trans. Roy. Soc. Trop. Med. Hyg.
    71, 338 (1977).
11. Olson, J. G., and Bourgeois, A. L., Am. J. Epidemiol. 106,
    172 (1977).
12. Elisberg, B. L., and Bozeman, F. M., in "Diagnostic Proce-
    dures for Viral Rickettsial and Chlamydial Infections"
    (E. H. Lennette and N. J. Schmidt, eds.), p. 1080. APHA,
    Washington, D.C. (1979).
13. Bozeman, F. M., and Elisberg B. L., Proc. Soc. Exp. Biol.
    Med. 112, 568 (1963).
14. Smadel, J. E., Woodward, T. E., Ley, H. L., Jr., Philip,
    C. B., Traub, R., Lewthwaite, R., and Savoor, S. R.,
    Science 108, 160 (1948).
15. Smadel, J. E., Am. J. Med. 17, 246 (1954).
16. Sheehy, T. W., Hazlett, D., and Turk, R. E., Arch. Intern.
    Med. 132, 77 (1973).

ULTRASTRUCTURE OF RICKETTSIAE

TECHNIQUES FOR ELECTRON MICROSCOPY OF RICKETTSIAE

Susumu Ito
Yasuko Rikihisa

Department of Anatomy
Harvard Medical School
Boston, Massachusetts

I. INTRODUCTION

Since the development of the electron microscope and the improved preparative techniques for biological materials, rickettsial ultrastructure has become an integral part of rickettsial research. The small size of rickettsiae which is near the limit of resolution of the light microscope makes the electron microscope useful and necessary for critical morphological studies. The precise intracellular localization of rickettsiae can be established with certainty by electron microscopy. Furthermore, the ultrastructure of rickettsiae can be used to distinguish them from other microorganisms of similar size.

Since a historical review of the numerous contributions of electron microscopy to rickettsiology is beyond the limitations of this paper, we present a synopsis of techniques useful for rickettsial electron microscopy.

Electron micrographs are images of heavy metal deposits in selective sites in fixed or denatured cells. The specimens have been impregnated, dehydrated, infiltrated, heated, cooled, sliced, and irradiated so that they are far from being anything like the living microorganism. The images that the microscopist selects to illustrate the observations are based upon the investigators' interpretation that the images are representative of rickettsiae in the living state.

With these reservations we will present methods that have been employed in studying rickettsial ultrastructure. We will not attempt to describe every method that has been tried but will concentrate on those accepted as being appropriate for our objectives.

RICKETTSIAE AND RICKETTSIAL DISEASES

213

II. SPECIFIC TECHNIQUES

A. Thin Section Transmission Electron Microscopy

Although whole rickettsiae were among the earliest biological specimens examined with the electron microscope (1-3), thin
sections have given considerably more information on rickettsial ultrastructure (Fig. 1). The early demonstration that
rickettsiae were enclosed by two membranes (4-7) similar to
gram-negative bacteria was an important finding as was their
definitive identification in thin sections as an intracellular
parasite (8-10).

1. Fixation Methods. As with most aspects of biological
microscopy the initial fixation of the rickettsiae is a very
crucial step. A fixative found useful for many biological
samples including rickettsiae is a trinitro-containing solution
which was described some years ago (24). As used for rickettsiae, the final concentration of components are: 1.25% formaldehyde, 2.5% glutaraldehyde, 0.03% $CaCl_2$, and 0.03% trinitrocresol in 0.05 M cacodylate buffer, pH 7.4. Trinitrophenol or
picric acid may be substituted for the trinitrocresol which is
no longer available commercially. The stock solution of this
fixative without the glutaraldehyde is stable for months at
refrigerator temperature. The formaldehyde in the fixative is
made from paraformaldehyde by heating and adding sodium hydroxide. The glutaraldehyde that gives reproducible, acceptable
results is purified 25% glutaraldehyde purchased in sealed
ampoules.
Fixation is carried out at room temperature for about one
hour but specimens may be kept, stored, or mailed in this fixative and processed days later without apparent deleterious
effects.
There are many other routine and special fixation methods.
Among the most common are solutions of glutaraldehyde (21),
formaldehyde mixed with glutaraldehyde, permanganate, a mixture
of hydrogen peroxide and glutaraldehyde, a mixture of osmium
tetroxide and glutaraldehyde, or solutions of osmium tetroxide.
In our own experience the trinitro-containing fixative seems
to suit our purposes best.

2. Processing After Initial Fixation. After at least one
hour in the trinitro-fixative, the specimens are washed in
several changes of 0.2 M cacodylate buffer and osmicated with
1% OsO_4 in 0.1 M cacodylate buffer at pH 7.4 for one hour at
room temperature. With suspensions of isolated rickettsiae,
the specimens must be centrifuged at each solution change.
This step is followed by rinses in cacodylate buffer to wash

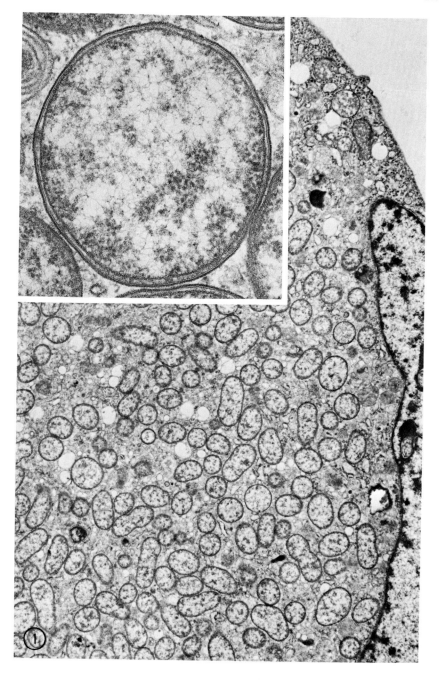

Fig. 1.   Electron micrograph of R. tsutsugamushi in a
BHK-21 cell, X6,500.   Inset: Enlarged rickettsiae showing trilaminar membranes, ribosomes and DNA filaments.   X100,000.

out unreacted osmium and then in a 0.1 M maleate buffer,
pH 5.2. The samples are then treated with 1% uranyl acetate
in maleate buffer, pH 5.2, for 1 hr at room temperature.

The uranium treatment appears to be essential to observe
two important ultrastructural characteristics of rickettsiae
(and other gram-negative microorganisms). Without the uranium
treatment the inner membrane is frequently unseen or not clear.
Another feature of this procedure is the preservation of rickettsial DNA as fine intermeshing filaments rather than as a
clumped mass seen after no uranium treatment. The procedure
must be carried out before dehydration of the tissue with alcohol. Although the chemical basis for these effects is not
clear, it appears that the uranium acts as some means of further fixing the inner membrane and the DNA filaments.

The next step is to make certain that the unreacted uranyl
acetate is washed out of the sample before dehydration. Several changes of maleate buffer, pH 5.2, are used for at least
several hours or even overnight. The reason for this careful
washout is that the dehydration process may precipitate the
uranium.

Dehydration with graded (50, 75, 95%) ethanol follows.
These alcohols are kept at 4°C. The solutions are added to the
tubes or vials containing the rickettsiae and changed as rapidly as is convenient and then allowed to warm up to room temperature in a sealed tube. Afterwards several changes of absolute
alcohol dehydration at room temperature are made and followed
by two or three changes in propylene oxide.

Several other practical points should be mentioned at this
stage. First, the use of minimal quantities of reagents is
needed for each solution change. For the usual pelleted sample
no more than 2 to 5 ml solutions need be used. When centrifugation is routinely done for concentrating specimens, the presence of ground glass in solutions should be avoided. All
solutions should be millipore-filtered prior to use.

The only step in our procedure for which we use cold solutions is the acohol dehydration step. All others are at room
temperature. The rationale for the cold alcohol is as follows:
ethanol at 50% dilution has at 0°C a rather high viscosity.
Therefore, dehydration by ethanol at lowered temperatures is
relatively slow. Furthermore, the low temperature tends to
minimize the heating caused by mixing ethanol with water.
These two aspects are believed to be beneficial in minimizing
possible damage to specimen ultrastructures.

The final step is plastic embedding. The most favorable
medium for rickettsial studies has been a very low viscosity
epon, 1,2,7,8-diepoxyoctane as described by Luft (16). When
mixed in a proportion of 18 parts diepoxyoctane to 32 parts
nonenyl succinic anhydride, it is a very fluid mixture even at
refrigerator temperature. To this mixture 2 to 3% DMP30

catalyst is added for both the propylene oxide-plastic infiltration step and the final embedding mixture. Since this epoxy
is designated as a possible carcinogen, and because it is rather expensive, we use it in minute quantities; only a few
tenths of one ml is adequate per embedding capsule. The remaining block is made by adding ordinary epoxy or quick-setting
dental mold material.

Most of the ordinary epoxy embedding substances have been
tried but the low viscosity diepoxyoctane is superior to others
because it seems to prevent the shrinkage of rickettsiae as indicated by the crinkled limiting membranes. It also minimizes
the presence of the clear halo surrounding intracellular organisms. This effect is presumed to be due to the more freely
penetrating plastic into the fixed rickettsiae.

After infiltration in the mixture of equal parts propylene
oxide with the low viscosity epon mixture, the samples are
placed in conical capsules with about 0.1 ml of the plastic
mixture and centrifuged into the tip with a clinical table centrifuge. The plastic is hardened at 60°C for about 12 hrs and
is then ready for thin sectioning.

The procedure for the preparation of thin sections is quite
standard; glass or diamond knives are used and thin sections on
bare grids are stained first with an equal volume of saturated
uranyl acetate and acetone for 10 to 15 seconds, rinsed with
water and then stained with lead citrate for an equal period.

B. Labeling of Antigenic Sites

The ultrastructural localization of antigenic sites with
conjugates of electron dense markers or enzymes to antibodies
has revealed much information on localizing immunologically
active sites. A sizable number of electron dense markers or
enzymes have been attached to specific antibodies for antigen
localization (23). In this paper, we will describe only the
immunoferritin technique which we have found to be most useful
since the ferritin is precisely localized and is characteristically dense. Anacker et al. described the first immunoferritin
label of Coxiella burnetii (25). In general, most immunolabeling methods share common basic principles. Two key factors for
the consistent and precise immunoferritin labeling are the removal of nonspecific label binding and the adequate penetration
of antibodies into the specimens to the antigenic site (except
when dealing with the easily approachable superficial antigens). The method routinely used in our laboratory for obtaining ferritin-conjugated antibodies is as follows: commercial
ferritin (twice recrystallized) from horse spleen is further
purified by four additional cycles of crystallization with
$CdSO_4$ and three cycles of precipitation with 50% saturated
$(NH_4)_2SO_4$. This ferritin is dialyzed extensively against

distilled water to remove the $(NH_4)_2SO_4$ which otherwise inhibits the reaction of conjugation. Contaminating apoferritin is removed by three centrifugations at 100,000g for 3 hrs. This step is important, since apoferritin (ferritin with low iron content) cannot be seen by electron microscopy. The purified ferritin is then suspended in 0.05 M potassium phosphate buffer pH 7.4 and stored at 4°C.

Goat antiserum against rabbit Fc fraction of IgG or goat antiserum against rabbit IgG can be used (both work equally well). Antiserum is purified to obtain the IgG fraction and the anti-rabbit Fc goat-IgG is conjugated with the purified ferritin particles. The bifunctional reagent, P,P'-difluoro-m, m'-dinitrodiphenylsulfone according to the procedure of Sri Ram et al. (14) is used. An appropriate volume of an acetone solution of the reagent (5 mg/ml) is added to a final concentration of 0.3 mg/ml of the conjugating reagent in a mixture of 4% protein of ferritin and IgG of the same molar ratio. The reaction is done in 2% Na_2CO_3 (pH 10.5) at 0°C for 24 hrs. The quantity and quality of the ferritin-labeled antibody is then determined by cellulose acetate membrane electrophoresis on a Microzone Electrophoresis System as described previously (11). Unlabeled IgG and nonspecific binding substances are removed from the ferritin-labeled antibody preparation by the method of Rikihisa et al. (11). This purification is essential because the non-reacted IgG inhibits the specific binding of ferritin antibody. Furthermore, nonspecific binding substances (denatured and highly anionic ferritin) produce a high background of ferritin and inhibit specific binding.

Once a good, clean, specific labeled antibody has been made, the next step is to get the immunolabel to the antigenic site while maintaining good cell ultrastructure. Although cells may be labeled before fixation after some kind of permeabilization procedure, cell structures tend to suffer during the immunolabeling procedure. On the other hand, good or complete fixation may render the antigenic sites unrecognizable to the labeled antigen. To preserve structural details and also to label intracellular sites, the following procedure has been adapted for rickettsial studies.

The infected host cells or the isolated rickettsial preparations are fixed in 2% formaldehyde in PBS at room temperature for 10 min and washed in PBS three times. This minimizes the degeneration of cells during subsequent incubations with antibodies and does not reduce the antigenicity determined by using ^{125}I-labeled antibodies.

To make the rickettsiae-infected host cells readily permeable to labeled antibodies, the cells are frozen in phosphate-buffered saline (PBS), pH 7.4, by immersing vials in a dry ice-alcohol mixture, and thawed in a 37°C water bath. This ruptures the host cell membranes.

The immunolabeling with antibodies is carried out with about 3×10^6 formaldehyde-fixed, infected host cells in 0.2 to 0.5 ml PBS. To each of these batches a final concentration of 7 mg/ml of the IgG fraction of following antibodies is added: antibody against rickettsiae grown in yolk sac or BHK cell culture or non-immunized rabbit IgG as a control. The mixtures are reacted for 15 min at room temperature, washed twice with PBS and reacted with a final concentration of 10 mg/ml of ferritin-labeled goat anti-rabbit Fc for 15 min at room temperature. An excess of antibodies is used to insure that all available antigens are reacted. After washing in PBS to remove as much of the non-reacted ferritin-labeled antibody as possible, the samples are fixed and processed as pellets as described above for thin section electron microscopy. Specimens are then examined for sites with ferritin-labeled particles (Fig. 2).

Although it is possible to employ the direct immunoferritin technique, the indirect technique has the advantage that any antibody made in the same species (in this case the rabbit) may be used. It also avoids the decrease in titer of the specific antibody during the direct conjugation step and amplifies the labeling of antigenic sites. It should be cautioned, however, that there is an increased possibility of nonspecific binding and requires increased reaction time.

III. OTHER TECHNIQUES

Space, time, and editorial restrictions do not allow more than brief descriptions of the seven remaining common electron microscope techniques.

1. _Negative Staining._ The simplest method of examining rickettsiae in the electron microscope is to dry the microorganisms onto film-coated grids and use the inherent electron absorbing and scattering characteristics to study their morphology. However, this has many limitations and a more useful method is negative staining with uranyl acetate or phosphotungstic acid. By this technique, the biological specimen is revealed in negative contrast because the background is made dense by the stain (Fig. 3).

For the rickettsial negative staining the infected host cells are disrupted by freezing and thawing and a small drop of diluted specimen is placed on a carbon-coated celloidin or formvar-coated grid. The surface of the grid is then washed with three successive drops of 1% uranyl acetate in water. Care must be taken to avoid wetting the under surface of the grids. The fluid is drawn off the grid by touching the edge

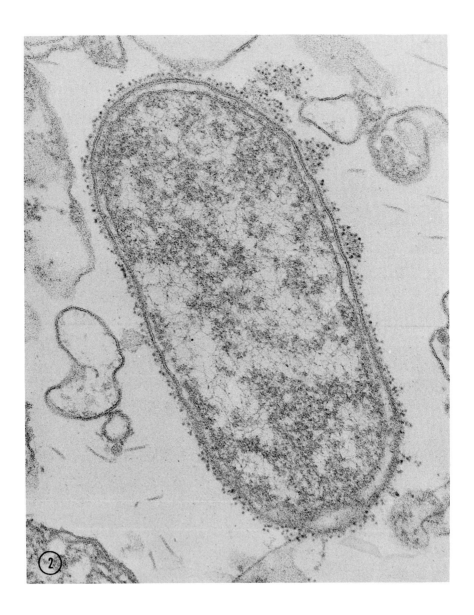

Fig. 2. R. tsutsugamushi in a BHK-21 cell immunolabeled
with rabbit anti-R. tsutsugamushi IgG and ferritin conjugated
goat anti-rabbit Fc fraction of IgG. The ferritin label is
present only on the surface of the rickettsiae. X99,000.

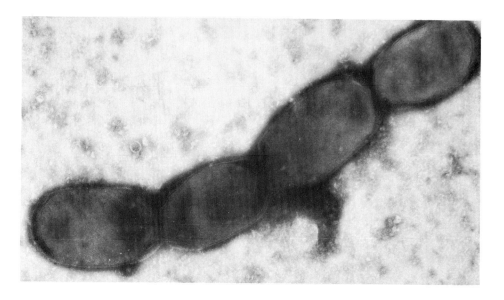

Fig. 3.   A chain of four R. rickettsii negatively stained with uranyl acetate.   X32,400.

of the drop with the edge of a filter paper. Grids are then air dried and treated under UV light to inactivate the rickett-siae before examination.

    2. Freeze-Fracture Replicas. This technique has been used to relatively little advantage in rickettsial studies but has become a primary method for studying the internal structure of membranes in general. These replicas give little information on cellular structures other than membranes (Fig. 4). For general information the reader is referred to reference 17.
    For rickettsial freeze-fracture replicas, heavily infected cell cultures or isolated pellets are good sources of material. The samples are fixed in the standard fixative or one of the other glutaraldehyde-containing fixatives for 30 min. The specimens are washed in a buffer solution and then treated with 20% glycerol buffer, pH 7.4, for 2 hrs. Concentrated suspen-sions of cells or rickettsiae are placed on gold disks and fro-zen rapidly in liquid freon 22 cooled with liquid nitrogen. These samples are stored in liquid nitrogen until replicas are to be made. The fracturing and coating techniques will not be described because they are related to the specific equipment employed.
    After the specimens are platinum-shadowed and carbon-coated, they are removed and digested with 4-6% sodium hypo-chloride to remove the organic material. Washing in distilled

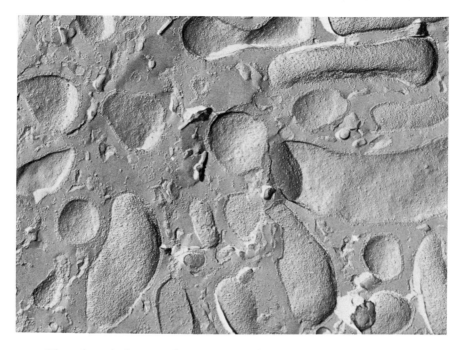

Fig. 4. A freeze fracture replica of R. mooseri in louse
intestinal epithelium. X32,900.

water and collecting the replicas on copper grids complete the
procedure.

  3. Scanning Electron Microscopy. This technique limits
observatioṇ to the very outer surface of biological specimens.
It also has somewhat limited resolution when compared to transmission electron microscopy. The advantage of scanning electron microscopy is that it visualizes large surface areas and
has a great depth of field (see reference 19 for general information).
  In infected host cells, rickettsiae are revealed only when
they protrude from the cells (Fig. 5) or when the cytoplasm of
the host cell is exposed.
  To prepare such specimens, infected cells grown in plastic
culture dishes are fixed and dehydrated in situ by standard
methods. The dishes are then cut or cracked into 1 cm squares,
dried by the critical point technique and coated with a thin
layer of gold or gold-palladium.
  In the scanning electron microscope, the only part of the
specimens revealed is the metal coating over the biological
sample. Thus, projecting rickettsiae are visible due to their
shape and the gold coating.

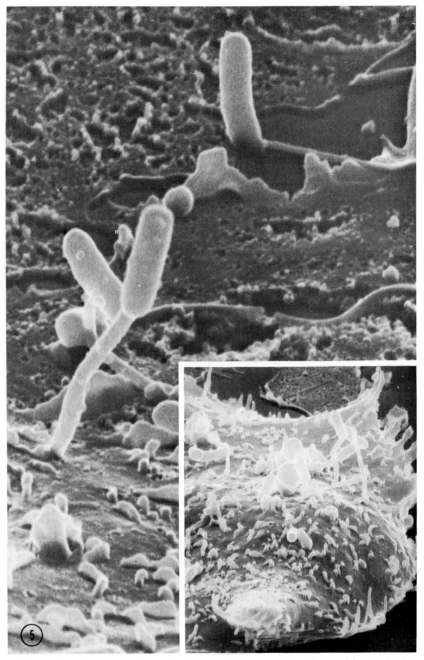

Fig. 5. A scanning electron micrograph of BT-20 cell infected with R. rickettsii protruding at the tip of stalks. X27,000. Inset: A rotated low power view of the same cell. X7,000.

    4. Electron Microscope Autoradiography. This technique
localizes the site of incorporated radioactive precursors to
sites less than 0.1 μm (18,23). The usual procedure is to
grow rickettsiae in a medium containing maximal amounts of
the labeled precursor that the cells will tolerate. The isotope of choice is tritium-labeled compounds but other isotopes
may also be used.

    In the examples provided (Figs. 6A,B) rickettsiae growing
in cultured cells were given ^{3}H-thymidine or ^{3}H-uridine at a
dose of about 25 μCi/ml. The cells were harvested at appropriate intervals and processed as described earlier for transmission electron microscopy. Both light microscope and electron microscope autoradiography may be made for the same specimens. For light microscopy, 0.5 or 1.0 μm thick sections are
cut and dried onto gelatinized glass slides. These slides are
coated by dipping them into Ilford L4 emulsion diluted two
times with water. After drying, the slides are stored in the
dark and developed for 5 min in Kodak D-19 developer. Very
radioactive specimens may be developed in one day but the usual
exposure period is several days to weeks.

    The emulsion is cleared in an acid-fixing solution and the
slides are stained for 30 min in 1% toluidine blue, pH 7.2, in
0.15 M phosphate buffer. The dried slides are then mounted in
immersion oil and cover-glassed.

    For electron microscopy autoradiography, the same blocks
may be thin-sectioned and picked up on bare copper grids.
These sections are coated with a thin layer of Ilford L4 emulsion applied with a wire loop. After exposure of 2 weeks or
more the grids are stained with standard alkaline lead citrate
stain used for thin sections for 10 min and viewed in the electron microscope after washing with water.

    The light microscope autoradiographs reveal much about the
level of radioactivity and the areas of localization. However,
the electron microscope can show the detailed localization of
the radioactive sites and provide a means for identifying the
ultrastructural sites of substrate incorporation.

    5. High Voltage, Electron Probe and Rapid Freeze Electron
Microscopy. High voltage microscopy is characterized by the
greater penetrating power of the electron beam. The commonly
used acceleration voltage is one million volts compared to the
one hundred thousand volts or less used in conventional electron microscopy. Ordinary plastic embedded sections may be cut
at up to several micrometers in thickness and viewed directly
in the microscope (20). These sections would be virtually
opaque in the conventional electron microscope. The major
problem with thick specimens is that there is too much information and much confusing overlapping of structural components.
Some of this disadvantage can be overcome by employing stereo

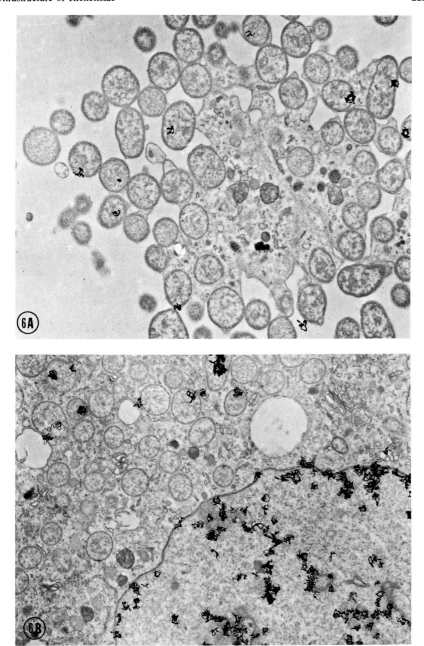

Fig. 6A. R. tsutsugamushi in BHK-21 cells incubated with 25 μCi/ml ³H-uridine, 5 d. Few grains on some rickettsiae. X9,000. Fig. 6B. Similar rickettsiae incubated with 25 μCi/ml ³H-thymidine show limited uptake. Host cell nucleus is very radioactive. X7,400.

pairs. Another major limitation is that structures must be
selectively stained or contrasted to reveal rickettsiae or
other components.

Electron probe analysis is a technique that allows the determination of elements in the specimen in areas restricted to
less than one micrometer in diameter. There are two types of
electron probes and both use electrons to excite x-rays from
the specimen. The most common type is the energy dispersive
x-ray analysis which results in the display of the spectrum of
x-rays so that the range of elements above the atomic number
of 6, carbon is detectable. A major disadvantage of this
method is that fewer elements can be quantified than by the
wavelength dispersive spectrometers. In this type of electron
probe analysis, the x-rays being emitted by the specimens are
specifically detected and readily quantitated (22).

The rapid freezing technique to immobilize living cells
offers an interesting approach to the study of rickettsiae.
This method employs a metal surface such as pure copper or
silver cooled with liquid nitrogen or, more recently, with
liquid helium. Cells or tissues in the living state are frozen
as rapidly as possible so that the ice crystals which are
formed are very small. The ice should be so fine that the
cellular structures should be comparable with specimens fixed
by the best of the chemical methods. The early liquid nitrogen freezing device of van Harrevald (12) has been modified by
the Heuser and Reese (13) apparatus which employs liquid
helium. The results are more reproducible and the depth of
good freezing is increased from a few micrometers to 10 or 15
μm by the improved, though expensive, method using liquid
helium.

Once frozen, the samples may be fixed with 2 to 4% osmium
tetroxide in acetone at -79°C by freeze substitution fixation.
After several hours or days at this temperature, the tissues
are gradually warmed, dehydration is completed in absolute acetone and the sample is embedded in plastic and examined, as
described for thin section transmission electron microscopy.
Alternatively, the frozen samples may be kept cold, fractured
and coated for freeze-fracture replica information. Both methods have their distinct advantages and limitations. In
either case, however, it is imperative that the freezing quality must be very good or the specimens become a useless mass of
small ice crystals.

REFERENCES

1. Plotz, H., Smadel, J. E., Anderson, T. F., and Chambers,
    L. A., J. Exp. Med. 77, 355 (1943).

2. Shepard, C. C., and Wyckoff, R.W.G., Public Health Rep. 61, 761 (1946).
3. Van Rooyten, C. E., and Scott, G. D., Can. J. Res. 26E, 250 (1949).
4. Schaechter, M., Tousimis, A. J., Cohn, Z. A., Rosen, H., Campbell, J., and Hahn, F. E., J. Bacteriol. 74, 822 (1957).
5. Higashi, N., in "Recent Advances in Studies of Tsutsuga-mushi Disease in Japan" (T. Tamiya, ed.), p. 145. Medical Culture, Inc., Tokyo (1962).
6. Anacker, R. L., Pickens, E. G., and Lackman, D. B., J. Bacteriol. 94, 260 (1967).
7. Shkolnick, L. Y., Zatulousky, B. G., and Shestopalova, N. M., Acta Virol. 10, 260 (1966).
8. Wissig, S. L., Caro, L. G., Jackson, E. B., and Smadel, J. E., Amer. J. Pathol. 32, 1117 (1956).
9. Anderson, D. R., Hopps, H. E., Barile, M. F., and Bernheim, B. C., J. Bacteriol. 90, 1387 (1965).
10. Jadin, J., Greemers, J., Jain, J. M., and Giroud, P., Acta Virol. 12, 7 (1968).
11. Rikihisa, Y., Ohkuma, S., and Mizuno, D., Cell Struct. Func. 1, 251 (1976).
12. Van Harrevald, A., and Crowell, J., Anat. Rec. 149, 381 (1964).
13. Heuser, J. E., Reese, T. S., Dennis, M. J., Jan, Y., Jan, L., and Evans, L., J. Cell Biol. 81, 275 (1979).
14. Sri Ram, J., Tawde, S. S., Pierce, G. B., and Midgley, A. R., J. Cell Biol. 17, 673 (1963).
15. Rogers, A. W., in "Techniques of Autoradiography" Elevier/North-Holland, New York (1979).
16. Luft, J. H., in "Advanced Techniques in Biological Electron Microscopy" (J. K. Koehler, ed.), p. 1. Springer-Verlag, New York (1973).
17. Bullivant, S., ibid. p. 67.
18. Salpeter, M. M., and McHenry, F. A., ibid. p. 113.
19. Hayes, T. L., ibid. p. 153.
20. Hama, K., ibid. p. 153.
21. Glauert, A. M., in "Practical Methods in Electron Microscopy" (A. M. Glauert, ed.), Vol 3, p. 1. North-Holland Publishing Co., New York (1975).
22. Chandler, J. A., ibid., Vol. 5, p. 313 (1977).
23. Williams, M. A., ibid., Vol. 6, p. 1 (1977).
24. Ito, S., and Karnovsky, M. L., J. Cell Biol. 51, 146a (1971).
25. Anacker, R. L., Fukushi, K., Pickens, E. G., and Lackman, D. B., J. Bacteriol. 88, 1130 (1964).

OUTER MEMBRANE VESICLES
OF RICKETTSIA TSUTSUGAMUSHI

Yasuko Rikihisa
Susumu Ito

Department of Anatomy
Harvard Medical School
Boston, Massachusetts

I. INTRODUCTION

During the course of a study on the immunolabeling
characteristics of Rickettsia tsutsugamushi (1), small vesicles containing flocculent material were found labeled with
immunoferritin in the host cell cytoplasm. The present report is an attempt to determine the source and to define some
of the characteristics of these vesicles. They appear to be
outer membrane vesicles of rickettsia and share similar features with outer membrane vesicles excreted from E. coli. In
a mutant of E. coli it was found that under certain conditions
there was an excretion of diaminopimelic acid as well as lipid
and carbohydrates which were identified as a lipopolysaccharide (LPS) (2,3). Electron microscopic observations revealed
that these vesicles were formed from blebs which pinched off
from the outer bacterial membrane (4). Analysis of these
outer membrane vesicles showed 60% LPS, 26% lipid (mostly
phosphatidyl ethanolamine), and 11% protein (5). More recently (6), it was reported that these vesicles were formed and
excreted by any strain of E. coli or Salmonella when protein
synthesis was inhibited by chloramphenicol or when certain required amino acids were restricted.

Supported in part by NIH grant R01 AI 11508 and NSF
grant DCM 78-16158.

The experimental conditions favoring the formation of the outer membrane vesicles of R. tsutsugamushi were not investigated in detail and the isolation of these vesicles for chemical analysis was not attempted. The present study reports some observations on the immunolabeling characteristics, reaction to antibodies, labeling with cationized ferritin, and the ultrastructural features of the outer membrane vesicles. These observations are directed toward comparing the relationship and properties of these vesicles with the outer rickettsial membrane on intact microorganisms.

II. MATERIALS AND METHODS

Rickettsia tsutsugamushi, Gilliam strain used for this study was obtained from the Walter Reed Army Institute of Research, Washington, D.C., and propagated in BHK-21 cells, clone 13 (Lister Institute, London) as described in previous studies (1). Cultures were grown in a modified Rubella medium (7) and rickettsiae in infected BHK-21 cells were screened with Gram or Giemsa stain as well as by fluorescent antibody techniques (1). The antiserum to rickettsiae was raised in rabbits as described previously in detail (1), and the immunolabeling technique employed goat anti-rabbit IgG which was ferritin labeled (9).

Rickettsiae were labeled with cationized ferritin (Miles Labs, Inc., Kankakee, IL) by incubation with 2 mg of the ferritin solution per ml of PBS for 30 min at room temperature. Some microorganisms were left intact while other samples were disrupted by freezing to -20°C and thawing, or by sonication (1). Electron microscope preparations were made as previously described (1). The rickettsial pellets were fixed in formaldehyde and trinitrocresol (8), and embedded in a low viscosity epon. Acrolein fixation was according to Silverman et al. (10). Thin sections were stained with uranyl acetate and lead citrate and examined in a JEOL 100B, 100CX or 100S electron microscope.

III. RESULTS

A. Immunoferritin Label of Intracellular Rickettsiae

When heavily infected BHK-21 cells were frozen and thawed, fixed with 2% formaldehyde, and immunolabeled with anti-rickettsiae IgG and ferritin-labeled goat anti-rabbit Fc, rickettsial surfaces were heavily and specifically labeled with

ferritin. With nonimmune rabbit IgG instead of anti-rickettsiae IgG, no immunoferritin label was observed (1). The cytoplasmic components of BHK-21 cells remained unlabeled, but some
small vesicles were heavily labeled (Fig. 1). The ferritin
labeling of these vesicles was usually more prominent and
thicker than that on the intact rickettsiae (Fig. 1 Inset).
The thickness of vesicle membrane is about 13nm and is similar
to the outer rickettsial membrane and is distinctly different
from the inner rickettsial membranes which are about 6nm thick
as well as from the host cell cytoplasmic membranes.

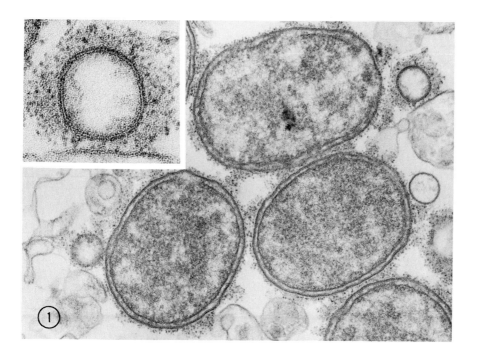

Fig. 1. Immunoferritin-labeled R. tsutsugamushi in the
cytoplasm of BHK-21 cells. Infected cells were reacted with
anti-rickettsiae IgG and ferritin-conjugated goat anti-rabbit
Fc IgG. Note thicker ferritin label on the outer membrane
vesicles X 89,300. Figure 1 inset is a higher magnification of
one of vesicles labeled with immunoferritin. Note that the
thickness of the membrane resembles the outer rickettsial membrane and the amorphous material contained within the vesicle
X 233,000.

When formaldehyde-glutaraldehyde-trinitrocresol (FGC)-fixed
BHK-21 cells infected with R. tsutsugamushi for 6 to 8 days
were examined, characteristic vesicles ranging from 0.10 to
0.30 nm in diameter and either round or slightly elongated in
sectioned profiles were found in the BHK-21 cell cytoplasm.
These vesicles were relatively homogenous in size and measured
$0.15 \pm 0.02 \, \mu m$ (N = 32) in diameter. At this stage, most BHK-
21 cells were heavily infected with rickettsiae and contained
randomly distributed outer membrane vesicles. Some vesicles
were adjacent to the inner surface of the host cell plasma membrane (Fig. 2) but none were observed to protrude from the surface like intact rickettsiae.

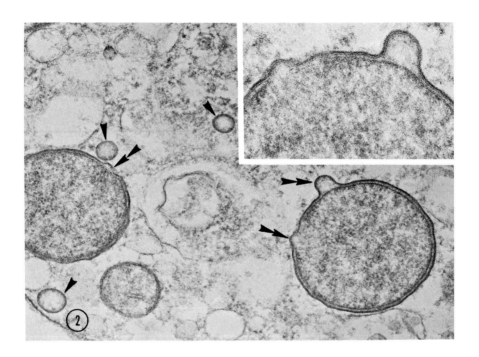

Fig. 2. A part of a FGC-fixed BHK-21 cell infected with
rickettsiae. There are three outer membrane vesicles (arrows)
and two rickettsiae with small protrusions of their outer membranes (double arrows). X47,000. Figure 2 inset is a higher
magnification of the protrusions. The outer rickettsial membrane forms the blebs while the inner membrane maintains a flat
contour. Note the presence of an amorphous lining in the outer
membrane protrusion. X94,000.

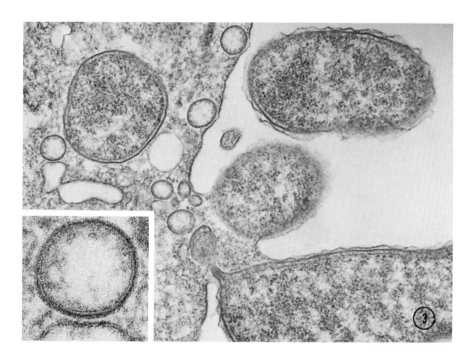

Fig. 3. A part of acrolein fixed BHK-21 cell infected with rickettsiae. The outer membrane vesicles appear similar to those in Fig. 2. Rickettsiae often protrude from the surface of BHK-21 cells still tightly surrounded with the host cell membrane. Some outer membrane vesicles are located adjacent to the inner surface of the plasma membrane. X62,000.
Fig. 3 Inset. A vesicle at higher magnification. Note that the thick outer leaflet of the vesicle membrane is clearly distinct from neighboring host cell membranes. X250,000.

The vesicles always consisted of a single enveloping membrane. The thick outer leaflet of these vesicle membranes was about 8.5 nm while the inner leaflet at 2.4 nm was considerably thinner. These leaflets were separated by a uniformly thin clear space of about 2.5 nm so that the total thickness of this membrane was about 13 nm as shown in Fig. 2.
Similar dimensions for the enclosing membrane were found after acrolein-glutaraldehyde fixation (Fig. 3). The appearance and thickness of this membrane were very similar to the outer membrane of intact rickettsiae and clearly different from vesicles formed from host cell membranes or the inner membrane of rickettsiae. After acrolein-glutaraldehyde fixation, rickettsial ribosomes were more discrete than after

FGC fixation, but the inner rickettsial membrane was more distinct after FGC fixation. In general, there was no great difference in the number or appearance of these vesicles after
either of the fixation methods (Figs. 2 and 3). The inner
surface of the outer membrane vesicles was lined with amorphous material similar in appearance to material present between the inner and outer membranes of rickettsiae (Figs. 1,
2,3,4, insets). The central region of these vesicles contained a small amount of low density flocculent material and
no ribosomes, DNA filaments, nor membranous structures were
found in any outer membrane vesicle.

     Occasional rickettsiae had blebs or protrusions of the
outer membranes as shown in Fig. 2 and inset. These protrusions contained some amorphous material similar to the contents of outer membrane vesicles. The inner rickettsiae membrane under the blebs maintained the normal contour of the
microorganism.

     In the samples of heavily infected BHK-21 cells there
were always a number of damaged, disrupted host cells. Outer
membrane vesicles of R. tsutsugamushi were also present within
remnants of these BHK-21 cells among the rickettsiae.

     B. Membrane Vesicles Reacted With Anti-Rickettsia IgG

     When heavily rickettsia-infected BHK-21 cells were incu-
bated with IgG fraction of rabbit antiserum against live
rickettsiae grown in yolk sac or grown in BHK-21 cell cultures,
these membrane vesicles as well as the rickettsiae were coated
with a prominent fuzzy coat (Fig. 4). When nonimmunized
rabbit IgG was used as a control, this coating was not seen.
The thickness of the fuzzy coat varied from 20 to 100 nm and
was usually thicker on the vesicles than that on the rickettsiae. After treatment with antisera, the thickness of the
outer leaflet of the vesicle membrane was reduced to about
5 nm (Fig. 4, inset), but the thickness of outer leaflet of
outer membrane of intact rickettsiae was not affected by the
incubation with the antibody.

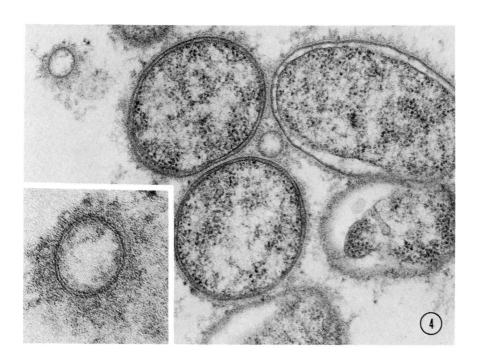

Fig. 4. R. tsutsugamushi from disrupted BHK-21 cells incubated with antibody against rickettsiae. Rickettsiae as
well as vesicles are coated with a layer of antibody which
appears fuzzy. X58,000. Fig. 4 Inset. An outer membrane
vesicle at higher magnification. There is a thick, fuzzy
coat of antibody on the leaflet. In these preparations, the
outer leaflet is thinner than on rickettsiae not exposed to
antibody. X145,000.

C. Cationized Ferritin Label of Rickettsiae

To localize the negative charged sites on rickettsiae,
cationized ferritin labeling was used. Rickettsiae often protrude from the surface of BHK-21 cells, tightly surrounded
with the host cell plasma membrane. Cationized ferritin
labeled the entire surface of BHK-21 cells including rickettsial protrusions (Fig. 5). In disrupted, infected BHK cells,
cytoplasmic membranes such as mitochondria and endoplasmic
reticulum were labeled with cationized ferritin but the
rickettsial surface was not labeled (Fig. 6). To expose the
interior of rickettsiae to cationized ferritin, the rickettsiae were first fixed and then mildly disrupted by sonication.

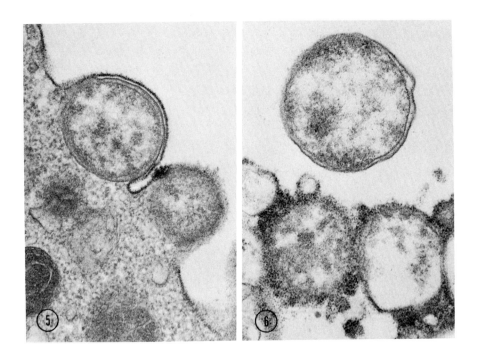

Fig. 5. Cationized ferritin label of infected BHK-21
cells. The entire cell surface including the area of rickettsial protrusion is homogeneously labeled with cationized
ferritin. X48,700.

Fig. 6. Cationized ferritin label of disrupted BHK-21
cells infected with rickettsiae. While the host cell cytoplasmic membranes is heavily labeled, there is absence of
labeling on the surface of rickettsia. X60,000.

Cationized ferritin still did not label the outer surface of
rickettsiae, but the inner surface of the outer membrane and
the outerside of inner membrane were labeled by a monolayer of
ferritin (Fig. 7). When the inner surface of the inner membrane was exposed to the label, in well disrupted specimens,
this surface was also labeled. Bits of fragmented outer membranes also labeled on their innerside which could be distinguished by the thick outlayer. When antibody-reacted rickettsiae with a coating of antibody were incubated with cationized ferritin, rickettsiae as well as the outer membrane vesicles were moderately labeled with cationized ferritin (Fig.
8).

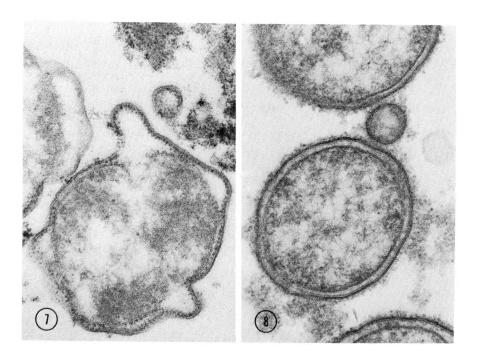

Fig. 7. Cationized ferritin labeling of rickettsiae disrupted by sonication. Innerside of the outer membrane and outer surface of inner membrane are labeled while the free surface of the rickettsia is not labeled. Note that the labeling is limited to the inner side of the vesicle membrane. X88,700.

Fig. 8. Cationized ferritin label of rickettsiae reacted with anti-rickettsial IgG. Rickettsiae as well as the vesicles are coated with a fuzzy material and are labeled with cationized ferritin. X103,000.

IV. DISCUSSION

This study provides the first detailed description of the small outer membrane vesicles of R. tsutsugamushi in the cytoplasm of infected BHK-21 cells. Since both acrolein-glutaraldehyde as well as glutaraldehyde-formaldehyde-trinitrocresol fixation resulted in the similar numbers of these vesicles, and because similar vesicles are not found in noninfected BHK-21 cells, it seems reasonable to attribute them to be normally occurring structures and not due to the preparation technique. The presence of evagination or protrusions from the outer membrane suggest that the vesicles originate from these blebs. In free living E. coli, outer membrane vesicles 12-200 nm in diameter are excreted when protein synthesis is inhibited with antibiotics or by amino acid depletion. These excreted vesicles were found to contain more lipid and less glycoprotein than the E. coli outer membrane. The origin of these vesicles have been attributed to the many small blebs on the surface of E. coli (4). The rickettsial outer membrane vesicles are consistently larger (100-300 nm) than the E. coli vesicles and more uniform in size.

The factors which bring about the formation of the rickettsial outer membrane vesicles is not known but may be due to some unbalance of rickettsial outer membrane synthesis in heavily infected BHK-21 cells.

The physiological role of these vesicles is also unknown. However, some of these vesicles have been observed in close opposition to the innerside of the plasma membrane of BHK-21 cells and may be exteriorized by some mechanism. The immuno-labeling characteristics of these vesicles indicate that they have similar or more enhanced surface immunoreactivity than whole rickettsiae. Thus, it seems possible that extracellular rickettsial vesicles may interact with other potential host cells as smaller units of rickettsiae. However, we have not observed any outer membrane vesicles in phagosomes or in the process of invading the cytoplasm of new host cells.

Cationized ferritin labeling indicates the absence of negative charges on the outer surface of rickettsiae. However, negatively charged sites as indicated by the labeling of this marker are found on the innerside of the outer membrane and outer surface of inner membrane surrounding rickettsiae. After rickettsiae are reacted with antibody, their outer surfaces were labeled with cationized ferritin. Silverman et al. also reported ruthenium red labeling after antibody treatment of rickettsiae (10). It is not clear whether the substances with negative charges are not present on the outer surface or

whether they are easily sloughed off during specimen preparation and that the addition of antibodies stabilizes these
sites. These anionic sites may be lipopolysaccharide or its
precursor as observed on Salmonella typhimurium with immunoferritin technique by Shandes (11) using antibody against
lipopolysaccharide.

Much further clarification of the role and significance
of rickettsial outer membrane vesicles is needed. However,
the present observation on the high density of antigenic
sites on these vesicles may make their isolation and purification in large quantities feasible. If this is possible,
these vesicle preparations may be used for the effective
production of surface antigens for possible use as source
of rickettsial vaccines.

V. SUMMARY

When R. tsutsugamushi infected BHK-21 cells were
reacted with rabbit anti-rickettsia IgG and ferritin conjugated goat anti-rabbit IgG, the outer surface of the rickettsiae and vesicles about 150 nm in diameter were specifically
labeled with immunoferritin. These vesicles appear to be
formed by blebbing of the outer membrane of intact rickettsiae and retain the ultrastructural features of the outer
rickettsial membrane. The rickettsial outer membrane vesicles are not found in uninfected BHK-21 cells but are present in rickettsiae infected host cells after different fixation methods and are presumed to be naturally occurring
structures. Further indication that the outer membrane vesicles are of rickettsial origin is that neither intact rickettsiae nor these vesicles are labeled with cationized ferritin.
After mild disruption with sonication the inner surfaces of
both the rickettsial outer membrane and the outer membrane
vesicles are cationized ferritin labeled. In addition, after
incubation with anti-rickettsia IgG, outer surfaces of both
the rickettsial outer membrane and the vesicles are cationized ferritin labeled. Since the rickettsial outer membrane
vesicles have similar immunolabeling characteristics with the
rickettsial outer membrane, the possibility that they may be
useful as a source of specific rickettsial surface antigens
is suggested by this study.

ACKNOWLEDGMENTS

The skilled assistance of Louise Aulenbach is gratefully acknowledged. The cultivation of rickettsiae was done in the Department of Microbiology at the Harvard School of Public Health. The use of their facilities for this purpose is greatly appreciated.

REFERENCES

1. Rikihisa, Y., Rota, T., Lee, T. H., MacDonald, A. B., and Ito, S., Infect. Immun. 26, 638 (1979).
2. Bishop, D. G., and Work, E., Biochem. J. 96, 567 (1965).
3. Taylor, A., Knox, K. W., and Work, E., Biochem. J. 99, 53 (1966).
4. Knox, K. W., Vesk, M., and Work, E., J. Bacteriol. 92, 1206 (1966).
5. Knox, K. W., Cullen, J., and Work, E., Biochem. J. 103, 192 (1967).
6. Rothfield, L., and Pearlman-Kothenez, M., J. Molec. Biol. 44, 477 (1969).
7. Rikihisa, Y., and Ito, S., J. Exp. Med. 150, 703 (1979).
8. Ito, S., and Karnovsky, M. J., J. Cell Biol. 39, 1968a (1968).
9. Rikihisa, Y., Ohkuma, S., and Mizuno, D., Cell Struct. Func. 1, 251 (1976).
10. Silverman, D. J., Wisseman, C. L., Jr., Waddell, A. D., and Jones, M., Infect. Immun. 22, 233 (1978).
11. Shands, J. W., Ann. New York Acad. Sci. 133, 292 (1966).

ENVELOPMENT AND ESCAPE OF <u>RICKETTSIA RICKETTSII</u> FROM HOST MEMBRANES

David J. Silverman
Charles L. Wisseman, Jr.
Anna Waddell

Department of Microbiology
University of Maryland School of Medicine
Baltimore, Maryland

I.   INTRODUCTION

Recent comparative electron microscopic studies of the intracellular growth of <u>Rickettsia prowazekii</u> and <u>Rickettsia rickettsii</u> in chicken embryo fibroblasts (1, 2) have revealed striking differences in these two organisms' capacity for producing visible cytopathology of the infected host cell. <u>R. prowazekii</u>, on the one hand, which multiplies free only in the cytoplasm, produces no significant demonstrable cytopathic changes in the host until late in infection, despite the accumulation of large numbers of intracellular rickettsiae (2). <u>R. rickettsii</u>, on the other hand, multiplies in both nucleus and cytoplasm, has the capacity for bidirectional movement into and out of cells, and causes early cytopathic changes in the form of widespread dilatation of the outer nuclear envelope and rough-surfaced endoplasmic reticulum (1, 3). The dilatation of these membranes eventually is followed by the appearance of small islets of host cell cytoplasm within the swollen cisternae. These islets presumably are created by fusion of adjacent cisternal membranes and

---

[1]   Supported by contract DADA 17-71-C-1007 with the U.S. Army Medical Research and Development Command, and the Pangborn Fund, University of Maryland School of Medicine.

entrapment of interceding cytoplasmic matrix. As the extent
of internal membrane dilatation increases, rickettsiae also
become entrapped within these membranes, and at terminal
stages of infection, membrane-bound rickettsiae appear to
comprise 40%-50% of the total cytoplasmic rickettsial
population (1). Rickettsiae in the nucleus, however, seem to
be unaffected.

The purpose of this study is to examine the supernatant
culture fluids of R. rickettsii-infected chicken embryo cells
to determine whether these rickettsiae are released from
infected cells in a membrane-bound state, as suggested by
their intracellular appearance late in the infection cycle.

II. METHODS

Plaque purified seeds of the Sheila Smith strain of
Rickettsia rickettsii and the Breinl strain of Rickettsia
prowazekii were used throughout this study. Secondary chicken
embryo fibroblasts, prepared from specific-pathogen free eggs
(SPAFAS, Norwich, Conn.) were employed exclusively as the host
cell system. Dulbecco's medium, diluted 1:1 with Earle's salt
solution, containing 0.1% glucose and supplemented with 10%
fetal calf serum, was used to culture the cells.

Chicken embryo cells were infected in suspension according
to the method of Wisseman and Waddell (manuscript in preparation). The infected cell suspensions were washed 3x by
centrifugation in tissue culture medium to remove unadsorbed
organisms, and then grown as monolayers in 75 cm^2 Falcon
flasks at $32^{\circ}C$, in an atmosphere of 5% CO_2 in air. Chamber
slides (Lab Tek, Napierville, Ill.), containing aliquots of
the same infected cell cultures, were incubated as above, and
Giménez-stained (4) slides were prepared and examined at daily
intervals to monitor the growth of the rickettsiae.

The supernatant fluids from flasks of infected cells were
harvested at 24, 36, 48, 72, 96 and 120 hr. post infection,
and centrifuged at 12,000 x g for 30 min at $4^{\circ}C$ in a Sorvall
RC2-B centrifuge. The pellets were resuspended in a fixative
solution containing 3% acrolein and 2% glutaraldehyde in 0.1 M
cacodylate buffer, pH 7.3. In one experiment, the supernatant
fluid removed from R. rickettsii-infected cells at 72 hr was
transferred to a similar vessel and incubated for an
additional 48 hr at $32^{\circ}C$ in an atmosphere of 5% CO_2 in air
prior to centrifugation and fixation. Infected cells were
removed from the plastic surface at similar time points with
trypsin-EDTA, washed in tissue culture medium, and also fixed
in acrolein-glutaraldehyde.

Infected cells and the pelleted supernatant fractions were fixed for either 1 hr at room temperature (22°C) or overnight at 4°C, washed in buffer, post-fixed for 1 hr in 1% osmium tetroxide, and embedded in Epon 812 by the method of Luft (5). There were no detectable differences between samples fixed at either of the two temperatures. Ultrathin sections were cut on a Sorvall MT-2 ultramicrotome with a diamond knife, picked up on collodion and carbon-coated copper grids and examined in a Siemens IA electron microscope. Since the fine structural details of infection of chicken embryo cells with both R. rickettsii and R. prowazekii have been characterized previously in our laboratories (1, 2), primary emphasis was placed on examination of pellets from the supernatant culture fluids. Examination of cells infected with both organisms was used only to confirm previous knowledge concerning the status of cells and rickettsiae during the infection.

III. RESULTS

The extensive dilatation of the rough-surfaced endoplasmic reticulum (ER) of secondary chicken embryo fibroblasts beginning about 48 h after infection with R. rickettsii is shown in Figure 1. When the swelling of ER occurs in regions of the cell occupied by the infecting rickettsiae, the organisms together with small portions of host cytosol apparently are subject to circumscription by cisternal membranes (Figure 2). It was shown in previous studies in our laboratory that these membrane-bound rickettsiae persisted in the infected host cells until cell lysis, and it was assumed that some rickettsiae were released in that state. To determine the comparative frequency of "free" rickettsiae and host membrane-associated organisms released during a typical infection cycle, supernatant fluids from infected cultures were collected, pelleted by centrifugation, and examined by transmission electron microscopy. R. prowazekii, which causes no substantial morphological alteration to the internal membranes of infected cells, was used as a control.

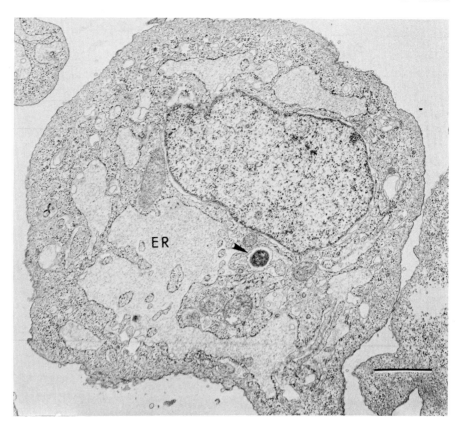

Fig. 1. Ultrathin section of a secondary chicken embryo
fibroblast infected with R. rickettsii showing widespread
dilatation of the rough-surfaced endoplasmic reticulum (ER).
Arrow denotes membrane-bound rickettsia. Bar = 0.5 μm.

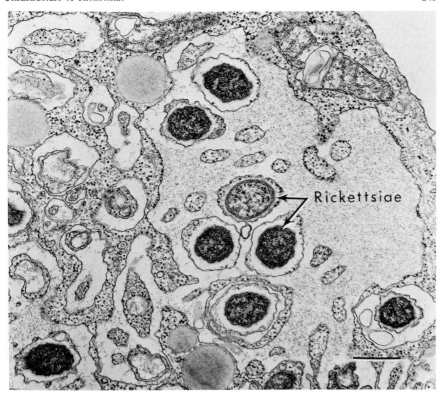

Fig. 2. Portion of infected chicken embryo cell 72 h post infection showing rickettsiae enveloped with host membranes. In some instances only a rickettsia appears to have been trapped, while in others both host cytosol and rickettsiae are included in the envelopment process. Fragments of host cytosol containing no rickettsiae are also present within the ER cisternae. Bar = 0.5 μm.

Table 1 depicts the results of these experiments. Free R. prowazekii were detected in the supernatant fraction of infected chicken embryo cells beginning at 48 h. No host membrane-associated organisms were found. The supernatant fractions from R. rickettsii-infected cells also yielded numerous free rickettsiae. At 48 h post infection, however, 2% of the rickettsiae examined in pelleted supernatant fractions from R. rickettsii-infected cells were found to be host membrane-associated. This percentage increased to 42% at 72 h, and then dropped to 31% at 96 h and to less than 1% at 120 h. Supernatant fractions removed at 72 h and reincubated free of infected monolayer cells for an additional 48 h period also showed that less than 1% of the rickettsiae were

associated with host cell membrane. Figure 3 (A & B) are
representative of thin sections through a 72 h pelleted
supernatant fraction from an R. rickettsii-infected culture of
secondary chicken embryo fibroblasts, showing both free
rickettsiae and also those bounded by host cytosol and

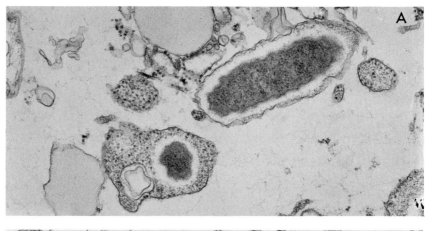

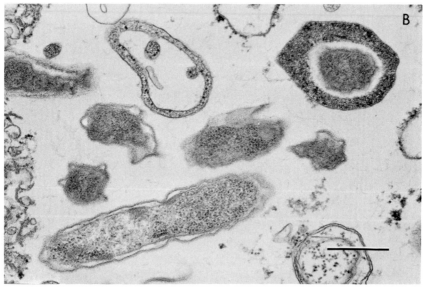

Fig. 3 A & B.   Pelleted supernatant fraction from a 72 h
infected chicken embryo cell culture showing both free and
host membrane-bound R. rickettsii.   Bar = 0.5 µm.

membranes. Ninety-six hour samples were similar except for a
slightly higher ratio of free to membrane-associated
rickettsiae (Table 1). Thin sections through samples
harvested at 120 h, or those harvested at 72 h and incubated
for an additional 48 h period, were typical of those seen in
Figure 4. The number of rickettsiae present in such samples
taken late in the infection was substantially greater than in
earlier samples, and nearly all of the organisms were free of
detectable host cell membranes. Morphologically, many of the
organisms were plasmolyzed, and some had uncharacteristic
shapes and forms, possibly reflecting prolonged extracellular
exposure in the culture medium. The pH of the supernatant
fluids was measured at all time intervals beginning at 48 h,
and ranged from pH 7.1 to pH 6.8.

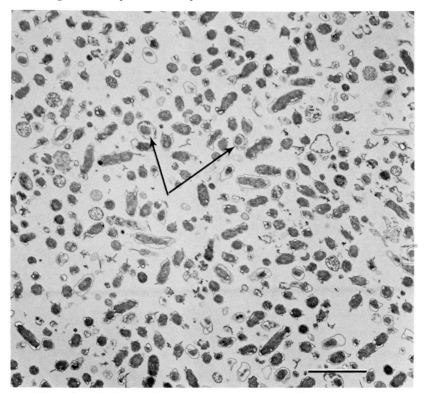

Fig. 4. Thin section through pelleted supernatant
fraction 120 h post infection with R. rickettsii. Note: most
rickettsiae free of host membranes. Arrows show some of
remaining rickettsiae enveloped with membrane. Bar = 2 μm.

Figure 5 represents a selected area from a sample of the 120 h supernatant fraction showing a rickettsia partially enveloped by host membrane. Few organisms were found in this state, suggesting that membrane shedding takes place relatively rapidly, and that to demonstrate larger populations in the escape process would necessitate the harvest of samples at shorter time intervals.

TABLE 1. Electron Microscopic Observations on the Relationship of Rickettsia prowazekii and Rickettsia rickettsii to Host Cell Membranes in the Supernatant Fluids Collected from Infected Chicken Embryo Fibroblasts in Monolayer Culture

Organism	Time Post Infection	Free Rickettsiae	Membrane-Bound Rickettsiae	% Membrane- Bound Rickettsiae
R. prowazekii				
	24	0	0	0
	48	52	0	0
	72	112	0	0
	120	221	0	0
R. rickettsii				
	24	125	0	0
	36	115	1	1
	48	276	6	2
	72	343	248	42
	96	644	284	31
	120	938	5	1
	120[a]	902	7	1

[a] Supernatant fluid removed at 72 h and reincubated for an additional 48 h at 32°C in an atmosphere of 5% CO_2 in air.

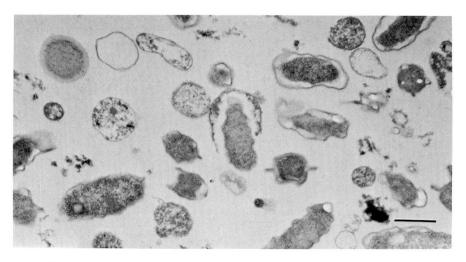

Fig. 5. Partially enveloped rickettsia in process of escaping from host membrane. Bar = 0.5 μm.

IV. DISCUSSION

The mechanism of escape of rickettsiae from infected host cells is poorly understood. The variation which occurs, even within the same species of organism in different cell types, makes it difficult to propose a single model for the escape process. For example, R. tsutsugamushi exits mouse mesothelial cells enveloped in plasma membrane and is subsequently phagocytosed by another mesothelial cell, while still retaining previously acquired host cell membrane (6). Ito, on the other hand, (personal communication) has successfully harvested large numbers of R. tsutsugamushi from the supernatant fraction of infected baby hamster kidney cells. These rickettsiae were entirely free of host membrane material, suggesting that release in this system is quite different from that observed in the mouse mesothelial cell model.
     Previous studies in our laboratory with R. prowazekii in a chicken embryo cell system, as well as the data presented in this report, suggest that R. prowazekii is also released without acquiring host cell membranes. Exceptions seem to be the occasional autophagosomes within some cells which may be released upon lysis of the host cell late in infection (Silverman, personal observation).
     The mechanism of release of R. rickettsii from infected chicken embryo cells is more diverse than that of both R.

<u>prowazekii</u> and <u>R</u>. <u>tsutsugamushi</u> in that the organisms are
capable of exiting similar host cells in either a free state or
circumscribed by host membranes. The degree to which these two
distinct modes of release occur appears to be directly related
to the stage of growth and to the cytopathic changes occurring
within the infected cell. Early in the infection of susceptible cells there are virtually no detectable cytopathic
effects, and it is at this time that organisms collected from
the supernatant fractions are free of host membrane. However,
as marked cytopathology in the chicken cells becomes evident,
as seen by extensive dilatation of internal membranes, many
rickettsiae collected in the supernatant fractions are bounded
by membranes of host cell origin.
     In the early phases of infection the presence of free rick-
ettsiae in the supernatant fraction can perhaps be attributed
to two distinct escape or release mechanisms: (a) the capacity
for early bidirectional movement of the rickettsiae through
plasma membranes as demonstrated earlier by Wisseman et al.
(3).; and (b) premature lysis of a small sensitive population
of host cells.
     As dilatation of the rough-surfaced endoplasmic reticulum
becomes pronounced at approximately 48 h, there is a corresponding increase in the number of membrane-bound rickettsiae
collected in the supernatant fractions (Table 1). Although
membranes of the endoplasmic reticulum probably constitute the
majority of those membranes associated with the rickettsiae,
plasma membrane-bound organisms are likely to contribute as
well. Wisseman et al. (3) have reported previously in a light-
microscopic study the movement of <u>R</u>. <u>rickettsii</u> into narrow
cytoplasmic extensions of cells, and Whitescarver et al. (unpublished observations) have shown by scanning electron microscopy the presence of <u>R</u>. <u>rickettsii</u> on "stalks" protruding from
the host cell body. Walker and Cain (7) have recently shown by
transmission electron microscopy <u>R</u>. <u>rickettsii</u> in cytoplasmic
projections, which appear to be attached precariously to the
cell body, and perhaps subject to being pinched off.
     The acquisition by <u>R</u>. <u>rickettsii</u> of membranes of host cell
origin is a fascinating and, to date, unique observation. The
exact mechanism(s) by which this occurs is unclear, although
it is legitimate to speculate that dilatation of the endoplasmic reticulum, with subsequent fusion of adjacent membranes,
results in the formation of small islets of host cytosol, some
of which contain rickettsiae.
     Just as fascinating as the acquisition of membranes around
rickettsiae, however, is the organisms' ability to shed these
membranes once they are released from the host cell. The time
after release of the organisms at which this is initiated is
unknown. However, it appears to approach totality by 120 h

postinfection, and seems not to require the presence of the
infected host cell monolayer.

   Winkler (8) has postulated a role for phospholipase in the
entry of rickettsiae into susceptible host cells. It is conceivable that a similar enzyme might also be involved in the
escape of rickettsiae from infected cells, and possibly from
acquired internal host membranes as well. However, further studies are necessary to confirm this hypothesis.

V. SUMMARY

   When Rickettsia rickettsii infect and grow in chicken
embryo fibroblasts, they cause widespread dilatation of the
outer nuclear envelope and rough-surfaced endoplasmic reticulum. Although many of the rickettsiae remain free in the cytoplasmic matrix until the infected cell is totally destroyed,
some rickettsiae become enveloped within these dilating membranes along with portions of the host cell cytoplasm, and are
eventually released from damaged cells in this state. Once
free in the culture fluid, however, membrane-bound R. rickettsii seem to have the capacity for shedding these membranes, an
interesting phenomenon which may relate to the mechanism of
entry and release of rickettsiae in the intact susceptible host
cell.

ACKNOWLEDGMENTS

   We acknowledge the excellent technical assistance of Chris
Kunze and thank Cecilia Queen for typing the manuscript.

REFERENCES

1. Silverman, D. J., and Wisseman, C. L., Jr., Infect. Immun.
    26: 714 (1979).
2. Silverman, D. J., Wisseman, C. L., Jr., and Waddell, A.,
    Infect. Immun. 29: 778 (1980).
3. Wisseman, C. L., Jr., Edlinger, E. A., Waddell, A. D., and
    Jones, M. R., Infect. Immun. 14: 1052 (1976).
4. Giménez, D. F., Stain Tech. 39: 135 (1964).
5. Luft, J. H., J. Biophys. Biochem. Cytol. 9: 409 (1961).
6. Ewing, E. P., Jr., Takeuchi, A., Shirai, A., and Osterman,
    J. V., Infect. Immun. 19: 1068 (1978).

7. Walker, D. H., and Cain, B. G., <u>Lab. Invest.</u> <u>43</u>: 388
    (1980).
8. Winkler, H., <u>in</u> "Rickettsiae and Rickettsial Diseases"
    (W. Burgdorfer and R. L. Anacker, eds.), p.   . Academic
    Press, New York (1981).

ULTRASTRUCTURAL ANALYSIS OF <u>RICKETTSIA RICKETTSII</u> IN CULTURES OF PERSISTENTLY INFECTED VOLE CELLS

William J. Todd[1]

Department of Anatomy
Colorado State University
Fort Collins, Colorado

Willy Burgdorfer
Anthony J. Mavros

Epidemiology Branch
Rocky Mountain Laboratories
Hamilton, Montana

George P. Wray

Department of Molecular, Cellular,
and Developmental Biology
University of Colorado
Boulder, Colorado

I.   INTRODUCTION

Persistent infection of host cells is required to insure survival of <u>R. rickettsii</u> in nature. Such persistent infection of host cells was recently obtained in cell cultures established from the tunica vaginalis of the meadow vole, <u>Microtus pennsylvanicus</u>. These cultures provide a model to investigate the establishment and maintenance of nonlytic

---

[1]Presently on assignment to the Rocky Mountain Laboratories, under the Intergovernmental Personnel Act.

infections, and to determine how the lytic cycle of this pathogen is induced to kill the host cells. This paper describes
the ultrastructural features of interactions between rickettsiae and host cells in persistent and lytic infections of
cultured cells.

II. MATERIALS AND METHODS

A. Biologicals

The Wachsmuth strain of R. rickettsii used in this study
was isolated in 1974 from a Dermacentor andersoni female tick
removed from a Rocky Mountain spotted fever patient in Hamilton, MT.
Vole cell cultures were established from the tunica vaginalis of a laboratory reared meadow vole, Microtus pennsylvanicus as described elsewhere (1). Cultures of Vero cells used
for lytic infections were propagated according to the method
of Yunker and Cory (2). Both cell types were passaged in minimal essential medium (MEM) containing 10% foetal calf serum
(FCS). To initially infect both vole and Vero cells, 10^{-3}
to 10^{-4} dilutions of yolk sac suspensions containing R. rickettsii were used. Persistent infections of vole cells were
established by serial passage of infected cultures. Infected
cells were in the 5th to 17th passage when fixed for microscopic studies. Vero cells used for microscopy were infected
with aliquots of R. rickettsii freshly harvested from infected
Vero cell monolayers.

B. Electron Microscopy

For electron microscopy (EM) all samples were fixed as described by Ito (6). For standard transmission electron microscopy (TEM), fixed cells were stained "en block" in uranyl
acetate and embedded in Spurr's medium. Silver sections cut
with a Reichert ultramicrotome were stained with uranyl acetate followed by lead citrate, and examined in a Hitachi HU-11
electron microscope. For scanning electron microscopy (SEM),
fixed cells were dried at the critical point in freon, sputter
coated with gold and examined in an ETEC electron microscope.
For high voltage electron microscopy (HVEM), cells were grown
on formvar-coated gold grids, fixed, stained with uranyl acetate, dried by the critical point method (7), carbon coated,
and examined in a 1000 KV JEOL electron microscope.

III. RESULTS

A. Location of R. rickettsii within Infected Cells

Rickettsiae were present within all vole cells where they
were observed throughout the host cell, sometimes in clusters,
but usually dispersed within the cytoplasm. Occasionally,
organisms were inside the nucleus. Within both the cytoplasm
and the nucleus, the rickettsiae were found free and were not
within membrane-bound vacuoles. When the persistently infected cultures were examined by SEM, bulges were observed within
plasmodesmata (Fig. la). When cross-sectioned and examined by
TEM, these bulges frequently contained rickettsiae (Fig. lb).
Bulges were also present at the tips of microvilli-like processes and close to the surface of the infected cell (Fig. 2a).
When cross-sectioned, rickettsiae were also found within these
membrane-limited protrusions (Fig. 2b). Further documentation
of the presence of rickettsiae within membrane-limited protrusions was obtained by HVEM and is presented as a stereo image
in Fig. 3. In this stereo pair the host plasmalemma closely
follows the contour of the rickettsial organism.

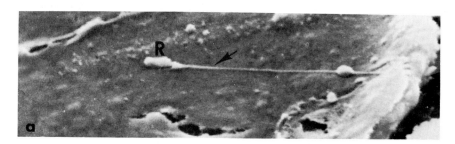

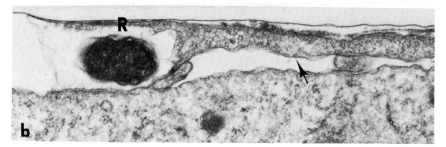

Fig. 1. Detection of rickettsiae (R) within thin extensions of host cell cytoplasm (arrows). (a) SEM 10,000X.
(b) TEM 35,000X.

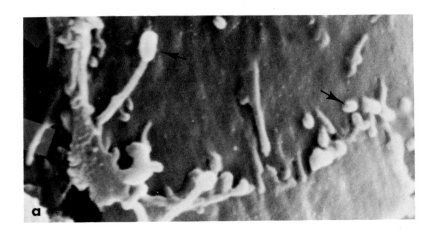

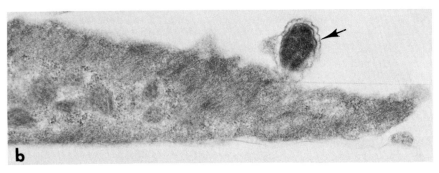

Fig. 2. Budding of rickettsiae (R) from the surface of
persistently infected cells. (a) SEM buds (arrows) 20,000X.
(b) TEM host cell membrane (arrow) 29,000X.

For comparison, Vero cells were infected with the same
strain of R. rickettsii and examined by EM. By 36 h postinoculation, rickettsiae were found within the microvilli-like
processes of infected cells (Fig. 4a) from where they appeared
to be released (Fig. 4b) into the tissue culture fluid.

B. Ultrastructure of R. rickettsii in Persistently
Infected Cells

When thin sections of rickettsiae were examined by TEM,
the electron density of the cytoplasm and the amount of electron translucent coat or halozone surrounding the cell wall
were found to vary (Fig. 5). Within the same host cell, rickettsiae containing electron-dense cytoplasm were present along

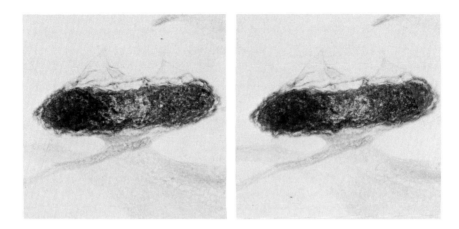

Fig. 3. The budding of R. rickettsii is apparent when
the HVEM images are fused using a two-lens viewer. 50,000X

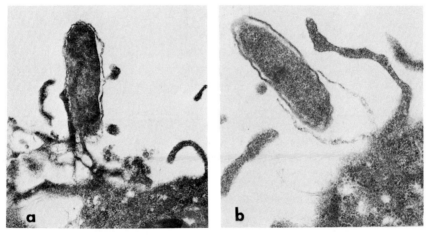

Fig. 4. Budding and release of rickettsiae from Vero
cells. (a) R. rickettsii surrounded by the plasmalemma of
the host cell.   25,000X. (b) Release of R. rickettsii.
33,000X

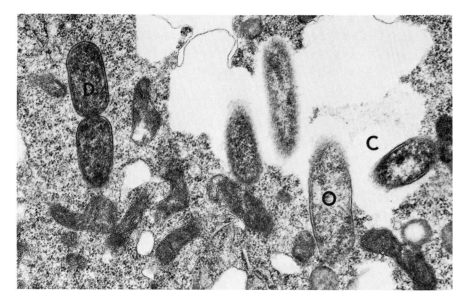

Fig. 5. TEM of rickettsial infected vole cell including
dense (D) and open (O) forms of R. rickettsii and electron
translucent coat (C). 35,000X

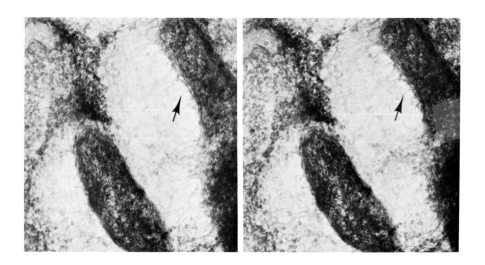

Fig. 6. When HVEM micrographs of R. rickettsii within
whole cells are fused, fibers extending from the rickettsial
cell wall are detected (arrows). 50,000X

with rickettsiae containing electron-translucent cytoplasm,
and organisms without any apparent coat were present along
with organisms surrounded by copious amounts of electron translucent coat. At high magnification, thin sections of rickettsiae-infected vole cells revealed the possible existence of
fibers or tubules that formed connecting bridges from one
rickettsia to another and possibly to structural fibers of the
host cell. The existence of such tubules was also documented
by HVEM of whole infected cells. Numerous tubules connected
to the cell wall of the rickettsiae traverse the clear halo-
zone which appears pressed against the cytoplasm of the host
(Fig. 6).

C. Cytopathic Effect of R. rickettsii

The principal ultrastructural alteration attributed to
rickettsiae within persistently infected cells was the formation of membrane bound vacuoles (Fig. 7a). The number of

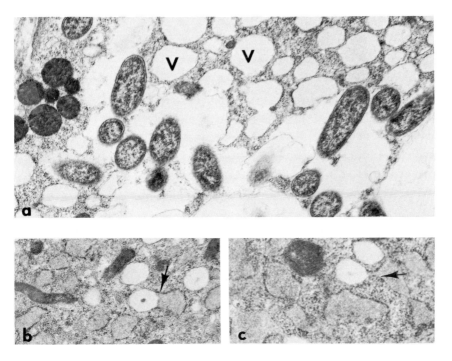

Fig. 7. Cytopathic effect of R. rickettsii in vole cells.
(a) vacuoles (V) 20,000X. (b) and (c) vacuoles continuous
with rough endoplasmic reticulum (arrows). 29,000X

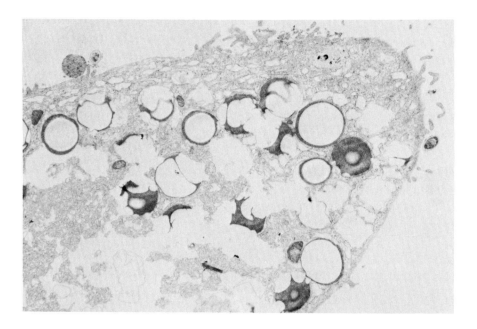

Fig. 8.   Cytopathic effect of R. rickettsii in Vero cells.
7,800X

electron translucent vacuoles formed correlated directly with
the number of rickettsiae present within each cell.   These
vacuoles appeared to be continuous with rough endoplasmic reticulum (Figs. 7b, 7c).
     For purpose of comparison, ultrastructural features of
Vero cells were examined 96 h postinfection (Fig. 8).   At this
stage practically all Vero cells were in advanced stages of
degeneration characterized by debris of membranes, amorphous
electron-dense material and vacuoles.   Vero cells were uniformly unable to survive infection with R. rickettsii.

IV. DISCUSSION

     Establishment of persistent rickettsial infections in
cells cultured from the tunica vaginalis of a meadow vole, an
important and possibly primary host of R. rickettsii in nature,
provided a model to study the fine structural features of
rickettsiae and their interactions with host cells.   The presence of rickettsiae dispersed throughout the host cell cytoplasm and on occasion within the nucleus is consistent with

previous reports (5, 6). The mechanism of entry into the nucleus is not established. We hypothesize rickettsiae are simply trapped within the nucleus during reformation of the nuclear membrane which occurs at the terminal stage of nuclear division.

The presence of rickettsiae within plasmadesmata and within thin stalks formed by the plasmalemma of the host cell is characteristic of the genus Rickettsia (7-9), and may provide a mechanism for the direct transfer of rickettsiae from infected to uninfected cells. Electron microscopic evidence for the direct transfer of R. tsutsugamushi from thin stalks of BHK-21 cells to polymorphonuclear leukocytes was reported by Rikihisa and Ito (9). In addition, the formation of well-defined plaques by R. rickettsii in monolayers of chick embryo fibroblasts and Vero cells, without agar overlay, supports the phenomenon of direct transfer of these organisms between adjacent cells. If rickettsiae were first released into the tissue culture fluid before they could infect other cells, plaque formation would not be expected. It is not established how the rickettsiae reach the restricted locations within plasmodesmata and cytoplasmic stalks. Either they are capable of moving into or are incorporated inside during formation of these structures. The movement of rickettsiae inside of host cells, in nonrandom fashion, has long been documented by time-lapse microscopy (10). This movement appears to be independent of cytoplasmic flow and is frequently linear as though the rickettsiae were traveling back and forth along subcellular tracks.

The detection by HVEM of tubules or fibers that appear to connect rickettsiae to structural fibers of the host cell provides some evidence for directed interactions between rickettsiae and their host cells. Whether these tubules are rickettsial products attached to host constituents, or are host cell structures attached to the rickettsiae has not as yet been established. We speculate that rickettsiae are attached by these tubules to the contractile elements of the host cell such as microfilaments, microtubules or microtrabeculae. This attachment to contractile elements could explain the nonrandom movement of rickettsiae referred to above.

The most obvious ultrastructural alteration attributed to the presence of rickettsiae within persistently infected vole cells was dilation of rough endoplasmic reticulum and loss of electron-opaque constituents to form electron translucent vesicles (Fig. 7). Whether these vesicles remain continuous with the network of rough endoplasmic reticulum or form separate vacuoles was not determined. In cells containing few rickettsiae, the amount of vesicle formation was insignificant; in cells containing large numbers of organisms, vesicles

occupied the major portion of the cytoplasmic space. The
ultrastructural disintegration, as commonly occurs when Vero
cells are infected with R. rickettsii, was not observed in the
persistently infected vole cell cultures. In Vero cells, the
depletion of host cell constituents by rickettsiae appeared to
progress gradually as multiplication of rickettsiae continued.
All Vero cells present in the cultures were killed.

V. SUMMARY

Fine structural features of rickettsial infected host
cells were investigated. Host cells cultured from the tunica
vaginalis of Microtus pennsylvanicus were established as a
cell line persistently infected with a virulent strain of R.
rickettsii. All cells contained rickettsiae. The surface
features of cells from confluent monolayers examined by SEM
included the presence of bulges extending from the cell surfaces from microvilli-like stalks and from within plasmodesmata. The presence of rickettsiae within bulges was confirmed
by TEM and HVEM. By HVEM, existence of fibers or tubules connected to the cell walls of rickettsiae was established. On
occasion, adjacent rickettsiae were observed connected to each
other as well as to the fine structural features of the host
cell through the fibers. We speculate that some fibers are
important to the movement of rickettsiae within the host cell.
The ultrastructural pathology induced by the presence of rickettsiae within persistently infected vole cells was limited
primarily to dilitation of the rough endoplasmic reticulum
compared to the complete disintegration of host cell constituents which occurred in Vero cells. Understanding the fine
structural features of interactions between rickettsiae and
cultured cells provides a basis for understanding both persistent and lytic infections induced by R. rickettsii in nature.

ACKNOWLEDGMENTS

The authors appreciate the advice and assistance given by
Dan Corwin with SEM. Opportunity to use HVEM for this investigation was provided by the Department of Molecular, Cellular,
and Developmental Biology, University of Colorado, Boulder, CO.

I

REFERENCES

1. Todd, W. J., Mavros, A. J., and Burgdorfer, W., in preparation.
2. Yunker, C. E., and Cory, J., TCA Manual 5, 1077 (1979).
3. Ito, S., Vinson, J. W., and McGuire, T. J., Jr., in "Pathobiology of Invertebrate Vectors of Disease" (L. A. Bulla and T. C. Chen, eds.), p. 35. The New York Academy of Sciences, New York (1975).
4. Wolosewick, J. J., and Porter, K. R., in "Practical Tissue Culture Applications", (K. Maramarosch and H. Hirumi, eds.), p. 59. Academic Press, New York (1979).
5. Burgdorfer, W., Anacker, R. L., Bird, R. G., and Bertram, D. S., J. Bacteriol. 96, 1415 (1968).
6. Wisseman, C. L., Jr., Edlinger, E. A., Waddell, A. D., and Jones, M. R., Infect. Immun. 14, 1052 (1976).
7. Vinson, J. W. and Whitescarver, J., personal communication.
8. Ewing, E. P., Jr., Takeuchi, A., Shirai, A., and Osterman, J. V., Infect. Immun. 19, 1068 (1978).
9. Rikihisa, Y., and Ito, S., Infect. Immun. 30, 231 (1980).
10. Kokorin, I. N., Miskarova, E. O., Gudima, O. S., Kabanova, E. A., and Truong, K., in "Rickettsiae and Rickettsial Diseases" (J. Kazar, R. Ormsbee and I. Tarasevich, eds.), p. 197, VEDA, Bratislava (1976).

ULTRASTRUCTURAL AND BIOLOGICAL ASPECTS
OF COXIELLA BURNETII UNDER PHYSICAL DISRUPTIONS

Thomas F. McCaul
Ted Hackstadt
Jim C. Williams

Laboratory of Microbial Structure and Function
Rocky Mountain Laboratories
Hamilton, Montana

I. INTRODUCTION

Coxiella burnetii, the etiologic agent of Q fever, exhibits similar properties with other members of the family Rickettsiaceae in that they are obligate intracellular prokaryotic parasites. Initially, C. burnetii was placed in a separate genus (1, 2), because of its filterability, a characteristic not shared by other members of the family Rickettsiaceae. The filterability of C. burnetii was explained by the existence of two cell types (3-9) which could be separated into two bands when centrifuged to equilibrium in density gradients (10, 11). An important difference between the members of the family Rickettsiaceae is the ability of C. burnetii to resist physical and chemical agents, more so than any other pathogenic rickettsia (12). C. burnetii has the capacity to survive in the environment (summarized in Table 1), where the microbe is generally transmitted aerogenically to domestic animals and man. Thus many problems have been encountered regarding disinfection of objects in the external environment and the sterilization of dairy products infected by this agent.

A previous study has demonstrated the occurrence of "endospore-like" forms during the developmental cycle of Q fever (8); analogous to the bacterial endospore formation of Gram-positive bacteria. Since an important aspect of the Gram-positive bacterial endospore is its resistance to

TABLE 1.   Survival Sites of Coxiella burnetii

Apart from its residence in the phagocytic vacuoles of
eukaryotic host cells, Coxiella burnetii has the ability to
survive in extreme adverse environments.

Waste products   a) Feces of tick, lice, fleas, and bedbugs.
                     Survive in feces of tick for 586 days.
                     (13, 14)
                  b) Human sputum and nasal discharges.   (15)

Secretions   a) Milk – skimmed milk for 42 months at
                     4–6°C.   (16)
                  b) Milk – 63°C for 30 mins; 74°C for 15
                     secs.   (17)
                  c) Butter – prepared from unpasteurized
                     milk.   (18)

Vestiture   a) Wool of sheep – 12 to 16 months at 4–6°C.
                     (19)
                  b) Wool processing plant.   (20)

Dust   a) Surfaces of animals, floors of animal
                     quarters, roadways used by domestic
                     animals, clothing of shepherds and other
                     handlers of livestock.   (17)

Soil   a) Sheep pastures readily contaminated
                     following lambing time.   (21)
                  b) Sandy and clay soil – 4–6°C for 9 months.
                     (19)

Meat   a) Cold storage conditions – 30 days (fresh
                     meat), 150 days (salted meat).   (22)

adverse conditions, the knowledge, gained from the effect of
physical disruptions on the cell variants of C. burnetii may
provide some understanding of the pleomorphism of C. burnetii.
The effect of physical extremities on C. burnetii was studied
by subjecting suspensions of Renografin purified (Phase I)
cells to osmotic shock in water followed by incubation at
different temperatures, sonication, and finally centrifugation
through 40 to 70% sucrose density gradients.   Ultrastructural
and metabolic analyses carried out on the final fractions
indicated that the small cell variants, or endospores, were
extremely resistant to adverse conditions.

II. MATERIALS AND METHODS

A. Propagation, Harvest and Purification of C. burnetii

   The Ohio strain of C. burnetii (Phase I) was used in this
study (23). This strain had been passed 5 times in the yolk
sac of embryonated hen eggs (5EP), 2 times in guinea pigs
(Hartley strain) (2GP), and then 2 more egg passages (2EP)
were carried out. Thus, the passage history is described as
5EP/2GP/2EP. C. burnetii were propagated in 6-day specific
pathogen-free (SPF) type 5, antibiotic-free, fertile hen egg
yolk sacs (H & N Hatchery, Redmond, Wash.).
   On the 7th day postinfection, the yolk sacs from viable
embryos were harvested and stored at -70°C. The rickettsiae
from the infected yolk sac material were purified by isopyknic
Renografin gradients, and the steps in the procedure of separation were carried out as described by Williams et al. (23).
The purified rickettsiae were resuspended in phosphate-
buffered saline (PBS, pH 7.35) containing 0.25 M sucrose
(PBSS) (23).

B. Physical Treatments

   The treatments consisted mainly of a) osmotic shock, b)
temperature variation, c) sonication, and d) centrifugation
through linear sucrose density gradient (40 to 70%). A flow
chart showing the steps in the preparation of rickettsial
suspensions as a result of such treatments is shown in
Figure 1.

C. Electron Microscopy

   1. Thin Sectioning. Pellets from each fraction were
resuspended in 9 volumes of 3% glutaraldehyde, 2.5 mM $CaCl_2$
in 66 mM cacodylate buffer (pH 6.8) overnight at 4°C. The
remaining procedures for all fractions were carried out as
described by McCaul and Williams (8). The pellets were pre-
embedded in 2% Difco Noble Agar (24) before postfixation in
1% Osmium tetroxide buffered with 66 mM cacodylate buffer for
1 hr at 4°C. After a further rinse with buffer, the blocks
were dehydrated through graded methanol washes. Uranyl
acetate staining was carried out as 0.5% in 30% methanol during
dehydration for 1 hr at room temperature. All blocks were
embedded in Spurr epoxy resin (25). Ultrathin sections were
cut on a Reichert OMU2 microtome, collected on uncoated Pelco

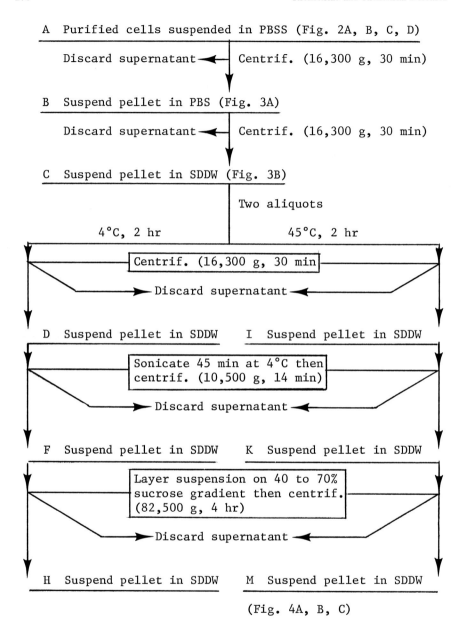

Fig. 1. Flow chart of technique for isolating small
cell variants of C. burnetii Selected fractions were
assayed for metabolic and biological activities (Table 2).
Some fractions were examined by electron microscopic
techniques (Fig. 2, 3 and 4).

200 grids, stained with potassium permanganate (26, 27) and
examined in an Hitachi EM HU-11E-1 operated at 75 Kv.

    2. Negative Staining. A 3% ammonium molybdate solution
adjusted to pH 6.5 with 1 M NH_4OH was used as a negative
stain. Fifty μl of this solution was added to the rickettsial
suspension (50 μl). The mixture was then placed on carbon and
parlodion-coated 400 mesh grids. After 30 seconds, the
excess fluid was removed and the grids were dried before examination in the electron microscope.

    3. Measurement of Glutamate and Glucose Metabolism. The
production of CO_2 from both [U-^{14}C]-glutamate and [U-^{14}C]-
glucose was measured as described previously (28) with the
exception that the final concentration of labeled glutamate
used in this experiment was 1.0 mM [U-^{14}C]-glutamate (0.1 μCi/
μMol). The incorporation of substrate into the TCA insoluble
material was also determined as described previously. The
reaction mixture was maintained at pH 4.5. Protein was determined by the Lowry method (29). Results are expressed as the
amount of substrate (nMol) metabolized per mg of protein.

                        III. RESULTS

            A. Ultrastructure of Selected Fractions

    A heterogenous population of large and small cell variants
(LCV and SCV) was suspended in different diluents so that the
effects of decreasing osmolarities on cell morphology could
be determined. Although all of the fractions were analyzed,
only selected fractions which show distinct ultrastructural
characteristics are presented for the purpose of clarity and
brevity.
    Fraction A. Cells suspended in PBSS contained a popula-
tion of both LCV and SCV (Fig. 2). The LCV exhibited extreme
pleomorphism, and the multilayered cytoplasmic membranes, a
common feature in the SCV, were not observed in the LCV. However, some of the LCV appeared to be plasmolyzed as evidenced
by the shrinkage of cell contents which appeared as though the
outer membrane was distended thereby increasing the volume of
the periplasmic space between the cytoplasmic and outer membranes (Fig. 2A and B). Development of an endospore (8)
within one pole of the LCV was observed in this preparation
(Fig. 2C). The SCV was recognized by a dense central nucleoid
region surrounded by granular material, probably ribonucleoprotein (Fig. 2D). The trilaminar cytoplasmic and outer

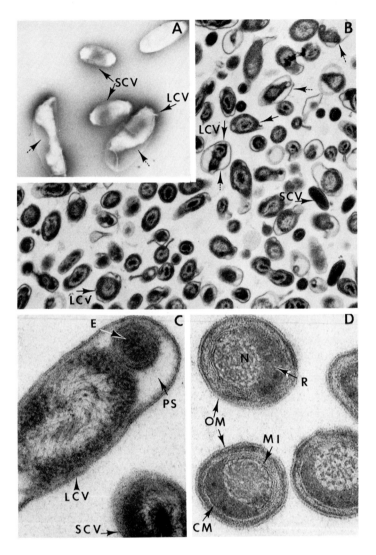

Fig. 2. Electron micrographs of purified cells of C. burnetii showing the pleomorphic nature of the organism. Fraction A of Fig. 1: (A) Negative staining (X 28,700). (B) Thin section (X 24,600). (C) LCV containing an endospore (X 144,000). (D) SCV of C. burnetii (X 192,000). SCV = small cell variant, LCV = large cell variant, some of which showed plasmolysis (broken arrows). Cytoplasmic membranous intrusions (MI), outer (OM) and cytoplasmic (CM) membranes, dense periplasmic space (PS), nucleoplasm (N), ribonucleoprotein (R), and endospore (E).

membranes of the SCV were separated by an electron-dense
periplasmic space.

Fraction B. Cells suspended in PBS were comprised of two
cell variants. The periplasmic space between the cytoplasmic
and the outer membrane of the LCV was, however, reduced (Fig.
3A) in PBS as compared to that observed with the cells in PBSS
(Fig. 2A and B). The central nucleoid filaments in the LCV
(Fig. 3A) were more dispersed than those described in Fraction
A. LCV containing endospores within the pole of the cell were
not commonly observed in this preparation which had undergone
slight osmotic shock after resuspension of PBSS pellets in
PBS.

Fraction C. Resuspension of cells from Fraction B in SDDW
caused drastic changes in the morphology of the LCV. Osmotic
shock in water caused, in some cells, lysis as evidenced by an
aggregation of ribonucleoprotein particles and loss of cytoplasmic components (Fig. 3B). Although cell wall fragments of
the LCV were observed, the SCV appeared unaffected by this
osmotic shock procedure.

Fraction H. Suspensions of the sonicated and differentially centrifuged cells were pelleted in 40 to 70% sucrose
gradients so that a pure population of SCV might be obtained.
This preparation still contained aggregated cytoplasmic components as well as SCV (data not shown).

Fraction M. This fraction contained SCV similar to
Fraction H which were observed by both thin sectioning and
negative staining (Fig. 4A and B). However, aggregated cytoplasmic components observed in Fraction H (data not shown)
were not observed. Some SCV appeared morphologically unaffected by the harsh physical treatments (Fig. 4C).

The final products of the series (Fractions H and M) were
inoculated into 6-day-old chicken embryos (23) and mice
(C57B/10 strain) (30). The chicken embryos died on the 7th
day post-inoculation which suggests that the rickettsiae were
present in large numbers (i.e., $\geq 1 \times 10^8$ organisms per ml)
(23). Rickettsiae were detected by both Giménez staining and
direct fluorescence antibody prepared against C. burnetii as
previously described (31). The mice developed splenomegaly
and liver lesions, and C. burnetii were isolated from the
spleens of infected mice as previously described (30). By
microagglutination test, the sera were positive for C.
burnetii anti-Phase I and Phase II antibodies.

B. Measurement of Glutamate and Glucose Metabolism

The results of metabolism studies carried out on selected
fractions are presented in Table 2. Metabolism of both

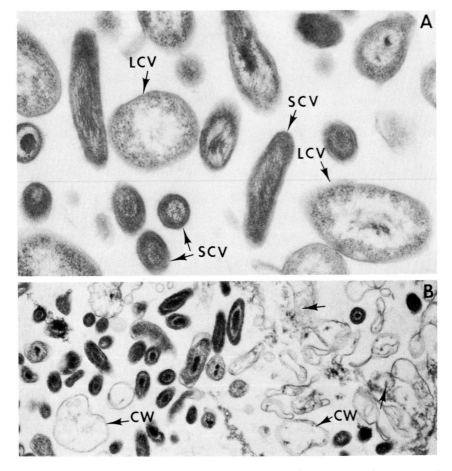

Fig. 3. Effect of osmotic shock on the two cell types of
C. burnetii. Fraction B of Fig. 1: (A) Ultrasection of C.
burnetii after osmotic shock in PBS. (SCV = small cell
variants, LCV = large cell variants) (X 66,300). Fraction C
of Fig. 1: (B) Ultrasection of C. burnetii suspended in SDDW
showing the effect of osmotic shock in water. Note cell wall
fragments (CW) and cytoplasmic contents (arrows) (X 24,600).

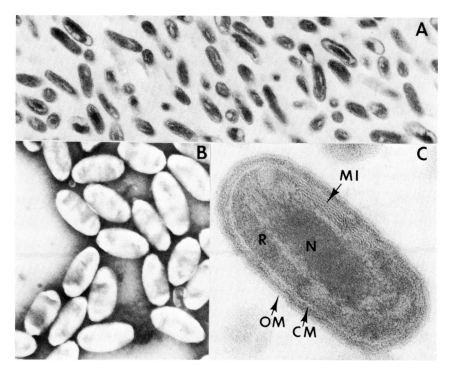

Fig. 4.   Electron micrographs of the purified SCV of C. burnetii. Fraction M of Fig. 1:   (A) Thin sectioning (X 24,600).   (B) Negative staining (X 28,700).   (C) Higher magnification illustrating cytoplasmic membrane (CM), membranous intrusions (MI), outer membrane (OM), nucleoplasm (N), periplasmic space (PS), ribonucleoprotein (R) (X 192,000).

TABLE 2. Metabolic Activity of _Coxiella burnetii_ Fractions Following Physical Disruption

Fraction	nMol glutamate / mg protein / hr		nMol glucose / mg protein / hr	
	CO_2	Incorporated	CO_2	Incorporated
A	438.06	18.01	1.55	0.005
C	101.19	0.53	0.45	UD[a]
D	74.71	UD	0.41	UD
F	61.82	16.97	0.10	UD
H	24.72	7.80	0.077	UD
I	26.40	UD	0.069	UD
K	43.63	8.24	0.041	UD
M	30.29	UD	0.036	UD

[a]Undetectable.

[U-^{14}C]-glucose and [U-^{14}C]-glutamate was carried out as previously described by Hackstadt and Williams (28). The results
are presented as specific activities (i.e., nMol/hr/mg protein), thus each fraction has been compared on the basis of
mg protein per sample. Osmotic shock greatly reduced the
metabolic capability of the respective fractions. Fraction C
showed a sharp decrease in metabolic activity compared to
Fraction A illustrating the effect of osmotic shock on C.
burnetii. However, Fractions H and M, which contained solely
SCV, metabolized both substrates at relatively slower rates
when compared with that recorded for Fraction A. More important is the observation that the SCV rich fractions were
capable of metabolizing glucose and glutamate.

IV. DISCUSSION

The pleomorphic nature and the relationship between the 2
cell variants, LCV and SCV, of C. burnetii have been the subject of this investigation. Previous investigations have
suggested that physical stresses associated with storage, purification and preparation of samples for electron microscopy
were contributing factors in generating LCV from SCV (11).
Our studies of C. burnetii cells by transmission electron
microscopy clearly revealed that the SCV, or endospore, has
the ability to withstand physical changes, whereas the LCV,
possibly due to the labile nature of the peptidoglycan and
the distensible outer membrane, is susceptible to osmotic
shock. Physical disruption caused by osmotic stress associated with storage and purification may lead to lysis of the
LCV. Induction of lysis of the LCV can be reduced to a minimum by resuspending the Renografin-purified rickettsiae in
PBSS as demonstrated in a previous study (23).
Other investigators have suggested that the LCV was a
degraded SCV, formed by host-mediated digestion of the peptidoglycan of the cell wall (32, 33). Since C. burnetii proliferate within the phagolysosomes of host cells, the LCV were
regarded as end-products of Q fever infection as a result of
lysosomal enzymatic degradations of the host cells. However,
this study has shown that both the LCV and SCV were metabolically active. In Fractions H and M, which consisted
solely of SCV, there was a 14-fold reduction in metabolic
activity of glutamate compared to Fraction A, which contained
a mixture of both SCV and LCV. By quantitative digital image
analysis, Fraction A contained 35% LCV (McCaul and Williams,
in preparation). Although metabolically active, the susceptibility of the LCV to physical stresses suggests that the

LCV may play a minor role in withstanding extracellular environments. The low metabolic activity and resistance to physical stresses exhibited by the SCV suggest that this cell may be derived from the endospore of C. burnetii (8). Furthermore, the SCV or endospore (8) may be the filterable cell which has been described by Rosenberg and Kordova (9). However, the description of the SCV in a previous (8) and the present study fits the descriptions of the term spore defined by Cross and Attwell (34) for specialized structures occurring in both eukaryotes and prokaryotes.

Man is probably an incidental host (35) for C. burnetii; therefore, man is not necessary for the propagation and survival of the parasite in nature. However, Q fever infections in man are usually acute, ranging from mild to severe. In some individuals, however, chronic infections may lead to eventual valvular heart disease, hepatitis, splenomegaly and hepatomegaly (36). The knowledge of the persistence of C. burnetii following recovery of acute infections still remains obscure. The endurance of the SCV to resist adverse physical extremities may, however, relate to the capacity both to combat immunological defenses and to persist in individuals with chronic infections. The evidence reported herein implicating the SCV as a heat-resistant relatively dormant spore-like structure should facilitate future studies on the physiological, biochemical and immunological factors of the surface-antigenic determinants of SCV and their role in acute and chronic infections.

V. SUMMARY

C. burnetii, the etiologic agent of Q fever, shares a common characteristic with other members of the genus Rickettsia in being an obligate intracellular parasite. C. burnetii is unique in that two cell types, large and small cell variants, are present which contribute to some unusual characteristics. The effect of physical conditions on C. burnetii was studied by subjecting suspensions of Renografin purified C. burnetii (Phase I) to osmotic shock in water, incubation at elevated temperatures followed by sonication and finally centrifugation through 40 to 70% sucrose density gradients. Examination of the cells by scanning and transmission electron microscopy revealed that the large cell variant was osmotically sensitive. The final fraction contained rickettsiae of small variant form which were shown to retain metabolic activity as demonstrated by the metabolism of radiolabeled glutamate and glucose. The small cell variant or endospore rickettsiae, were also found to be infectious in chick embryonated eggs and mice. In conclusion, these data suggest that the small cell variant which has been described previously in the sporogenic developmental cycle of C. burnetii retains its morphology and viability during exposure to extreme environmental conditions.

ACKNOWLEDGMENTS

The technical assistance of E. Davis and the expert secretarial preparation of S. Smaus are gratefully acknowledged.

REFERENCES

1. Philip, C. B., Am. J. Hyg. 37, 301 (1943).
2. Philip, C. B., Public Health Rept. 63, 58 (1948).
3. Anacker, R. L., Fukushi, K., Pickens, E. G., and Lackman, D. B., J. Bact. 88, 1130 (1964).
4. Ariel, B. M., Khavkin, T. N., and Amosenkova, N. I., Path. Microbiol. 39, 412 (1973).
5. Handley, J., Paretsky, D., and Stueckemann, J., J. Bact. 94, 263 (1967).
6. Kishimoto, R. A., Veltri, B. J., Canonico, P. G., Shirey, F. G., and Walker, J. S., Infect. Immun. 14, 1087 (1976).
7. Kishimoto, R. A,, Veltri, B. J., Shirey, F. G., Canonico, P. G., and Walker, J. S., Infect. Immun. 15, 601' (1977).
8. McCaul, T. F. and Williams, J. C., J. Bact. in press (1981).
9. Rosenberg, M. and Kordova, N., Acta Virol. 4, 52 (1960).
10. Canonico, P. G., Van Zwieten, M. J., and Christmas, W. A., Appl. Microbiol. 23, 1015 (1972).
11. Wiebe, M. E., Burton, P. R., and Shankel, D. M., J. Bact. 110, 368 (1972).
12. Ormsbee, R. A., in "Viral and Rickettsial Diseases of Man" (F. L. Horsfall and I. Tamm, eds.), p. 1144. J. B. Lippincott, PA, (1965).
13. Philip, C. B., J. Parasitol. 34, 457 (1948).
14. Stocker, M. G. P. and Marmion, B. P., Bull. Wld. Health Org. 13, 781 (1955).
15. Steinmann, J., Ann. Inst. Pasteur 81, 109 (1951).

16. Ignatovich, V. F., J. Microbiol. Epidemiol. Immunol.
    30, 134 (1959).
17. Babudieri, B., Adv. Vet. Sci. 5, 81 (1959).
18. Jellison, W. L., Huebner, R. J., Beck, M. D., Parker,
    R. R., and Bell, E. J., Public Health Rept. 63, 1712
    (1948).
19. Ignatovich, V. F., J. Microbiol. Epidemiol. Immunol.
    30, 156 (1959).
20. Sigel, M. M., Scott, T. F. M., and Henle, W., Am. J.
    Public Health 40, 524 (1950).
21. Silich, V. A., J. Microbiol. Epidemiol. Immunol. 28,
    816 (1957).
22. Welsh, H. H., Lennette, E. H., Abinanti, F. R., Winn,
    J. F., and Kaplan, W., Am. J. Hyg. 70, 14 (1959).
23. Williams, J. C., Peacock, M., and McCaul, T. F., Infect.
    Immun. in press (1981).
24. Gowans, E. J., Med. Lab. Technol. 30, 113, (1973).
25. Spurr, A. R., J. Ultrastruct. Res. 26, 31 (1969).
26. Lawn, A. M., J. Biophys. Biochem. Cytol. 7, 197 (1960).
27. Sutton, J. R., J. Ultrastruct. Res. 21, 424 (1968).
28. Hackstadt, T. and Williams, J. C., Proc. Natl. Acad.
    Sci. U.S.A. in press (1981).
29. Lowry, O. H., Rosebrough, N. J., Farr, A. L., and
    Randall, R. J., J. Biol. Chem. 193, 267 (1951).
30. Cantrell, J. L. and Williams, J. C., Infect. Immun.
    in press (1981).
31. Peacock, M., Burgdorfer, W., and Ormsbee, R. A., Infect.
    Immun. 3, 355 (1971).
32. Burton, P. R., Kordova, N., and Paretsky, D., Can. J.
    Microbiol. 17, 143 (1971).
33. Nermut, M. V., Schramek, S., and Brezina, R., Acta
    Virol. 12, 446 (1968).
34. Cross, T. and Attwell, R. W., in "Spores" (P. Gerhardt,
    R. N. Costilow, and H. L. Sadoff, eds.), Vol. VI, p. 3.
    Am. Soc. Microbiology, Washington, D.C. (1975).
35. Huebner, R. J. and Bell, J. A., J. Am. Med. Assn. 145,
    301 (1951).
36. Turck, W. P. G., Howitt, G., Turnberg, L. A., Fox, H.,
    Longson, M., Matthews, M. B., and Das Gupta, R., Quart.
    J. Med. New Series 65, 193 (1976).

ULTRASTRUCTURAL COMPARISONS OF WOLBACHIA-LIKE
SYMBIOTES OF TICKS (ACARI: IXODIDAE)

Stanley F. Hayes
Willy Burgdorfer

Epidemiology Branch
Rocky Mountain Laboratories
Hamilton, Montana

I. INTRODUCTION

Pleomorphic, bacteria-like tick symbiotes, first observed
by Cowdry (1) in 16 species of ixodid ticks and called wolbachia by Hertig (2), have since been encountered in all species of ticks examined (3). They grow intracellularly and
without exception are found in ovarial tissues of females that
pass them via eggs to their progeny. Depending upon the species of tick, certain tissues of other organs, such as the
midgut, small intestine, and malpighian tubules, may also be
infected.

The first isolation of such a symbiote was reported by
Suitor and Weiss (4) from ovarian and malpighian tubule tissues of <u>Argas persicus</u> (later determined to be <u>A. arboreus</u>),
collected from heron rookeries near Cairo, Egypt. Because of
its similarity to rickettsial agents (size, intracellular
growth, susceptibility to broad spectrum antibiotics) this
symbiote was classified as a member of Rickettsiaceae and was
included in the genus <u>Wolbachia</u> of the tribe Wolbachieae.
This tribe contains organisms adapted to existence in arthropods as symbiotes, but not in vertebrates as highly pathogenic
parasites (5).

A similar symbiote has since been isolated from the wood
tick, <u>Dermacentor andersoni</u> (6).

Most symbiotes studied so far stain best by Giemsa's method although they occasionally retain the basic fuchsin and
carbol fuchsin of Macchiavello's and Giménez' stains, respectively (7). On the other hand, certain symbiotes like those

of <u>Rhipicephalus</u> <u>sanguineus</u>, stain best by the Giménez method.
In such cases, the differentiation by conventional light
microscopy of symbiotes and rickettsiae may be difficult.
Therefore, morphologic characterization of wolbachiae is just
as essential as that of the true rickettsiae that may occur in
the same tissues of the tick. This paper describes the ultrastructure and morphology of symbiotes in 5 species of ticks,
whose roles as vectors of spotted fever group rickettsiae are
now the subjects of our investigations. These ticks include
the Rocky Mountain wood tick, <u>D</u>. <u>andersoni</u>, the American dog
tick, <u>D</u>. <u>variabilis</u>, the rabbit tick, <u>Haemaphysalis</u> <u>leporis-</u>
<u>palustris</u>, the brown dog tick, <u>R</u>. <u>sanguineus</u>, and the lone
star tick, <u>Amblyomma</u> <u>americanum</u>.

II. METHODS

   To determine, by conventional microscopy, the distribution
of wolbachiae within the various tick vectors, adult ticks
from colonies maintained at Rocky Mountain Laboratories were
dissected, and smears prepared from the various tissues were
stained either by Giemsa or by Giménez methods.
   For electron microscopy, tissues of half-engorged adult
ticks were fixed in a modified Ito's fixative (8). The tissues were treated with osmium, dehydrated in acetone, embedded
in Spurr's resin and polymerized. Blocks were sectioned with
a duPont diamond knife. Sections were picked up on naked 300
mesh copper grids, poststained with aqueous 2% uranyl acetate
and lead citrate, and examined in a Hitachi HU-11E electron
microscope at 75 kV. Size and morphologic comparisons between
the various wolbachiae were determined directly from micrographs obtained from the examination of multiple section profiles of several preparations per tick species. All micrographs were enlarged 3X. Maximum length vs width measurements were recorded and averaged to obtain the values reported. No effort was made to eliminate tangential or oblique
profiles.

III. RESULTS

A. Distribution of wolbachiae

   The organ and regional distribution of the symbiotes within the 5 tick species studied is summarized in Table I and
graphically illustrated in Fig. 1. Organisms were present in

TABLE 1.

Tick species		MT	T OV	MGS	L#1	L#2	SI
D. andersoni	♂	−	−	−	+++	+++	+++
	♀	−	+++	+	++	++	+
D. variabilis	♂	−	−	+	W(+)	+++	++
	♀	−	+++	+	++	++	++
R. sanguineus	♂	+++	−	−	−	−	−
	♀	+++	+++	−	−	−	−
H. leporispalustris	♂	−	+	++	++	++	+++
	♀	+	++	++	++	++	+++
A. americanum	♂	++	−	−	−	−	−
	♀	++	+++	−	−	−	−

MT = malpighian tubules, T = testes, OV = ovary, MGS = midgut stalk, L#1 and L#2 = lobes of the posterior diverticula, and SI = small intestines (see Fig. 1 also). The degree of infection is indicated as + = light, ++ = moderate, and +++ = heavy, − indicates not detected, W(+) = weak positive.

the ovarial tissues in both the germinative cells and the supporting epithelium, within the epithelium of malpighian tubules in R. sanguineus and A. americanum, or in the posterior parts of the midgut and small intestine of D. andersoni, D. variabilis, and H. leporispalustris. In the midgut, wolbachiae were limited to the two posterior lobes (L#1, L#2), the posterior part of the stomach (MGS), and the small intestine (SI). In male ticks, the symbiotes occurred either in the posterior lobes of midgut (D. andersoni, D. variabilis, H. leporispalustris) or in the distal portions of the blind-ending malpighian tubules (R. sanguineus and A. americanum).

B.   Electron microscopic Characterization of Wolbachiae

The fine structure of the symbiotes of the 5 ticks studied was much the same. The organisms were diverse in size and pleomorphic, ranging from small coccoid or rodlike bacillary to large pleomorphic forms. Single organisms range from 0.3 to 6.5 μ in diameter. Average width and length measurements usually fall within the range of 0.6 to 4.0 μ. The wolbachiae

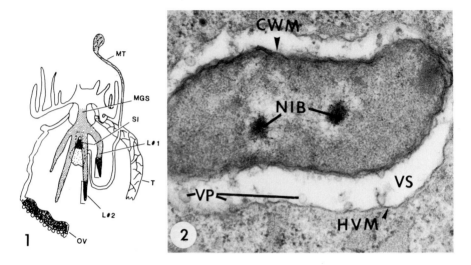

Fig. 1. Graphic illustration of wolbachia distribution
in ticks studied. Shading depicts areas and degree of infection.

Fig. 2. R. sanguineus wolbachia - used to depict general
ultrastructure. HVM - host vacuolar membrane, VS - vacuolar
space, CWM - cell wall membrane, NIB - nucleoid inclusion bodies, and VP - vesicle or viroid particles. 55,500X

of A. americanum and R. sanguineus represent the largest end
of this range, while those of H. leporispalustris represent
the smallest. Between these extremes are the symbiotes of D.
andersoni and D. variabilis。 The organisms are located in
the cytoplasm of host cells, usually within a vacuole either
singly or in coalescent colonylike nests. There is no particular association with any specific cellular organelle, i.e.,
mitochondria, Golgi apparatus, endoplasmic reticulum, and they
do not invade the nucleus.

Fig. 2, showing the wolbachia of R. sanguineus, is representative of the general ultrastructure and morphology of
these tick symbiotes. They have one or more cell-wall membranes (CWM) that are usually very flaccid and sinuous, often
giving the organism a spheroplastic appearance. The CWM of
wolbachiae, about 10 μm in width, is distinct from the vacuolar membrane. In some instances, the vacuolar membrane was
absent or difficult to discern, as in H. leporispalustris
(Fig. 5). Often there is a periplasmic space that may be
filled with an electron-dense, fine granular, homogenous material. The plasma membrane is of typical unit membrane construction and often lies closely apposed to the cell wall.

In this configuration, it appears to be one of the cell wall
membranes per se. The nucleus and cytoplasm are typical of
procaryotic organisms. They have a dense-appearing cortical
region that contains prominent ribosomes randomly dispersed
in a homogenous, electron-dense ground substance. They also
possess a medullary or nuclear region which is electron-lucent
and essentially free of ribosomes. Frequently within this
medullary region were dense nucleoid bodies that have the appearance of whorls with anastomosing fibrils. A variable
space between the symbiote and the host vacuolar membrane is
always seen, but is particularly pronounced in the symbiote
vacuole of R. sanguineus. Also observed within this space,
in R. sanguineus and A. americanum, were small vesicles or
viroid-like particles (Figs. 6, 7).

The fine structure of the H. leporispalustris wolbachia
deviates somewhat from that of the other symbiotes in that it
possesses a rather rigid cell wall consisting of a single CW
membrane and appears to be free in the cytoplasm, i.e., not
within a vacuole.

A halo zone surrounding the organisms in "nests" of symbiotes was seen in D. andersoni, D. variabilis and H. leporispalustris but not in the other ticks (Figs. 3, 4, 5).

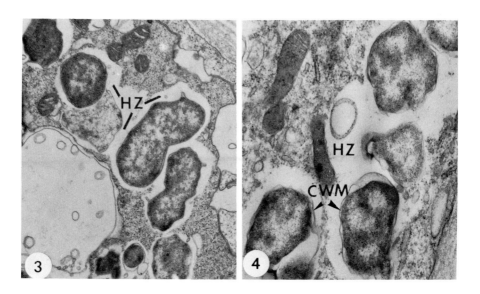

Fig. 3. D. andersoni wolbachiae in cytoplasm of undiffer-
entiated oogonial cell. Halo-zone (HZ). 16,500X

Fig. 4. D. variabilis wolbachiae in cytoplasm of ovarial
interstitial cell. Note the flaccid CWM and the HZ around
these organisms. 28,500X

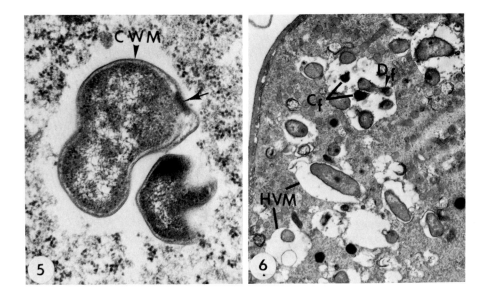

Fig. 5. H. leporispalustris wolbachiae in developing
oocyte. Note rigidity of CWM and the lack of a HVM. An electron dense material in the periplasmic space may be seen
(arrow). 45,000X
Fig. 6. R. sanguineus wolbachiae within vacuoles in developing oocyte. Note the D_f, dividing form, C_f condensing
form and the HVM around the nests of wolbachiae containing
all developmental forms. 8,700X

Occasionally, in R. sanguineus and A. americanum, wolbachiae were seen within autophagosomes, where they appear to
undergo degeneration. The organisms seemed to have lost their
differentiated morphology and were of condensed crystalline
form (Figures 6, 7). Reduction in volume and increase in
density gave them the appearance of chlamydial elementary
bodies (9, 10).
Multiplication of wolbachiae is by binary fission without
formation of transverse septa. Frequently the organisms take
on a leaflet or pinched dough appearance that seems to result
from the pulling or pinching apart of the daughter units.
Although ovarial tissues were often heavily infected with
symbiotes, there was no evidence of histopathologic changes.

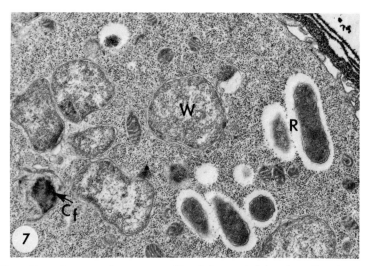

Fig. 7. <u>A</u>. <u>americanum</u> wolbachiae within developing oocyte infected with spotted fever group rickettsiae. W = wolbachiae, C_f = condensing form, and R = rickettsiae. 12,300X

IV. DISCUSSION

Differentiation of tick-borne wolbachiae from spotted fever group rickettsiae, often difficult by conventional microscopy, can readily be accomplished by electron microscopy. Most characteristic of these symbiotes is the differentiation of their cytoplasm into an electron-dense cortical region and an electron-lucent medullary or nuclear region. The cytoplasm of RMSF rickettsiae, on the other hand, consists of a more or less finely amorphous ground substance that contains ribosomes of various sizes but no reticulate fibrillar matrix or nucleoid inclusion bodies (6, 13, 14). Other differences include the development of wolbachiae in vacuoles (with the exception of those in <u>H</u>. <u>leporispalustris</u>), the absence of a microcapsular layer, and their limited distribution within the ticks (8, 11, 12, 15, 16).

Despite morphologic similarities, wolbachiae of the 5 tick species studied represent a highly heterogenous group not only in their sizes but also in their fine structure. Thus, the symbiote of <u>H</u>. <u>leporispalustris</u> has a cell wall different from those of the other symbiotes, and exists free of a vacuolar environment in the cytoplasm of its host tissues.

The presence of a halo zone or slime layer, commonly associated with pathogenic rickettsiae (8, 13, 14), surrounding

"nests" of wolbachiae in D. andersoni, D. variabilis, and
H. leporispalustris has not previously been alluded to. We
do not feel that this halo zone represents an artifact but
rather a phenomenon associated with the respective symbiotes.

The viroidal particles within the vacuolar space of symbiotes in R. sanguineus and A. americanum have never been
found in the wolbachiae of the other three ticks studied.
Similar bodies have been observed in Wolbachia pipientis of
Culex pipiens by Wright et al. (12) who suggested that they
may represent phage or turoidal virus particles.

The presence of wolbachiae within certain parts of the
digestive system of ticks, particularly males, is a new finding. Previous failure by Burgdorfer et al. (6) to detect
them in the posterior lobes of the midgut and in the small
intestine may have been due to the possibility that only anterior lobes were examined. Trager (17) reported wolbachiae
within the anterior lobes of the diverticula of larval and
nymphal D. variabilis. The finding of wolbachiae in the lobes
of the posterior diverticula of adult ticks suggests migration
of the symbiotes during ecdysis.

Hecker et al. (15) and Rheinhart et al. (16) studied the
wolbachiae of the African argasid tick, Ornithodoros moubata,
and described two distinct morphologic forms. A round form
whose ultrastructure is similar to those observed in the present study was found within vacuoles in tissues of the ovary
and malpighian tubule. A larger, typically rickettsialike
form was said to occur within the salivary gland, coxal organs,
central ganglion, rectal ampule, and midgut. Existence of
two different morphotypes of the same symbiote in the same
tick was discussed, but the possibility that the larger symbiote represented a secondarily acquired rickettsia was not
considered.

Lastly, we now have studies in progress to characterize
the wolbachiae of the various tick vectors in an effort to
establish their antigenic relatedness and to determine possible interactions between symbiotes and secondarily acquired
pathogens.

V.   SUMMARY

This paper describes the morphology and ultrastructure of
wolbachia-like organisms in D. andersoni, D. variabilis, R.
sanguineus, H. leporispalustris and A. americanum. Morphologically, these symbiotes are highly pleomorphic and vary in
size from 0.3 to 4 μm in diameter. They occur singly and/or
in colony-like coalescent groups within vacuoles of the host

tissues with the exception of the Hlp wolbachia which can
exist outside a vacuole. Ultrastructurally, they have a mul-
tilamellar, sinuous, membrane-type cell wall, a periplasmic
space of uniform dimension, and a well-differentiated cytoplasm which consists of a medullary region and a dense appearing cortical region containing prominent, but randomly distributed, ribosomes. The medullary region is electron lucent
and devoid of ribosomes or granular ground substance but contains a reticular, fibrous matrix, which sometimes appears as
whorls or dense nucleoid masses. Division appears to be by
binary fission.

REFERENCES

1. Cowdry, E. V., J. Exp. Med. 41, 817 (1925).
2. Hertig, M., Parasitol. 28, 453 (1936).
3. Roshdy, M. A., J. Invert. Path. 2, 155 (1968).
4. Suitor, E. C., Jr., and Weiss, E., J. Infect. Dis. 108,
    95 (1961).
5. Philip, C. B., in "Bergey's Manual of Determinative
    Bacteriology", 7th ed. (Breed et al., eds.), p. 952.
    Williams & Wilkins Co., Baltimore (1957).
6. Burgdorfer, W., Brinton, L. P., and Hughes, L. E.,
    J. Invert. Path. 22, 424 (1973).
7. Weiss, E., in "Bergey's Manual of Determinative Bacteri-
    ology", 8th Ed. (Buchanan et al., eds.), p. 898.
    Williams & Wilkins Co., Baltimore (1974).
8. Hayes, S. F., and Burgdorfer, W., J. Bacteriol. 137,
    605 (1979).
9. Anderson, D. R., Hopps, H. E., Barile, M. F., and
    Bernheim, B. C., J. Bacteriol. 90, 1387 (1965).
10. Costerton, J. W., Poffenroth, L., Wilt, J. C., and
    Kordova, N., Can. J. Microbiol. 21, 1433 (1975).
11. Wright, J. D., and Barr, A. R., J. Ultrastruct. Res. 72,
    52 (1980).
12. Wright, J. D., Sjostrand, F. S., Portaro, J. K., and
    Barr, A. R., J. Ultrastruct. Res. 63, 79 (1978).
13. Burgdorfer, W., Aeschlimann, A., Peter, O., Hayes, S. F.,
    and Philip, R. N., Acta Tropica 36, 357 (1979).
14. Hayes, S. F., and Burgdorfer, W., Infect. Immun. 27,
    638 (1980).
15. Hecker, H., Aeschlimann, A., and Burkhardt, M. J., Acta
    Tropica 25, 256 (1968).
16. Rheinhardt, C., Aeschlimann, A., and Hecker, H., Z.
    Parasitenk. 39, 201 (1972).
17. Trager, W., J. Parasitol. 25, 233 (1939).

BIOLOGY OF RICKETTSIAE

SOME BIOLOGICAL PROPERTIES OF RICKETTSIAE PATHOGENIC FOR MAN

Charles L. Wisseman, Jr.

Department of Microbiology
University of Maryland
School of Medicine
Baltimore, Maryland

I.   INTRODUCTION

My previous review of biological properties of rickettsiae pathogenic for Man in 1967 at the International Symposium on Rickettsiae and Rickettsial Diseases at Smolenice (1) dealt with a portion of the evolving, but limited, body of information that was permitting rickettsiae to be accepted fully as bacteria, as previously suggested by Moulder (2). In support of this basic concept, broad similarities and a few special differences among "the rickettsiae" were stressed. The importance of this conceptual advance cannot be stressed too strongly, for it brought to bear on rickettsiology the enormous conceptual framework of the science of bacteriology.

Since that time, there have been enormous advances in methodologies for studying rickettsiae, which had previously presented so many technical obstacles - e.g., improved methods for preparing purified suspensions of rickettsiae with high viability, simple methods for counting the number of rickettsial bodies in a suspension, methods for quantitating viable rickettsiae and of cloning rickettsiae by now simple routine plaque techniques, highly reproducible, quantitative cell culture methods and many others, including those of electron microscopy. This technological revolution has literally unshackled the rickettsiologist in the laboratory, introduced an unprecedented level of quantitation, and permitted rickettsiae to be examined by the most sophisticated methods of modern microbiology and molecular biology. An enormous

amount of new information has accumulated, but the information
gap between rickettsiae and other bacteria is so great that
many great deficits still exist. Some of these advances were
reviewed by Weiss (3) at the Second International Symposium on
Rickettsiae and Rickettsial Diseases also held at Smolenice in
1976 and, in an unpublished review presented at the ASM
Conference on Mechanisms of Microbial Virulence held at
Clearwater Beach, Florida in 1977, I developed in abbreviated
historical perspective some of the concepts which I include in
brief updated form here.

The accumulating evidence strongly suggests that we are
not dealing simply with a group of closely related microorganisms that differ from one another in only minor ways, but
instead are finding that these organisms display such an array
of properties that diverse origins must be considered as
highly likely. Indeed, these organisms, once lumped together
in the genus Rickettsia on the basis of some similarities in
size, shape and tinctorial properties, ill-defined host cell
association, arthropod transmission and characteristics of the
human disease, have already been redistributed by taxonomists
among the genera Rickettsia, Coxiella and Rochalimaea and
further reclassification can be expected. To account for the
observed diversity, it would not seem unreasonable to speculate that the organisms currently considered together on
traditional grounds as "rickettsiae pathogenic for Man" may
have arisen by two separate evolutionary processes. The first
is a process of convergent evolution in which procaryotic
organisms of diverse origin have adapted to occupy a series of
eukaryotic cell-associated niches in a sometimes alternating
arthropod-vertebrate cycle. This process has favored the
acquisition of some similar properties whose degree of
apparent similarity varies inversely with the observational
capabilities of the observer. Many apparent similarities,
which were a function of the limitations of light microscopy
but which were important in developing early ideas of
intracellular parasitism, are now rapidly giving way under the
scrutiny of more powerful tools to an appreciation that the
organisms under consideration actually display a broad range
of properties and types of host cell association. The second
major putative process is one of divergent evolution in which
some organisms of apparent common origin (a "group") have
evolved under selective influences into variants now known as
species, serotypes, etc. Though still incomplete, information
from studies on the genome and on phenotypic characteristics
seems to support this point of view.

In many ways, I would hope that this review might be the
last of those with a traditional, misleading, and now
anachronistic title of "The Biological Properties of the

Rickettsiae Pathogenic for Man". Although very important as a unifying mechanism in the evolution of knowledge about these organisms, the restrictions in thought imposed by this title have indeed hampered the smooth integration of rickettsiology into the more rapidly developing general field of microbiology and the fruitful comparison in pursuit of general principles of these organisms with the enormous range of cell-associated bacteria that exists in nature. Nevertheless, the uniqueness of these special organisms and the rich traditions associated with them will no doubt continue to captivate both the mind and heart of some investigators for years to come.

II. SELECTED OBSERVATIONS ON RICKETTSIAL BIOLOGY

In the short space available for this review, I have necessarily been highly selective. I have emphasized the long overdue application to rickettsiology of some of the simple, basic concepts of the kind that played such an important role in the development of bacteriology. Moreover, I stress some accumulating evidence for diversity of certain properties and kinds of interactions with host cells.

A. Pure Culture Methodology in Rickettsiology

The development of methods for obtaining pure cultures of bacteria was a hallmark event in the history of bacteriology. Refinement of the plaque technique for rickettsiae permitted only recently the ready application of the pure culture concept and practice to rickettsiology. The extent to which rickettsiologists have been working with impure or mixed cultures is now becoming evident and some aspects of rickettsiology may require re-examination or confirmation with the aid of pure cultures.

The critical need to apply pure culture practices to rickettsiae was recognized very early in our laboratories when we picked a low-frequency plaque from a chicken embryo cell monolayer inoculated with a conventional yolk sac seed of Rickettsia prowazekii, which had been incubated under selective conditions in search of antibiotic resistant mutants (Wisseman, C.L. Jr., and A. Waddell, unpublished data). Giménez-stained smears revealed organisms remarkably similar to R. prowazekii in size, shape and tinctorial properties. It grew in the yolk sac of embryonated chicken eggs producing a death pattern somewhat similar to that produced by R. prowazekii. But it was not R. prowazekii! Although the original

yolk sac seed from which it was derived had not shown any
bacterial contamination by routine sterility checks, the
organism was eventually coaxed to grow slowly in thiogly-
collate broth incubated at $32^{o}C$ in an atmosphere containing 5%
CO_2. Subsequently, it was found that the yolk sac seeds of
many rickettsiae, especially those in long yolk sac passage in
conventional eggs and those which required relatively concentrated infected yolk sac inocula in passage, contained
various extraneous agents, some bacterial and some possibly
viral, yielding plaques that ranged from very rare to numbers
that equalled those of the rickettsiae themselves. Detection
of extraneous plaque-forming agents, including some bacterial
agents, was facilitated by the fact that some were not
inhibited by concentrations of doxycycline (1 µg/ml) or
rifampin (1 µg/ml) which inhibited rickettsial growth.
Moreover, occasionally a bacterial microcolony could be
detected under magnification in the center of some extraneous
plaques. Finally, from time to time, uninoculated monolayers
of chicken embryo cells from conventional eggs, but very
rarely from specific pathogen-free (SPAFAS) eggs, showed
variable small numbers of spurious plaques.

Accordingly, we have applied the principles of the pure
culture technique to all of our strains of R. prowazekii, R.
mooseri, R. canada and all established and field isolates of
the spotted fever group in our possession. This has consisted
of three serial clonings of single plaques in monolayers of
chicken embryo cells from specific pathogen-free eggs,
followed by seed production in the yolk sac of specific
pathogen-free eggs. These seeds are now free of extraneous
agents detectable by the methods described above. One seed of
R. rickettsii, prepared in such a manner for use in a
vaccination-challenge study in human beings, was found to be
free of bacteria, mycoplasmas, fowl leukosis viruses and many
other agents in a special extensive safety testing. The
practice of using plaque-purified seeds of rickettsiae is now
widespread among rickettsiologists. It has also been applied
to serotypes of R. tsutsugamushi (Bozeman, F.M., personal
communication; 4) and to phase variants of Coxiella burnetii
(Ormsbee, R.A., personal communication).

One can only speculate about the aberrations in rickettsial research which might have been caused by the presence of
extraneous agents in rickettsial preparations. In preliminary
studies in our laboratories on immunity to R. mooseri in
guinea pigs, inoculation with conventional yolk sac seeds
produced some confusing results attributed to extraneous
agents. Certainly, studies on metabolism, DNA composition,
polypeptide analysis, etc., could be severely distorted by a

high proportion of extraneous bacterial organisms in the
rickettsial preparation approaching that of the rickettsiae.

The plaque cloning technique also offers the opportunity
to resolve several potential problems associated with the
possible admixture of species, strains, serotypes or phase
variants among the rickettsiae themselves. For example, in
our laboratories we have been able to isolate multiple pure
cultures of R. prowazekii from the blood of typhus patients in
the Burundi epidemic, of R. mooseri from the tissues of small
mammals from Ethiopia and Burma and of R. rickettsii from the
blood of patients with Rocky Mountain spotted fever.
Rickettsial isolates from the field may in fact consist of
mixtures of strains, serotypes or even species. Accordingly,
we have been able to plaque-purify the spotted fever group
isolates from pools of ticks from Pakistan (5) and have begun
to plaque purify some of the isolates of R. tsutsugamushi from
pools of small mammal tissues and chiggers from Pakistan
(6). Moreover, some of the perplexing observations on scrub
typhus in human beings and in chiggers in Malaysia (7, 8),
which involve such major basic issues as variable transmission
of mixtures of serotypes vs. variation in phenotypic expression of antigenic determinants, likely will be resolved by
application of the pure culture techniques. Finally, the
study of rickettsial genetics has been facilitated, although
there remain some major technical problems which limit the
capacity to detect low frequency mutants (Wisseman, C.L. Jr.,
and A. Waddell, unpublished observations).

Plaque purification, however, is not without certain
theoretical disadvantages. The clone selected might differ in
significant properties from those dominant in the wild
population and must be carefully characterized to assure that
the clone selected retains the desired characteristics. This
has not yet been a problem in our laboratory with respect to
those characteristics which we have examined in detail.
Moreover, such purified seeds of R. prowazekii (Breinl), R.
mooseri (Wilmington) and R. rickettsii retain the capacity to
produce disease in human beings. Finally, attempts to select
stable plaque-size variants from a spotted fever group isolate
from Pakistan failed. Clones derived from small and large
plaques gave indistinguishable distributions of plaque size
(Wisseman, C.L. Jr., and M.R. Jones, unpublished observations). Nevertheless, the need for caution remains and the
necessity of preserving "wild" stocks of rickettsiae as a
source for the full range of genetic information is evident.

B. Very Selected Observations on the
    Nature of the Organisms

Although the ghost of a special status of rickettsiae
somewhere between viruses and bacteria still haunts some
textbooks, electron microscope studies by a number of
investigators have revealed that members of the genus
Rickettsia and Rochalimaea have many ultrastructural features
in common with other gram negative bacteria (9-14). The outer
envelope of Rickettsia tsutsugamushi, however, differs
substantially in ultrastructural detail from the outer
envelopes of R. prowazekii and R. rickettsii (11). The nature
and function of the microcapsular layer (12-14) and the slime
layer (10) that have been demonstrated on some members of the
genus Rickettsia remain to be clarified.
     Studies of the rickettsial genome are beginning to yield
important information. The existence of a compact nucleoid,
first suggested by Ris and Fox (15) on the basis of Feulgen-
positive spherical structures in R. prowazekii, has been
confirmed for this organism by fluorescence microscopy of
DAPI-and ethidium bromide-stained organisms (Wisseman, C.L.
Jr., D.J. Silverman and A. Waddell, unpublished observations). The same studies demonstrated by the Kleinschmidt
technique existence of a single chromosome organized as in
other bacteria and suggested the existence of plasmids in the
form of 2-3 size ranges of apparent minicircular DNA. The
genome size is considerable, varying between about 1.0 and 1.5
x 10^9 daltons, depending upon the rickettsial species and
subgroup (16-19). As with other bacteria, the number of
polypeptides of average molecular weight theoretically coded
for by a genome of this size far exceeds the number actually
found by SDS-PAGE electrophoresis, isoelectric focussing or 2-
dimensional electrophoresis. The different genera and
subgroups studied to date have distinctive nucleotide
compositions (%G+C) (17-21). DNA hybridization studies in
progress are beginning to yield important information about
the natural groupings of rickettsial organisms, the degree of
relatedness within groups and the probabilities of common or
diverse origins (18, 19; Myers, W.F., and Wisseman, C.L. Jr.,
this volume). On a practical plane, these studies have
already yielded information which strongly points to the
improbability of rapid interconversions between R. mooseri and
R. prowazekii in a simple selective process or between R.
mooseri and R. conori (22).
     Finally, studies on the nutritional requirements of
members of the genus Rickettsia and the nature of the host
cell dependence have progressed little beyond those reported
by Hopps et al. (23) over two decades ago. However, advances

in quantitative methodology and in knowledge of growth cycles
(vide infra) have made possible a few additional observations. Thus, the lack of immediate direct dependence of
rickettsial growth on the host cell nucleus that was suggested
by the observations of Hopps et al. (23) on the growth of R.
tsutsugamushi and other members of the genus in host cells
arrested in the metaphase by colchicine has been amply
confirmed by demonstration of growth of different members of
the genus (1) in x-irradiated host cells (24-26), (2) in
enucleated host cells (27) and (3) in host cells in which DNA
synthesis has been inhibited by pretreatment with Mitomycin C
(Wisseman, C. L., Jr., A. Waddell and M. L. Cremer, unpublished
observations). The independence of the growth of R. mooseri
and R. akari from host cell protein synthesis described by
Weiss' group (24, 28) in cycloheximide-inhibited cells has
been amply confirmed by similar observations with R.
prowazekii, R. rickettsii and R. tsutsugamushi grown in
cycloheximide- or emetine-inhibited host cells (28; Oaks,
E. V., Wisseman, C. L., Jr., Smith, J. F., this volume)
(Hanson, B., and Wisseman, C. L., Jr., this volume). Diversity among groups within the genus, however, has been detected
in the requirement for growth on atmosphere enriched in CO_2 by
species of the typhus and spotted fever groups but not by
strains of R. tsutsugamushi (29). A systematic study of
rickettsial nutritional requirements might now yield much
useful information.

>   C.   Where Rickettsiae Grow: Morphologic Clues from
>   Major Replication Sites to Diversity in
>   Rickettsia-Host Cell Interactions

    Light and electron microscope studies of cultures of
rickettsia-infected host cells have revealed a considerable
diversity in detail of the association with host cells among
the various rickettsiae pathogenic for man. Some major
categories of host association among these are described
below. Whether these reflect physiological differences among
these organisms is unknown.

    1. Replication "Free" in Cytoplasm. All members of genus
Rickettsia replicate free in the cytoplasm of their host cell,
not surrounded by a vacuolar membrane (9, 30, 31). The
density to which they accumulate, the tendency to grow in
compact masses or to be diffusely distributed in the cytoplasm
or an apparent predilection for one portion of the cytoplasm
or another, e.g., the perinuclear region with R. tsutsugamushi
(32) and cytoplasmic processes with R. rickettsii (26, 33),

seem to be functions in part of the rickettsial species but
also may be influenced by other factors, such as the kind of
host cell and conditions and stage of growth. This bears
further systematic and controlled study.

    2. Replication Within the Host Cell Nucleus. Rickettsia
canada (34), all established species of the spotted fever
group of rickettsiae and many as yet unnamed or provisionally
named recent spotted fever group isolates (35, 36; Wisseman,
C. L., Jr., Steiman, I., and Jones, M. R., unpublished data)
may also grow within the host cell nucleus. In this site, the
organisms often appear as compact masses, free in the nucleoplasm.
    A systematic comparative study in CE cell cultures of
growth characteristics of established spotted fever group
species and of various field isolates revealed that intranuclear growth was detectable relatively late in the life of
the culture and was present in only a minority (usually <5%)
of the infected cells (Wisseman, C. L., Jr., Steiman, I., and
Jones, M. R., unpublished data).

    3. Replication Within Cytoplasmic Membrane-Bound Vacuole.
In contrast, Coxiella burnetii, which most likely enters the
host cell passively by endocytosis, replicates within
membrane-bound cytoplasmic vacuoles or vesicles, which may
occupy much of the host cell cytoplasm (37). The significance
of the occasional organism free in the cytoplasm is not
known.

    4. Pericellular Association. Finally, Rochalimaea
quintana and the related Baker's vole agent, both capable of
growth in artificial, cell-free medium, grow in cell cultures
in close association with the external surface of the "host
cell" plasma membrane (38) -- i.e., a pericellular
predilection. R. quintana also shows a close extracellular
association with brush border of the midgut cells of its louse
vector (39).

    D. Intracellular Growth Cycle: Emerging Patterns
                 Among Rickettsia Spp.

    Simplified, quantitative in vitro methods, employing
cultures of infected relatively isolated non-replicating host
cells, have permitted confirmation and extension of the
observations on intracellular rickettsial growth begun some

years ago by the Walter Reed group (23, 32, 40) and have led
to the recognition of distinctive growth patterns among
members of the genus Rickettsia.

All adequately studied members of the genera Rickettsia
and Rochalimaea replicate by binary fission. In contrast, at
this meeting McCaul et al. reported the formation by
Coxiella burnetii of minute, dense, multilamellate forms and
Khavkin showed putative minute forms in infected tissues.

Two distinct growth cycle patterns in chicken embryo cells
in culture, which reflect quite different associations with
host cells, have emerged among Rickettsia species. These
patterns appear to be broadly applicable to the extent that
observations have been extended to other host cell types.

No evidence for the existence of an "eclipse phase", as
proposed earlier by Kordova (41), has been encountered in any
of the many organisms observed to date, rickettsiae being
continuously visible through all stages of infection.
However, the possible occurrence of unusual forms under some
circumstances has not been excluded, as the recent experience
with C. burnetii illustrates.

Type 1 (R. prowazekii prototype) (25, 31, 42). Upon entry
into the host cell cytoplasm, the organisms replicate by
binary fission and undergo a growth cycle, with attendant
morphologic changes, similar to that of a classical bacterium
in a fluid medium. The presence or absence of a lag phase is
dependent upon the physiological state of the infecting
organisms. The organisms are retained within the host cell
until it eventually breaks down to release the contained
organisms, upon which new infection cycles are initiated in
previously uninfected cells. The host cell shows very little
evidence of ultrastructural damage almost up to the time it
breaks down. This growth cycle pattern, originally
demonstrated with the Breinl and E strains of R. prowazekii,
has also been observed with recent R. prowazekii isolates,
such as from typhus patients in Burundi and the strains from
flying squirrels, and hence may be a constant or dominant
species characteristic (Wisseman, C.L. Jr., and A. Waddell,
unpublished results). In contrast to the in vivo observations
reported by Osterman's group (43), results obtained to date in
our laboratories with prototype serotypes of R. tsutsugamushi
in vitro suggest, not yet published, that these follow a
similar growth cycle pattern. Certain unresolved technical
problems with the quantitation of R. tsutsugamushi, with
evaluation of detailed morphology and with its state of
adaptation to growth in CE cells leave some aspects of its
growth cycle unresolved.

Type 2. (R. rickettsii prototype) (26, 30, 33, 35, 44).
From the earliest time points after infection that

statistically significant changes can be measured, organisms
showing this spreading type of growth cycle show evidence of
escaping from infected cells without causing detectable damage
and infect other cells in the culture so that most cells in
the culture are soon infected with small numbers of
organisms. Although the organisms have been found in fine
cell processes, suggesting the possibility that the pinching
off of host cell membrane-bound organisms might be the
mechanism of escape, evidence presented at this meeting by
Silverman and Wisseman supports the idea that in the early
spreading stages of infection the organisms which escape from
host cells are not surrounded by a membrane. Only later,
after the host cells show damage and breakdown, are membrane-
bound organisms transiently present. The organisms do not
accumulate in quantity in cells until late, when they seem to
be trapped by the enormous vesicle formation by endoplasmic
reticulum characteristic of late stages of infection by R.
rickettsii. In a minority of the infected cell population,
the nucleus is invaded where the organisms accumulate in
compact masses. Originally described for the Sheila Smith
strain of R. rickettsii, this growth pattern has now been
demonstrated for recent isolates of R. rickettsii from
Maryland and Costa Rica and, in similar form for all
established species of the spotted fever group and for recent
field isolates of spotted fever group rickettsiae from
Pakistan, Czechoslovakia and Israel (Wisseman, C.L. Jr., I.
Steiman and M.R. Jones, unpublished results). Hence, it
appears to be a characteristic of the spotted fever group.

A similar spreading type of infection, but without nuclear
invasion and not yet subjected to detailed ultrastructural
study, has been found with all strains of R. mooseri (R.
typhi) tested to date -- viz., the classical Wilmington strain
and recent field isolates from Ethiopia and Pakistan
(Wisseman, C.L. Jr., et al., unpublished observations).

Type 3. This type of growth cycle has tentatively been
applied to that exhibited by Coxiella burnetii, which grows
intracellularly in membrane bound vesicles.

In addition to the general biological significance of
these reproducible growth patterns, which seem to be stable
characteristics of strains of rickettsial species and of some,
but not all (e.g., the typhus group), groups, detailed
information about the quantitative aspects of rickettsial
uptake and of growth cycles of the different rickettsiae has
permitted an unprecedented capacity, with great predictability
and reliability, to produce in cell cultures any desired
degree of infection, to provide organisms in any desired

physiological state related to growth cycle and to perform an
enormous variety of quantitative studies which require
measurement of rickettsial growth.

E. Host Cell Range

Despite the fact that the host cell range (i.e., "target
cells") appears to be sharply restricted in natural rickettsial infections of Man and certain other mammals largely to
endothelial cells of small blood vessels in infections caused
by members of the genus Rickettsia and to phagocytic cells of
the monocyte-macrophage-histiocyte series in Coxiella burnetii
infections, an extremely broad range of cells support the
growth of these organisms in culture in vitro.
Probably, best studied is the host cell range of
Rickettsia prowazekii. A broad range of cells permissive for
growth, of reptilian, avian and mammalian origin, was
documented in the 1967 review (1). Since that time, partly
through studies performed for other purposes, a large list of
cells which support the growth of R. prowazekii strains has
accumulated in our laboratories (Dalton, D., A. Waddell and
C.L. Wisseman, Jr., unpublished observations). These include
cells of fish and mammalian (human, sub-human primate, mouse,
hamster) origin, fibroblast and epithelial types, and primary,
diploid, virus-transformed and malignant states. In addition,
we have observed growth in the following cells of human origin
related to the vascular, inflammatory and immune systems:
umbilical cord endothelial cells (Wisseman, C.L. Jr. and A.
Waddell, unpublished observations), peripheral monocytes and
monocyte-derived macrophages (45, 46) and peripheral blood
lymphocytes (Stork, E. and C.L. Wisseman, Jr., unpublished
observations). Finally, we (Beaman, L., D. Dalton and C.L.
Wisseman, Jr., unpublished observations) have found that fresh
resident (unstimulated) peritoneal macrophages from outbred
Swiss mice, a host relatively resistant to virulent R.
prowazekii infection, did not support the growth of R.
prowazekii in culture but that such cells in culture for 6
days supported rich rickettsial growth, as did a continuous
line of SV-40-transformed mouse macrophages.
These accumulated observations suggest that R. prowazekii
is remarkably catholic in the range of eukaryotic cells of
vertebrate origin which, in culture, it will infect and within
which it will grow. Such cells, permissive in culture, must
therefore possess and express those factors, processes and
conditions essential for this rickettsia to enter the host
cell and to grow within it. Little has yet been done to apply
modern methods of cell biology or even to use the existing

valuable collections of cell cultures with defined,
genetically determined metabolic and other lesions to the
study of the nature(s) of rickettsia-host cell interactions.
Knowledge of the "biology" of an obligate intracellular parasite cannot be complete without also considering the biology
of the host cell.

In contrast, the dominant host cell range expressed during
natural typhus infection within the intact mammalian host or
arthropod vector (louse midgut epithelial cells) is by
comparison severely restricted, despite the fact that other
cell types may become infected with different routes of
inoculation -- e.g., intraperitoneal or intranasal routes in
mammals and into the hemocoele of lice (47). The factors
responsible for "targeting" rickettsiae to selected cell types
in intact animals are not clear at this time. Nor is it known
how the different growth cycles observed in vitro are
expressed in vivo infection and how they might be related to
pathogenesis of disease and to the way these microorganisms
interact with both innate and acquired immune systems in the
animal host.

F. Interaction of Rickettsiae with Host Cell Membranes

As obligate intracellular parasites of eukaryotic cells,
members of the genus Rickettsia must possess mechanisms by
which they can enter into the appropriate intracellular micro-
habitat and subsequently escape from it. This implies some
means for passing across the plasma membrane and, perhaps, of
interacting with other membranous host cell structures. Some
aspects of the entry of rickettsiae into host cells, and the
two related paraphenomena of rickettsia-induced hemolysis and
mouse lethal toxic action, have received considerable attention by investigators over many years. During our studies on
rickettsial infection cycles (vide supra), however, certain
patterns began to emerge which suggested the concept of an
array of interactions between various members of the genus
Rickettsia and different host cell membranous structures.
This includes such considerations as similarities and
differences among members of the genus, concepts of direction
of transit and possible differential susceptibility of outer
and inner membrane leaflets to rickettsial action and differential susceptibility of different kinds of host cell
membranous structures to rickettsial action. The evolving
conceptual framework, first presented at the 1977 ASM
Conference on Mechanisms of Microbial Virulence, is outlined
briefly below, along with some selected supporting detail.
1. All members of the genus Rickettsia have the capacity

to pass through the host cell plasma membrane in the direction
from an extracellular site to an intracytoplasmic site where
they replicate "free" in the cytoplasm.

This directional transit of rickettsiae across the plasma
membrane into the host cell has been the most studied of all
rickettsia-host cell membrane interactions. According to the
early observations of Cohn et al. (48) with R. tsutsugamushi
and more recently of Winkler and his associates (49) with R.
prowazekii, uptake, which requires metabolically competent
rickettsiae and host cells, involves at least two steps, i.e.,
attachment to the plasma membrane and subsequent passage
through it, both of which are temperature dependent. Our own
studies on R. prowazekii uptake (Wisseman, C.L. Jr., D. Dalton
and A. Waddell, unpublished data) suggest that the influence
of temperature is complex, probably involving differential
effects on both rickettsia and host cell.

The nature of the receptors and substrates on the host
cell has begun to yield to investigation. Several years ago,
as some of the implications of the extra-ordinarily broad host
cell range for R. prowazekii (vide supra) began to surface
into conscious thought, it became apparent to me that the
receptors and substrates for "penetration" in the outer
leaflet of the plasma membrane were likely to be constituents
common to a very wide range of vertebrate cells, possibly
lipid in nature. Indeed, some preliminary inhibition
experiments with n-butanol extracts of isolated plasma
membranes from several types of cells were just beginning to
show promising results when Winkler and his associates (50;
elsewhere in this volume) began to publish papers implicating
cholesterol and phospholipids and, more recently, to show the
accumulation of products of phospholipase activity.

The exact mechanism by which the rickettsiae physically
cross the plasma membrane remains speculative. Concepts have
ranged between the extremes of the creation of a physical
defect in the plasma membrane with the passage of the
rickettsia through this defect by some ill-defined means,
possibly involving sublemmal contractile fibrils, to
phagocytosis with subsequent escape from the phagosome, with
"induced phagocytosis" in between. This has been complicated
by the fact that investigators rarely have presented
quantitative data on the innate phagocytic activity of the
host cells employed under the conditions of experiment.

Although the molecular approach, often relying upon
indirect methods, has yielded important results, classical
methods of observing processes with the aid of the light and
electron microscope can yield additional perspectives.
Accordingly, I take the liberty to recount some observations
made over the last two decades, mostly unpublished, which may

have a bearing on the two extreme poles identified above.

In historical sequence, in the early 1960's when I was
studying phagocytosis and opsonization of typhus rickettsiae,
I observed under phase microscopy the interaction of viable
rickettsial preparations with different cell types from human
peripheral blood. The many hours of observation with erythrocytes were not fruitful but, with certain nucleated cell types
which generated quantities of microfibrils, it was possible to
observe a mechanism of entry which differed sharply from
classical phagocytosis. An extracellular rickettsia in the
absence of antiserum lying in contact with a microfibril one
instant would be translocated into the microfibril so rapidly
that the details of the process could not be observed and the
bulge in the microfibril caused by the rickettsia could be
seen moving centripetally towards the cell cytoplasm. This
was clearly not the classical mechanism of phagocytosis.

Then, when the concentration of extracellular rickettsiae
was increased sharply, cells clearly identified as
polymorphonuclear leukocytes rapidly and literally exploded,
releasing cytoplasmic granules, and the nucleus promptly
stained with trypan blue. Almost a decade later, in
collaboration with Dr. Dennis T. Brown, then on the faculty of
our Department of Pharmacology and Cell Biology, we attempted
to catch R. prowazekii in the act of entering the relatively
nonphagocytic chicken embryo fibroblast by gently centrifuging
the CE cells onto a layer of rickettsiae in the cold, warming
the tube to 37° C and fixing for electron microscopy after
short intervals (the "Mohammed" experiment). After only 1.5
to 2 minutes of warming, the CE cells were already reduced to
disorganized rubble, with prominent membrane fragments.

Then, when Ms. Waddell joined my group, we began the
development of methods for the precise, reproducible infection
of cells (Wisseman, C.L. Jr., and A. Waddell, in preparation),
along with appropriate statistical models. We observed that,
at very high rickettsial concentrations, when the probabilities were very high for a single host cell to have multiple
interactions with rickettsiae within a very short period of
time, there was progressive host cell lysis without significant antecedant accumulation of trypan blue positive cells.
These same studies showed that, under the conditions of these
experiments, the CE cells displayed a negligible, statistically insignificant degree of phagocytosis of dead rickettsiae.

These studies clearly indicated that typhus rickettsiae
could (1) gain entry into eukaryotic cells by a process which
differed from classical phagocytosis and (2) cause rapid loss
of the integrity of the plasma membrane and disruption of the
cell when large numbers of rickettsiae interacted with cells

within a short period of time, i.e., can cause defects in the
plasma membrane. It is conceivable that defects in the plasma
membrane produced by one or a few rickettsiae can be sealed
over quickly and preserve the host cell integrity but that,
when multiple defects are produced above a critical rate, the
plasma membrane loses its integrity and the cells disrupt.
There is no slow increase in cell permeability. As a result
of this series of observations, I introduced the concept of
"lysis from without" at the 1977 ASM Conference, recently
adopted by Walker and Winkler (51) in their studies with polymorphonuclear leukocytes.

At the opposite extreme are the observations by Meyer and
Wisseman (46) on the mechanism of entry of R. prowazekii into
the cytoplasm of human macrophages in culture in the absence
of immune serum where they multiply free of a phagosomal
membrane as they do in other cells which are not professional
phagocytes. In this case, initial entry of the rickettsia
into the macrophage cytoplasm is largely by phagocytosis.
Within a very few minutes, however, an easily observed
enlarging defect regularly appears in the phagosomal membrane
and very soon the still viable rickettsia is free in the
cytoplasm. This constitutes the best direct evidence that R.
prowazekii can cause a visible physical defect in a host cell
plasma membrane-derived structure.

It is unknown at this time if simple creation of a defect
in the plasma membrane will permit otherwise non-motile
rickettsiae to move through the plasma membrane to an intracytoplasmic site. It is conceivable that the process involves
a very local progressive change in the plasma membrane under
the attached rickettsia resulting in a rapid, transient local
invagination of the plasma membrane as its integrity is being
breached, thus in effect "pulling" the rickettsia into the
cell and leaving the rickettsia "free" in the cytoplasm when
the defect reseals. A process of this kind would be compatible with the observations currently available. There is no
doubt that entry occurs very rapidly and by a process unlike
classical phagocytosis. Whether or not this is "induced
phagocytosis" is a matter of definition. Nevertheless, in
studies of this kind, it is crucial to define the innate
phagocytic capacity of the host cell employed, for one can
envision a whole range of results, depending upon the level of
innate phagocytic activity of the host cell, between the two
extremes described above.

2. Some rickettsiae in vitro, such as R. mooseri and
members of the spotted fever group, have the capacity to
escape from their host cells without visible damage to that
host cell whereas others, such as R. prowazekii and possibly
R. tsutsugamushi, do not and must await ultimate physical

disruption of the plasma membrane (25, 26; Wisseman, C.L. Jr., et al., unpublished observations). Indeed, Schaechter et al. (40) described the release of R. rickettsii from infected host cell processes in cultures observed continuously under phase contrast microscopy. This suggests that, whereas all Rickettsia spp. have the capacity to recognize and interact with components of the outer leaf of the host cell plasma membrane, only some have this capacity with respect to the inner surface of the plasma membrane.

This concept has been complicated by the fact that some non-quantitative and non-kinetic electron microscope studies have shown some rickettsiae, like R. rickettsii and R. tsutsugamushi, in host cell cytoplasmic processes (Whitescarver et al., unpublished observations; 33, 43). The investigators speculated that these organisms might escape by pinching off and that they might exist in the extracellular state as host cell membrane-bound organisms which could enter new cells by simple fusion of the membranes of host cell origin. In the case of R. rickettsii, however, the study by Silverman and Wisseman reported elsewhere in this volume suggested that this is not the case, in vitro at least, in the early spreading stages of the infection cycle. Moreover, our failure to detect spread of R. tsutsugamushi in culture until late in the growth cycle suggests that this does not occur as a significant mechanism with this organism in vitro either (vide supra). Whether or not such processes are involved in cell to cell spread in vivo in tissues composed of contiguous cells, as suggested by Ewing et al. (43) for R. tsutsugamushi, does not detract from the principle of differential capacity to escape as free organisms from host cells through the plasma membrane.

3. Members of the spotted fever group and R. canada have the capacity to pass through the nuclear membrane, at least in the direction from outside to inside the nucleus, whereas R. prowazekii, R. mooseri and R. tsutsugamushi do not. However, even with the spotted fever group, this is a relatively rare event.

4. Other intracellular membranes, such as those of the mitochondria and the endoplasmic reticulum, do not seem to be susceptible to the kind of action associated with passage of the organisms through the plasma membrane (30, 31, 33). Despite the apparent close association possible between rickettsiae and these intracellular membranes, there does not seem to be an early lytic action or substantial decrease in number of mitochondria. Especially late in the infection cycle of both R. prowazekii and R. rickettsii, mitochondria may show some relatively mild changes and, with R. rickettsii, the endoplasmic reticulum may show extensive vesicle

formation. However, even with the close physical association
of R. rickettsii with the outer surface of the endoplasmic
reticulum, the rickettsiae do not seem to pass through it.
Since the changes seen in both mitochondria and endoplasmic
reticulum are similar to those which are well-known early
responses of cells to a variety of types of cell injury, it is
not possible at this time to ascribe them either to direct
action of the rickettsiae or to a nonspecific response to cell
injury.

The plasma membrane and those of various intracellular
organelles, as well as the outer and inner leaflets of a given
membrane, may differ in composition. It may not be surprising
that different rickettsiae, which may vary in their capacity
to act upon different membrane components, should vary in
their capacity to pass through or to damage the different
membranous structure of their host cells.

REFERENCES

1. Wisseman, C.L. Jr. Zentralbl. f. Bakt., Parasitenk.,
    Infektionskr. u. Hyg. 206, 299 (1968).
2. Moulder, J.W. (1962). "The Biochemistry of Intracellular
    Parasites". Univ. of Chicago Press, Chicago.
3. Weiss, E. In "Rickettsiae and Rickettsial Diseases" (J.
    Kazar, R.A. Ormsbee and I.N. Tarasevich, eds), p. 137.
    VEDA Publ. House of the Slovak Acad. Sci., Bratislava.
4. Oaks, S.C. Jr., Osterman, J.V., and Hetrick, F.M. J.
    Clin. Microbiol. 6, 76 (1977).
5. Robertson, R.G., and Wisseman, C.L. Jr. Am. J.
    Epidemiol. 97, 55 (1973).
6. Traub, R., Wisseman, C.L. Jr., and Ahmad, N. Trans. Roy.
    Soc. Trop. Med. Hyg. 61, 23 (1967).
7. Shirai, A., Robinson, D.M., Brown, G.W., Gan, E., and
    Huxsoll, D.L. Japan. J. Med. Sci. Biol. 32, 337 (1979).
8. Robinson, D.M., Roberts, L.W., Dohany, A.L., Gan, E.,
    Chan, T.C., and Huxsoll, D.L. S.E. Asian J. Trop. Med.
    Publ. Hlth. 8, 227.
9. Anderson, D.R., Hopps, H.E., Barile, M.F., and Bernheim,
    B.C. J. Bacteriol. 90, 1387 (1965).
10. Silverman, D.J., Wisseman, C.L. Jr., Waddell, A.D., and
    Jones, M.R. Infect. Immun. 22, 233 (1978).
11. Silverman, D.J., and Wisseman, C.L. Jr. Infect. Immun.
    21, 1020 (1978).
12. Anacker, R.L., Pickens, E.G., and Lackman, D.B. J.
    Bacteriol. 94, 260 (1967).

13. Avakyan, A.A. In "Rickettsiae and Rickettsial Diseases" (J. Kazar, R.A Ormsbee and I.N. Tarasevich, eds), p. 21, VEDA Publ. House of the Slovak Acad. Sci., Bratislava.
14. Palmer, E.L., Martin, M.L., and Mallavia, L. Appl. Microbiol. 28, 713 (1974).
15. Ris, H., and Fox, J.P. J. Exper. Med. 89, 681 (1949).
16. Kingsbury, D.T. J. Bacteriol. 98, 1400 (1969).
17. Tyeryar, F.J. Jr., Weiss, E., Millar, D.B., Bozeman, F.M. and Ormsbee, R.A. Science 180, 415 (1973).
18. Myers, W.F., Wisseman, C.L. Jr., Fiset, P., Oaks, E.V., and Smith, J.F. Infect. Immun. 26, 976 (1979).
19. Myers, W.F., and Wisseman, C.L. Jr. J. Systematic Bacteriol. 30, 143 (1980).
20. Myers, W.F., Baca, O.G., and Wisseman, C.L. Jr. J. Bacteriol. 144, 460 (1980).
21. Wisseman, C.L. Jr. Acta Virol. 17, 443 (1973).
22. Giroud, P., and Jadin, J. Bull. Acad. Nat. Med. 164, 415 (1980).
23. Hopps, H.E., Jackson, E.B., Danauskas, J.X. and Smadel, J.E. J. Immunol. 82, 161 (1959).
24. Weiss, E., Newman, L.R., Grays, R., and Green, A.E. Infect. Immun. 6, 50 (1972).
25. Wisseman, C.L. Jr., and Waddell, A.D. Infect. Immun. 11, 1391 (1975).
26. Wisseman, C.L. Jr., Edlinger, E.A., Waddell, A.D., and Jones, M.R. Infect. Immun. 14, 1052 (1976).
27. Stork, E., and Wisseman, C.L. Jr. Infect. Immun. 13, 1743 (1976).
28. Weiss, E., Green, A.E., Grays, R., and Newman, L.M. Infect. Immun. 8, 4 (1973).
29. Kopmans-Gargantiel, A.E., and Wisseman, C.L. Jr. Infect. Immun. 31, 1277 (1981).
30. Silverman, D.J., and Wisseman, C.L. Jr. Infect. Immun. 26, 714 (1979).
31. Silverman, D.J., Wisseman, C.L. Jr., and Waddell, A. Infect. Immun. 29, 778 (1980).
32. Bozeman, F.M., Hopps, H.E., Danauskas, J.X., Jackson, E.B., and Smadel, J.E. J. Immunol. 76, 475 (1956).
33. Walker, D.H., and Cain, B.G. Lab. Invest. 43, 388 (1980).
34. Brinton, L.P., and Burgdorfer, W. J. Bacteriol. 105, 1149 (1971).
35. Pinkerton, H., and Hass, G.M. J. Exper. Med. 56, 151 (1932).
36. Burgdorfer, W., Anacker, R.L., Bird, R.G., and Bertram, D.S. J. Bacteriol. 96, 1415 (1968).

37. Burton, P.R., Stueckemann, J., Welsh, R.M., and Paretsky, D. Infect. Immun. 21, 556 (1978).
38. Merrell, B.R., Weiss, E., and Dasch, G.A. J. Bacteriol. 135, 633 (1978).
39. Ito, S., and Vinson, J.W. J. Bacteriol. 89, 481 (1965).
40. Schaechter, M., Bozeman, F.M., and Smadel, J.E. Virology 3, 160 (1957).
41. Kordova, N., and Kovacova, E. Acta Virol. 11, 252 (1967).
42. Wisseman, C.L. Jr., Waddell, A.D., and Silverman, D.J. Infect. Immun. 13, 1749 (1976).
43. Ewing, E.P. Jr., Takeuchi, A., Shirai, A., and Osterman, J.V. Infect. Immun. 19, 1068 (1978).
44. Kokorin, I.N. Acta Virol. 12, 31 (1968).
45. Gambrill, M.R., and Wisseman, C.L. Jr. Infect. Immun. 8, 519 (1973).
46. Meyer, W.A. III, and Wisseman, C.L. Jr. Amer. Soc. for Microbiology Abstracts, p. 39 (1980).
47. Weyer, F. In "Rickettsiae and Rickettsial Diseases" (J. Kazar, R.A. Ormsbee and I.N. Tarasevich, eds), p. 515, VEDA Publ. House of the Slovak Acad. Sci., Bratislava.
48. Cohn, Z.A., Bozeman, F.M., Campbell, J.M., Humphries, J.W. and Sawyer, T.K. J. Exp. Med. 109, 271 (1959).
49. Walker, T.S., and Winkler, H.H. Infect. Immun. 22, 200 (1978).
50. Ramm, L.E., and Winkler, H.H. Infect. Immun. 13, 550 (1976).
51. Walker, T.S., and Winkler, H.H. Infect. Immun. 31, 289 (1981).

THE TAXONOMIC RELATIONSHIP OF RICKETTSIA CANADA TO THE TYPHUS AND SPOTTED FEVER GROUPS OF THE GENUS RICKETTSIA

William F. Myers
Charles L. Wisseman, Jr.

Department of Microbiology
University of Maryland
School of Medicine
Baltimore, Maryland

I. INTRODUCTION

The genus Rickettsia is comprised of a number of species which are divided into the typhus, spotted fever, and scrub typhus groups. The groups were established on the basis of the human disease patterns produced as well as other significant biological and ecological differences. The typhus group contains currently three recognized species: R. prowazekii, R. mooseri (R. typhi), and R. canada. The classification is based on serological cross-reactions within the group as well as on other biological characteristics (1). The third species, R. canada, was added to the typhus group of rickettsiae following its isolation by McKiel, Bell, and Lackman in 1967 (2). This new agent was isolated from Haemaphysalis leporispalustris ticks removed from rabbits near Richmond, Ontario. It was found to possess antigens in common with R. prowazekii and R. mooseri as shown by complement fixation cross-reactions with antisera prepared in guinea pigs, rabbits, and hamsters. However, tests with mouse antisera suggested that it was different from the two known species, R. prowazekii and R. mooseri. In 1968, acute and early convalescent serum specimens from a patient suspected of having Rocky Mountain spotted fever (RMSF) were submitted to Walter Reed Army Institute for Research for confirmatory serology. Complement-fixation tests with soluble antigens prepared from the spotted fever group failed to demonstrate antibodies, but tests with group and specific antigens from the typhus group established a relationship with R. canada. As a result of this finding, a follow-up study was done on some 70 sera where RMSF was diagnosed clinically; 10 of these could not be confirmed earlier by serology (3). The new serological data developed indicated the possibility that 4 of these patients may have experienced a severe febrile illness due to R. canada. In this new study positive complement-fixation titers were not found when the sera from these 4 patients were reacted with specific antigens from R. prowazekii or R. mooseri.

The biological properties of R. canada are, in several ways, more attuned to the spotted fever group. Burgdorfer and Brinton (4) showed that when R. canda was grown in several species of ticks, the rickettsiae were noted not only in the cytoplasm but also in the nuclei of infected cells. It was noted also that infection with R. canada could be transmitted transovarially since larvae were observed to be infected. Rickettsial growth within the host nucleus and transovarial passage are biological properties associated with neither R. prowazekii nor R. mooseri but are found with members of the spotted fever group. The taxonomic relationship of R. canada to the typhus group and/or the spotted fever group is con-founded, however, by the fact that the guanine plus cytosine (G+C) content of its deoxyribonucleic acid (DNA) (30%) coincides with the values reported for the other members of the typhus group rather than with those found (32%) in the spotted fever group.

Thus, in an effort to clarify this issue, taxonomic relationships between R. canada, R. prowazekii, R. mooseri, and the prototype species of the spotted fever group, R. rickettsii, were determined on the basis of percent G+C content, genome size, and DNA-DNA hybridization.

II.   MATERIALS AND METHODS

A.   Rickettsial Strains

The designations, sources, passage histories, and other pertinent information on the strains used in this study are presented in Table 1.

TABLE 1. Sources and Passage History of the Strains
Employed in This Study

Organism/Strain	Source	Passage History	Reference
R. prowazekii (Breinl)	human	E155/TC3/E3	(5)
R. mooseri (Wilmington)	rat	E42/TC3/E3	(6)
R. canada (2678)	tick	E8/TC/E2	(2)
R. rickettsii (Sheila Smith)	human	E6/TC3/E2/TC4/E7	

B. Growth and Purification of Rickettsiae

Six-day-old eggs (Truslow Farms, Chestertown, MD) were inoculated via the yolk sac route with seed pool inoculum prepared
from plaque-purified rickettsiae, and diluted so that 30 to 50%
of the eggs were killed in 7 to 8 days. Only yolk sacs from
live embryos were harvested from eggs infected with R. prowazekii, R. mooseri and R canada. However, in the case of R.
rickettsii infected eggs, harvesting of the yolk sacs was delayed until 48 hrs after embryo death.

The rickettsiae were purified by both nonspecific and
immunologically specific precipitation of host cell contaminants combined with several procedures involving centrifugation. Further details regarding rickettsial growth and purification are found in an earlier publication (7).

C. Purification and Shearing of DNA

Cells were lysed in a solution of pronase and sodium dodecylsulfate, and the lysate was extracted with phenol. After
alcohol precipitation, the preparation was treated with ribo-
nuclease followed by adsorption to and elution from hydroxyapa-
tite. The DNA was sheared in a Ribi cell fractionator to a
fragment length of approximately 2.5×10^5 daltons. The purified DNA was stored in flame-sealed ampoules at $-70°C$. Further
details regarding DNA purification and assay methods for DNA
concentrations and purity can be found elsewhere (7).

D. Preparation of Radiolabeled Rickettsial DNA

Radiolabeled DNA was prepared using New England Nuclear's
(NEN) Nick Translation System Kit which was an adaptation of

the procedure described by Rigby et al. (8). It was modified,
however, by NEN to incorporate dTTP-^{3}H (specific activity, 97.8
Ci/m mol) instead of the usual dCTP-^{32}P. The deoxynucleoside
triphosphate mixture was changed, also, to reflect the change
in label employed. Fifty µCi of the dTTP-^{3}H were dried in a
siliconized Reacti-vial (Pierce Chemical Co.) followed immediately by the addition of nick translation buffer, deoxynucleoside triphosphate mixture, 0.5 µg rickettsial DNA, DNA polymerase I, and DNAase I (total volume of 20 µl). All additions
were carried out at 0°C in an ice bath. The reaction mixture
was then incubated in a constant temperature bath at 12 to 14°C
for 2 hrs. The level of incorporation was determined by removing two 2 1 samples which were added to tubes containing 0.2
ml of nick translation stop buffer (NEN). These samples were
stored on ice for later evaluation. To the remaining 16 µl of
nick translation reaction mixture were added 84 µl of Tris-EDTA
buffer (10 mM Tris, 1 mM EDTA), pH 8.1 to 8.3. An equal volume
(100 µl) of redistilled liquid phenol was added and the vial
was shaken by hand for 5 min. The bottom phenol layer was removed, using a capillary pipette, and the phenol extraction
process was once repeated. The DNA solution was then dialyzed
for 24 hrs through 3 changes (4 L) of 0.4 M NaCl at 4 to 6°C.
Its radioactivity was determined by liquid scintillation
counting and the DNA was stored at -70°C. The specific activity of the labeled DNA was determined by adding to the two
2 µl samples, which had been previously combined with the nick
translation stop buffer, 2 ml of cold 10% trichloracetic acid
(TCA). The preparation was allowed to set for 20 min, and the
precipitated DNA was then collected on membrane filters (Millipore HA). The filters were washed 7 to 10 times with 2 ml rinses of 5% TCA. The filters were then transferred to scintillation vials and 0.5 ml of 0.5 N HCl was added. The vials were
capped and heated on a steam bath (100°C) for 20 min. After
cooling, 1 ml of ethyl acetate was added and the filter was
dissolved within 5 to 10 min at room temperature. The vials
were vibrated to assist solution of the membranes. Ten ml of
PCS Solubilizer (Amersham Searle) were added and the sample was
counted.

E.   Determination of G+C Content of DNA

The G+C content (mole percent) of DNA was determined by the
method of Marmur and Doty (9). All assays were performed in a
Gilford spectrophotometer 2400-2 equipped with a thermo-
programmer unit and a reference compensator. After obtaining
base-line optical values at 25°C, the temperature was raised
to ca 10°C below the melting point and maintained there for 10
min to allow temperature equilibration. The temperature rise

was then set for 0.25°C/min, and temperature and OD changes
were recorded over a 20°C span.

F. Determination of Genome Size

Genome size determinations were performed by using the initial rate of renaturation method of Gillis (10), which is based
on measuring the rate of reduction in optical density at 260 nm
during an initial 30-min period of DNA renaturation. After
heat denaturation, the DNA solutions were allowed to renature
at the optimal renaturation temperature (T_{OR}), as determined
from the following formula T_{OR} = 1.24 T_m - 38.8, where T_m is
the denaturation temperature. The reaction rate (k) is equal
to V/C^2, where V is the decrease in absorbance per min (260 nm)
and C is the DNA concentration expressed as millimolar nucleotide pairs. DNA molecular weight is related to k by the equation: molecular weight (X 10^7) = 98.37 - (0.91 x percent
G+C/k. Further details regarding this procedure can be found
in another publication (7).

G. Measurement of DNA-DNA Hybridization

Two different procedures were employed to measure the extent of DNA-DNA hybridization. Both procedures involved free-
solution reassociation.
The first procedure followed (11) was, in principle, very
similar to that involved in determining genome size. Four
cuvettes were required: an adenine blank, the two DNA samples
to be compared, and a cuvette containing a 1:1 mixture of the
two DNAs. In all other respects, the analytical procedure was
the same as described above for genome size determination. The
degree of hybridization (D) was determined by the following
equation when the genomes were of equal size: $D = 4V_m - (V_A + V_B) / 2 V_A V_B$, where V_m, V_A and V_B are the decrease in absorbance per min (260 nm) in the DNA mixture, sample A and sample
B, respectively. When the degree of hybridization was determined between genomes unequal in size, the following equations
were employed: $D_L = 4 V_m - (V_S + V_L) / 2 V_S$, and $D_S = 4 V_m - (V_S + V_L) / 2 V_L$, where D_L and D_S refer to the degree of hybridization to the larger or smaller genome, and V_m, V_L, and V_S
refer to the decrease in absorbance per min (260 nm) in the DNA
mixture, larger genome sample or smaller genome sample, respectively.
The second DNA-DNA hybridization procedure involved the
hybridization of a ^{3}H-labeled DNA present in low concentration
to unlabeled DNA present in much higher concentration followed
by single-stranded DNA removal by S_1 nuclease digestion (12,

13,14). Thus, 0.3 ng ^{3}H – DNA (specific activity of approximately 3×10^7 dpm/μg), was combined with unlabeled DNA (3 μg) in 0.4 M NaCl. The total volume was 50 μl. The reaction was carried out in 0.3 ml siliconized Reacti-vials (Pierce Chemical Co.). The vials were heated in an aluminum block at 95 to 100°C for 60 min to obtain complete denaturation. After denaturation the temperature was lowered to 62°C and maintained at this temperature during the hybridization period (4 hr).

At the completion of the hybridization period, the nuclease reaction was carried out as follows. The basal nuclease reaction mixture (Zn SO$_4$, 2 mM; Na acetate buffer, 0.06 M, pH 4.8) was pre-heated to the hybridization temperature (62°C), which was followed by the addition of nuclease S$_1$ (2000 units/ml) and sheared, denatured calf thymus DNA (20 μg/ml). The complete nuclease reaction mixture was then added to the completed hybridization reaction in a volume (50 μl) equal to that of the hybridization reaction. The resulting 2-fold dilution gave a final NaCl concentration of 0.2 M, which was the concentration found optimal for the nuclease reaction by other investigators (13,14). The samples were maintained at 62°C for 40 min. The reaction was then stopped by chilling in an ice bath. One hundred μg of sheared, denatured calf thymus DNA (1 mg/ml) were added followed by 1.0 ml of cold 10% TCA. The samples were allowed to stand in the ice bath for 10 to 15 min for DNA precipitation. The samples were then filtered through membrane filters and washed thoroughly with 5% TCA. The membranes were dissolved and counted for radioactivity as previously described.

III. RESULTS

Table 2 presents the G+C content and genome size in the four rickettsial species examined. The values obtained for the G+C content agree with previously published values (15), and differ by no more than 0.5% from these. The genome size values for R. prowazekii and R. mooseri were published by us previously (7). The genome size of R. canada (149 x 10^7 daltons) is distinctly larger than the genome sizes found in both other members of the typhus group (109-112 x 10^7 daltons) and that seen in R. rickettsii (130 x 10^7 daltons). The genome size of R. rickettsii is likewise distinctly larger than that found in R. prowazekii and R. mooseri.

TABLE 2.   G+C Content of the DNA and Genome Size of Strains
of R. prowazekii, R. mooseri, R. canada, and R. rickettsii

Organism	G+C content	Genome size Mol. wt. $(\times 10^{-7}) \pm SD$[a]
R. prowazekii	29.0	112 ± 9
R. mooseri	29.0	109 ± 8
R. canada	29.2	149 ± 4
R. rickettsii	32.6	130 ± 10

[a]Standard deviation.

Table 3 shows the results of DNA hybridizations between the
four rickettsial species as measured by the initial rate of renaturation (optical) and the radiolabel methods. The values
obtained by the optical method for the hybridization pair, R.
prowazekii-R. mooseri have been reported previously (7). There
is generally good agreement in the values obtained by the two
methods. Since the genomes involved differ in size, it is
necessary to give two sets of values for each hybridization
pair. In the optical procedure the two sets of values are
generated by mathematical manipulations of the raw data obtained in a single experiment, while in the radiolabel procedure
the two sets of values (genome A and genome B) are generated in
two separate experiments, where genomes A and B are separately
employed as radiolabels.

TABLE 3. Degree of Hybridization between R. prowazekii, R. mooseri, R. canada, and R. rickettsii as Measured by Initial Rate of Renaturation (Optical) and Radiolabel Methods

HYBRIDIZATION PAIRS (A + B)	HYBRIDIZATION METHOD	DEGREE OF HYBRIDIZATION			
		Genome A		Genome B	
		values	mean	values	mean
R. prowazekii (A) / R. mooseri (B)	optical	10 determinations	72 ± 3	10 determinations	72 ± 3
	radiolabel	69, 71	70	72	72
R. canada (A) / R. prowazekii (B)	optical	35, 35, 40	37	42, 43, 47	44
	radiolabel	45, 29	37	45	45
R. rickettsii (A) / R. prowazekii (B)	optical	38, 42, 35	38	47, 43, 60	53
	radiolabel			47	47
R. rickettsii (A) / R. mooseri (B)	optical	28, 26	27	36, 35	36
	radiolabel	20	20	42	42
R. canada (A) / R. mooseri (B)	optical	42, 41, 41, 40	41	48, 46, 45, 46	47
	radiolabel	43, 33	38	52	52
R. canada (A) / R. rickettsii (B)	optical	38, 39	39	43, 43	43
	radiolabel	37	37	47	47

IV. DISCUSSION

The genetic relatedness of R. canada to the typhus group of
rickettsiae (R. prowazekii and R. mooseri) and to a representative of the spotted fever group (R. rickettsii), as well as the
relationship of the latter to the typhus group, have been determined by obtaining data on (i) the %G+C of the rickettsial
DNA's, (ii) their genome size, and (iii) the degree of DNA-DNA
hybridization between various pairings of these four species.
The near identity in G+C content between R. prowazekii, R.
mooseri, and R. canada is compatible with a close relationship
between R. canada and the typhus group, but does not prove such
relationship because DNA's of the same overall nucleotide composition can have very different sequences. In a contrary manner, the 3 to 4% difference in G+C content seen when comparing
R. canada to R. rickettsii is not sufficiently great to exclude
the possibility of a relationship between these two (16). The
genome size of R. canada is significantly different from that
of the typhus group, and to a lesser extent, from that of R.
rickettsii. It is generally accepted that significant or large
differences in genome sizes between two microorganisms preclude
their having a close taxonomic relationship (17).
    While the degree of DNA-DNA hybridization between R. prowa-
zekii and R. mooseri is relatively high (70-77%), that seen between either of these two and R. canada or R. rickettsii is
somewhat lower, varying between 20 to 50%. This is in contrast
to the nearly 100% hybridization values found in a previous
study (7) when various strains within a species (R. prowazekii
or R. mooseri) were hybridized. Thus, the DNA-DNA hybridization studies establish neither a clear, close relationship of
R. canada to one group over the other, nor do the differences
observed exceed those commonly found among different species
of the same bacterial genus. Rickettsial taxonomy has been
based on a comparison of various phenotypic characteristics,
particularly those involving rickettsial interaction with its
environment: patterns of human disease and epidemiological,
ecological, and serological considerations. Thus, McKiel et
al. (2) suggested that R. canada belongs in the typhus group
of the genus Rickettsia on the basis of a strong cross reaction
when R. mooseri antigens (soluble and cellular) were employed
against R. canada antiserum (guinea pig) in the complement
fixation reaction. This occurred to a lesser extent against
R. prowazekii antigen, and the reciprocal reactions were much
weaker. When reciprocal cross-toxin neutralization tests were
performed in mice using R. prowazekii, R. mooseri, R. canada,
and R. rickettsii convalescent guinea pig sera, it was found,
however, that R. canada was distinctly different from the other
three species, since very little or no cross protection was

observed (2). Serological cross reactions involving surface
antigens of even somewhat remotely related microorganisms are
fairly common phenomena. Thus, recent studies have shown serological cross reactions between strains of enteric bacteria,
mainly Escherichia coli, and the capsular polysaccharides of
such invasive bacteria as Streptococcus pneumoniae, Hemophilus
influenzae, and Neisseria meningitidis, and there is evidence
that these heteroimmune anticapsular antibodies seem to be protective against the septicemic diseases caused by these encap-
sulated bacteria (18). A more pertinent example of such hete-
rophile systems is, of course, the Weil-Felix reaction, where
certain nonflagellated strains of Proteus vulgaris or P. mira-
bilis show bacterial agglutination in the presence of antibodies to R. prowazekii, R. mooseri, R. canada, R. rickettsii,
or R. tsutsugamushi (1). Such serological cross reactions
should be interpreted with caution, as in the case of R. canada
and its taxonomic relationship to the typhus group, since they
reflect the expression of only a small segment of the entire
genome.

    At the phenotypic level, R. canada differs from the typhus
group in a number of other ways, which include intranuclear
growth in the host cell (4), the tick as a vector (2), and the
presence of transovarial transmission within the tick (19).
It has not been conclusively proven that R. canada is a human
pathogen, since rickettsial isolation has not been accomplished
yet, but serological data suggesting an R. canada infection
(antibodies reacting to R. canada but not to R. rickettsii)
have been found in four patients with a Rocky Mountain spotted
fever-like illness; not an illness resembling those caused by
the typhus group (3).

    Other investigators have shown distinct phenotypic differ-
ences between R. canada and R. prowazekii or R. mooseri at the
molecular level. These differences have included protein patterns as observed by polyacrylamide gel electrophoresis, isoelectric focusing, and specific enzyme levels (20,21,22).

    R. canada appears, thus, to stand apart taxonomically from
the typhus group. At the genetic level there is a large difference in their genome sizes, a somewhat low percentage of
DNA-DNA hybridization is observed, and with the exception of
certain serological cross reactions, many phenotypic differences are observed.

    The genetic relatedness of R. prowazekii and R. mooseri to
R. rickettsii was examined also in this study. The G+C content
and genome size values between the two groups were shown to
have a small but significant difference. The hybridization
data indicated that the degree of hybridization between R.
prowazekii or R. mooseri to R. rickettsii is about on the order of what is seen between the former two and R. canada.
The degree of genetic relatedness observed here between

representatives of the typhus group (R. prowazekii and R. mooseri) and the spotted fever group (R. rickettsii) seem appropriate to their recognition as belonging to distinctly different biotypes within the genus Rickettsia, their separation into biotypes being based on such differences as intracellular location, cultivation in chick embryos, plaque formation, and soluble group antigens as well as differences in the human diseases produced and their means of transmission (1). Distinct differences have been observed also at the molecular level in the migration patterns of the proteins of R. prowazekii and R. mooseri vs. R. rickettsii as measured by polyacrylamide gel electrophoresis (21,22). It has been known for a long time that certain types of serological cross reactions can occur between antigens of R. prowazekii, R. mooseri, and R. rickettsii, and this is particularly true when these are analyzed by cross-immunity protection tests in guinea pigs or by rickettsial agglutination (23,24,25). Such serological relationships should be recognized as representing only one of many phenotypic expressions of the underlying genetic relatedness.

V. SUMMARY

The genetic relatedness of R. prowazekii and R. mooseri to R. canada and to R. rickettsii, a representative species of the spotted fever group, has been examined using the criteria of G+C content, genome size, and the degree of DNA-DNA hybridization, the latter determined by two independent methods. While the G+C content of R. canada DNA is closely similar to that of the typhus group, its genome is distinctly larger than those found in both the typhus group and in R. rickettsii. The degree of DNA hybridization found between R. canada and either R. prowazekii or R. mooseri is considerably lower than that seen between the latter two and is of the same order as that seen between R. canada and R. rickettsii. For these reasons and because of the phenotypic differences observed, we suggest that there is insufficient reason to consider R. canada as a member of the typhus biotype of the genus Rickettsia.

R. rickettsii differs significantly from both R. canada and the typhus group of rickettsiae (R. prowazekii and R. mooseri) at the genetic level. There is a distinct, albeit small, difference in G+C content, and its genome size is intermediate between that of R. canada and the typhus group. The degree of DNA hybridization between R. rickettsii and the typhus group is about equal to that observed between R. canada and the typhus group. Thus, while differences are observed at the genetic level between R. rickettsii and the typhus rickettsiae,

these do not seem incompatible with continued inclusion of all
within the genus <u>Rickettsia</u>.

ACKNOWLEDGMENTS

This study received support from contract DADA 17-71-C-1007
with the U.S. Army Medical Research and Development Command,
Office of the Surgeon General, Department of the Army.
We acknowledge the excellent technical assistance given by
Dena Grossman, Anna Waddell, and MayBritt Doelp and the super-
ior assistance given by Cecilia Queen in typing the manuscript.

REFERENCES

1. Weiss, E. and Moulder, J. W., <u>in</u> "Bergey's Manual of
    Determinative Bacteriology" (R. E. Buchanan and N. E.
    Gibbons, eds.), 8th ed., p. 882. The Williams and
    Wilkins Co., Baltimore (1974).
2. McKiel, J. A., Bell, E. J., and Lackman, D. B., <u>Canad. J.
    Microbiol.</u> <u>13</u>, 503 (1967).
3. Bozeman, F. M., Elisberg, B. L., Humphries, J. W., Runcik,
    K., and Palmer, D. B., Jr., <u>J. Infect. Dis.</u> <u>121</u>, 367
    (1970).
4. Burgdorfer, W., and Brinton, L. P., <u>Infect. Immun.</u> <u>2</u>, 112
    (1970).
5. Wolbach, S. B., Todd, J. L., and Palfrey, F. W., "The
    Etiology and Pathology of Typhus." Harvard University
    Press, Cambridge, MA (1922).
6. Maxcy, K. F., <u>Pub. Health Rep.</u> <u>44</u>, 598 (1929).
7. Myers, W. F., and Wisseman, C. L., Jr., <u>Int. J. Syst.
    Bacteriol.</u> <u>30</u>, 143 (1980).
8. Rigby, P.W.F., Dieckman, M., Rhodes, C., and Berg, P.,
    <u>J. Mol. Biol.</u> <u>113</u>, 237 (1977).
9. Marmur, J., and Doty, P., <u>J. Mol. Biol.</u> <u>5</u>, 109 (1962).
10. Gillis, M., DeLey, J., and DeCleene, M., <u>Eur. J. Biochem.</u>
    <u>12</u>, 143 (1970).
11. DeLey, J., Cattori, H., and Reynaerts, A., <u>Eur. J.
    Biochem.</u> 12, 133 (1970).
12. Sutton, N. D., <u>Biochem. Biophys. Acta</u> <u>240</u>, 522 (1971).
13. Crosa, J. H., Brenner, D. J., and Falkow, S., <u>J.
    Bacteriol.</u> <u>115</u>, 904 (1973).
14. Barth, P. T. and Grinter, N. J., <u>J. Bacteriol.</u> <u>121</u>, 434
    (1975).
15. Tyeryar, F. J., Weiss, E., Millar, D. B., Bozeman, F. M.,
    and Ormsbee, R. A., <u>Science</u> <u>180</u>, 415 (1973).

16. DeLey, J., J. Theor. Biol. 22, 89 (1969).
17. Mandel, M., Ann. Rev. Microbiol. 23, 239 (1969).
18. Robbins, J. B., Schneerson, R., Liu, T. Y., Schiffer,
    M. S., Schiffman, G., Myerowitz, R. L., McCracken, G. H.,
    Jr., Orskov, I., and Orskov, F., in "The Immune System
    and Infectious Diseases", 4th Int. Convoc. Immunol.,
    Buffalo, N.Y., 1974, p. 218. Karger, Basel (1975).
19. Burgdorfer, W., J. Hyg. Epidemiol. Microbiol. Immunol. 12,
    26 (1968).
20. Dasch, G. A., Samms, J. R., and Weiss, E., Infect. Immun.
    19, 676 (1978).
21. Obijeski, J. F., Palmer, E. L., and Tzinabos, T.,
    Microbios. 11, 61 (1974).
22. Eisemann, C. S., and Osterman, J. V., Infect. Immun. 14,
    155 (1976).
23. Castaneda, M. R., and Silva, R., J. Immunol. 42, 1 (1941).
24. Parker, R. R., Pub. Health Rep. 58, 721 (1943).
25. Plotz, H., Bennett, B., Wertman, K., and Snyder, M., Proc.
    Soc. Exp. Biol. Med. 57, 336 (1944).

IMMEDIATE CYTOTOXICITY AND PHOSPHOLIPASE A: THE ROLE OF PHOSPHOLIPASE A IN THE INTERACTION OF R. PROWAZEKI AND L-CELLS.

Herbert H. Winkler[1]
Elizabeth T. Miller

Department of Microbiology and Immunology
USA College of Medicine
Mobile, Alabama 36688

I. INTRODUCTION

The mechanism by which Rickettsia prowazeki enters its host cell has not been thoroughly characterized (1, 2, 3). However it is now clear from the work of Walker and Winkler (1) that entry of R. prowazeki into L-cells can be inhibited by metabolically poisoning either the host or parasite. Cytochalasin B, a classical inhibitor of phagocytosis, inhibits the uptake of rickettsiae when the L-cells are incubated with this inhibitor. Alkylation of either the rickettsiae or the L-cell with N-ethyl maleimide (NEM) also prevents the entry of the rickettsiae. Adsorption of the rickettsiae to the host was distinguished from the internalization of the rickettsiae by the L-cell in these experiments by taking advantage of the obligatory exchange system for the transport of ATP/ADP that R. prowazeki possesses (1, 4). A very small percentage of the rickettsiae associated with the L cells are adsorbed; the great majority of the rickettsia are actually internalized. Thus, the uptake process occurs very rapidly following the attachment of the rickettsia to the host cell membrane. The rickettsiae are clearly unable to penetrate a host cell that is incapable of phagocytosis and the L-cell is unable to phagocytize metabolically inactive rickettsiae. These facts lead to the

---

1. Supported by NIH AI-15035.

suggestion that R. prowazeki enters the L-cell through a
process of induced phagocytosis. Most likely, the rickettsia
interacting with the host membrane "tickles" the host in such
a way that the rickettsia is internalized in a microfilament
dependent fashion – presumably phagocytosis.

A similar process has been proposed for the bacterium
chlamydia (5), and the protozoan toxoplasma (6). However,
there is an important difference between these obligate
intracellular bacteria: the chlamydiae reside in a phagocytic
vacuole whereas the rickettsiae grow free in the host
cytoplasm. Therefore, the entry of rickettsiae requires an
extra step – the rickettsiae must escape from the phagosome.
At the international symposium on Rickettsiae and Rickettsial
Disease in 1976, we suggested (7) that R. prowazeki escapes
from the phagosome following induced phagocytosis by the same
mechanism used by the typhus rickettsiae to lyse erythrocytes.
This laboratory has shown that rickettsiae adsorb to a
cholesterol site on the erythrocyte membrane and then lyse
this membrane (8). These adsorptive and lytic processes can be
separated and both are dependent on metabolic energy in the
rickettsia (9, 10, 11). We postulated that the essential
difference between hemolysis and entry into host cells is the
fact that the erythrocyte cannot phagocytize the rickettsia.
Thus, in the erythrocyte, the plasma membrane would be lysed
while in the L-cell the phagosomal membrane would be lysed by
the adsorbed rickettsia. The lysis of the phagosome would
result in a rickettsia free in the cytoplasm.

Although the adsorptive step in hemolysis had been well
characterized, the lytic step has only recently been
characterized by Winkler and Miller (12). This study shows
that the breakdown of the erythrocyte membrane is due to a
phospholipase A activity. Lysophosphatides and free fatty
acids are formed from the phosphatides of the erythrocyte
membrane with a kinetic and inhibitor pattern similar to that
of hemolysis.

The detection of a similar phenomenon in L-cells required
an amplification of the usual uptake system. This was
accomplished by centrifuging (13, 14) rickettsiae onto a
monolayer of L-cells in which the phospholipids had been
labeled with ^{14}C-oleic acid . This resulted in a large number
of rickettsiae associated with each L-cell and a sensitive and
easily quantifiable signal. The situation with the L-cells is
clearly different from that with the erythrocyte where a
single rickettsia can lyse the cell. Preliminary results of
these studies are presented herein; a full study will be
published elsewhere.

II. METHODS

Rickettsia prowazeki, Madrid E strain, was purified from infected yolk sacs as previously described (12). L-cells were grown in 35 mm dishes so that they would be confluent on the day of the experiment. They were labeled with ^{14}C-oleic acid for 8 hrs the day before and then reincubated without label overnight. Rickettsiae were added to the dishes in 1.5 ml of SPGMg at the indicated multiplicities of infection (MOI) based on metabolically active (viable) rickettsiae as determined by the antibody-hemolysis method of Walker and Winkler (15). The dishes were centrifuged 15 min at 400 x g at 37°C to bring the rickettsiae into association with the L-cells. L-cell damage was accessed by release of lactate dehydrogenase (LDH) from the cells, by increased permeability to trypan blue or by release of ^{86}Rb from the cells. Fatty acid hydrolysis was measured by gas liquid chromatography as previously described (12) or by the percentage of ^{14}C-oleic acid present as free fatty acid relative to the total labeled phospholipids after separation of these species by thin layer chromatography.

III. RESULTS

When R. prowazeki at a MOI of 50 were centrifuged onto L-cells for 15 min at 37°C and then incubated at 34°C for another 45 min, there was obvious damage to and death of the L-cells. The L-cells became permeable to trypan blue, about 90% of the cytoplasmic LDH appeared in the medium and most of the ^{86}Rb of prelabeled cells was lost to the medium. This cytotoxicity was due to interaction of viable rickettsiae with the L-cells. If medium alone, heat-killed rickettsiae, KCN- or dinitrophenol-poisoned rickettsiae or NEM-inactivated rickettsiae were used in place of viable rickettsiae there was no cytotoxicity. Furthermore, if the viable rickettsiae at these MOI were incubated for 60 min with the L-cells but not centrifuged there was no cytotoxicity.

Cytotoxicity was nearly complete immediately after the 15 min centrifugation. To obtain a time course showing progressive cytotoxicity the rickettsiae were centrifuged at 2°C onto the L-cells. In this case, no cytotoxicity was apparent immediately after this centrifugation and cytotoxicity was initiated and plateaued during the subsequent 34°C incubation.

Analysis of the lipid composition of the L-cells showed that a phospholipase A activity was occuring concurrently with

the other markers of cytotoxicity. Approximately 20% of the
[14]C-oleic acid previously incorporated into the phospholipid
of the L-cell was cleaved from its glycerol backbone and
appeared as free fatty acid. Gas chromatographic analysis of
the total free fatty acids of control and rickettsiae-treated
L-cells showed that the major increase in free fatty acid
occurred in the 18:1 species. Separation of the phosphatides
and lysophosphatides of ^{32}P-labeled control and
rickettsiae-treated L-cells demonstrated a large decrease in
both phosphatidyl ethanolamine and phosphatidyl choline in the
treated cells. This decrease was accompanied by an increase of
the same magnitude in the corresponding lysophosphatide.

Both cytochalasin B and NEM treatments of the L-cell are
effective in preventing the internalization of rickettsiae (1)
since these agents inhibit phagocytosis. However, neither of
these agents inhibited the cytotoxicity or phospholipase A
activity that occurred when large numbers of rickettsiae were
associated with the L-cells (as long as rickettsial metabolism
remained intact). In fact these agents increased the amount of
[14]C-oleic acid released from phospholipid when non-saturating
multiplicities of rickettsiae were used. Thus, phagocytosis of
the rickettsiae was not necessary to elicit the breakdown of
the cell membrane through the action of this phospholipase A.
The enhancement of phospholipase activity probably results
from the rickettsiae remaining associated with the plasma
membrane.

IV. DISCUSSION

The results demonstrated that the lysis of both an
erythrocyte and an L-cell by R. prowazeki involves a
phospholipase A, probably A_2, since unsaturated fatty acids
rather than saturated fatty acids are seen as products. This
supports, but does not prove, our hypothesis that this
phospholipase is used to escape from the phagosome (Fig. 1).
However, at this time no alternate hypothesis has been
proposed.

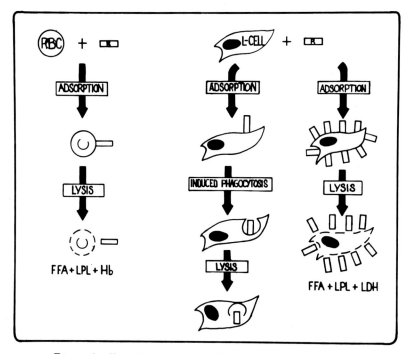

Fig. 1. Hypothesis for the role of phospholipase
activity in the lysis of erythrocytes and other cells
and the productive penetration of a host cell. Left
panel: the adsorption and lytic steps resulting in
hemolysis are shown. Right panel: the steps in the lysis
of an L-cell by a large number of rickettsiae are shown.
Middle panel: a productive infection is shown where the
rickettsia is phagocytized before lysis of the membrane
occurs. FFA=free fatty acid, LPL=lysophosphatides,
Hb=hemoglobin, LDH=lactic dehydrogenase.

There are many more questions than answers concerning this
phospholipase. Does the rickettsia have a phospholipase or
does it activate a latent host enzyme? What is the role of
rickettsial metabolic energy in this enzymatic or activation
activity? Does the phospholipase of the rickettsia-L-cell
interaction, like that involved in hemolysis, cleave the fatty
acids off the phospholipids of both the inner and outer
leaflets of the plasma membrane? What controls (turns off)
this phospholipase activity once the rickettsia is in the
cytoplasm? What is the nature of adherence of the rickettsiae
to the host membrane? Is the phospholipase involved in
adherence and is its activity the signal that induces

phagocytosis? How do the spotted fever group rickettsiae, which are not hemolytic, enter their host cells? We feel these are all fascinating questions some of which we are now investigating and some that will have to wait for appropriate methodology. As the answers to these questions are elucidated, the nature of one of the cardinal events in this highly evolved interaction of a eukaryotic host and a prokaryotic parasite – entry into that unique environmental niche, cytoplasm – will become clear and our understanding of rickettsiae and rickettsial diseases will be advanced, so that we are in a better position to attack the next set of questions.

V. SUMMARY

Phospholipase A has been shown (12) to cause the damage to the erythrocyte membrane that results in hemolysis by R. prowazeki. This phospholipase may also be the mechanism by which R. prowazeki gains entrance to the cytoplasm of its host cells and escapes from the phagolysosomes of professional phagocytes.

R. prowazeki at large multiplicities of infection (MOI>1000) on L-cell monolayers causes the rapid death of many of the L-cells and hydrolysis of fatty acids from the L-cell phospholipids. By centrifuging the rickettsiae onto L-cell monolayers this immediate cytotoxicity can be easily observed at MOI of less than 50. The activity of the phospholipase A can be monitored by using monolayers with ^{14}C-oleic acid incorporated into phospholipids. Hydrolysis of this ^{14}C-oleic acid is proportional to the MOI and the time-course of cytotoxicity can be followed by centrifuging at 0°C where no cytotoxicity occurs and then incubating the rickettsia-L-cell monolayers at 34°C . The cytotoxicity and concomitant phospholipase A activity can be inhibited by agents that prevent hemolysis and its associated phospholipase A activity. Cytochalasin B, a compound that prevents the internalization of R. prowazeki by L-cell monolayers, did not prevent the cytotoxicity phenomenon.

These results demonstrate that a phospholipase A activity is involved in both rickettsia-L-cell and rickettsia-erythrocyte interactions. The cytotoxicity phenomenon probably occurs when the number of rickettsiae associated with the surface membrane of the L-cell is too great to allow their induced phagocytosis so that the plasma membrane, instead of the phagosome membrane, is lysed.

REFERENCES

1. Walker, T. S. and Winkler, H. H., *Infect. Immun.* **22**, 200 (1978).
2. Cohn, Z. A., Bozeman, F. M., Campbell, J. M., Humphries, J. W., and Sawyer, T. K., *J. Exp. Med.* **109**, 271 (1959).
3. Wisseman, C. L., Jr., Waddell, A. D., and Silverman, D. J., *Infect. Immun.* **13**, 1749 (1976).
4. Winkler, H. H., *J. Biol. Chem.* **251**, 389 (1976).
5. Byrne, G. I., *Infect. Immun.* **14**, 645 (1976).
6. Jones, T. C., *in* "Mononuclear Phagocytes in Immunity, Infection, and Pathology" (R. van Furth, ed.), p. 269. Blackwell Scientific Publications, London, (1975).
7. Winkler, H. H., *in* "Rickettsiae and Rickettsial Diseases" (T. Kazar, R. A. Ormsbee, and I. N. Tarasevich, eds.), p. 95. Veda Publ. House, Bratislava, (1978).
8. Ramm, L. E., and Winkler, H. H., *Infect. Immun.* **13**, 120 (1976).
9. Ramm, L. E., and Winkler, H. H., *Infect. Immun.* **7**, 93 (1973).
10. Ramm, L. E., and Winkler, H. H., *Infect. Immun.* **7**, 550 (1973).
11. Winkler, H. H., *Infect. Immun.* **9**, 119 (1974).
12. Winkler, H. H., and Miller, E. T., *Infect. Immun.* **29**, 316 (1980).
13. Weiss, E., and Dressler, H. R., *Proc. Soc. Exp. Biol. Med.* **103**, 691 (1960).
14. Ormsbee, R., Peacock, M., Gerloff, R., Tallent, G., and Wike, D., *Infect. Immun.* **19**, 239 (1978).
15. Walker, T. S., and Winkler, H. H., *J. Clin. Microbiol.* **9**, 645 (1979).

RELEASE OF COXIELLA BURNETII FROM THE HOST CELL

Theodor Khavkin

Interferon Sciences, Inc.[1]
New Brunswick, New Jersey

Nina Amosenkova

Pasteur Institute of Epidemiology
and Microbiology
Leningrad, USSR

I. INTRODUCTION

Intracellular parasites consist of organisms of various
systematic positions. Under ordinary conditions of infection,
they all have the following features: they are able to a) enter host cells without noticeable damage and without being destroyed; b) multiply intracellularly; and c) escape the host
cell (1-3). These features insure survival of the parasites.
While considerable progress has been made in elucidation of a)
and b), the mechanism of release of intracellular organisms
from the host cell has been neglected (4). There is some evidence, however, of a variety of possible release mechanisms
among rickettsiae (5-7) and some other pathogens (1). The aim
of this work is a study of the cell-parasite interaction during
experimental infection with Coxiella burnetii with special reference to the release of organisms from the host cell.

C. burnetii resides inside intracellular vacuoles originating from phagosomes. It does not interfere with lysosome-
phagosome fusion (8), is resistant against lysosomal enzymes,
and until completion of the growth cycle causes no essential

---

[1]This work has been carried out partly at the Institute of
Experimental Medicine, Leningrad, USSR.

damage to the host cell. The mode of the release of C. burnetii from the host cell is not clear.

II. MATERIALS AND METHODS

Infection of cultured cells and intraperitoneal challenge
of albino mice with yolk sac culture of phase I C. burnetii,
strain Apodemus microtii-Luga were performed.

A. Cell Culture Experiments

An established line of monkey kidney epithelium (MK line)
was used. Twenty-four hour cultures were inoculated with
0.1 ml of 10^{-6} dilution of infected yolk sac and studied daily
for 4 weeks after inoculation. The culture medium was replaced every 3 days. Living cell cultures were examined by
means of time-lapse filming (intervals between shots 1-5 sec.),
and stained preparations were examined by light microscopy.

B. Animal Experiments

Forty-two albino mice were inoculated with 0.5 ml of 10^{-4}
dilution of a yolk sac suspension infected with C. burnetii.
Spread preparations of omentum and paraffin sections of spleen
were taken daily for 4 weeks postchallenge. Ultrathin araldite
sections of spleen taken from 20 mice 5 and 14 days post-
challenge were stained with uranyl acetate and lead citrate and
examined in an Hitachi electron microscope.

III. RESULTS

A. Infection of Cell Culture

The MK cell line used was characterized by slow growth and
delayed natural involution (18-20 days after the start of
growth). C. burnetii did not damage the infected cells and did
not interfere with cell division. Four or five divisions of
infected cells were observed in the course of continuous filming of the cell cultures during 4 days. The lack of damage of
infected cells and delayed involution of cell cultures enabled
us to trace cell-organism interaction for 3-4 weeks. As a
rule, organisms were either loosely suspended in a fluid of
well-known specific vacuoles (9) or formed compact

microcolonies.   Often organisms were unevenly distributed inside the same vacuole.   Motion picture studies revealed Brownian movement of C. burnetii of different intensity due to
changing viscosity of the vacuolar fluid (Fig. 1).   Most vacuoles became very large in the course of infection, but some
decreased in size.   In the latter case, the C. burnetii Brownian movement decelerated indicating condensation of the fluid
(Fig. 2).

   Observations of the same living cells showed fusion of some
of the vacuoles (Fig. 3).   Enhanced locomotor activity of infected cells - movement on a glass surface and periodical contractions lasting from several minutes to 3-4 hrs - were also
seen (Fig. 4).   Several mitotic divisions of neighbor cells,
requiring approximately 1 hr, could be observed during single
contraction.   During the contraction vacuoles with C. burnetii
were pushed out, but maintained a narrow bridge connection with
the cell.   Giant vacuoles often burst during the contraction
and released organisms into the culture medium.   Small vacuoles
returned to their initial position within the cell after the
cell relaxation.

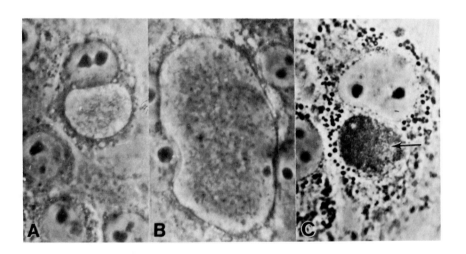

   Fig. 1.   A,B = medium and giant vacuoles with large amount
of fluid; organisms are not clearly resolved because of Brownian movement.   C = compact collection of C. burnetii (arrow) in
vacuole with small amount of fluid; no Brownian movement, 900x.

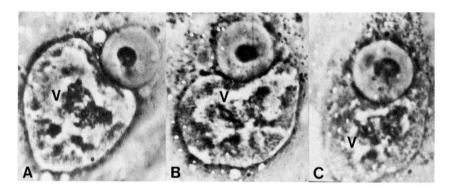

Fig. 2.   Infected cells (A-C) = 11-13 days after inoculation with C. burnetii.   Gradual reduction of vacuole (V),
uneven distribution of organisms.   1000x.

B.   Intraperitoneal Inoculation of Albino Mice

C. burnetii caused generalized infection of mice without
toxic effects and death.   Using total spread preparations of
omentum we could trace the infectious process in the peritoneum
from the first hours postchallenge.   The development of secondary infectious foci in the spleen was seen from 48 hrs after
inoculation.

In omentum, C. burnetii multiplied mostly in histiocytes,
as well as in mesothelial cells.   The organisms were either
loosely dispersed in the liquid contents of the vacuoles or
filled them tightly forming compact microcolonies, as those
seen in the cells growing in vitro.   Infected cells with com-
paratively large vacuoles prevailed in the omentum during the
first week postchallenge, but the number of such cells decreased during the 3rd week.   Few infected cells containing
small compact microcolonies were observed during the 4th week.

The development of the infectious foci in the spleen was
the same as described elsewhere (8).   C. burnetii multiplied
mostly in reticular cells inside typical vacuoles with the same
variability of the ratio between organisms and liquid contents,
as seen in the omentum and tissue cultures.   Electron microscopic studies showed that some vacuoles had one-membrane wall;
others, unlike the phagosomes, had two-membrane wall (Fig. 5).
Three and more membrane units were found in a limited area of
the wall of some giant vacuoles suggesting rupture of a membrane and restoration during growth of the vacuole.   Most of the
vacuoles containing organisms showed no signs of fusion with
each other even when the cell was heavily infected with C.
burnetii (Fig. 6).   Only rarely fusion of vacuoles was suggested by a separation of giant vacuoles by a single membrane.

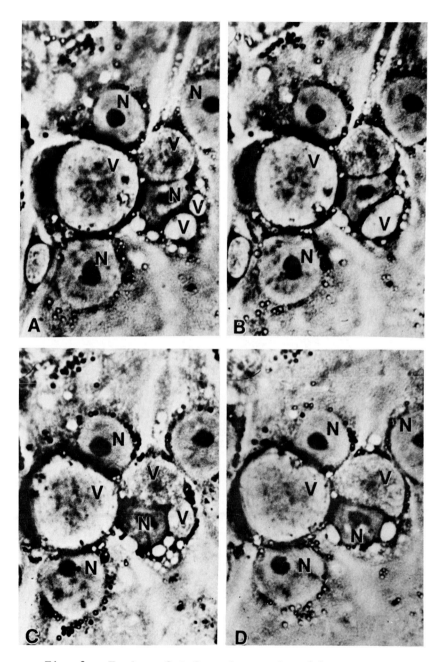

Fig. 3.   Fusion of infected vacuoles (V); A-D = 9-12 days after inoculation with C. burnetii. The images of organisms are faint because of Brownian movement.   N = nuclei of infected cells.   1200x.

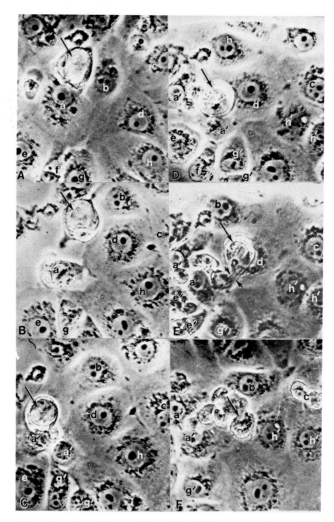

Fig. 4. Contraction of cell with extrusion of infected
vacuole (arrow) and mitotic divisions of neighboring cells.
A = spheric cell during contraction. B = beginning of vacuole
extrusion; division of (a) and (g) cells. C = continuation of
contraction, appearance of daughter cells (a') and (g'). D =
division of (e) cell; (h') = daughter cell of (h). E = cytoplasmic bridge (arrows) connecting vacuole to cell body; cell
(d) is seen through the vacuole. F = continuation of contraction, division of (c) cell. 400x.

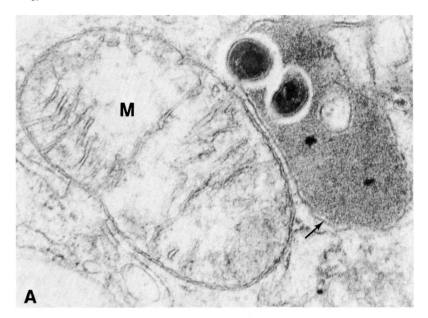

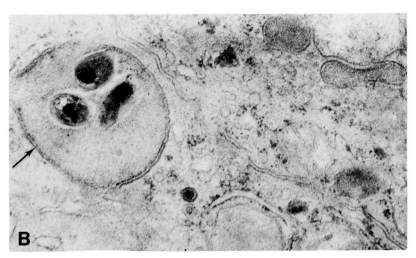

Fig. 5. Vacuoles (V) containing organisms, 5 days post-
challenge. A = wall of vacuole (arrow) consisting of one membrane unit, (M) mitochondrion. B = wall (arrow) of vacuole
consisting of two membrane units. 30,000x.

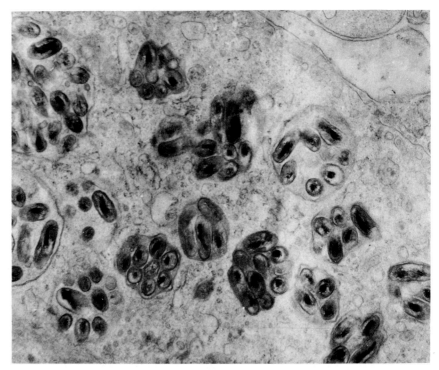

Fig. 6.   Numerous vacuoles with C. burnetii, 5 days post-
challenge.   The liquid contents of vacuoles display different
density.   23,000x.

        Infected cells with small and medium vacuoles often con-
tained numerous polyribosomes, lysosomes, and vesicles, well-
developed mitochondria, Golgi complexes and endoplasmic reticulum (Fig. 7), suggesting increased functional and metabolic
activities.   Some of the cells contained groups of Golgi complexes facing the vacuole (Fig. 8).   The cell with giant vacuoles exhibited gradual reduction of cytoplasm and organelles
without other signs of damage.   Such ring-like infected cells
with giant vacuoles, thinned out cytoplasm and displaced nucleus were also observed in lung and other internal organs (8,10).

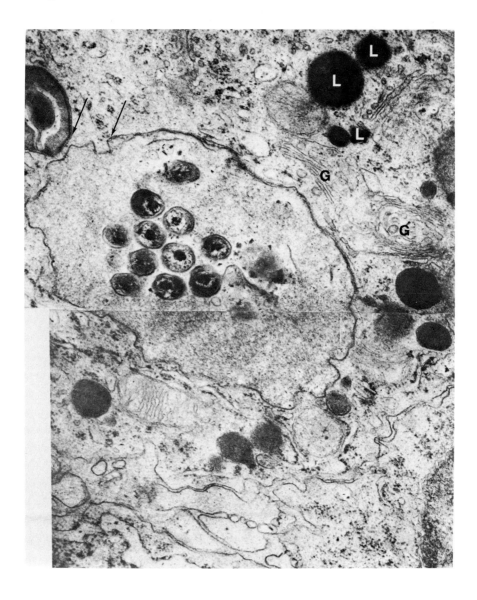

Fig. 7. Numerous lysosomes (L), polyribosomes, well-developed Golgi complexes (G) and mitochondria in vicinity of vacuoles (arrows) containing organisms. Different density of liquid contents of the small and large vacuoles. 36,000x.

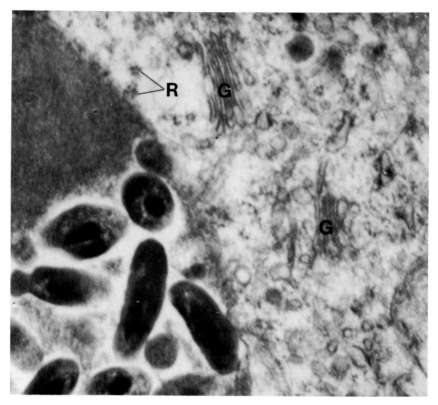

Fig. 8. Numerous vesicles and Golgi complexes (G) facing
vacuole with organisms. Liquid contents of vacuole are not
uniform, (R) polyribosomes. 52,000x.

IV.   DISCUSSION

Trager (1974) stated that parasitic protozoa inhabiting
intracellular vacuoles induced the host cell to assist actively
in the nutrition of the parasite. Trager's statement seems to
be valid for many other intracellular parasites including those
which inhabit a vacuole, like C. burnetii, and those which escape from the vacuole into the cytoplasm, as most of pathogenic
rickettsiae. For instance, morphologic signs of increased
energy production and protein synthesis were observed in early
infection of cells with Rickettsia prowazekii (5) and R. tsutsugamushi (6). In early C. burnetii infection such a nonspecific cell activation contributes both to the cell and parasite nutrition and to the cell contractions which can be regarded as a defense response.

The relations of the vacuoles containing C. burnetii with the host cell depend mostly on the fluid exchange between vacuole and cell. The growth of many vacuoles overtakes the multiplication of C. burnetii as the result of inflow of fluid. The presence of numerous vesicles and Golgi complexes around some of the vacuoles suggests that vesicular transport takes part in the fluid flow into the vacuole. Moreover, some vacuoles fuse, and the resulting giant vacuoles reduce the host cell cytoplasm without marked cell damage. The rupture of the vacuole overfilled with fluid is the final step of cell-C. burnetii interaction. Cell contractions promote the rupture of the giant vacuoles.

Some of the vacuoles display condensation of the liquid contents indicating outflow of the fluid. The fluid outflow and multiplication of C. burnetii result in formation of compact microcolonies. The rearrangement of the wall of some vacuoles (two-layered wall) makes them more resistant to cell contractions and may interfere with vacuole fusion.

Thus, the active fluid inflow with subsequent vacuole rupture can be considered as a main mode of the C. burnetii release without marked damage to the host cell itself. This view is supported by the observation that cells with giant vacuoles disappear from the mouse omentum by the end of acute stage of infection. One can speculate that outflow of the fluid and formation of compact microcolonies are steps to latent carrier state of C. burnetii.

V.   SUMMARY

The intracellular parasite, C. burnetii, residing in the phagolysosome causes nonspecific activation of early infected cell and simultaneous rearrangement of the vacuolar wall. Both cell activation and vacuolar rearrangement contribute to the survival of the pathogen and to vacuole strength. The cell responds during early infection with periodic contractions, but this response does not eliminate the pathogen. The activation is followed by alterations of the vacuole and host cell which facilitate the release of the infecting organisms. The main mechanism of the C. burnetii released from the cell is active fluid flow into the vacuole resulting in the cell rupture. The means of the organism release described here can be regarded as important determinant of pathogenicity of C. burnetii.

ACKNOWLEDGMENTS

The critical reading of manuscript by Emilio Weiss and his help in final edition are gratefully acknowledged. Valerian Bystrov is acknowledged for his assistance in the motion picture studies.

REFERENCES

1. Mims, C. A., "The Pathogenesis of Infectious Disease." Academic Press, London; Gruen & Stratton, New York (1976).
2. Moulder, J. W., J. Infect. Dis. 130, 300 (1974).
3. Trager, W., Science 183, 269 (1974).
4. Weiss, E., in "Microbiology 1979" (D. Schlesinger, ed.), p. 144. Am. Soc. Microbiol., Washington, D.C. (1979).
5. Khavkin, T. N., Ariel, B. M., Amosenkova, N. I., and Krasnik, F. I., Exp. Mol. Pathol. 22, 417 (1974).
6. Ewing, E. P., Jr., Takeuchi, A., Shirai, A., and Osterman, J. V., Infect. Immun. 19, 1068 (1978).
7. Wisseman, C. L., Jr., Edlinger, E. A., Waddell, A. D., and Jones, M. R., Infect. Immun. 14, 1052 (1976).
8. Ariel, B. M., Khavkin, T. N., and Amosenkova, N. I., Pathol. Microbiol. 39, 412 (1973).
9. Weiss, E., Bacteriol. Rev. 37, 259 (1973).
10. Khavkin, T. N., Arkh. Patol. (Mosk.) 1, 80 (1977).

PATHOLOGIC AND RICKETTSIAL EVENTS
IN TETRACYCLINE-TREATED EXPERIMENTAL
ROCKY MOUNTAIN SPOTTED FEVER

David H. Walker
Barbara G. Cain
James V. Lange

Department of Pathology
University of North Carolina
Chapel Hill, North Carolina

Alyne Harrison

Center for Disease Control
Atlanta, Georgia

I. INTRODUCTION

Rocky Mountain spotted fever (RMSF) is a disease with
specific injury to blood vessels caused by rickettsial infection of endothelium and vascular smooth muscle (1-5). Infection of the guinea pig with Rickettsia rickettsii offers
an excellent model of predictable acute vascular injury (6,7).
Treatment with tetracycline beginning on the third day of
fever effects a cure even with a highly virulent strain of
R. rickettsii. Previous studies of rickettsial pathogenesis
in animal models have concentrated on lesions at the peak of
illness with few observations of the healing phase (1,7-9).
Our early experience with diagnosis of RMSF by immunofluorescent examination of skin biopsies led us to the realization that rickettsiae are cleared from lesions over a period
of several days of rickettsiostatic treatment with tetracycline or chloramphenicol, often leading to false negative results (10).

RICKETTSIAE AND RICKETTSIAL DISEASES

Therefore, this investigation was undertaken 1) to determine the duration of persistence of R. rickettsii detected by immunofluorescence in lesions of tetracycline-treated experimental animals as a guide to rational timing of obtaining the skin biopsy for the diagnosis of RMSF, 2) to determine the inflammatory cell types present in lesions of RMSF during the course of rickettsial clearance and early tissue repair, and 3) to observe the histologic and ultrastructural events over the course of the early healing phase of RMSF, a specific model of injury to endothelium and vascular smooth muscle.

II. MATERIALS AND METHODS

A. Rickettsiae

R. rickettsii, Sheila Smith strain, was generously provided by Dr. Charles C. Shepard. The strain had been adapted to guinea pigs by numerous passages in that species and had acquired a fixed, high degree of virulence with onset of fever five days after inoculation in the vast majority of animals and death ten days after inoculation in all febrile animals (7). Stock inoculum was prepared by one further passage in guinea pigs with collection of spleen and blood on day 3 of fever. Pooled blood and spleen was stored frozen at -70°C until just prior to inoculation. Thawed stock was diluted 1:20 in sucrose-phosphate-glutamate (SPG) solution. This dilution had been titrated previously to contain approximately 10^4 plaque forming units per milliliter (11).

B. Experimental Design

Twenty-four adult male guinea pigs, Hartley strain, weighing >500 gm, were divided as shown in Table 1. The treated guinea pigs were administered tetracycline hydrochloride (10 mg/kg/day) intramuscularly in a divided dose twice daily beginning on the third day of fever. Daily rectal temperatures and body weights were recorded. At necropsy, samples of epididymis were collected for immunofluorescence, histology, and electron microscopy.

TABLE 1. Distribution of Guinea Pigs into Groups
by Rickettsial Infection, Treatment
Protocol, and Day of Sacrifice

	Days of treatment prior to sacrifice				
Protocol	1/2	1	2	3	7
Rickettsiae + tetracycline	4	3	3	2	2
Rickettsiae + saline	3	1	2	1	0
Uninfected, tetracycline	0	0	0	1	1
Uninfected, saline	0	0	0	1	0

C. Histology

Specimens of epididymis, testis, and cremaster muscle
were fixed in 4% neutral buffered formaldehyde, embedded in
paraffin, sectioned at 6 μm, and stained with hematoxylin and
eosin.

D. Immunofluorescence

Specimens of epididymis were embedded in polyethylene gly-
col compound (OCT, Ames Company, Division of Miles Laboratories Elkhart, Indiana) and frozen in a cryostat. Frozen sections (4 μm) were fixed in acetone for 20 minutes and stored
at -20°C. Fluorescein-conjugated rabbit anti-R. rickettsii
globulin fraction (Viral and Rickettsial Products Branch,
Center for Disease Control) was reacted with sections by direct immunofluorescent technique (7). Sections were washed
for 30 minutes in phosphate-buffered saline, dipped in distilled water, mounted in a 90% glycerol-10% saline solution,
and examined with a Leitz ultraviolet microscope using bar-
rier and exciter filters for fluorescein isothiocyanate.
Selected formalin-fixed, paraffin-embedded blocks were also
examined by the technique of deparaffinization, trypsin digestion, direct immunofluorescence (12). Tests for conjugate
specificity have been reported previously (2,3,7,10,12,13).

E. Electron Microscopy

Epididymis and cremaster muscle were dissected, fixed in
4% formaldehyde-1% glutaraldehyde, washed in 0.1 M Sorensen
phosphate buffer, postfixed in 2% osmium tetroxide, dehydrated in graded ethanol series, embedded in a mixture of Epon
and Araldite (14), sectioned on an ultramicrotome, stained
with uranyl acetate and lead citrate (15), and examined by
high resolution transmission electron microscopy.

F. Autoradiography

Four additional guinea pigs (400-600 gms) were inoculated intraperitoneally with R. rickettsii. Two control animals were inoculated with diluent. Animals were treated with
tetracycline hydrochloride according to the previous sched-
ule. At 48 and 72 hours after the first antibiotic injection, pairs of animals were sacrified and cremaster muscle
and epididymis were harvested for light microscopy and autoradiography. Thirty minutes prior to sacrifice animals were
injected intraperitoneally with ³H-thymidine, 1 μCi/gm of
body weight (Amersham Corporation, Arlington, Heights, IL),
specific activity 7.6 Ci/mM. Sections (5 μm) of tissue were

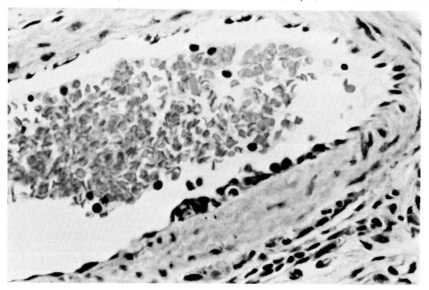

Fig. 1. Small artery in epididymis of guinea pig with
experimental RMSF after 48 hours of treatment with tetracycline. Endothelium is elevated focally by subendothelial
leukocytes. Hematoxylin-eosin stain. X440.

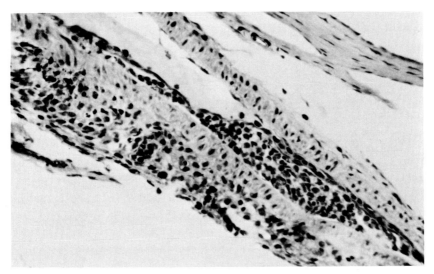

Fig. 2. Small artery in epididymis of guinea pig with
experimental RMSF after 72 hours of treatment with tetracycline. This longitudinal section reveals one normal endothelial surface and the opposite subendothelium markedly infiltrated by predominantly mononuclear leukocytes. Hematoxylin-
eosin stain. X280.

cut, mounted, deparaffinized, and processed for light microscopy and autoradiography. Autoradiographs were made by dipping slides with sections into undilute NTB-2 emulsion (East-
man Kodak, Rochester, N. Y.). Slides were exposed upright
for 4 weeks at 4°C and developed in Kodak Dektol developer
(1:1 in distilled water) and fixed in Kodak General Purpose
Fixer with hardener and then stained with hematoxylin and
eosin. All endothelial cells with identifiable nuclei and
within the walls of the capillaries, arterioles, venules,
arteries, and veins were counted in each tissue for each
animal using the oil immersion objective of a standard light
microscope (1000 X). A labeled cell was one which had five
or more exposed grains above its nucleus. Three hundred to
600 total cells were counted for each tissue per animal.
The percentage of labeled cells was calculated for each tissue for each animal and designated as the labeling index.

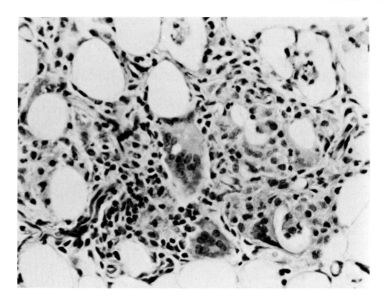

Fig. 3. Blood vessel from guinea pig with experimental
RMSF after 7 days of treatment with tetracycline. Eccentric
luminal narrowing with mural infiltration by macrophages and
fibroblasts is residual of vasculitis and thrombosis undergoing repair. Hematoxylin-eosin stain. X440.

III. RESULTS

A. Clinical and Gross Observations

Febrile guinea pigs in both tetracycline and placebo
groups exhibited the usual features of infection with R.
rickettsii with varying degrees of weight loss, scrotal
edema, congestion, and hemorrhage, conjunctivitis, and livor
of the footpads. One infected, placebo-treated animal died
on day 9 post-inoculation with R. rickettsii. Two animals
which were treated with tetracycline for 7 days became and
remained afebrile after 4 days of treatment.

B. Brightfield Microscopy

All groups of infected, febrile animals showed vascular
inflammatory lesions. In general, the pathologic lesions
had similar features over the first three days after initi-

ation of treatment whether animals were administered tetracycline or saline. A general tendency toward more severe
pathologic alterations was noted as the course of disease
progressed. Pathologic lesions included endothelial swelling; lining or pavementing of endothelial luminal surface
with leukocytes; subendothelial, intramural, and perivascular infiltrates of leukocytes (Figs. 1 and 2); focal
small hemorrhages; eccentric luminal, intramural, and perivascular deposition of fibrin; and adjacent fat necrosis.
Endothelial swelling and endothelial leukocytic pavementing
were relatively prominent early in the course. By day 7 of
treatment with tetracycline, endothelial leukocytic pavementing and subendothelial leukocytic infiltration were minimal
and evidence for repair of fibrin thrombi with infiltration
by macrophages was observed (Fig. 3). Pavementing was focal and often involved only a portion of the perimeter of the
lumen. Both mononuclear cells and polymorphonuclear (PMN)
leukocytes were observed in close apposition to vascular endothelium. Pavementing was often observed in association with
immediately adjacent subendothelial infiltration of leukocytes.

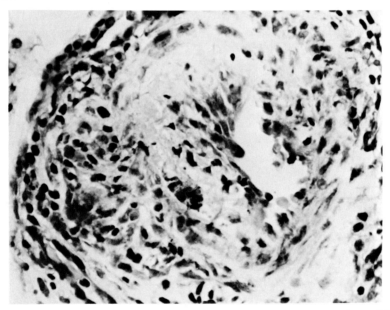

Fig. 4. Obliterative vasculitis in epididymis after 24
hours of tetracycline treatment. Central lumen containing
erythrocytes and overall ring outline of vessel wall are the
only landmarks remaining of the blood vessel morphology.
Vascular wall is infiltrated by many mononuclear and PMN leukocytes. Hematoxylin-eosin stain. X280

Subendothelial leukocytes were usually present in moderate
quantity, were contiguous to one another, and involved only a
portion of the circumference of the vessel with the uninvolved
endothelium appearing either normal or pavemented. Mononuclear leukocytes predominated over PMN leukocytes in the subendothelium. Intramural and perivascular leukocytic infiltrates were progressively more severe over the course of disease with many examples of virtual obliteration of the normal
mural architecture by infiltrates of large and small mononuclear cells and few PMN leukocytes (Fig. 4). Focal karyorrhexis of leukocytes was observed as well as rare intramural
giant cell formation. Extent of fibrin deposition in lumina,
vessel walls, and perivascular foci increased during the
course of the infection. No pathologic lesions were observed
in uninfected control experimental animals.

C. Rickettsial Immunofluorescence

The quantity of R. rickettsii increased progressively
over the course of infection in placebo-treated guinea pigs.
In contrast, tetracycline-treated animals continued to con-

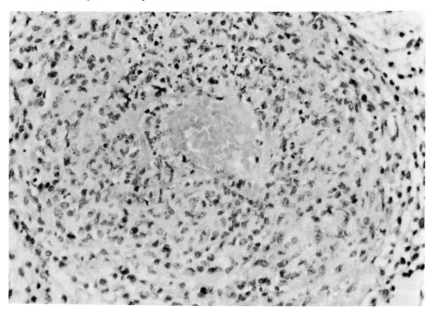

Fig. 5. Electron micrograph of epididymal capillary after 24 hours of tetracycline treatment. Endothelial cell injury is apparent from dilated endoplasmic reticulum and nuclear envelope (arrows) X5200

tain only a small number of rickettsiae for 48 hours after
initiation of therapy, and after 72 hours no rickettsiae
were detected. There also appeared to be a change in morphology of immunofluorescent rickettsial antigen with tetracycline treatment. Foci containing numerous fragments of
rickettsial antigen and morphologically intact rickettsiae
were observed in some tetracycline recipients, most promi-

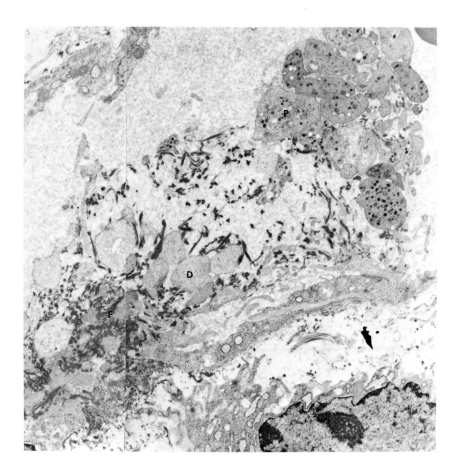

Fig. 6. Electron micrograph of a blood vessel from guinea pig with experimental RMSF treated with tetracycline for
24 hours. Separation of injured endothelial cells is plugged
by a fibrin thrombus (F) containing both degranulated platelets (D) and intact aggregated platelets (P) X5700.

nently after 48 hours of treatment. Furthermore, the focus
of infection appeared to be smaller with cytoplasmic accumulation of numerous rickettsiae. Often a single intensely
infected cell was observed in a vascular focus. On day 3
of treatment only minimal focal rickettsial antigen without
rickettsial morphology was detected.

D. Ultrastructural Observations

Vessels from animals sacrificed after 12 and 24 hours
of treatment showed similar findings including variable
degrees of endothelial cytopathology. Although the majority of endothelial cells were morphologically normal, many
contained profiles of dilated rough endoplasmic reticulum
and dilated nuclear envelope (Fig. 5). Focal separation of

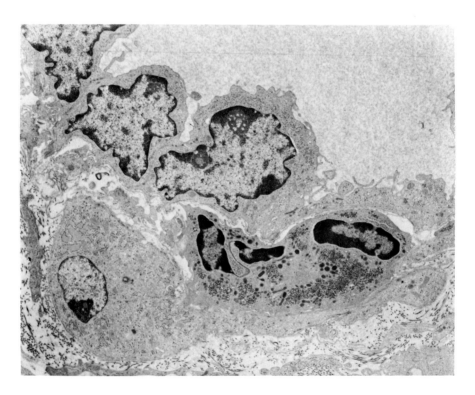

Fig. 7. Electron micrograph of a subendothelial PMN in
a guinea pig with experimental RMSF treated with tetracycline
for 12 hours. X4900.

endothelial cells was accompanied by platelet aggregates
and luminal and subendothelial fibrin (Fig. 6). Vasculitis
was manifest by subendothelial, intramural, and perivascular polymorphonuclear (PMN) leukocytes (Fig. 7), small lympho-

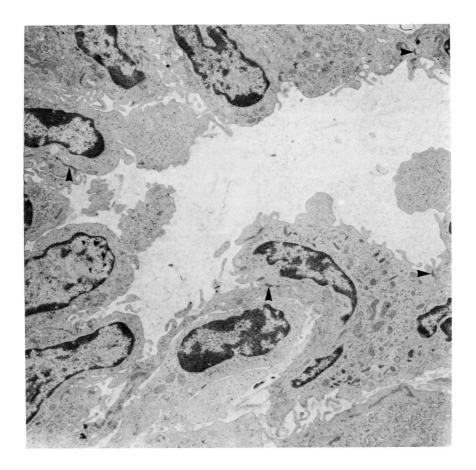

Fig. 8. Electron micrograph of a blood vessel from a
guinea pig with experimental RMSF treated with tetracycline
for 72 hours. Markedly hypertrophied endothelial cells with
characteristic intercellular junctions (arrows) form a continuous lining of the vessel lumen. A lymphocyte and electron lucent spaces are present in the subendothelium.   X6400.

cytes, large lymphocytes, and macrophages. Vascular permeability was demonstrated by perivascular and intramural erythrocytes, fibrin, and large clear intercellular spaces presumably representing edema. Following 48 hours of administration of tetracycline, endothelial cells showed morphologically similar cytopathology but of less extensive degree. Inflammatory and hemorrhagic phenomena were unchanged from the previous observations.

After 72 hours of treatment, the endothelial fine structure was remarkably altered. Dilatation of rough endoplasmic reticulum was rarely observed. Moreover, endothelial cells had undergone striking increase in mass with definite cellular hypertrophy (Fig. 8). These hypertrophied cells contained numerous organelles including many mitochondria and membrane-bound dense bodies. In addition, the endothelial cell membranes on the luminal surface had numerous thin projections resembling the filopodia of macrophages. Endothelium was distinguishable from mononuclear phagocytes by distinct tight junctions with neighboring endothelial cells but not with adjacent macrophages. Subendothelial electron lucent spaces were quite prominent. Foci of vascular smooth muscle showed dilated rough endoplasmic reticulum. Perivascular, intramural, and subendothelial inflammatory cell types consisted of macrophages, polymorphonuclear leukocytes, small and large lymphocytes, mast cells, and plasma cells. Rickettsiae were very rarely identified ultrastructurally at any time in the course of the study.

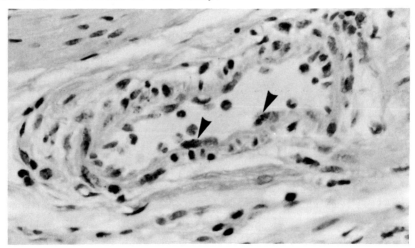

Fig. 9. Autoradiograph of a blood vessel after 72 hours of treatment. Dark grains overlie the nuclei of labelled endothelial cells (arrows) in the process of synthesis of DNA. Hematoxylin-eosin stain. X440.

TABLE 2. Labeling Indices of Endothelial Cells

Animal	Harvest[a]	Labeling Indices	
		Cremaster	Epididymis
A	48 hrs.	2.26%	1.80%
B	48 hrs.	1.06%	1.71%
C	72 hrs.	0.91%	1.24%
D	72 hrs.	–	1.85%
E	Control	0.63%	0.61%
F	Control	0.69%	0.75%

[a]Duration of treatment at time of sacrifice.

E. Autoradiography

The labeling indices of endothelial cells showed that the control animals had an index comparable to the accepted normal range for rodents and other small mammals (16–18) and that guinea pigs in the early healing phase of endothelial regeneration undergo definite endothelial cellular hyperplasia (Fig. 9) with labelling indices approximately double the resting rate (Table 2).

IV. DISCUSSION

The results of the immunofluorescent study of rickettsial antigen indicate that skin biopsy should never be used as an excuse to delay treatment with tetracycline since rickettsiae were detected easily after 24 hours. Further administration of tetracycline resulted in reduction in quantity of rickettsiae at 48 hours. Moreover, disrupted morphology was also observed. These factors make identification of rickettsiae less likely. It has been our experience with skin biopsies taken after 48 hours of tetracycline that in some cases a diagnosis is possible on the basis of the remaining morphologically intact rickettsiae despite their small numbers and the disrupted antigen. On the other hand, false negative results have also occurred at this stage of treatment. After 72 hours of treatment with tetracycline it is not worthwhile to search for immunofluorescent R. rickettsiae. It is interesting, however, to note that we have observed morphologically intact R. rickettsii in tissues of patients

treated for 4 days or more with chloramphenicol. We have
not examined tissues of guinea pigs with experimental RMSF
which were treated with chloramphenicol.

The identification of small lymphocytes, stimulated lymphocytes, macrophages, PMN's, and plasma cells in association
with the early healing phase of experimental RMSF suggests a
complex interaction of immunologic and inflammatory events
in vivo. The predominance of mononuclear leukocytes and the
remarkable localization of the cellular response such as was
observed in the subendothelial foci suggest the importance of
cell mediated immunity as a host defense as have other studies of rickettsial immunity (19-22). The pathologic morphology indicates the interaction of acute inflammatory processes,
humoral immunity, and cell mediated immunity in the clearance
of rickettsiae which were inhibited from further replication
by tetracycline. Determination of the contribution of each
element will be achieved only by further experiments which
delete or adoptively transfer these elements.

The endothelium itself exhibited remarkable alterations
in ultrastructural morphology during the course of rickettsiostatic treatment. The endothelial cytopathology observed 12
to 48 hours after onset of treatment or 7-1/2 to 9 days post-
inoculation differed somewhat from the previously described
terminal cytopathology. Dilated rough endoplasmic reticulum
and nuclear envelope suggest that injured endothelial cells
suffered increased permeability to water. Although this cyto-
pathologic lesion is not specific, it is similar to that seen
in cultured chick embryo cells infected by R. rickettsii (23,
24). An even more striking alteration was the apparently ab-
rupt transformation to endothelial hypertrophy observed after
72 hours of treatment. This regenerative response was accompanied by subendothelial electron lucent spaces and the
endothelium might not be functionally normal. However, 24
hours later the treated animals had become afebrile.

Furthermore, the labeling results indicate that the endothelium of the infected animals incorporated ^{3}H-T at a level
two to three times that for the controls (Table 2) and for
previously reported normal levels (16,17). This increased
level of mitotic activity was detected at both 2 and 3 days
after the initiation of antibiotic treatment and could be interpreted as a regenerative response on the part of the endothelium during the repair process after the initiation of
rickettsiostatic treatment. The observation that endothelial
regeneration was associated with the presence of leukocytic
margination, infiltration, and outright vessel wall obliteration parallels the results obtained in other models of endothelial damage and repair (25). Some authors have proposed

that the inflammatory cell plays a regulatory role in the process of endothelial regeneration (25,26), but the mechanism
involved remains to be elucidated. In the present study, the
autoradiographic data indicates that endothelial hyperplasia
is part of the early healing phase of vascular injury in the
RMSF guinea pig model.

REFERENCES

1. Wolbach, S. B., _J. Med. Res._ 41, 1 (1919).
2. Walker, D. H., Crawford, C. G., and Cain, B. G., _Human Path._ 11, 263 (1980).
3. Green, W. R., Walker, D. H., and Cain, B. G. _Am. J. Med._ 64, 523 (1978).
4. Walker, D. H., and Mattern, W. D., _Arch. Intern. Med._ 139, 443 (1979).
5. Walker, D. H., Paletta, C. E., and Cain, B. G., _Arch. Path. Lab. Med._ 104, 171 (1980).
6. Ricketts, H. T., _J. A. M. A._ 47, 33 (1906).
7. Walker, D. H., Harrison, A., Henderson, F., and Murphy, F. A., _Am. J. Path._ 86, 343 (1977).
8. de Brito, T., Hoshino-Shimizu, S., Pereira, M. O., and Rigolon, N., _Virchows Arch. Abt. A. Path._, _Anat._ 358, 205 (1973).
9. Moe, J. B., Mosher, D. F., Kenyon, R. H., White, J. D., Stookey, J. L., Bagley, L. R., and Fine, D. P., _Lab. Invest._ 35, 235 (1976).
10. Walker, D. H., Cain, B. G., and Olmstead, P. M., _Am. J. Clin. Path._ 69, 619 (1978).
11. Wike, D. A., and Burgdorfer, W., _Infect. Immun._ 6, 736 (1972).
12. Walker, D. H., and Cain, B. G., _J. Infect. Dis._ 137, 206 (1978).
13. Adams, J. S., and Walker, D. H., _Am. J. Clin. Path._, 75, 156 (1981).
14. Mollenhauer, H. H., _Stain Technol_ 39, 111 (1964).
15. Venable, J. H., and Coggeshall, R., _J. Cell Biol._ 25, 407 (1965).
16. Payling-Wright, H., _Nature_ 220, 78 (1968).
17. Payling-Wright, H., _J. Path._ 105, 65 (1971).
18. Polverini, P. J., Cotran, R. S., and Sholley, M. M., _J. Immunol._ 118, 529 (1977).
19. Walker, D. H., and Henderson, F. W., _Infect. Immun._ 20, 221 (1978).

20. Murphy, J. R., Wisseman, C. L., Jr., and Fiset, P., Infect. Immun. 27, 730 (1980).
21. Kenyon, R. H., and Pedersen, C. E., Jr., Infect. Immun. 28, 310 (1980).
22. Shirai, A., Catanzaro, P. J., Phillips, S. M., and Osterman, J. V., Infect. Immun. 14, 39 (1976).
23. Silverman, D. J., and Wisseman, C. L., Jr., Infect. Immun. 26, 714 (1979).
24. Walker, D. H., and Cain, B. G., Lab. Invest. 43, 388 (1980).
25. Sholley, M. M., Cavallo, T., and Cotran, R. S., Am. J. Path. 89, 277 (1977).
26. Sholley, M. M., and Cotran, R. S., Am. J. Path. 91, 229 (1978).

STUDIES ON MURINE TYPHUS RICKETTSIAE AND
XENOPSYLLA CHEOPIS FLEAS[1]

Abdulrahman Farhang-Azad
Charles L. Wisseman, Jr.
Robert Traub

University of Maryland
School of Medicine
Baltimore, Maryland

I. INTRODUCTION

Much remains to be learned about the ecology of murine typhus (1,2), especially concerning the interrelationships between Rickettsia mooseri (= R. typhi), the etiological agent;
the putative vector, the flea Xenopsylla cheopis; and rats of
the subgenus Rattus, commensal forms of which seem to be an
important but indirect source of human infection. The present
paper deals with the introductory phases of intensive investigations underway in our laboratory on 1) the capacity of X.
cheopis to acquire infection with R. mooseri after feeding on
rickettsemic hosts that had been inoculated with low levels of
rickettsiae, and 2) the distribution of R. mooseri within X.
cheopis at various periods after infection.
    Although lice, bloodsucking mites, trombiculid mites, and
ticks have been suggested as possible vectors of murine typhus,
the best evidence is for transmission by fleas to both rats
and man. As many as 7 genera and 8 species of fleas have been
implicated in various degrees as vectors, but on the basis of
epidemiological and experimental observations, the case is
strongest for the oriental rat flea, X. cheopis (1).

---

[1]Supported by contract N-000-14-76-C-0393 with Office of
Naval Research and Navy R&D Command and NIH Grant AI-04242.

Although there are limitations in the published data, as
indicated in our review (1), there is no doubt that: 1) X.
cheopis can readily acquire infection by feeding on rats that
have been inoculated with a large dose of R. mooseri; 2) the
rickettsiae can be found in large numbers in the midgut epithelium of the flea; 3) infective rickettsiae are shed in the
feces of the flea within less than 2 weeks; 4) transmission
to man or rats can occur after contact with these feces or
crushed fleas, but not by the bite of the flea; 5) X. cheopis
remains infected for life; and 6) the longevity of the flea is
not affected. The ultrastructural features of X. cheopis infected with R. mooseri have been well discussed and illustrated by Ito and colleagues (3,4). However, in previous studies, intraperitoneal inoculation of large doses of rickettsiae were given to the experimental hosts. In the present
study, in an effort to simulate natural conditions, where presumably a few rickettsiae may enter through a break in the
skin, we used a subcutaneous route of inoculation and a dose
of merely 100 plaque-forming units (PFU). By means of the direct fluorescent antibody technique on frozen sections and
whole smears of dissections of flea tissues, it was shown that
at even this low dose of inoculum, baby rats sustained a rickettsemia of 7-14 days duration and that all of the X. cheopis
that fed for a short period (e.g., overnight) on such hosts
acquired the infection.

II. MATERIALS AND METHODS

A. Rickettsiae

The recently isolated strain (AZ-332) of R. mooseri from
the kidney of an Ethiopian wild rat (Rattus rattus) used in
this study had been plaque-purified by three passages in tissue culture and amplified by two more passages in specific
pathogen-free eggs (SPAFAS). Seed B (2nd egg passage), characterized by Arango-Jaramillo et al. (in preparation), was
used after storage at -70°C as a 20% infected yolk sac suspension in brain heart infusion broth (BHI). The thawed seed was
diluted in BHI to obtain the desired dose.

B. Infection of Animals

Arango-Jaramillo et al. (in preparation) demonstrated that
baby rats inoculated subcutaneously (sc) with 100 PFU of seed
"B" displayed detectable rickettsemia between 8 and 16 days
after inoculation. In the present study, 3-day-old baby rats

were inoculated sc with 100 PFU (in a 0.1 ml volume) of the
rickettsiae and were permitted to remain with their mothers
for 7 days. The baby rats were then separated and used to
feed and infect X. cheopis.

C. Flea Colonies

Our cultures of X. cheopis are derived from stocks kindly
obtained from Dr. H. Krampitz in Germany in 1978. The rearing
procedure employed was that of Cole et al. (5), as modified in
our laboratory. The colonies were maintained at 24°C and a
relative humidity of 70%.

D. Infection of Fleas

Three types of experiments were conducted. In Series I,
designed to determine the ability of fleas to acquire R.
mooseri during a brief session of feeding, newly emerged adult
fleas were permitted to feed overnight on rickettsemic baby
rats (i.e., on day 8-9 postinoculation). After this infectious feeding, the fleas were transferred into special flea-
rearing jars and then fed twice weekly on normal baby rats.
Samples of 30 fleas were collected from this pool every other
day for 3 weeks and immobilized on crushed ice. Ten fleas
were then removed and screened by direct fluorescent antibody
test (DFA) and the rest stored at -70°C. In Series II, the
course of rickettsemia was followed, as determined by the acquisition of infection by X. cheopis. On each of alternate
days, commencing with day 3 after inoculation and continuing
for 40 days, infected baby rats were placed into jars, each
containing 50 newly emerged adult fleas. These rats had all
been infected simultaneously at 3 days of age. The infected
rats were removed from each jar after 48 hrs and the fleas
were thereafter fed only on normal baby rats. Seven days
after the infective feeding, a sample of 10 fleas was removed
for screening and the remainder stored at -70°C. Series III
dealt with the course of infection and the distribution of R.
mooseri in fleas at various intervals after the infectious
feeding. For this purpose, 300 fleas were exposed to rickettsemic baby rats for 36 hrs, after which the infected hosts
were replaced with normal baby rats. A sample of 10 fleas was
collected every other day for 40 days and stored at -70°C
until sectioned as indicated below.

E.   Examination of Fleas for R. mooseri Infection

Ten fleas from each group were checked for infection by
dissecting and excising the entire gut, which was then smeared
on a clean glass slide, air dried and fixed in cold acetone
(4°C) for 10 min. Smears of whole gut were examined after
staining by DFA, using high-titered anti-R. mooseri convalescent guinea pig serum conjugated with fluorescein isothiocyanate (FITC).

F.   Preparation and Staining of Flea Sections

Fleas collected at various intervals after the infectious
feeding were individually embedded in Tissue-Tex O.C.T. compound (Miles Laboratories) and sectioned in a cryostat at -10°C.
Serial sections (20-25 per flea), 4-6 μm in thickness, were
attached to clean microscopic slides, air dried and fixed in
cold acetone for 10 min. These sections were examined by DFA
for the presence and distribution of R. mooseri in various tissues. Controls included uninfected fleas sectioned and treated
in the same manner. For both test-fleas and controls, some
frozen sections that had been dried and fixed for DFA were
stained with hematoxylin and eosin for study by light microscopy to determine whether rickettsial infection caused gross
tissue damage.

III.   RESULTS

A.   Direct Staining of Flea Midgut Smears (Series I)

Smears of the gut of fleas which had been exposed overnight for feeding on rickettsemic baby rats showed no demonstrable rickettsiae for the first 4 days, as tested by DFA.
However, fluorescent rickettsial bodies appeared on day 5 and
increased in number daily. By day 6, 100% of the fleas were
positive, and all later samples were also positive until the
experiment was terminated on day 21. Later in the course of
infection (17-21 days), there was progressive increase of typical and "atypical" (dust-like) rickettsiae. No rickettsiae
were found in the fleas used as controls.

B.   The Course of R. mooseri Infection in the Rat as
     Measured by Infection in Fleas (Series II)

Figure 1 shows the capability of fleas to acquire R.
mooseri from the infected baby rat at different intervals after inoculation. Although 100% of the fleas became infected
after feeding on days 7-19 postinfection, 30% of the fleas fed
as early as the 5th day after infection were positive. Moreover, a comparable proportion of fleas acquired infection when
fed on rats 21 days postinfection. In contrast, when the
plaque assay method was used to detect rickettsiae in whole
blood (Fig. 1), R. mooseri was not demonstrable before day 7
nor after day 15. Thus, the "flea assay" was positive 2 days
earlier and 6 days later than the plaque method.

C.   Direct Fluorescent Antibody Tests on Frozen
     Sections of Infected Fleas (Series III)

Frozen sections of R. mooseri-infected X. cheopis revealed
no demonstrable fluorescent rickettsial bodies by DFA in the
samples collected during the first 3 days after the infectious
feeding. On day 4, only a small group of epithelial cells
mostly in the posterior region of the midgut, showed specific
fluorescence of R. mooseri. By 7 days postinfection, a larger
area of the midgut was involved. By 10 days, all portions of
the midgut epithelium contained intracellular rickettsiae,
essentially as shown in Figures 2 and 3, which are longitudinal sections of the midgut 13 days after infection. Although most of these epithelial cells contained masses of R.
mooseri, the intensity of the involvement of these cells
varied. As had been noted by Ito et al. (3,4), some cells
were packed with clumps of rickettsiae, while others had
scattered and fewer organisms. Similar observations were made
when sections were stained by the Giménez technique. The concentration and close packing of R. mooseri in the flea midgut
cells appears as a dense mass of fluorescence (Fig. 3). In
lightly infected cells the rickettsiae were localized in
densely packed but scattered clusters in the basal cytoplasm
or apical cytoplasm (Fig. 3). Although the infection was
widespread in the midgut epithelium and extended to the midgut cells at the junction with the proventriculus, there was
no evidence of R. mooseri in the proventriculus itself
throughout the course of the infection, nor in any of the
other structures tested by DFA, such as the salivary glands,
muscles, malpighian tubules, hindgut, or the reproductive
system (including the spermatheca, ovaries, eggs, or testes).
After the initial appearance of R. mooseri in the midgut
tissues, all subsequent examinations were positive for

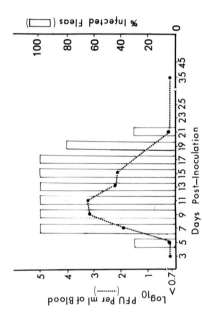

Fig. 1. Rickettsemia in R. mooseri-infected rats as indicated by plaque assay and acquisition by fleas.

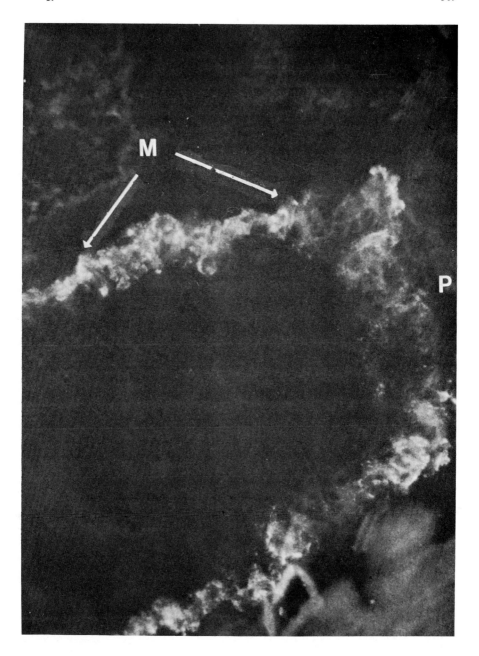

Fig. 2. A low power view of infected flea midgut. Specific fluorescence in cells throughout midgut (M) in contrast to its absence in the proventriculus (P).

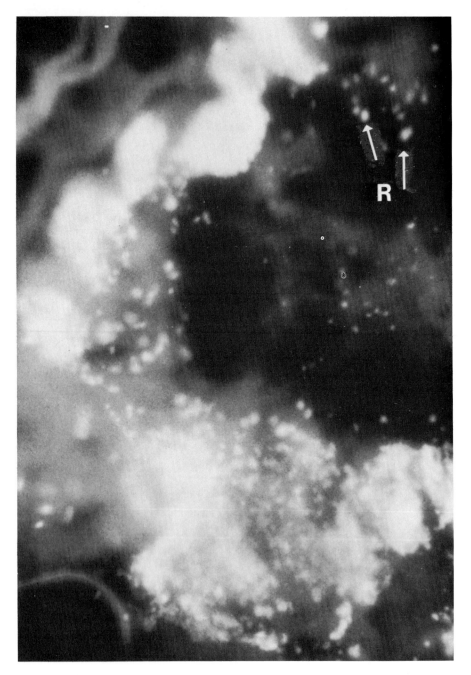

Fig. 3. Midgut epithelial cells of X. cheopis packed
with R. mooseri (white color), and some free rickettsiae
within the lumen (R).

fluorescence. As compared to infected epithelial cells, only
limited numbers of rickettsiae were observed in the lumen of
the midgut by day 10 and thereafter. The examination by DFA
of feces from the infected fleas on day 10 and thereafter dis-
closed the presence of R. mooseri from day 10 to 35, the last
date samples were collected. Large numbers of rickettsiae
were observed in the flea feces in the later stages of infection. On day 19, an increase in the amount of "dust-like"
rickettsiae in the midgut epithelial cells became noticeable
and these gradually became widespread in the cell lining of
the midgut epithelium. All tests with controls failed to show
presence of rickettsiae. No significant histological changes,
which differed from the control fleas, nor overt signs of damage were noted in sections of midgut of the infected fleas at
any time.

VI. DISCUSSION

The following observations are especially worthy of note.
1) Subcutaneous inoculation of R. mooseri at as low a dose as
100 PFU resulted in a rickettsemia of 7-14 days duration, with
a mean of 1.3×10^3 PFU (range: 4.5×10^2 to 2.9×10^3 PFU/ml
of whole heart blood). 2) This level of rickettsemia sufficed
to infect 100% of the X. cheopis exposed merely overnight to
such rickettsemic baby rats. 3) Some fleas became infected
when fed on rats as soon as 5 and as long as 21 days after inoculation. 4) The flea-feeding technique was significantly more
sensitive in demonstrating rickettsemia than was the plaque
assay method. The findings suggest that xenodiagnosis by X.
cheopis may be a useful tool in studies on experimental R.
mooseri infection. 5) The fleas remained infected and shed
feces containing masses of R. mooseri during the entire subsequent course of the experiment.

Data on the presence of rickettsiae in the lumen of the
gut and in the feces of the fleas suggest that about 10 days
must elapse before the fleas can transmit infection by means
of infective feces. Because there was no evidence for the
presence of R. mooseri in the proventriculus, salivary glands,
genital system or any other organs and tissues besides the
midgut in the long series examined, our observations support
the existing impression in the literature (1) that it is highly unlikely that X. cheopis can transmit R. mooseri by bite or
infect its eggs by transovarian transmission.

The cuticular (exoskeletal) nature of the lining of the
foregut, proventriculus and hindgut in X. cheopis may preclude
penetration by R. mooseri into those organs. Further study
should be made regarding the features of the midgut in fleas.
For example, this organ in a species of Ctenophthalmus was

found to be highly unusual in several respects as compared to
other insects (6,7). Since our histological study was based
upon frozen sections, details regarding changes in the tissues
could not be observed. However, it seems significant that we
could discern no loss of epithelial cells by this technique
during the course of infection. Ito et al. (3,4) in their
study of the ultrastructure of X. cheopis infected with R.
mooseri failed to observe any damage to the midgut cells.
How R. mooseri enters the midgut epithelium and how it later
escapes into the lumen of the gut has not yet been determined.
The impression gained from the literature (1) is that R.
mooseri infection in X. cheopis does not affect the longevity
of the fleas. This point, coupled with the ability of X.
cheopis to acquire R. mooseri from rickettsemic rats and
excrete the rickettsiae for long periods, if not for life,
suggests that this species of flea plays an important role in
the transmission of murine typhus, at least in certain areas.
Moreover, the life of the infective flea is apparently sufficiently long to ensure that R. mooseri infection can survive
outside the commensal rat until the next generation of rats
appear. The absence in the flea of untoward effects as a result of the infection strongly suggests a long-standing association between R. mooseri and fleas.

   This study has also demonstrated the utility of the
fluorescent antibody techniques, both for smears of dissected
tissues and for frozen sections, in studying this infection.

                              V. SUMMARY

   X. cheopis fleas can readily become infected with R.
mooseri by feeding on rickettsemic baby rats that had been inoculated subcutaneously with the low dose of rickettsiae (100
PFU). Infection of rats was more readily demonstrable by employing this technique than by employing standard plaque assay
tests. Infection was detectable by immunofluorescence as early as 5 days after the infectious feeding and persisted for at
least the course of the experiment (35 days). By the 10th day,
R. mooseri was detected in the flea feces and excretion of the
rickettsiae persisted thereafter throughout the period of observation. R. mooseri in flea tissues were strictly limited
to the midgut; all other tissues and organs, including the
salivary glands and genital system, were consistently free of
demonstrable rickettsiae. Transmission by bite or via eggs
therefore seems highly unlikely. The infection did not cause
any detectable histological damage to X. cheopis, nor produce
any observable difference from controls in behavior, reproductive capacity or longevity. In general, the findings confirm,
refine or extend reports in the literature.

REFERENCES

1. Traub, R., Wisseman, C. L., Jr., and Farhang-Azad, A.,
   Trop. Dis. Bull. 75, 237 (1978).
2. Traub, R., Wisseman, C. L., Jr., and Farhang-Azad, A.,
   in "Fleas" (R. Traub & H. Starcke, eds.), p. 283. A. A.
   Balkema, Rotterdam (1980).
3. Ito, S., Vinson, J. W., and McGuire, T. J., Jr., Ann. N.Y.
   Acad. Sci. 266, 35 (1975).
4. Ito, S., and Vinson, J. W., in "Fleas" (R. Traub &
   H. Starcke, eds.), p. 277. A. A. Balkema, Rotterdam
   (1980).
5. Cole, M. M., VanNatta, D. L., Ellerbe, W., and Washington,
   F., J. Econ. Ent. 65, 1495 (1972).
6. Richards, A. G., and Richards, P. A., Science 160, 423
   (1968).
7. Richards, P. A., and Richards, A. G., Ann. Ent. Soc. Amer.
   62, 249 (1969).

EFFECTIVENESS OF SEVERAL ANTIBIOTICS
IN SUPPRESSING CHICK EMBRYO LETHALITY
DURING EXPERIMENTAL INFECTIONS
BY COXIELLA BURNETII,
RICKETTSIA TYPHI AND R. RICKETTSII

Alan J. Spicer

Royal Army Medical Corp.
British Military Hospital
Munster, West Germany

Marius G. Peacock
Jim C. Williams

Laboratory of Microbial Structure and Function
Rocky Mountain Laboratories
Hamilton, Montana

I. INTRODUCTION

The effect of antibiotics on rickettsiae during experimental infection has been studied in animal models (1), fertile hens' eggs (2, 3, 4) and tissue culture (5). All of these studies have indicated that Coxiella burnetii, the etiologic agent of Q fever, was more resistant to antibiotics than other rickettsiae. C. burnetii was shown to be relatively resistant to the effects of chloramphenicol and erythromycin (2, 3) and streptomycin (1) in experimental infections in chick embryos. Other rickettsial species have been shown to be highly susceptible to chloramphenicol, streptomycin, tetracycline, doxycycline, minocycline, erythromycin and rifampin (2-5). However, tetracycline antibiotics are generally considered the most efficacious drugs against rickettsial infections in experimental models (2-5).

RICKETTSIAE AND RICKETTSIAL DISEASES

375

A review of these results suggested to us that a more
effective antibiotic against C. burnetii should be sought.
We, therefore, tested the effect of various antibiotics on
four strains of C. burnetii, one strain of Rickettsia
rickettsii, and one of R. typhi.

II. MATERIALS AND METHODS

A. Bacterial Strains and Preparation of Seed Stocks

C. burnetii strains used in this study were in various
passage levels in guinea pigs (GP), chicken embryo fibroblast
tissue culture (TC) and chicken embryo yolk sac (YS). Previous
studies had shown that Phase I C. burnetii are selected when
strains were isolated from the spleens of infected guinea pigs
during the febrile response, whereas Phase II strains were
obtained by repeated egg passage (EP) in YS (2, 7).   Clones
used in this study were isolated by selecting plaques on
chicken embryo fibroblast monolayers (22).   The five strains
of C. burnetii (CB) used in this study were from various geographical regions: i) CB 9 Mile Phase I (CB9MI, 307GP/1TC/1EP,
clone 7) was isolated in 1935 from Dermacentor andersoni in
western Montana (9, 10); ii) CB 9 Mile Phase II (CB9MII, 90EP/
1TC/4EP, clone 4) was derived from CB9MI; iii) CB Ohio Phase I
(CBOI, 5EP/2GP/2EP) was isolated from raw milk obtained from
Ohio (11); iv) CB Cyprus Phase I (CBCYPI, 1GP/4EP) was isolated
from an aborting sheep in 1975 (12) by injecting homogenized
splenic tissue into guinea pigs.   Guinea pig spleens were harvested and stored at -20°C.   In 1979 the splenic tissue was
passed four times in the YS of fertile chicken eggs; v) CB
Scottish Phase I and II (CBSCOI-II, 1GP/14EP) was isolated
from sheep placenta as described above and passed 14 times in
the YS of fertile chicken eggs.   The culture was lyophilized
in 1979.
R. typhi (RTWIL, Wilmington strain) and R. rickettsii
(RRSS, Sheila Smith strain) were propagated in chicken embryo
YS as previously described (13, 14).   Each of the rickettsial
seed pools was prepared as a 50% suspension of YS and brain
heart infusion broth (BHI, Difco) and stored at -70°C.

B. Preparation of Antibiotics and Inoculation of Yolk Sacs

Nine antibiotics were used in this study: Cephalothin,
sodium for injection, Eli Lilly and Co., Indianapolis, IN;
Clindamycin HCl, Upjohn LTD; D-Cycloserine, Sigma Chemical Co.,

S t. Louis, MO; Doxycycline Hyclate, Chas. Pfizer and Co. Inc.,
Brooklyn, NY; Erythromycin and Oxytetracycline, Sigma Chemical
Co., St. Louis, MO; Rifampin, Dow Pharmaceuticals, The Dow
Chemical Co., Indianapolis, IN; Trimethoprim, Burroughs
Wellcome Co., Research Triangle Park, NC and Viomycin sulfate,
Pfizer Inc., Groton, CT. Eight of the antibiotics were dis-
solved separately at 1 mg per ml in sterile demineralized and
distilled water (SDDW). Trimethoprim was first suspended in
dimethyl sulfoxide at 10 mg per 0.1 ml and then mixed with
9.9 ml of SDDW.

Solutions of the antibiotics were prepared in BHI broth
immediately before use and sterilized by filtration through
0.22 μm Millipore filters. Stock solutions of antibiotics
were diluted to the appropriate concentrations in BHI broth
and then injected as 0.25 ml volumes into each YS of batches
of 36 5-day-old chicken embryos. Thirty minutes later the YSs
were injected with 0.2 ml volumes of the rickettsiae which
had been diluted in BHI broth. Plaque-forming units (pfu's)
inoculated into each YS were 1.1×10^9 for CBOI, 1.5×10^7 for
CB9MI, 5.6×10^7 for CB9MII, 1.1×10^7 for CBCYPI, 1.1×10^8
for CBSCOI-II, 8.1×10^1 for RRSS and 1.4×10^2 for RTWIL
strains (see Table 1).

In calculating the mean survival time (MST), all embryos
alive at the end of the experiment were considered to have
died on the 14th day (15). The mean day protection (MDP) was
calculated by subtracting the MST with antibiotic from the MST
without antibiotics. Percentage survival and MDP were used as
the parameters of assessment. Weighted mean plus or minus
standard error (SE) was determined for each group. The level
of statistical significance was determined by the student t-
test using the weighted mean $\pm$ SE values.

C. Efficacy of Antibiotics

Evaluation of statistical significance of antibiotics and
the criterion of efficacy against rickettsiae in embryonated
eggs was determined from the MST and MDP (15). The rickettsiocidal and/or-static activity of the antibiotics were
evaluated from the subculture of surviving embryo YSs on day 14
postinfection. Fifty percent YS suspensions were prepared,
and 0.2 ml was injected into 5-day-old embryos. Embryo
deaths were evaluated as described above.

III.   RESULTS

A.   Toxicity of Rickettsial Strains for Embryos

Some strains of C. burnetii were more toxic for embryos
as determined by the pfu's required to consistently kill
embryos with a 7-day MST. Titration of seed stocks indicated
that CB9MI was 10- and 100-fold more toxic for embryos than
CBSCOI-II and CBOI; whereas, CB9MI, CB9MII and CBCYPI were
approximately equally toxic for embryos (Table 1). Therefore,
each antibiotic was tested in embryos receiving the above
pfu's so that the MST, percentage survival and MDP could be
evaluated with consistency.

The titration of R. rickettsii and R. typhi seed stocks
indicated that the RRSS and RTWIL strains were highly toxic
for embryos (Table 1). A MST of 5.7 ± 0.1 and 7.7 ± 0.2 days
was found to be optimal for evaluating the effect of antibiotics on the RRSS and RTWIL strains.

TABLE 1. Toxicity of Rickettsial Strains for Chick Embryos

Rickettsial strains[a]	Dosage of organisms (pfu's/embryo)	Mean survival time in days (MST $\pm$ SE)
C. burnetii		
CB9MI	1.5×10^7	7.8 ± 0.8
CB9MII	5.6×10^7	7.4 ± 0.2
CBCYPI	1.1×10^7	7.5 ± 0.6
CBSCOI-II	1.1×10^8	7.4 ± 0.4
CBOI	1.1×10^9	7.4 ± 0.2
R. rickettsii		
RRSS	8.1×10^1	5.7 ± 0.1
R. typhi		
RTWIL	1.4×10^2	7.7 ± 0.2

[a]See Materials and Methods.

TABLE 2. Effect of Antibiotics on the Suppression of Embryo Mortality During C. burnetii Infections

Antibiotic[a]	Concentration μg/embryo	Mean day protection (percentage survival)				
		CB9MI	CB9MII	CBCYPI	CBSCOI-II	CBOI
Rifampin	250	4.8(64)[b]	5.7(87)[b]	3.4(46)[b]	4.2(50)[b]	5.5(75)[b]
	125	4.7(70)[b]	4.8(62)[b]	2.2(33)[b]	4.5(48)[b]	3.6(43)[b]
	50	4.8(71)[b]	5.2(71)[b]	2.6(34)[c]	4.2(48)[b]	3.7(37)[b]
Trimethoprim	250	4.1(53)[b]	5.8(80)[b]	3.3(30)[c]	1.8(12)[d]	5.3(66)[b]
	125	5.0(62)[b]	4.7(67)[b]	4.0(38)[b]	2.9(20)[b]	3.6(21)[b]
	50	4.0(7)[b]	4.4(38)[b]	3.4(6)[c]	1.3(0)[d]	2.5(3)[b]
Doxycycline	250	2.7(36)[d]	5.5(81)[b]	1.9(23)	2.6(19)[b]	4.5(70)[b]
	125	5.3(86)[b]	4.4(56)[b]	1.7(12)	2.9(27)[b]	3.0(26)[b]
	50	5.2(73)[b]	4.2(45)[b]	1.7(9)	4.1(38)[b]	3.2(6)[b]
Oxytetracycline	250	3.4(41)[b]	4.8(72)[b]	1.8(16)	3.1(23)[b]	5.1(60)[b]
	125	5.7(75)[b]	3.8(45)[b]	0.5(7)	2.2(11)[b]	4.6(58)[b]
	50	4.2(58)[b]	3.8(38)[b]	1.3(11)	3.8(33)[b]	4.5(20)[b]

[a] Clindamycin, Erythromycin, Viomycin, Cycloserine and Cephalothin were not effective in increasing the MST of treated embryos.

[b] Statistical significance ρ value as compared to a control group without antibiotic.

[b] ρ value <0.001.
[c] ρ value <0.025.
[d] ρ value <0.05.

B. Suppression of Embryo Lethality by Antibiotics During Experimental Rickettsial Infections

The comparative effectiveness of nine antibiotics in suppressing experimental C. burnetii infections in embryos is presented in Table 2. Antibiotics were tested at 250, 125 and 50 μg per embryo. The average volume of the eggs was 40 ml, therefore each antibiotic was tested at 6.25, 3.12 and 1.25 μg per ml. The MDP and percentage survival of embryos on day 14 postinfection were used to evaluate the efficacy of each anti-biotic. Statistical analysis of the MDP indicated that rifampin, trimethoprim, doxycycline and oxytetracycline were highly effective against four of the C. burnetii strains tested, whereas only rifampin and trimethoprim were effective against CBCYPI. Thus, CBCYPI was more resistant to tetracyclines than the other strains. Clindamycin, erythromycin, viomycin, cycloserine and cephalothin were not efficacious in suppressing embryo mortality during C. burnetii infection. Thus, these antibiotics produced no significant increase in the MST of infected embryos as compared to no antibiotic treatment.

When these nine antibiotics were tested during experimental R. rickettsii and R. typhi infections in embryos, marked dif-ferences were noted between the genera Rickettsia and Coxiella (Table 3). Rifampin, doxycycline, oxytetracycline and eryth-romycin were highly efficacious in suppressing R. rickettsii and R. typhi infections, whereas trimethoprim, viomycin, cycloserine and cephalothin were not efficacious in suppressing embryo mortality during rickettsial infections.

Examination of YS tissues of surviving embryos by the Giménez staining procedures (16) and fluorescein-conjugated anti-rickettsial antibody (17) indicated that numerous C. burnetii cells could be seen, whereas R. rickettsii and R. typhi microorganisms were rarely observed. We tested the ability of antibiotic-treated rickettsiae to infect and kill fresh embryos by subculturing the YS tissue of surviving embryos (see Materials and Methods). The results of this study indicated that members of the genera Coxiella were extremely resistant to prior exposure to rifampin, doxycycline, oxytetracycline and trimethoprim (data not shown). Although these antibiotics were efficacious in prolonging the MST and generating survivors on the initial exposure of C. burnetii to antibiotics, they appeared to be without effect in the subculture study. R. typhi and R. rickettsii were eliminated by doxycycline, whereas a significant percentage of surviving embryos was noted with erythromycin, rifampin and oxytetra-cycline. Microscopic examination of the YS tissue from dead embryos revealed numerous microorganisms, whereas an occasional organism was observed in the surviving embryo YSs.

TABLE 3. Effect of Antibiotics on the Suppression of Embryo
Mortality During R. rickettsii and R. typhi Infections

Antibiotics[a]	Concentration µg/embryo	Mean day protection (percentage survival)	
		R. rickettsii	R. typhi
Rifampin	250	$6.5(75)^b$	$3.8(63)^b$
	125	$5.7(55)^b$	$4.3(64)^b$
	50	$5.3(58)^b$	$4.5(63)^b$
Doxycycline	250	$4.1(48)^b$	$3.2(53)^b$
	125	$5.1(51)^b$	$4.8(70)^b$
	50	$4.8(51)^b$	$4.3(65)^b$
Oxytetracycline	250	$4.9(45)^b$	$5.5(83)^b$
	125	$5.3(56)^b$	$5.8(85)^b$
	50	$5.9(57)^b$	$4.9(76)^b$
Erythromycin	250	$6.5(64)^b$	$4.8(78)^b$
	125	$4.8(13)^b$	$3.7(66)^b$
	50	$1.4(3)$	$3.0(55)^b$

[a]Trimethoprim, Viomycin, Cycloserine, and Cephalothin were
not effective in increasing the MST of treated embryos.

[b]ρ value <0.001. Statistically significant ρ value as
compared to a control group without antibiotic.

IV. DISCUSSION

Antibiotics effective against experimental Q fever in
embryonated eggs were rifampin, trimethoprim, doxycycline and
oxytetracycline, whereas clindamycin, erythromycin, viomycin,
cycloserine and cephalothin were not effective. These effective antibiotics were rickettsiostatic as determined by subculture of treated rickettsiae into fresh YSs in the absence
of additional antibiotics. The most striking result was the
observation that the recently isolated Cyprus strain of C.
burnetii (12) was more resistant to the tetracyclines than
laboratory strains. Other investigators have isolated chloro-
tetracyline resistant strains of C. burnetii by serial culture
in the presence of low concentrations of antibiotic in chick

embryo YSs (18). However, this is the first report of a
recently isolated C. burnetii strain with enhanced resistance
to tetracyclines. Previous reports (12, 19, 20, 21, 22) of
equivocal results during various Q fever epidemics may be a
real indication of enhanced antibiotic resistance of C.
burnetii strains.

Rifampin, doxycycline, oxytetracycline and erythromycin
were effective and rickettsiocidal against R. typhi and R.
rickettsii infections. These results were expected since
other investigators have shown the drugs to be highly efficacious. A surprising result was the observation that trimethoprim was completely ineffective against R. typhi and R.
rickettsii. These results suggest a basic difference in the
folate metabolism of these rickettsiae. Further studies in
rickettsial plaque assay and animal models are required to
determine the relative effectiveness of these antibiotics
against Q fever infections.

V.   SUMMARY

We have tested the potencies of several antibiotics on the
inhibition of Coxiella burnetii, Rickettsia typhi and R.
rickettsii multiplication in ovo. Rifampin, doxycycline,
oxytetracycline and trimethoprim were effective against C.
burnetii infections. Whereas, doxycycline, erythromycin,
rifampin and oxytetracycline were highly efficacious against
R. typhi and R. rickettsii infections. Therefore, a marked
difference between the antibiotic sensitivities of these
rickettsiae was noted since erythromycin was not effective
against C. burnetii and trimethroprim was not effective against
R. typhi and R. rickettsii infections. Although some of the
antibiotics were effective in increasing the mean survival time
and percentage survival of embryos, the effective antibiotics
were rickettsiostatic for C. burnetii, but they were rickettsiocidal for R. typhi and R. rickettsii. The recently isolated
Cyprus strain of C. burnetii was more resistant to the tetracyclines tested, but rifampin and trimethoprim were efficacious.

ACKNOWLEDGMENTS

The technical assistance of E. Davis and the expert secretarial assistance of S. Smaus are gratefully acknowledged.

REFERENCES

1. Huebner, R. J., Hottle, G. A., and Robinson, E. B.,
    Public Health Rept. 63, 357 (1948).
2. Smadel, J. E., Jackson, E. B., and Gauld, R. L., J.
    Immunol. 57, 273 (1947).
3. Ormsbee, R. A., and Pickens, E. G., J. Immunol. 67,
    437 (1951).
4. Ormsbee, R. A., Parker, H., and Pickens, E., J. Infect.
    Dis. 96, 162 (1955).
5. Wisseman, C. L. Jr., Waddell, A. D., and Walsh, W. T.,
    J. Infect. Dis. 130, 564 (1974).
6. Stoker, M. G. P., J. Hyg. 51, 311 (1953).
7. Stoker, M. G. P., Can. J. Microbiol. 2, 310 (1956).
8. Ormsbee, R., and Peacock, M. G., Tissue Culture Assoc.
    2, 475 (1976).
9. Davis, G. E., and Cox, H. R., Public Health Rept.
    53, 2259 (1938).
10. Cox, H. R., and Bell, E. J., Public Health Rept. 54,
    2171 (1939).
11. Reed, C. F., and Wentworth, B. B., J. Am. Vet. Med.
    Assoc. 130, 458 (1957).
12. Spicer, A. J., Crowther, R. W., Vella, E. E., Bengsston,
    E., Miles, R., and Pitzolis, G., Trans. Royal Soc. Trop.
    Med. Hyg. 71, 16 (1977).
13. Weiss, E., Coolbaugh, J. C., and Williams, J. C.,
    Appl. Microbiol. 39, 456 (1975).
14. Anacker, R. L., McCaul, T. F., Burgdorfer, W., and
    Gerloff, R. K., Infect. Immun. 27, 468 (1980).
15. Dougherty, R. M., in "Techniques in Experimental
    Virology" (R. J. C. Harris, ed.), p. 169. Academic
    Press, New York (1964).
16. Giménez, D. F., J. Bact. 90, 834 (1965).
17. Peacock, M., Burgdorfer, W., and Ormsbee, R. A.,
    Infect. Immun. 3, 355 (1971).
18. Brezina, R., Schramek, S., and Kazar, J., Acta Virol.
    19, 496 (1975).
19. Tigertt, W. G., and Benenson, A. J., Trans. Assoc. Am.
    Physicians 69, 98 (1956).
20. Powell, O. W., Kennedy, K. P., McIver, M., and
    Silverstone, H., Australasian Ann. Med. 11, 184 (1962).
21. Clark, W. H., and Lennette, E. H., Ann. N.Y. Acad.
    Sci. 55, 1004 (1952).
22. Powell, O., Australasian Ann. Med. 9, 214 (1960).

BIOCHEMISTRY AND METABOLISM OF RICKETTSIAE

BIOCHEMISTRY AND METABOLISM OF RICKETTSIAE: CURRENT TRENDS

Emilio Weiss[1]

Naval Medical Research Institute
Bethesda, Maryland

I.   INTRODUCTION TO PAPERS PRESENTED AT THIS CONFERENCE

When an obligate intracellular bacterium is about to parasitize a eukaryotic cell, the first successful encounter almost invariably results in phagocytosis or induced phagocytosis. This event leads to one of the following developments:
parasite type I quickly gains entrance into the cytoplasm and,
sometimes, nucleus of the host cell; parasite type II remains
in the phagosome, which is prevented from developing into a
phagolysosome; parasite type III does not prevent phagolysosome formation (1). The investigation of the biochemistry and
metabolism of these parasitic bacteria must take into account
these major differences.

The genus Rickettsia is the most prominent, if not the only, member of parasite type I. Winkler and Miller (2, 3[a])
have identified phospholipase A activity involved in the hemolysis of sheep and human erythrocytes and in the immediate
toxicity on L-cells by R. prowazekii. The phospholipase may
well represent the mechanism by which R. prowazekii escapes
from the phagosome and gains access to the cytoplasm. The
ownership of this enzyme has not been established: It could
be a rickettsial enzyme, but it could also be a host enzyme
activated by the rickettsiae.

---

[1]Supported by the Naval Medical Research and Development
Command, Work Unit No. MR00001.001.1251.
[a]Paper presented at this conference.

Inside the cytoplasm the rickettsiae find a great number of metabolic intermediates not encountered elsewhere. It has been recognized for some time that rickettsiae would not go through the trouble of entering the cytoplasm, if they had not learnt to transport some of these metabolites, including phosphorylated compounds, for their own use (4,5). Unusual transport properties of R. prowazekii are discussed by Atkinson and Winkler (6[a]). Rickettsiae, unlike Chlamydia (7), are not energy parasites, however, and produce their own ATP (4,8,9[a]). Just as important as transport and metabolism is enzyme regulation for the orderly development of energy and biosynthesis from the resources of the cytoplasm. This is a much neglected topic. Phibbs and Winkler (10[a]) examine the properties of some enzymes of the tricarboxylic acid cycle for evidence that they might reflect regulation in this unusual environment.

Type II parasitism is a highly sophisticated one. The parasite avoids digestion not by escaping from the phagosome, but by preventing phagosome-lysosome fusion. This phenomenon has been described in detail in Chlamydia (7), but the mechanism of phagolysosome inhibition has not been elucidated. Rickettsiae in the narrow sense (genera Rickettsia, Coxiella, Rochalimaea) do not include parasites in this category. However, the rickettsias, as defined in Bergey's Manual of Determinative Bacteriology (11) provide several examples of type II parasitism, such as Ehrlichia (12).

Type III parasites manage to survive and thrive in the highly hostile environment of the phagolysosome, in the presence of hydrolytic enzymes and low pH. To this group belong Coxiella burnetii and some of the Mycobacteria. John Hanks has often emphasized that, if we want to grow bacteria that normally reside in the macrophage, we must adjust the pH of the medium to that of the phagocytic vacuoles, which is 4.5 to 5.5. At these pHs, Morrison (13) and Wheeler and Hanks (14) obtained good growth of Johne's bacillus, Mycobacterium paratuberculosis, a pathogen of cows and sheep, and the mycobacterium of the wood pigeon. At neutral pH growth was poor. This is not true of all mycobacteria. The Nakamura media for the growth of M. lepraemurium have a pH close to neutrality (15).

Hackstadt and Williams (16[a]) show that Coxiella burnetii, too, metabolizes a number of substrates efficiently, provided the pH is lowered to 4.5. This finding explains an apparent discrepancy seen in previous experiments. Paretsky and his associates (4,17) have demonstrated the presence of numerous enzymes in cell extracts of C. burnetii, but not in whole cells suspended in commonly used physiologic buffers. Ormsbee and Peacock (18) obtained only low levels of activity. In the experiments of Hackstadt and Williams the low pH requirement appears to involve primarily transport. This represents an exquisite adaptation to the phagolysosomal environment: outside this environment C. burnetii cells are metabolically inert and protected from unbalanced growth. The enzymes themselves, including those described at this conference (19[a], 20[a]), do not appear to have highly unusual properties. Paretsky, who has pioneered the study of the metabolism of C. burnetii, is now focusing his attention on the biochemical changes that occur in the infected animal model (21[a]).

The assumption is justifiably made that host-dependent bacteria have unusual membrane components reflecting either special transport properties or mechanisms of interaction with the host cells. Two papers at this conference deal with membranes, one on C. burnetii (22[a]) and one on the rickettsia-like bacterium of Pierce's disease of grape (23[a]). We do not know whether or not the Pierce's disease agent is truly akin to rickettsiae, but comparisons of results obtained with two bacteria parasitizing two entirely different host cells can only be beneficial.

Wisseman (24[a]) emphasizes that rickettsiae, in addition to being highly sophisticated parasites, have most of the attributes of ordinary bacteria. Two papers at this conference deal with investigations commonly applied to host-independent bacteria: Oaks et al. (25[a]) illustrate the two-dimensional electrophoretic patterns of the proteins of R. prowazekii; Hanson and Wisseman (26[a]) provide much needed data on the protein migration patterns of Rickettsia tsutsugamushi. Wisseman (24[a]) also emphasizes differences among rickettsial species as indicated by the extent of DNA-DNA hybridization. This is important in the study of evolution. Differences in nucleotide base sequence between R. prowazekii and Rickettsia typhi, as indicated by 70-77% DNA-DNA hybridization (27), are just too great for an explanation of origin of one species from the other by a few mutational steps. From the point of view of biochemistry and metabolism, however, stressing similarities is just as important. In fact, Brenner et al. (28,29) and Hebert et al. (30) placed Legionella pneumophila, L. micdadei, L. bozemanni, and L. dumoffii in the same genus, although in some of the DNA-DNA crosses the extent of hybridization was insignificant[2]. As Brenner et al. (29) aptly put it, "ideally, a genus should contain a group of genetically and phenotypically related species. When both criteria cannot be met, phenotypic relatedness should take precedence to ensure that the genus designation is of practical use at the bench."

---

[2] Two of the above species designations honor Joseph E. McDade and F. Marilyn Bozeman, who have successfully applied rickettsial methodology to Legionella.

    With rickettsiae we might be confronted with the opposite
situation. Myers and Wisseman (27) made the remarkable observation that the DNAs of the typhus group of rickettsiae
hybridize to the extent of 25-33% with the DNA of Rochalimaea
quintana. This is surprising because the DNA base ratios of
typhus rickettsiae and Rochalimaea differ by 8% (30 and 38%
molar guanine plus cytosine, respectively) and Rochalimaea
can readily be grown in bacteriologic media. These results
suggest that some phenotypic similarities between the two
genera might have been overlooked.

                    II. The genus Rochalimaea

    About two years ago we showed that the vole agent (31)
greatly resembled the Fuller strain (32) of Rochalimaea
quintana in cultural and biochemical properties (33,34).[3]
Subsequent work has confirmed that the two microorganisms are
similar, although they are not identical. Cross reactions
with hyperimmune rabbit sera, determined in indirect fluorescent antibody tests (IFA), are illustrated in Table 1. The
Guadalupe strain, of human Mexican origin (35) appears to be
identical to the Fuller strain. The vole strain reacts moderately well with antisera prepared against the Fuller and Guadalupe strains, but these strains react weakly with vole antiserum. Myers et al. (36) showed that Henry S. Fuller developed antibodies against both agents following his historic
self-induced R. quintana experimental infection, although the
titers against the infecting strain were higher.
    Myers et al. (36) also showed that the extent of DNA-DNA
hybridization between R. quintana and the vole agent ranged
from 31 to 42% and that their protein migration patterns were
similar but not identical. Fig. 1 illustrates the protein migration patterns of the Fuller, Guadalupe, and vole strains in
comparison with those of R. prowazekii, R. typhi, and R. canada. As shown previously (37), the polypeptide patterns of the
rickettsial species are quite similar, but there are distinct
differences, especially between R. canada and the other two
species. The Fuller and Guadalupe migration patterns appear
to be identical and to differ from those of the vole agent to

-----

    [3] At the time we were unaware that J. W. Vinson had previ-
ously recognized the basic similarity and some of the differ-
erences between the two agents (Annual Report to the U.S. Army
Medical Research and Development Command, 1 September 1968).

Table 1. Serological Cross-reactions among <u>Rochalimaea</u> Strains[a]

Antisera	Antigens		
	Fuller	Guadalupe	Vole
Fuller	<u>500</u>	500	200
Guadalupe	500	<u>500</u>	200
Vole	25	25-50	<u>500</u>

[a]By IFA. The titers are the means of observations on 11-12 colonies of each strain and are expressed as the inverse of the serum dilution. The homologous titers are underlined.

approximately the same extent as those of <u>R. prowazekii</u> and <u>R. typhi</u>. From the results of DNA-DNA hybridization (27) some similarity in protein migration patterns should be expected between the <u>Rickettsia</u> species and <u>Rochalimaea quintana</u>. The results shown in Fig. 1 are compatible with this expectation.

We have recently cultivated the two strains of <u>R. quintana</u> and the vole agent in a liquid medium in bottles in an incubator shaker at 35°C. The composition of the medium is shown in Table 2. The use of hematin, rather than fetal calf serum (FCS), is necessary for the demonstration that both casamino acids (CAA) and yeast extract (YE) are essential and that the concentrations shown are approximately optimal. For routine cultivation of cells for metabolic experiments, FCS is more convenient to use than hematin, because hematin produces a black precipitate that adheres to the cells. An absolute need for succinate was not shown, but this metabolite is used at a rapid rate. All three strains grow well in this medium, except that the vole agent multiplies somewhat faster when the medium contains FCS (generation time 4.5 h instead of 6 h), does not require CO_2, and readily settles to the bottom of the vessel.

These results clearly indicate that the vole agent might be regarded as a new species of the genus <u>Rochalimaea</u>, rather than a strain of <u>R. quintana</u>, as we had previously suggested (33). The study of <u>Rochalimaea</u> by conventional bacteriological and biochemical methods is thus facilitated by the availability of more than one strain and more than one species.

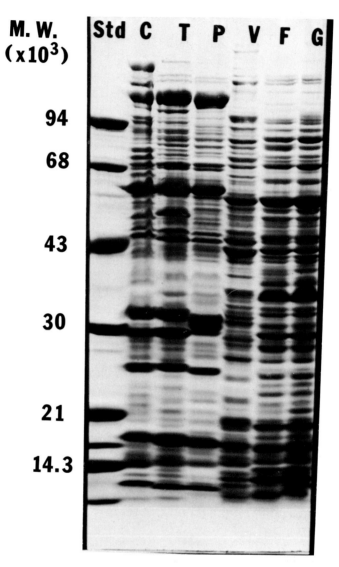

Fig. 1. Discontinuous sodium dodecyl sulfate-polyacrylamide gel electrophoretic patterns of solubilized proteins
from whole cells of Rickettsia and Rochalimaea. The gel was
prepared with a 10-20% acrylamide gradient. Abbreviations:
C = Rickettsia canada; T = R. typhi (Wilmington strain);
P = R. prowazekii (Breinl strain); V = vole agent; F = Fuller
strain of Rochalimaea quintana; G = Guadalupe strain of R.
quintana. This experiment was kindly performed by Gregory
A. Dasch.

Table 2. Medium for the Cultivation of Rochalimaea Strains

Autoclaved reagents	Filter sterilized reagents
1. Hanks BSS without glucose, $CaCl_2$, with HEPES buffer, 25 mM, final pH 7.2 2. Casamino acids (Difco), 0.8%	3. Yeast extract (Difco), 0.1% 4. Succinate, 2 mM 5. Fetal calf serum, 10% or hematin, 0.02 mM 6. $NaHCO_3$, 4.5 mM

III. Biochemical Reactions of Rochalimaea

For Enterobacteriaceae and for other bacteria a number of multi-test systems have been developed, which facilitate the study of their biochemical reactions. The Micro-ID system (General Diagnostics, Warner-Lambert Company, Morris Plains, NJ 07950) does not depend upon growth of the organism, but detects the presence of constitutive enzymes in a bacterial suspension incubated for 4 h. This system has been used for the characterization of strains, such as Haemophilus, which are not expected to grow in media intended for Enterobacteriaceae (38). We applied the Micro-ID system to the study of Rochalimaea.

The 15 reactions of the Micro-ID system were generally negative for the three strains of Rochalimaea, but three reactions were on occasion weakly positive: Voges-Proskauer, malonate utilization, and ornithine decarboxylase. The Voges-Proskauer reaction, as originally described, involves the fermentation of glucose with production of acetoin (39), sometimes as a major by-product (40). Rochalimaea does not utilize glucose, but metabolizes pyruvate quite well (33,41). Pyruvate is a close precursor of acetoin and it is not surprising, therefore, that the Voges-Proskauer reaction is weakly positive in Rochalimaea, since the Micro-ID system contains both glucose and pyruvate. Neither is the utilization of trace amounts of malonate surprising, since exogeneous succinate is avidly metabolized (33,41). There is no obvious explanation for ornithine decarboxylase activity, except that a non-glycolytic organism can be expected to utilize exogenous amino acids. The test for lysine decarboxylase was consistently negative.

The results of the ornithine decarboxylase reaction in the
Micro-ID system were quite puzzling. When the cells were
washed well and suspended in physiologic saline the results
were negative. However, when the medium was removed but the
cells were not washed, the test was often positive. Control
tests of saline plus an amount of medium matching that of un-
washed cells were also negative. We studied the reaction,
therefore, with ornithine labeled with ^{14}C in the carboxylic
position. The results of preliminary experiments with the
three strains appeared to be qualitatively comparable, but the
greatest activity was shown with the vole agent. Thus, the
vole agent was selected for more detailed experiments.

Fig. 2 illustrates the reaction with various components of
the medium. There was little activity when the cells were
suspended in buffer, or when succinate or FCS was added. The
reaction was enhanced by the addition of casamino acids and
yeast extract, even more when succinate was added to it, and
still more in the complete medium. These results suggest
that ornithine decarboxylase or the transport of ornithine--
the experiments done thus far do not distinguish between the
two--is an inducible activity. To prove this hypothesis, it
is necessary to show that there is a lag period before ornithine is utilized in the complete medium and that the activity does not develop in the presence of chloramphenicol. Fig.
3 shows that the reaction has both of these characteristics.
Chloramphenicol reduced the reaction to the level obtained in
buffer. The reaction appeared to be linear for the period 15
to 90 min. A regression line drawn for this period indicates
that there is a lag period of 5-7 min. Fig. 4 illustrates the
effect of substrate concentration on the reaction. The Lineweaver-Burke plot indicates that the concentration for half-
maximal activity is 1/0.77 or 1.3 mmolar.

Fig. 5 illustrates the ornithine decarboxylase reaction
with the Fuller strain. Compared to the reaction of the vole
agent, the lag period was longer (20 min) and the activity was
not enhanced as much by medium, while the effect of chloramphenicol was similar. More recent work indicates that there
are other differences in the activities of the two strains.

IV. CONCLUSIONS

It is obvious that the genus Rochalimaea is amenable to
investigations by techniques commonly employed in microbial
physiology. The principal value of such studies lies in their
applicability to the understanding of Rickettsia, which can
only be studied with much greater difficulty. During the past

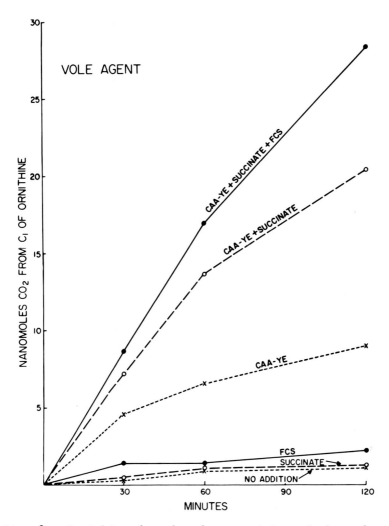

Fig. 2. Ornithine decarboxylase activity of the vole agent measured by evolution of $^{14}CO_2$ from ornithine-1-^{14}C. The experiment was performed in triplicate flasks, as described previously (42). Medium constituents were added to Hanks BSS-HEPES buffer at one fourth the final concentrations shown in Table 2. The cells (protein content: 0.63 mg/flask) were preincubated for about 0.5 h with the various medium constituents, prior to the addition of ornithine (final concentration, 1 mM) containing 0.1 μCi/flask. The total volume in each flask was 2 ml. The temperature of incubation was $35^{\circ}C$. CO_2 produced is expressed as nanomoles per mg protein. Abbreviations: FCS = fetal calf serum; CAA = casamino acids; YE = yeast extract.

several decades a number of phenotypic similarities, such as,
morphology and staining properties, association with similar
arthropod and vertebrate hosts, and lack of glycolytic pathways, have been identified (4,11,33,41,43). Since we know now
that a portion of the genome of the genera is similar (27),
other important phenotypic similarities may yet be uncovered.

As clearly demonstrated at this conference, several metabolic activities and unusual transport properties have been
found in Rickettsia and Coxiella. Ornithine metabolism has
been investigated previously in C. burnetii (44), but not in
Rickettsia or Rochalimaea. Although many of the features of
ornithine decarboxylase activity in Rochalimaea need to be
further elucidated, the results reported here indicate that

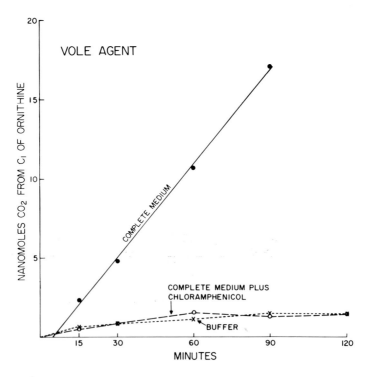

Fig. 3. Ornithine decarboxylase activity of the vole
agent. The cells (protein content: 0.62 mg/flask) were thermoequilibrated for 10 min prior to the addition of a mixture
of the other reagents, and for 1 min thereafter. The final
concentration of chloramphenicol was 0.2 mg/ml. Determinations were made in duplicate flasks. For other detail see
the legend for Figure 2.

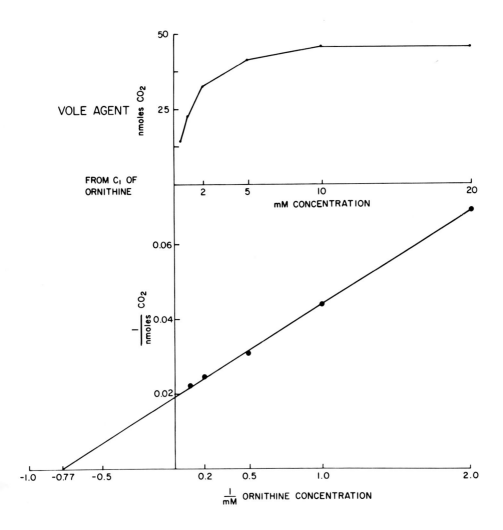

Fig. 4. Ornithine decarboxylase activity of the vole agent. The cells (protein content: 0.4 mg/flask) were maintained on ice water while mixed with medium, varying amounts of ornithine to give the final concentrations shown, and constant amounts of labeled ornithine (0.1 μCi/flask). The reaction mixtures were incubated for 2 h plus 10 min for thermoequilibration. For other detail see legend for Figure 2. Top section: CO_2 produced. Bottom section: Lineweaver-Burke plot calculated from the results shown in the top section.

this reaction has the earmarks of an inducible activity. If
such an activity, or comparable activity, can be demonstrated
in Rickettsia, it would offer obvious advantages: It would
provide a simple procedure for the identification of conditions that permit protein synthesis and it would provide a
start towards the study of enzyme regulation. It remains to
be determined whether or not ornithine decarboxylase activity
can be demonstrated in Rickettsia. In any case, the exploration of Rochalimaea as a model for the biochemistry and metabolism of Rickettsia well deserves further exploration.

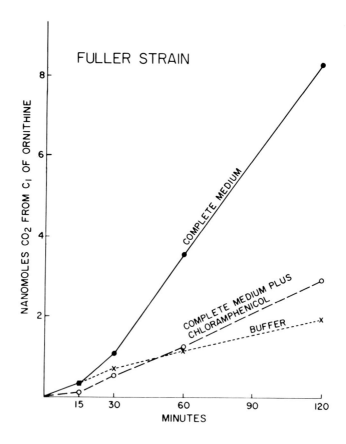

Fig. 5. Ornithine decarboxylase activity of the Fuller
strain. The cells (protein content: 1.06 mg/flask) and the
other reagents were thermoequilibrated separately prior to the
start of the reaction. For other detail see previous legends.

ACKNOWLEDGMENTS

The excellent technical assistance of Byron L. Ward and
Hermoise K. Mamay is gratefully acknowledged. I am also in-
debted to my colleagues, Gregory A. Dasch and A. Louis
Bourgeois, for stimulating discussions.

REFERENCES

1. Weiss, E., in "Rickettsiae and Rickettsial Diseases"
    (J. Kazar, R. A. Ormsbee, and I. N. Tarasevich, eds.),
    p. 137. VEDA, Bratislava (1978).
2. Winkler, H. H., and Miller, E. T., Infect. Immun. 29,
    316 (1980).
3. Winkler, H. H., and Miller, E. T., in "Rickettsiae and
    Rickettsial Diseases" (W. Burgdorfer, and R. L. Anacker,
    eds.), p. 327. Academic Press, New York (1981).
4. Weiss, E., Bacteriol. Rev. 37, 259 (1973).
5. Winkler, H. H., J. Biol. Chem. 251, 389 (1976).
6. Atkinson, W. H., and Winkler, H. H., in "Rickettsiae
    and Rickettsial Diseases" (W. Burgdorfer, and R. L.
    Anacker, eds.), p. 411. Academic Press, New York (1981).
7. Moulder, J. W., J. Infect. Dis. 130, 300 (1974).
8. Williams, J. C., and Weiss, E., J. Bact. 134, 884 (1978).
9. Zahorchak, R. J., and Winkler, H. H., in "Rickettsiae
    and Rickettsial Diseases" (W. Burgdorfer, and R. L.
    Anacker, eds.), p. 401. Academic Press, New York (1981).
10. Phibbs, P. V., and Winkler, H. H., Ibid., p. 421.
11. Buchanan, R. E., and Gibbons, N. E., eds., Bergey's
    Manual of Determinative Bacteriology, 8th ed. The
    Williams & Wilkins Company, Baltimore (1974).
12. Ristic, M., Vet. Parasitol. 2, 31 (1976).
13. Morrison, N. E., J. Bact. 89, 762 (1965).
14. Wheeler, W. C., and Hanks, J. H., J. Bact. 89, 889 (1965).
15. Dhople, A. M., and Hanks, J. H., Science 197, 379 (1977).
16. Hackstadt, T., and Williams, J. C., in "Rickettsiae and
    Rickettsial Diseases" (W. Burgdorfer, and R. L. Anacker,
    eds.), p. 431. Academic Press, New York (1981).
17. Paretsky, D., Zentralb. Bakteriol. Parasitenk. Infek-
    tionkr. Hyg. Abt. Orig. 206, 284 (1968).

18. Ormsbee, R. A., and Peacock, M. G., J. Bact. 88, 1205 (1964).
19. Donahue, J. P., and Thompson, H. A., in "Rickettsiae and Rickettsial Diseases" (W. Burgdorfer and R. L. Anacker, eds.), p. 441. Academic Press, New York (1981).
20. Gonzales, F., and Paretsky, D., Ibid., p. 493.
21. Paretsky, D., and Gonzales, F., Ibid., p. 453.
22. Williams, J. C., Ibid., p. 473.
23. Kuriger, W. E., and Schaad, N. W., Ibid., p. 483.
24. Wisseman, C. L., Jr., Ibid., p. 293.
25. Oaks, E. V., Wisseman, C. L., Jr., and Smith, J. F., Ibid., p. 461.
26. Hanson, B., and Wisseman, C. L., Jr., Ibid., p. 503.
27. Myers, W. F., and Wisseman, C. L., Jr., Int. J. Syst. Bact. 30, 143 (1980).
28. Brenner, D. J., Steigerwalt, A. G., Weaver, R. E., McDade, J. E., Feeley, J. C., and Mandel, M., Curr. Microbiol. 1, 71 (1978).
29. Brenner, D. J., Steigerwalt, A. G., Gorman, G. W., et al., Curr. Microbiol. 4, 111 (1980).
30. Hebert, G. A., Steigerwalt, A. G., and Brenner, D. J., Curr. Microbiol. 3, 225 (1980).
31. Baker, J. A., J. Exp. Med. 84, 37 (1946).
32. Vinson, J. W., and Fuller, H. S., Pathol. Microbiol. Suppl., 24, 152 (1961).
33. Weiss, E., Dasch, G. A., Woodman, D. R., and Williams, J. C., Infect. Immun. 19, 1013 (1978).
34. Merrell, B. R., Weiss, E., and Dasch, G. A., J. Bact. 135, 633 (1978).
35. Varela, G., Vinson, J. W., and Molina-Pasquel, C., Amer. J. Trop. Med. Hyg. 18, 708 (1969).
36. Myers, W. F., Wisseman, C. L., Jr., Fiset, P., Oaks, E. V., and Smith, J. F., Infect. Immun. 26, 976 (1979).
37. Dasch, G. A., Samms, J. R., and Weiss, E., Infect. Immun. 19, 676 (1978).
38. Edberg, S. C., Melton, E., and Singer, J. M., J. Clin. Microbiol. 11, 22 (1980).
39. Eddy, B. P., J. Appl. Bact. 24, 27 (1961).
40. Paretsky, D. and Werkman, C. H., Arch. Biochem. Biophys. 14, 11 (1947).
41. Huang, K., J. Bact. 93, 853 (1967).
42. Weiss, E., Peacock, M. G., and Williams, J. C., Curr. Microbiol. 4, 1 (1980).
43. Coolbaugh, J. C., Progar, J. J., and Weiss, E., Infect. Immun. 14, 298 (1976).
44. Mallavia, L., and Paretsky, D., J. Bact. 86, 232 (1963).

HYDROLYSIS AND SYNTHESIS OF ATP
BY RICKETTSIA PROWAZEKII [1]

Robert J. Zahorchak[2]
Herbert H. Winkler

Department of Microbiology and Immunology
University of South Alabama College of Medicine
Mobile, Alabama

I. INTRODUCTION

The coupling of the energy released during the catabolism of various compounds to the synthesis of ATP appears to be a general biologic phenomenon. An organism unable to synthesize ATP would be dependent upon both an environment from which to obtain the compound and a mechanism by which to transport it into the cytoplasm. Rickettsia prowazekii, like other species in its genus, are obligate intracellular parasites. Assessments of the ability of rickettsiae to synthesize ATP have been made in order to determine whether these organisms are essentially energy parasites and whether this characteristic accounts in part for their requirement for the host cell. Although the evidence clearly demonstrates that rickettsiae do possess the endogenous capability to synthesize ATP at the expense of glutamate oxidation (1,2,3), detailed analyses of the components involved in this process in these bacteria are lacking.

ATP may be synthesized via the action of a variety of cytoplasmic kinases in a process known as substrate level phosphorylation. These reactions require ADP, a phosphate donor, the appropriate kinase and Mg^{+2} but do not require

[1]Supported by NIH grant AI-15035.
[2]Supported by National Research Service award 3 F32 AI 05991-105.

the presence of a unit membrane. Alternatively, ATP may be
synthesized in conjunction with the oxidation of various
compounds (NADH, succinate, etc.). In addition to a complex
system of cytochromes, quinones, flavoproteins, non-heme
iron sulfur proteins, and a proton-impermeable membrane,
this process, known as oxidative phosphorylation, requires a
multiunit membrane-bound ATP phosphohydrolase (4).

The observation that the ATP synthetic capability of R.
prowazekii (1) and R. typhi (2) is drastically reduced by
uncouplers and inhibitors of respiration suggest that
oxidative phosphorylation accounts for the majority of the
ATP synthesized in these bacteria. Logically then, it would
be expected that rickettsiae possess an electron transport
system, a proton impermeable membrane, and a membrane-bound
ATPase.

There is one report of the detection of cytochromes in
R. typhi (mooseri) (5). No information is available
concerning the permeability of the rickettsial cytoplasmic
membrane to protons. ATP hydrolytic activity has been
observed by Williams (6) in R. typhi but there was no
examination of its relationship to energy transduction in
this study. Smith and Winkler (7) have demonstrated that
exogenous ATP can "energize" lysine transport in R.
prowazekii by a mechanism sensitive to dinitrophenol. These
results were interpreted as meaning that lysine transport
was linked to a proton-motive-force (PMF). The PMF could be
maintained either by electron transport or by ATP
hydrolysis. In rickettsiae exogenous ATP could serve as a
substrate for an internally oriented ATPase because these
organisms have an ATP/ADP transport system (8). Exogenously
supplied ATP also appears to be capable of energizing
rickettsial hemolysis (9). Although these observations
strongly indicate the presence of a membrane-bound ATPase in
rickettsiae, there has been no published study demonstrating
a functional, i.e. energy coupling ATPase in rickettsiae. In
this report we describe the effects of
dicyclohexylcarbodiimide on rickettsial ATPase, ATP
synthesis, and on processes energized by exogenous ATP.

II. MATERIALS AND METHODS

Rickettsia prowazekii, Madrid E strain, was cultivated
and purified as previously described (8). All assays were
performed in Buffer A(7), pH7.0 at $34^{\circ}C$.

ATPase activity was determined by monitoring the release
of radioactive phosphate from [γ -^{32}P]ATP. [γ -^{32}P] ATP was

enzymatically synthesized according to the method of Glynn
and Chappell (10). Rickettsial cells were incubated in
buffer containing 4 mM [γ -^{32}P]ATP (10^6cpm/ml). At ten
minute intervals 0.15 ml aliquots were removed and the
reaction was stopped with 7% PCA. Each aliquot was reacted
with 1.0 ml of 1.25% (NH$_4$)Mo$_7$4H$_2$O in 1 N HCl and extracted
with 500 μl isobutanol:benzene:acetone (3:3:1). The amount
of ^{32}P in the extract, representing the inorganic phosphate
released, was determined by liquid scintillation counting.
Corrections were made for rickettsial independent release of
inorganic phosphate from ATP.

Previously described methods were employed to monitor
ATP transport (8), lysine transport (7) and hemolytic
activity (9).

ATP synthesis was monitored by determining the
incorporation of ^{32}PO$_4$ into ATP. Rickettsiae (1.6 mg/ml)
were incubated in buffer A containing 5 mM ADP and ^{32}PO$_4$ (2
x 10^7cpm/ml). Aliquots of 150 μl were removed and the
reaction was stopped with 7% PCA. After neutralization with
KOH/KHCO$_3$ samples were chromatographed on PEI in the
discontinuous formate system described by Randerath and
Randerath (11). The ATP spot was cut out and the
radioactivity was determined by liquid scintillation
counting.

Oxygen consumption was monitored at 34°C with a YSI
Model 53 Oxygen Monitor (Yellow Springs Instrument Co.,
Yellow Springs, Ohio, 45387). Protein was determined by the
modified Lowry method described by Markwell et al. (12)
after precipitation with 7% trichloroacetic acid.

III. RESULTS

When whole cells of R. prowazekii were incubated with
ATP the nucleotide was cleaved to ADP and inorganic
phosphate at a rate of about 30 nmoles/min/mg protein (Table
1). Dicyclohexylcarbodiimide (DCCD) is an inhibitor of
membrane-bound ATPase in bacterial, mitochondrial, and
chloroplast systems. ATP hydrolysis by R. prowazekii cells
was inhibited by DCCD. (Table 1).

In order to determine whether or not ATP hydrolysis
occurred within the rickettsial cell, rickettsiae were
loaded with ATP labeled with tritium at the 2 and 8
positions in the adenine moiety and with ^{32}P in the gamma
phosphate position. Both tracers were internalized with
similar kinetics indicating that the molecule was
transported intact (data not shown). After exogenous

nucleotide was removed the fate of the two tracers was
followed (Table 2). Tritium remained associated with the
cells with little loss to the medium as expected due to the
obligatory exchange nature of the ATP/ADP transporter.
Throughout the experiment most (>60%) of the cell associated
^{32}P was organic in nature. In contrast to the slow rate of
loss of the tritium tracer, ^{32}P was rapidly released from
the cell and appeared in the surrounding medium as inorganic
phosphate.

TABLE 1.   DCCD Inhibition of Rickettsial ATPase

DCCD (mM)	ATPase (mIU/mg protein)	% Inhibition
0	34.9, 32.2, 30.5, 29.7	0
0.002	16.5	35
0.02	15.2	49
0.2	8.5	72
2.0	5.2, 11.9, 11.0	82, 66, 63
20	7.3	75

TABLE 2.   Release of Terminal Phosphate from ATP Internalized by R. prowazekii.[a]

Time	% of label remaining associated with rickettsial cells	
	^{3}H	^{32}P
-10	(100)	(100)
2	86	86
10	91	73
20	86	56
30	85	46
45	86	33
60	81	24
90	75	11

[a]Rickettsiae were loaded with ATP by incubation for 10 min
at 34°C in buffer A containing 40μM ATP, [^{3}H]ATP (1.2 x 10^6
cpm/ml, [γ-^{32}P]ATP (5.7 x 10^5 cpm/ml). Cells were washed
and resuspended (zero time) at a density of approximately
0.5 mg protein/ml. Cell associated radioactivity was
determined by filtration.

TABLE 3.   DCCD Inhibition of ATP Driven Lysine Uptake in
R. prowazekii.

Treatment	Lysine uptake (5 min) (pmoles lysine/mg protein)
Control	648
1mM KCN	88
+mM KCN + 1mM ATP	512
+200μM DCCD + 1mM ATP	488
+200μM DCCD + 1mM ATP + 1mM KCN	144

The fact that ATP hydrolysis could support energy
dependent processes was determined by assessing the effect
of DCCD on ATP driven lysine uptake and ATP driven
hemolysis. As previously reported by Smith and Winkler (7),
R. prowazekii could transport and accumulate lysine (Table
3). 1 mM KCN inhibited lysine uptake. The addition of 1 mM
ATP to cyanide poisoned cells restored uptake to the levels
observed in control cells. Lysine uptake in the presence of
1 mM ATP and 200 uM DCCD was determined. Uptake under these
conditions was unaffected if no KCN was present. However, if
KCN was present lysine uptake was inhibited. Thus, it is
clear that, in cells that are unable to respire, DCCD
inhibits ATP-dependent lysine uptake. Similar results were
obtained when examining the effect of DCCD on ATP driven
hemolysis (data not shown). These results indicate that the
inhibition of ATP hydrolysis prevents the ability of ATP to
support certain energy dependent processes in rickettsiae
and strongly implicates the involvement of a membrane-bound
ATPase.
      In addition to the involvement of a membrane-bound
ATPase in ATP hydrolysis, a very important function of the
enzyme is the catalysis of ATP synthesis. Table 4 shows the
incorporation of ^{32}P labelled inorganic phosphate into ATP
by cells of R. prowazekii. ATP synthesis is inhibited by the
ATPase inhibitor, DCCD, as well as KCN, an inhibitor of
respiration, and AsO_2 and inhibitor of α-keto-glutarate
dehydrogenase. This suggests that, in addition to glutamate
catabolism and respiration, ATPase activity is necessary in
the coupling of energy to ATP synthesis in R. prowazekii.

We have evaluated the efficiency of ATP synthesis
coupled to respiration in R. prowazekii. The rickettsial
cells at various concentrations were incubated with 5 mM ADP
and 10 mM phosphate containing $^{32}PO_4$ as a tracer. The
incorporation of inorganic phosphate into ATP was determined
as well as the amount of O_2 consumed. Table 5 shows the
calculated P:O ratios to be in the vicinity of 1.3.

TABLE 4. Effect of Various Inhibitors on the Synthesis
of ATP by R. prowazekii.

Treatment	Net ATP synthesized (nmoles ATP/mg rickettsial protein/30 min)
Control	60
1mM KCN	0
100μM NaAsO$_2$	0
50μM DCCD	2

TABLE 5. Efficiency of Oxidative Phosphorylation in
R. prowazekii.

Rickettsial protein (mg)	Time (min)	P$_i$ incorporated into ATP (nmoles)	O consumed (nmoles)	P:O
0.11	15	75	58	1.30
0.21	15	161	140	1.15
	45	249	306	0.81
0.07	15	115	87	1.33
	30	195	162	1.20
0.04	15	26	14	1.83

IV. DISCUSSION

The results presented in this report demonstrate the
involvement of a membrane-bound ATPase in various energy
coupling processes in R. prowazekii. DCCD prevented both
ATP-driven lysine uptake and ATP synthesis. Both processes
therefore most likely involve a membrane-bound ATPase.

The membrane-bound ATPase is a key enzyme in many
bacterial systems. The enzyme can function to couple
respiration to ATP synthesis as well as coupling ATP
hydrolysis to the transport of various compounds (4). The
results presented here indicate that rickettsiae are not
unlike free-living bacteria with respect to possessing an
energy-transducing ATPase. One might wonder what advantage
this capability would provide, since these organisms are
able to transport ATP and reside predominantly in an
environment where they are bathed in this important
metabolite. Three possible advantages quickly come to mind.
Firstly, it must be remembered that rickettsiae must for
some amount of time be able to survive outside the host
cell, e.g. the time to transit from the previously infected
and destroyed cell to a new host cell. Indeed, Williams and
Weiss (2) observed a drastic decrease in the adenylate
energy change in R. typhi in vitro if no glutamate was
available. It may be an advantage to the rickettsiae to be
able to maintain a high adenylate energy charge during this
time. The coupling of glutamate oxidation to ATP synthesis
via an ATPase could accomplish the maintenance of a high
energy change. Secondly, a similar type of advantage would
be offered if the host cell energy charge were affected by
the invasion and growth of the rickettsiae. It has been
pointed out that the obligatory exchange nature of the
ADP/ATP porter would tend to equalize the rickettsial and
host cell adenylate energy charges (8). If the host cell
energy charge was adversely affected by the infection, a
rickettsial oxidative phosphorylation system may aid in
maintaining the rickettsial energy charge. Thirdly. a
membrane-bound energy-coupling ATPase could function to
couple the energy released upon ATP hydrolysis to the
transport of a variety of metabolites. This may be an
important advantage for the rickettsiae in competing with
the host cell for certain metabolites. The demonstration of
such coupling in vitro to lysine transport certainly makes
this possibility appealing.
     The following model is consistent with results presented
here and elsewhere, and can be used to describe the
interactions of ATPase with other processes in the
rickettsial cell. Glutamate enters the cell and is
catabolized by the TCA cycle which results in the production
of NADH. This can then serve as a substrate for electron
transport which generates a proton motive force that can
drive lysine transport, hemolysis, and ATP synthesis. DCCD
prevents ATP synthesis by its interaction with the ATPase.
If glutamate is removed, or its catabolism is prevented by
inhibitors such as arsenite, or if electron transport is

inhibited by CN, no PMF is generated. Therefore, no lysine can be transported, no hemolysis occurs, and no ATP is synthesized. However, in the absence of glutamate catabolism and/or respiration, exogenous ATP can support the two former processes by entering the cells in exchange for an endogenous nucleotide and, upon hydrolysis by the ATPase, a PMF can be generated which could then serve to drive lysine uptake or hemolysis. Again the generation of a PMF via the ATPase is inhibited by DCCD.

The efficiency of ATP synthesis was determined to be in the range of 1.3. These values are much higher than the P:O ratio of 0.3 reported by Bovarnick (1). The differences may be explained by the fact that we have used only fresh, unfrozen rickettsiae, whereas the previously mentioned study routinely employed frozen rickettsiae.

V. SUMMARY

1. R. prowazekii hydrolize exogenously supplied ATP with the subsequent release of inorganic phosphate from the cell.
2. ATP hydrolysis by rickettsiae is inhibited by DCCD.
3. Energy dependent processes (lysine transport, hemolysis) are also inhibited by DCCD when exogenous ATP is the energy supply.
4. ATP synthesis is inhibited by arsenite, cyanide, or DCCD.
5. All the above support the conclusion that rickettsiae contain a classical membrane-bound, energy-transducing ATPase that couples respiration to ATP synthesis.

REFERENCES

1. Bovarnick, M.R. J. Biol. Chem. 220:353(1956).
2. Williams, J.C. and Weiss, E. J. Bacteriol. 134:884(1978).
3. Williams, J.C., Peterson, J.C., and Coolbaugh, J.C.,in "Rickettsiae and Rickettsial Diseases" (Kazar, J., Ormsbee, R.Z., and Tarasevich, I.N. ed.), p. 99, VEDA, Bratislava(1978).
4. Harold, F.M. Bacteriol. Rev. 36:172(1972).
5. Hayes, J.E., Hahn, F.E., Cohn, Z.A., Jackson, E.B., and Smadel, J.E. Biochim. Biophys. Acta 26:570(1957).
6. Williams, J.C. Infect. Immunity 28:74(1980).
7. Smith, D.K. and Winkler, H.H. J. Bacteriol. 29:1349(1977).

8. Winkler, H.H. J. Biol. Chem. 251:389(1976).
9. Winkler, H.H. Infect. Immunity 9:119(1974).
10. Glynn, I.M. and Chappell, J.B. Biochem. J.
    90:147(1964).
11. Randerath, K., and Randerath, E., Methods Enzymol
    12:323(1967).
12. Markwell, M.A.K., Haas, S.M., Bieber, L.L., and
    Tolbert, N.E. Anal. Biochem. 87:206(1978).

A CENTRIFUGAL FILTRATION METHOD FOR THE STUDY OF TRANSPORT OF NICOTINAMIDE-ADENINE DINUCLEOTIDE AND PYRUVATE BY RICKETTSIA PROWAZEKI[1]

William H. Atkinson
Herbert H. Winkler

Department of Microbiology and Immunology
University of South Alabama College of Medicine
Mobile, Alabama

I. INTRODUCTION

The nature of the obligate intracellular existence of
Rickettsia prowazeki remains a mystery. The availability of
specific metabolic compounds may be one of the factors
limiting the successful cultivation of these organisms in a
defined medium. Rickettsial suspensions do not metabolize
glucose but do exhibit metabolic activity in the presence
of glutamate (1). The list of substances taken up and
utilized by rickettsiae is growing but there are still
gaps. Metabolic activity supported by glutamate raises
questions about anaplerotic pathways in the tricarboxylic
acid cycle (TCA).
The pathways by which nicotinamide adenine dinucleotide
(NAD) is utilized by rickettsiae are not known. Bovarnick
and Allen described the reactivation of rickettsiae by NAD
following freezing and thawing in isotonic salt solution
(2). Inactivation was demonstrated by loss of infectivity
for eggs, hemolytic activity, and respiration. All of these
properties could be partially restored by incubation of
rickettsiae with NAD.
Metabolite transport by microorganisms is usually
determined by membrane filtration methods that remove cells

---

[1]Supported by NIH grant AI-15035.

from the radiolabeled compound in the incubation reaction
medium. This method is of limited value when measuring the
transport of substances that only equilibrate across the
cell membrane or are concentrated only slightly. Filtration
methodologies require a wash to remove extracellular
metabolite. However, washing of cells often leads to the
loss of accumulated substances. These problems can be
circumvented by using centrifugal filtration for separating
cells from incubation media. The extracellular adherent
media is removed as the cells are pelleted through a
nonaqueous phase. Analyses and applications of this method,
described by Werkheiser and Bartley (3), have been reviewed
(4). This paper describes the application of a centrifugal
filtration methodology for quantitating the uptake of NAD
and pyruvate by Rickettsia prowazeki. Utilization of NAD
and its catabolites is discussed.

II. METHODS

Rickettsia prowazeki was purified from infected yolk
sacs of embryonated chicken eggs as previously described
(5). Rickettsial uptake of NAD and pyruvate was determined
by a centrifugal filtration method modified from Werkheiser
and Bartley (3). Purified rickettsiae were placed in an
incubation mixture composed of SPG-Mg and the radiolabeled
substance being assayed for uptake. This procedure is
outlined in Figure 1. Following an incubation period, 55 μl
were layered onto the prepared 250 μl microcentrifuge tube.
The tube contained, from the bottom up, 25 μl of 14% $HClO_4$
aqueous solution, 100 μl dibutyl phthalate, 30 μl silicone
oil (Dow Corning 560 silicone fluid, density = 1.040 at
25°C) and finally 55 μl of rickettsial incubation mixture.
Triplicate tubes were prepared for each determination. The
microtubes were centrifuged at 11,000 x g for ten minutes
at 4°C. All incubations of rickettsiae with the
radiolabeled compound were at 25°C. Upon centrifugation the
rickettsiae entered the silicone oil and were stripped of
most of the extracellular incubation medium. As the cells
enter the acid layer at the bottom of the tube they are
lysed and all soluble constituents are extracted. Following
centrifugation, the tubes were frozen at -80°C. While still
frozen, the tube bottom containing the acid extract was
sliced off with a razor blade just above the acid-dibutyl
phthalate interface. The portion of the tube sliced off was
placed in a scintillation vial containing 5 ml of

scintillation fluid. The volumes of the intracellular,
periplasmic, and extracellular spaces were determined from
the distributions of ^3H_2O, [^{14}C]sucrose and [^{14}C]inulin. The
intracellular volume was calculated by subtracting the
sucrose space from the total water space of the pellet.
These spaces represent the periplasmic volume plus any
adherent media and total cell water, respectively. These
space determinations permit calculations of uptake by
assaying for the intracellular space occupied by any
radiolabeled substrate (4). Equilibrium with intracellular
constituents was indicated if a compound occupied a space
equal to the intracellular water. Substances that were not
transported into a cell did not have an intracellular
space. Those that were actively transported had
intracellular spaces greater than that of water. From these
values of intracellular space, the intracellular
concentration could be calculated.

A CENTRIFUGAL FILTRATION METHOD

FOR DETERMINING RICKETTSIAL MICROSPACE

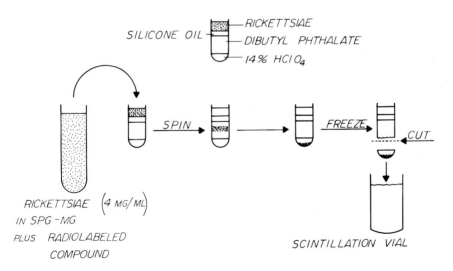

Fig. 1. A centrifugal filtration method for determining
rickettsial microspaces.

The composition of the cell extracts and the incubation medium was determined by polyethyleneimine-cellulose thin layer chromatography. NAD and adenylate standards were chromatographed with the samples. Thin-layer plates were developed in 0.5 M LiCl using the system described by Randerath and Randerath (6). Identification of unknowns was based on co-migration with known standards. Confirmation of the identity of these compounds was achieved by enzymatic conversion to some other product which also co-chromatographed with standards. Cell extracts were prepared by centrifuging 100 μl of rickettsiae in incubation medium through silicone oil. The resulting cell pellet was added to 400 μl of 65% ethanol. This was vortexed and freeze-thawed twice. This extract was centrifuged at 11,000 x g for 15 minutes to remove residual silicone oil and cell remnants. The supernatant fraction was collected and concentrated to 25 μl by vacuum evaporation. Twenty μl of this cell extract was spotted onto the thin-layer plates. Incubation medium was spotted directly onto the plates. All samples had standards included so that after chromatography, the R_f values could be ascertained. Standards were visualized under short wave ultraviolet light, marked with a soft lead pencil and scraped into scintillation vials containing 10 ml of scintillation fluid.

Pyruvate metabolism was determined by incubating rickettsiae in SPG-Mg containing either [1-^{14}C]pyruvate or [2-^{14}C]pyruvate in a flask containing a center cup. The center cup contained a CO_2 trap consisting of a filter paper strip saturated with Hyamine hydrochloride. The incubation was terminated by injecting 0.25 ml of 30% HClO$_4$ into the flask with a syringe. The apparatus was further incubated for 30 minutes at 37^{0}C. After this period of time, the center cup was removed and placed into a scintillation vial containing 10 ml of scintillation fluid. Controls consisted of a similar treatment but with no rickettsiae added to the flask.

III. RESULTS

Initial uptake studies utilizing centrifugal filtration methodology demonstrated that when rickettsiae were incubated with [^{32}P] or [^{3}H] NAD (labeled in the adenosine monophosphate (AMP) moiety), radioactivity appeared intracellularly and increased as a function of incubation time. When these cells were extracted, the intracellular radioactivity was distributed in both NAD and adenine nucleotide pools. The radioactivity associated with the adenine nucleotides was primarily present as AMP. Cell-free incubation media and cell extracts were prepared for chromatographic analysis at varying times after addition of rickettsiae to radiolabeled NAD. Both the incubation media and the cell extracts contained radiolabeled compounds in addition to the original NAD. This conversion was not observed in controls without rickettsiae. The rickettsiae acted upon the NAD in such a way that, as NAD was consumed, adenylates appeared. Intracellular levels of both NAD and adenylates continued to accumulate throughout a 60 minute period. When excess unlabeled AMP was included in the incubation mixture along with NAD, the appearance of labeled AMP in both cell extracts and media was inhibited by at least 30%. Under these conditions the radioactivity associated with the cells was largely found as NAD. The excess AMP may interfere with the enzymatic conversion of NAD to AMP but the site of this inhibition has not been determined.

Preliminary studies have indicated that R. prowazeki can transport and metabolize pyruvate. Pyruvate has been shown to prevent the loss of activity of rickettsiae that were starved for glutamate (7). The oxidation of pyruvate by rickettsiae was demonstrated by Bovarnick and Miller (8). Our data taken from both uptake and CO_2 production studies suggest that metabolism occurs via a decarboxylation step which is probably mediated by a pyruvate dehydrogenase complex. This enzymatic activity has been demonstrated (see Phibbs and Winkler, this volume). The apparent uptake of $[2-^{14}C]$pyruvate was greater than that of $[1-^{14}C]$pyruvate when measured by centrifugal filtration. In metabolic assays the amount of CO_2 produced by rickettsiae was greater with $[1-^{14}C]$ pyruvate than with $[2-^{14}C]$pyruvate. The uptake and metabolism of pyruvate by rickettsiae may represent the source of anaplerotic carbons required for a TCA cycle functioning with glutamate as carbon source.

IV. DISCUSSION

The centrifugal filtration method for separating rickettsiae from incubation mixtures is useful when assaying for the uptake of compounds that are only slightly accumulated. The advantages of this method over membrane filtration methods is that no washing of the cells is

required to remove extracellular media. By pelleting
rickettsiae through a nonaqueous phase, most of the
adherent media is striped away. This type of separation
procedure is useful when intracellular substrates are
easily washed out and the membrane filtration procedures
are of little use. By selecting proper isotopes, the total
cell water space, periplasmic space, and extracellular
space can be calculated. By correcting for periplasmic and
adherent volumes, the correct intracellular or cytoplasmic
space can be determined. These studies showed that R.
prowazeki has an intracellular volume of approximately
3μl/mg of cell protein. This space represents about 45% of
the total water brought down with the cells. By comparing
the space occupied by any given radiolabeled compound with
that of sucrose and water, the degree of accumulation can
be calculated. Spaces can be determined in the system
described, using less than 200 μg of rickettsial protein
per microcentrifuge tube. This method requires much less
rickettsiae and is easier to use than the micro-space
method in capillary tubes (9). Disadvantages of this system
are that incubation times of less than one minute are not
possible. Therefore, kinetic studies of compounds that are
rapidly accumulated are not possible.

The results described suggest that R. prowazeki
accumulates both NAD and AMP when exposed to media
containing NAD. AMP appears in the incubation medium
rapidly after addition of rickettsiae. Two of our working
hypotheses for the accumulation of radioactivity from NAD
are shown in Figure 2. Both models are consistent with our
preliminary results. Model 1 shows the transport of NAD
into the cell followed by an intracellular enzymatic
cleavage yielding AMP. Some of this AMP moves out of the
cell and back into the medium. Model 2 differs both in the
site of enzymatic activity and in the origin of
intracellular AMP. In this model, NAD is cleaved both
outside the cell proper and inside, thus giving rise to AMP
both extracellularly and intracellularly. Williams has
shown that extracellular AMP can be transported by R. typhi
(10). Our studies showed that R. prowazeki also accumulates
AMP.

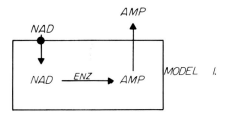

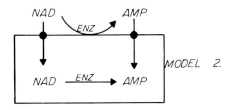

Fig. 2. Working hypotheses for uptake and enzymatic
hydrolysis of NAD by rickettsiae.

The mechanism by which NAD causes reactivation of
rickettsiae (2) is not known. The studies presented here
demonstrate that rickettsiae take up NAD and also hydrolyse
it, forming adenine nucleotides and presumably some
nicotinamide containing byproduct. These results are
preliminary observations and we are currently investigating
the nature and cellular location of the enzyme that
hydrolyses NAD and the fate of the nicotinamide portion of
the NAD molecules that are cleaved.

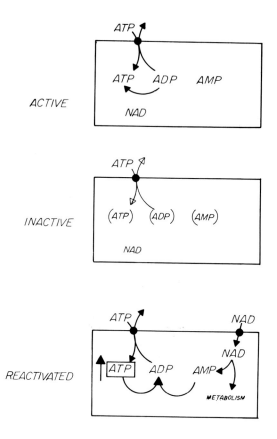

Fig. 3. A possible scheme for the reactivation of
rickettsiae by NAD.

    One scheme by which NAD may reactivate rickettsiae is
depicted in Figure 3. Active rickettsiae (top) have
adequate intracellular levels of ATP and NAD and possess a
high energy charge. Inactive rickettsiae (middle) have low
levels of adenylates and NAD, and have a low energy charge.
Williams discussed the lack of degradative pathways in R.
typhi for AMP (10). The adenylate energy charge falls as
ATP and ADP are dephosphorylated to AMP. This AMP increases
because there are no degradative pathways. Inactive
rickettsiae may have low total adenylate levels because of

loss of adenylates from the cell. NAD levels could also
fall as a result of diffusion from the cell. Reactivation
of rickettsiae by NAD (bottom) may result from the
accumulation of both NAD and AMP derived from it. The
intracellular NAD could be utilized in oxidative metabolism
and the AMP might aid in the regeneration of an adequate
energy charge if extracellular ATP were available. In this
reactivation scheme, AMP could react with ATP via adenylate
kinase and generate ADP. The enhanced levels of ADP could
then serve to promote the uptake of extracellular ATP.
Rickettsiae possess an ADP-ATP exchange transport system
(11). This system does not function to increase the total
adenylate pool, but if cellular levels of ATP are
depressed, it will exchange intracellular ADP for
extracellular ATP. The resulting intracellular increase in
ATP would reestablish a high energy charge which may
account for the reactivation phenomena observed by
Bovarnick.

V. SUMMARY

A centrifugal filtration method for determining
rickettsial metabolite transport is described. This method
was used to demonstrate the uptake of NAD and pyruvate by
Rickettsia prowazeki. Rickettsiae hydrolyse NAD and
accumulate both NAD and the hydrolytic product AMP. The
role of NAD in rickettsial reactivation is discussed.

REFERENCES

1. Bovarnick, M.R., and Snyder, J.C., J. Exp. Med.
   89:561(1949).
2. Bovarnick, M.R., and Allen, E.G., J. Gen. Physiol.
   38:169 (1954).
3. Werkheiser, W.C., and Bartley, W., Biochem. J.
   66:79(1957).
4. Palmieri, F., and Klingenberg, M., Methods Enzymol.
   56:279(1979).
5. Winkler, H.H., and Miller, E.T., Infect. Immun.
   29:316(1980).
6. Randerath, K., and Randerath, E., Methods Enzymol.
   12:323(1967).
7. Bovarnick, M.R., and Allen, E.G., J. Bacteriol.
   74:637(1957).

8. Bovarnick, M.R., and Miller, J.C., *J. Biol. Chem.*
184:661(1950).
9. Winkler, H.H., *Appl. Environ. Microbiol.* 31:146(1976).
10. Williams, J.C., *Infect. Immun.* 28:74(1980).
11. Winkler, H.H., *J. Biol. Chem.* 251:389(1976).

REGULATORY PROPERTIES OF PARTIALLY PURIFIED
ENZYMES OF THE TRICARBOXYLIC ACID CYCLE OF
RICKETTSIA PROWAZEKII

Paul V. Phibbs, Jr.[1]
Herbert H. Winkler[2]

Department of Microbiology and Immunology
College of Medicine
University of South Alabama
Mobile, Alabama

I. INTRODUCTION

There has been considerable experimental evidence that
purified cells of species of Rickettsia respire CO_2 from exogenously supplied glutamate, presumably through the action of
an oxidative tricarboxylic acid (TCA) cycle (1-3). Coolbaugh,
Progar and Weiss (4) have demonstrated the presence of selected
TCA cycle and peripherally associated enzyme activities in
crude, cell-free extracts of Rickettsia typhi using direct enzyme assay techniques. These extracts were shown to contain
citrate synthase, first enzyme unique to the pathway, and several other activities, but neither pyruvate dehydrogenase nor
2-oxoglutarate dehydrogenase complex activities were mentioned.
However, uniformly negative results were obtained in assays for
several glycolytic/gluconeogenic enzymes of the Embden-Meyerhof
pathway (4).
    Rickettsiae are known to contain an ADP-ATP transport sys-
tem that allows these obligate intracellular bacteria to

[1]Present address: Department of Microbiology, Medical
College of Virginia, Virginia Commonwealth University,
Richmond, Virginia 23298.
[2]Research supported by NIAID grant AI 15035.

accumulate ATP from their environment via exchange with intra-
rickettsial ADP (5).   These bacteria also are believed capable
of generating ATP during glutamate oxidation, but the biochemical mechanisms for coupling of ATP formation to oxidative metabolism have not been described (reviewed in reference 2).   More
recently, Williams and Weiss (6) described the effects of exogenously provided glutamate and adenine nucleotides on the
endogenous adenylate pools (energy charge) in suspensions of
purified R. typhi.   Little additional information has been published on the regulation of metabolism in rickettsiae and no
efforts have been made to purify key enzymes or to characterize their catalytic regulatory properties.

     In this report, we provide evidence for the presence of
pyruvate dehydrogenase and 2-oxoglutarate dehydrogenase complex activities in cell extracts of purified R. prowazekii and
describe procedures for the partial purification of citrate
synthase, malate dehydrogenase (MDH), and pyruvate dehydrogenase complex (PDHC).   Moreover, some catalytic regulatory properties of partially purified citrate synthase and PDHC from
R. prowazekii are described for the first time.

II.   MATERIALS AND METHODS

     R. prowazekii, Madrid E strain, was propagated and purified
as described previously (5).   The resultant bacterial suspension was passed through type AP20 glass filters (7) and was
further purified by Renografin density gradient centrifugation
according to a variation (8) of the method of Weiss et al. (7).
These suspensions contained undetectable or insignificant
traces of contaminating yolk sac enzyme activities.

     Crude extracts were prepared by passing a suspension of
purified rickettsiae through a prechilled miniature French
pressure cell twice.   The soluble cytoplasmic fraction, containing all enzyme activities described in tis study, was obtained by centrifuging crude extract at 105,000 x g for 2 hr.
The supernatant fluid was concentrated and used immediately or
stored overnight at -70°C, with little loss of enzyme activities.   In a typical experiment, approximately 1 gram (wet wt.)
of purified rickettsiae in 11.2 ml of suspension yielded 9.5 ml
crude extract (76 mg protein); this resulted in 2.3 ml of
final concentrated soluble fraction containing 37 mg protein.

     Concentrated soluble fractions were applied to a column of
Sephacryl S-200 (Pharmacia) and fractions were assayed immediately for protein (A_{280}), citrate synthase and MDH activities.   Fractions containing enzyme activities were pooled, concentrated by ultrafiltration and stored overnight.   Citrate

synthase and MDH were separated and further purified by Immobilized Cibacron Blue F3GA chromatography (9).

PDHC activity was assayed by trapping $^{14}CO_2$ released from
[1-^{14}C]pyruvate (10) or by a direct spectrophotometric (340 nm)
method (11). A similar assay procedure was employed to assay
2-oxoglutarate dehydrogenase complex (ODHC) activity. Citrate
synthase activity was determined spectrophotometrically at 412
nm (12) and MDH was determined spectrophotometrically at 340 nm
(13). Previously described procedures were employed for protein determination (14,15).

III. RESULTS

A. Partial Purification of Enzyme Activities

Citrate synthase and MDH activities were separated from
approximately 90% of concentrated soluble fraction protein by
Sephacryl S-200 column chromatography, but eluted unresolved
from each other in markedly asymmetrical, multi-shouldered
peaks. Citrate synthase and MDH activities were purified by
3.6-fold (32% recovery) and 17-fold (105% recovery) respectively. PDHC activity applied to the column was recovered with
the voided protein. This enzyme activity was sedimented from
pooled fractions at 156,000 x g and stored at -70°C. The final
preparation contained 1.25 mg protein and PDHC activity was
purified by approximately 33-fold.

Complete separation and further purification of citrate
synthase and MDH by Cibacron Blue affinity chromatography is
shown in Figure 1. Most of the protein applied to the column
was eluted with the rinsing buffer (2.5 mM PEM). Citrate synthase eluted in a sharp, symmetrical peak when the buffer was
made to contain 0.35 M KCl. A major peak of MDH activity,
followed by several minor, trailing peaks, were eluted when the
KCl concentration was increased from 0.35 M to 0.75 M. The
sharp increase in A_{280} beginning in fraction 32 was due to the
elution of NADH that was added as indicated to the final, high-
salt buffer. Fractions 10-13 contained approximately 780 μg
protein, 81% of the applied enzyme activity, and no detectable
MDH. Fractions 20-36 contained 99% of the applied MDH activity.

Preparations of citrate synthase and MDH similar to those described above were chromatographed individually on a calibrated, 1.5 x 87 cm column of Sephacryl S-200. Partially purified (90-fold) citrate synthase activity eluted in one major, symmetrical peak with a relative molecular weight of about 65,000. Partially purified (∿200-fold) MDH activity eluted in a major peak, with a relative molecular weight of 55,000 to 60,000; however, several smaller peaks of activity with apparently lower molecular weights also were eluted.

B.   Pyruvate Dehydrogenase Complex Activity

Low specific activities of PDHC were detected in preliminary determinations with crude and soluble fraction extracts using the $^{14}CO_2$-release assay. These results were confirmed with the spectrophotometric assay, which was also employed to characterize further the activity present in partially purified preparations described above. Activity was dependent on extract, proportional to protein concentration, and the specific activity was 30 to 35-fold higher in the partially purified preparation. Activity was greatly reduced in the absence of cofactors (coenzyme A, thiamine-pyrophosphate, NAD) known to be required by this enzyme from other biological sources and was

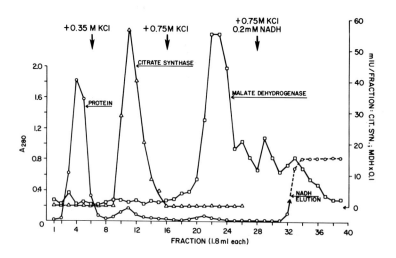

Fig. 1.   Resolution of citrate synthase and MDH by Cibacron Blue column chromatography. The 1.6 ml sample applied to the column (5 ml bed volume) contained 159 mIU citrate synthase and 2,840 mIU MDH. Proteins were eluted by step gradients of KCl in 2.5 mM PEM buffer (9) as indicated by arrows.

saturable with respect to pyruvate concentration (apparent
Km < 0.5 mM).

A more highly purified preparation of PDHC was employed
to examine NAD saturation kinetics and the effects of reduced
pyridine nucleotides on enzyme complex activity (Fig. 2). The
activity was saturable with respect to NAD concentration and
maximum velocity was achieved with >50 μM NAD. NADH caused a
powerful inhibition of enzyme activity, shown here as the
effect of the mole fraction of NAD (NAD/[NAD + NADH]) on reaction velocity when the sum of [NAD] + [NADH] was held constant
at 250 μM. Thus, when the mole fraction of NAD fell below 0.5,
activity was completely inhibited. NADP was an ineffective
substrate/co-factor for the enzyme complex, but NADPH appeared
to exert a modest inhibitory effect (Fig. 2). Modest inhibition (20-25%) also was observed in the presence of 100 μM
acetyl coenzyme A; but 5 mM adenylates (ATP, ADP, and AMP) had
little or no effect on reaction velocity when added individually or in combinations (results not shown).

C.   2-Oxoglutarate Dehydrogenase Complex Activity

Preliminary evidence for the presence of a sedimentable,
high molecular weight ODHC activity was obtained in these

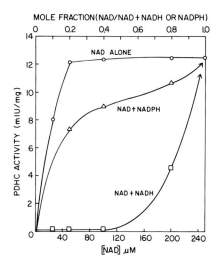

Fig. 2. NAD saturation kinetics and effects of the NAD
mole fraction on activity of partially purified PDHC from R.
prowazekii. The total pyridine nucleotide pool was constant
(250 μM) in determinations of the effects of NAD mole fraction
(i.e., at mole fraction of 0.5, both NAD and NADH were 125 μM).

studies (Table 1). Release of $^{14}CO_2$ from $[1-^{14}C]$2-osogluta-
rate was dependent on extract. Activity was diminished by 64%
and 79%, respectively, by deletion of the cofactors NAD and
coenzyme A; the undialyzed extract preparation employed in
these assays may contain trace amounts of these metabolites.
Curiously, the addition of unlabelled pyruvate (14.7-fold
higher than 2-oxoglutarate concentration) to the complete
reaction mixture caused a 76% loss in activity, presumably by
either competitive or non-competitive effects on the enzyme
complex. Low levels of PDHC activity (179 pmoles x min^{-1} x
mg^{-1}) also were present in the extract preparation and $^{14}CO_2$
release from $[1-^{14}C]$pyruvate was inhibited by 96% in the
presence of 14.7-fold excess unlabelled 2-oxoglutarate.

D. Some Characteristics of Citrate Synthase

Partially purified citrate synthase preparations exhibited
hyperbolic saturation curves for acetyl-CoA and oxalacetate
(OAA) from which apparent Km values of approximately 5-10 μM
for each substrate were estimated. The effects of metabolite
effectors (known to inhibit the enzyme from other bacteria;
see reference 16) on partially purified citrate synthase from
R. prowazekii are summarized in Table 2. Adenylates were
strongly inhibitory with sub-saturating concentrations of
acetyl-CoA, in the order ATP > ADP >> AMP, but appeared not to

TABLE 1. Evidence for 2-Oxoglutarate Dehydrogenase
Complex Activity in Extracts of R. prowazekii[a]

Reaction conditions[b]	$^{14}CO_2$/30 min (cpm)	pmoles/min mg protein
Complete control	14,732	415
delete extract	268	7
delete NAD	5,322	150
delete coenzyme A	3,086	87
add 5 mM ^{12}C-pyruvate	3,481	98

[a]Undialyzed resuspended 156,000 x g sediment of
soluble enzyme fraction of crude extract.

[b]$^{14}CO_2$-release assay (see METHODS) with 0.34 mM
$[1-^{14}C]$2-oxoglutarate (14,940 cpm/mmole) and 79 μg
extract protein.

be inhibitory when reaction rate was limited by sub-saturating concentrations of OAA. Neither NADH nor 2-oxoglutarate affected citrate synthase activity under the conditions described here.

IV. DISCUSSION

Conventional protein purification procedures were employed successfully for partial purification of catalytically active citrate synthase, MDH, and PDHC from large batches (0.5 to >1 gm wet weight) of Renografin-purified R. prowazekii. The resultant enzyme preparations made it possible to originate

TABLE 2.   Effects of Selected Metabolites on Activity of R. prowazekii Citrate Synthase[a]

Metabolite added (concn.)	Spec. Activity[b] (% of control)
Complete with 10 μM acetyl-CoA + 500 μM OAA	
no addition control	100
AMP (5 mM)	76
ADP (5 mM)	21
ATP (1 mM)	45
(5 mM)	19
NADH (0.25 mM)	94
2-oxoglutarate (1 mM)	100
Complete with 10 μM OAA + 50 μM Acetyl-CoA	
no addition control	100
ATP (1 mM)	98
NADH (0.25 mM)	103
2-oxoglutarate (2 mM)	100

[a]Standard spectrophotometric assay (12) was employed with partially purified (MDH-free) citrate synthase preparations (1-5 μg protein used/reaction).

[b]Results represent a composite of 3 separate experiments, using different batches of enzyme; thus, the actual control specific activities varied (0.41 to 0.55 IU/mg). Data are expressed as percent of appropriate control specific activity for greater clarity.

studies of the catalytic regulatory properties of these enzymes
for comparison with the known properties of enzymes from free-
living cells. Thus far, metabolic studies of these obligate
intracellular bacteria have been limited primarily to determination of the physiological activities of whole cell suspensions
and of enzyme activity in crude extracts of rickettsiae (1-7).
     Citrate synthases isolated from a large number of biologi-
cal sources have been classified as being of either the "large"
(MW $\sim$ 230,000) or "small" (MW $\sim$ 100,000) type, which correlates
highly with regulatory properties of these enzymes (16). The
relative molecular weight of citrate synthase from R. prowazekii (about 65,000), its hyperbolic saturation kinetics, and
its sensitivity to inhibition by adenylates (but not by NADH
or 2-oxoglutarate) are similar to properties of the "small"
type enzyme that is widely distributed among gram-positive
bacteria and most eukaryotic cells (16). With few exceptions,
gram-negative bacteria are reported to contain the "large" type
enzyme that is inhibited by NADH. To our knowledge, there have
been no previous studies of the enzyme from obligate intracellular bacteria.
     MDH from R. prowazekii was purified greater than 200-fold
in some preparations, but these still contained 4-7 polypeptide
bands when examined by sodium dodecylsulfate polyacrylamide
disc gel electrophoresis according to the method of Fairbanks
et al. (17). Most of the catalytically active MDH in these
preparations exhibited a relative molecular weight of 55,000-
60,000; but there appeared to be several other molecular forms
of active enzyme in these preparations, based on elution profiles in both exclusion and affinity chromatography. This was
consistent with the repeated observation of numerous catalytically active forms in disc gel electropherograms that were prepared and stained for activity according to methods nearly
identical to those employed by Coolbaugh et al. (4). Large
amounts of substrate-dependent activity remained atop (and
throughout) the 3% stacking gels and multiple bands appeared
in the resolving gels. We conclude that R. prowazekii MDH
exists in multiple active forms in cell-free extract that may
include large, complex aggregates of the predominant 55,000-
60,000 MW form. In contrast, MDH prepared from several representative free-living bacteria, by essentially the same purification procedure, appeared to exist entirely in monomeric or
dimeric forms (9).
     The demonstration of PDHC activity in extracts of R. prowa-
zekii provides original evidence that these bacteria are
capable of oxidizing pyruvate to acetyl-coenzyme A. Therefore,
rickettsiae may not be dependent on the eukaryotic host cell
for the continuous supply of acetyl-CoA that is essential for
a complete functional, oxidative TCA cycle. The partially
purified activity was similar to PDHC from other sources (18),

with respect to cofactor requirements and its apparent very
high molecular weight. Moreover, the enzyme complex exhibited
exquisite sensitivity to regulation by the oxidation/reduction
state of the NAD + NADH pool, such that activity rose most
steeply with the NAD mole fraction (NAD/[NAD + NADH]) at around
0.8. A similar regulatory property has been reported for the
PDHC in E. coli (11).

Glutamate presumably is converted to the intermediate 2-
oxoglutarate and oxidized completely to CO_2 via enzymes of the
TCA cycle in Rickettsia (1-4, 6); but there has been no direct
evidence that these bacteria contain the crucial 2-oxyglutarate
dehydrogenase complex. Preliminary results obtained in this
study provide evidence for a high molecular weight ODHC activity in extracts of R. prowazekii that was dependent on NAD and
coenzyme A, but the enzyme was not further characterized. The
possibility that pyruvate and 2-oxoglutarate may be substrates
for the same dehydrogenase complex should be explored.

V. SUMMARY

These results demonstrate the feasibility of obtaining partially purified preparations of rickettsial enzymes that are
suitable for use in studies of their catalytic regulatory properties. Evidence was obtained in this study that the activity
of PDHC and citrate synthase (two essential enzymes of a complete oxidative TCA cycle) are highly modulated by metabolites
that reflect cellular energy economy, but not by metabolites
that are indicators of carbon skeleton economy. Therefore, it
is plausible to suggest that metabolic flux through the TCA
cycle may be minimal when R. prowazekii is in an ATP-rich environment, such as host cell cytoplasm. When cells are de-
prived of abundant exogenous ATP (i.e., outside the healthy
host cell), inhibition of TCA cycle function should be re-
lieved, allowing increased rates of glutamate oxidation and
subsequent endogenous generation of reducing power and ATP required for the maintenance of cellular proton motive force and
viability. Continued study of the biochemical regulatory properties of these bacteria may provide a better understanding
of the molecular basis for their obligatory existence as intracellular parasites.

REFERENCES

1. Bovarnick, M. R., and Snyder, J. C., J. Exp. Med. 89, 561 (1949).
2. Weiss, E., Bacteriol. Rev. 37, 259 (1973).
3. Wisseman, C. L., Jr., Hahn, F. E., Jackson, E. B., Bozeman, F. M., and Smadel, J. E., J. Immunol. 68, 251 (1952).
4. Coolbaugh, J. C., Progar, J. J., and Weiss, E., Infect. Immun. 14, 298 (1976).
5. Winkler, H. H., J. Biol. Chem. 251, 389 (1976).
6. Williams, J. C., and Weiss, E., J. Bacteriol. 134, 884 (1978).
7. Weiss, E., Coolbaugh, J. C., and Williams, J. C., Appl. Microbiol. 30, 456 (1975).
8. Smith, D. K., and Winkler, H. H., J. Bacteriol. 137, 963 (1979).
9. Kay, W. W., and Down, J. A., Current Microbiol. 1, 293 ((1978).
10. Chulavatnatol, M., and Atkinson, D. E., J. Biol. Chem. 248, 2716 (1973).
11. Shen, L. C., and Atkinson, D, E., J. Biol. Chem. 245, 5974 (1970).
12. Srere, P. A., in "Methods in Enzymology" (J. M. Lowenstein, ed.), Vol. XIII, p. 3. Academic Press, New York (1969).
13. Reeves, H. C., Rabin, R., Wegener, W. S., and Ajl, S. J., in "Methods in Microbiology" (J. R. Norris and D. W. Ribbons, eds.), Vol. 6A, p. 435. Academic Press, New York (1971).
14. Kalb, V. F., Jr., and Bernlohr, R. W., Anal. Biochem. 82, 362 (1977).
15. Lowry, O. H., Rosebrough, N. J., Farr, A. L., and Randall, R. J., J. Biol. Chem. 193, 265 (1951).
16. Weitzman, P.D.J., and Danson, M. J., in "Current Topics in Cellular Regulation" (B. L. Horecker and E. R. Stadtman, eds.), Vol. 10, p. 161, Academic Press, New York (1976).
17. Fairbanks, G., Steck, T. L., and Wallach, D.F.H., Biochemistry 10, 1606 (1971).
18. Reed, L. F., and Willms, C. R., in "Methods in Enzymology" (W. A. Wood, ed.), Vol. IX, p. 247. Academic Press, New York (1969).

INCORPORATION OF MACROMOLECULAR PRECURSORS BY COXIELLA BURNETII IN AN AXENIC MEDIUM

Ted Hackstadt
Jim C. Williams

Laboratory of Microbial Structure and Function
Rocky Mountain Laboratories
Hamilton, Montana

I. INTRODUCTION

Coxiella burnetii differs in many respects from other members of the family Rickettsiales. Unlike members of the genus Rickettsia, which replicate primarily within the cytoplasm of eukaryotic cells, C. burnetii progresses through its entire developmental cycle within phagolysosomes (1, 2). C. burnetii is also unique among Gram-negative intracellular parasites in that its developmental cycle includes a sequence comparable to endospore formation (3, McCaul and Williams, submitted). The intracellular environment in which C. burnetii replicates is considered a hostile environment to most bacteria due to the hydrolytic enzymes (4), low pH (5), and other microbicidal mechanisms (6). Until recently, the metabolic capabilities of C. burnetii in the extracellular environment have been considered minimal (7, 8, 9). This is despite the demonstration of a number of enzymes of key metabolic sequences in cell-free extracts of this organism (9, 10). We have recently demonstrated, however, that the transport, catabolism, and incorporation of both glutamate and glucose by C. burnetii are highly stimulated under hydrogen ion concentrations reflective of the intraphagosomal space (11). Here we present evidence that purine and pyrimidine nucleosides are both catabolized and/or incorporated better at acidic pH than at neutrality. Thus, it appears that both deoxyribonucleic acid and ribonucleic acid are synthesized by C. burnetii at pH 4.5 in the presence of an energy source.

II. MATERIALS AND METHODS

A. Organisms

    Plaque purified (12) 9-mile strain of C. burnetii, Phase
I, (9miI/c17) was propagated in SPF type IV embryonated hens'
eggs as previously described (13). Purification of C.
burnetii from host material by isopyknic Renografin centrifugation was also as described (13).
    R. typhi, Wilmington strain, was also propagated in SPF
type IV embryonated hens' eggs (14). Yolk sacs were harvested
at 7 days postinoculation and organisms purified by Renografin
density gradient centrifugation (13). C. psittaci, strain
6BC, was grown and purified by the same procedures.

B. Metabolism Studies

    Whole cell metabolism studies were carried out as de-
scribed previously (11).
    Radiolabeled substrates were purchased from Amersham
(Arlington Hts, Ill.). Other chemicals were from Sigma (St.
Louis, Mo.).

III. RESULTS

    Although the organisms used in these studies were highly
purified through two cycles of Renografin gradient centrifugation and no yolk sac antigen was detectable in complement
fixation tests, the question of enzymatic activity due to
contamination by host cellular material is always a consideration. We, therefore, examined the pH optima of glucose
metabolism of a crude suspension of yolk sac cells. As shown
in Figure 1, both the catabolism and incorporation of glucose
by yolk sac cells exhibited a pH optimum of approximately
7.0. In contrast, the optimal pH for glucose metabolism by
C. burnetii was 4.8 (11). Further, the specific activities
of 0.822 nMol/mg protein/hr and 0.250 nMol/mg protein/hr for
glucose catabolism and incorporation, respectively, by yolk
sac cell suspensions differ from the specific activities of
3.32 and 0.130 nMol/mg protein/hr for glucose catabolism
and incorporation determined for whole cells of C. burnetii.
These results indicate that it is unlikely that glucose
metabolism by C. burnetii is due to contamination by cellular
enzymes.

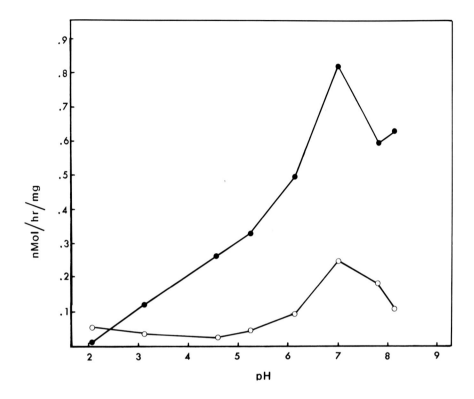

Fig. 1.   Glucose metabolism by normal yolk sac cells. Catabolism of [U-^{14}C]-glucose to $^{14}CO_2$ (●) and incorporation of [U-^{14}C]-glucose into a trichloroacetic acid insoluble product (○); both expressed as nMol substrate per hr per mg protein.

The pH optima for substrate metabolism was studied for representative members of the two orders of Rickettsias, Rickettsia typhi and Chlamydia psittaci.   Unlike C. burnetii, neither of these organisms replicates within phagolysosomes (9, 15).   As shown in Figure 2, metabolism of glutamate by R. typhi is optimal at about pH 7.0.   In agreement with previous reports of lack of glycolytic enzymes in R. typhi (16), glucose was not catabolized at any pH examined.   Similarly, C. psittaci metabolized glutamate optimally at approximately pH 7.0 but not glucose at any pH examined (Fig. 3).   Collectively these data suggest that the optimal pH for metabolism by intracellular parasites is reflective of the sub-cellular compartment in which the organism replicates.

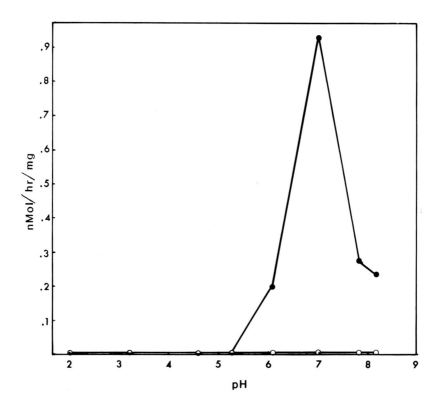

Fig. 2. Catabolism of glutamate and glucose by Rickettsia typhi. Results expressed as nMol [U-^{14}C]-glutamate (●), or [U-^{14}C]-glucose (○) recovered as $^{14}CO_2$ per hr per mg dry wgt. [U-^{14}C]-glutamate was at 1 mM final concentration in the reaction mixture (1 μCi/0.1 μMol); [U-^{14}C]-glucose was 0.1 mM (1 μCi/μMol).

While pH of the suspending medium appears to be a critical factor in the stimulation of metabolism by C. burnetii, that alone does not appear to be the singular factor restricting growth of this organism to the intracellular environment. To determine if metabolic activity by C. burnetii could be en-hanced by the addition of any exogenous metabolite to the axenic reaction mixture, the effect of non-radiolabeled metab-olites on the catabolism and incorporation of glutamate and glucose was examined. Both the total amount of substrate catabolized to $^{14}CO_2$ or incorporated into a trichloroacetic acid (TCA) precipitable product as well as the relative pro-portions into each product may be altered by the presence of

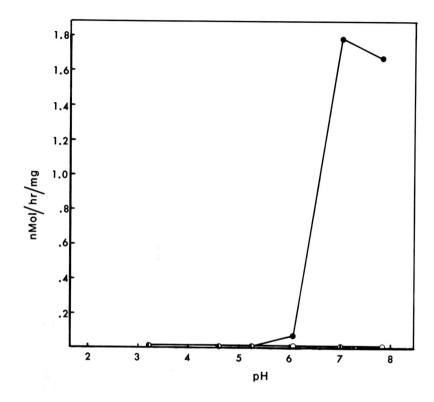

Fig. 3.   Catabolism of glutamate and glucose by Chlamydia psittaci.   Results expressed as nMol $[U-^{14}C]$-glutamate (●) or $[U-^{14}C]$-glucose (○) recovered as $^{14}CO_2$ per hr per mg dry wgt.   Reaction conditions as in Fig. 2.

additional substrates (Table 1).   Both pyruvate and succinate, which are metabolized preferentially over glutamate (in preparation), reduce the amount of glutamate catabolized or incorporated.   NAD, NADP, or ATP did not enhance either catabolism of glutamate to $^{14}CO_2$ or the incorporation of glutamate. Addition of the remaining 19 amino acids to the concentrations of Eagle's minimum essential medium (MEM) or addition of MEM vitamins appears to enhance incorporation of glutamate into a TCA insoluble product.   Incorporation of glucose is markedly enhanced in the presence of 5 mM glutamate.   Both the glycolytic and pentose phosphate pathways of glucose metabolism (17) appear to be active in C. burnetii at pH 4.5 as shown by the evolution of $^{14}CO_2$ from glucose labeled in the 1 or 6 positions (Table 2).

TABLE 1.   Effect of Exogenous Metabolites on Glutamate
and Glucose Metabolism by C. burnetii

Substrate	Additions	Catabolism[a]	Incorporation[a]
[U-^{14}C]-glutamate	-	(100)%	(100)%
"	Glucose (5mM)	93.9	59.0
"	Citrate (5mM)	101.2	93.4
"	Pyruvate (5mM)	42.4	16.4
"	α-ketoglutarate (5mM)	109.9	80.3
"	Succinate (5mM)	27.2	8.2
"	NAD (1.5 μM)	97.2	85.2
"	NADP (1.5 μM)	105.6	83.6
"	ATP (10 μM)	92.2	86.9
"	MEM amino acids[b]	86.6	145.9
"	MEM vitamins	90.0	133.9
"	MEM amino acids + vitamins	87.1	147.9
[U-^{14}C]-glucose	-	(100)	(100)
"	Glutamate (5mM)	369.9	5635.3

[a]Catabolism and incorporation are expressed as percent of
that substrate catabolized or incorporated in the absence
of any addition. Specific activities for glutamate
catabolism and incorporation were 111.14 nMol/mg/hr and
6.07 nMol/mg/hr, respectively, in the absence of additional
substrates. Specific activities for glucose catabolism
and incorporation were 6.45 nMol/mg/hr and 59.8 pMol/hr/mg,
respectively, in the absence of glutamate.

[b]Eagle's minimum essential medium (MEM), essential and non-
essential amino acids, and vitamins were added to the concentrations of Eagle's MEM.

The incorporation of glutamate into a TCA insoluble
product indicates a functional protein synthetic mechanism
in C. burnetii. To examine the ability of C. burnetii to
synthesize other macromolecules in an axenic medium, the
metabolism of [U-^{14}C]-thymidine and [U-^{14}C]-uridine was
examined (Table 3). Thymidine was not catabolized to CO_2
under any of the conditions examined, i.e., with or without
a metabolizable substrate or at pH 4.5 or 7. It is notable
that thymidine was not incorporated into a TCA insoluble
product in the absence of an energy source. Similarly,

TABLE 2. Metabolism of Glucose Labeled in Different
Positions by C. burnetii

Substrate	$^{14}CO_2$[a]	Incorporated[b]
[U-^{14}C]-glucose	3935	12
[1-^{14}C]-glucose	7664	228
[6-^{14}C]-glucose	2297	65
[2-^{14}C]-glucose	3849	69

[a]Results expressed as counts per minute (CPM) above background as $^{14}CO_2$ per mg dry wgt C. burnetii following 2 hr
incubation at 37°C. All substrates were at 1.0 mM final
concentration (0.1 μCi/μMol).

[b]Results expressed as CPM above background incorporated into
a trichloroacetic acid insoluble product.

TABLE 3. Pyrimidine and Purine Nucleoside Metabolism
by C. burnetii at pH 4.5

Substrate[a]	Glutamate[b]	Sp. Act. (pMol/mg/hr)	
		Catabolism	Incorporation
[U-^{14}C]-thymidine	−	UD[c]	UD
	+	UD	450.4
[U-^{14}C]-uridine	−	UD	UD
	+	UD	267.7
[U-^{14}C]-guanosine	−	UD	UD
	+	843.7	1686.5

[a]All substrates were added to 0.1 mM final concentration
[1 μCi/μMol].

[b]Reactions were carried out in the presence or absence of
5 mM glutamate.

[c]Undetectable.

uridine was not catabolized to a detectable level under any
of the conditions examined. Again, no incorporation was
detected in the absence of glutamate as an energy source or
at pH 7.0 (data not shown). The metabolism of the purine
ribonucleoside, guanosine, was also examined. Again, incorporation was only detectable in the presence of an energy
source, but in the presence of glutamate, however, guanosine
was catabolized to $^{14}CO_2$.

IV. DISCUSSION

The metabolic capabilities of C. burnetii have long been
considered to be minimal in the extracellular environment.
Glucose had been reported not be to utilized by this organism
and glutamate only minimally (7, 8). The limited metabolism
by C. burnetii in a cell-free environment led to the approach
of analyzing cell-free extracts for key enzymes of metabolic
sequences in an attempt to demonstrate an enzymatic deficiency
leading to the obligate intracellular nature of this organism
(9, 10). The results of these types of studies have thus far
failed to demonstrate an obvious biochemical lesion restricting growth of C. burnetii to an intracellular environment (9,
10, 18). Because of the disparity between enzymatic capabilities and activity displayed by intact C. burnetii in an
axenic reaction mixture, we sought to reexamine the metabolic
capabilities of this organism. We found that transport,
catabolism, and incorporation of both glucose and glutamate
were highly stimulated by hydrogen ion concentrations designed
to reflect the intravacuolar environment inhabited by C.
burnetii (11). The results presented here extend those observations to a number of substrates and clearly demonstrate the
acidophilic nature of C. burnetii.
The pH dependence of metabolism of members of the two
orders of Rickettsias, R. typhi and C. psittaci, was examined.
These organisms replicate in the cytoplasm and phagosomes,
respectively, of infected cells, but unlike C. burnetii, are
degraded within phagolysosomes (15, 19). In contrast to C.
burnetii, R. typhi and C. psittaci did not metabolize glucose
to a detectable level, and both metabolized glutamate optimally at about pH 7. Therefore, the activation of intracellular
parasites by acidic pH does not appear to be a general phenomenon as shown by neutral pH optima of R. typhi and C.
psittaci. Rather the optimal pH for metabolism of these
parasites appears to reflect the intracellular microenviron-
ment in which they replicate.

While attempts to demonstrate growth of C. burnetii in
an axenic medium have so far been inconclusive, the incorporation of glutamate, uridine and thymidine into TCA precipitable products indicates macromolecular synthesis in the
axenic reaction mixture. Hence, pH alone is not the only
factor which restricts growth of C. burnetii to the phagolysosome. Preliminary attempts to identify a nutritional requirement which could trigger cell-free growth of C. burnetii
were designed to detect the effect of exogenous metabolites
on glutamate, glucose, or nucleoside catabolism and incorporation. While none of the exogenous metabolites demonstrated
an outstanding stimulation of metabolism, the following observations are of importance: i) The relative proportion of
glutamate or glucose catabolized or incorporated was modulated
by the presence of added metabolites. These results demonstrate that C. burnetii possesses some of the metabolic
regulatory mechanisms typical of autonomously growing microorganisms. ii) An energy source, such as glutamate, is
required for the synthesis of macromolecules. Thus, a sufficient energy charge (20) appears to be a requirement for
macromolecular synthesis. This requirement is satisfied in
the axenic reaction medium utilized in these studies.

V.   SUMMARY

The pH dependent activation of substrate transport and
metabolism by Coxiella burnetii represents a unique pathogenic
mechanism by which this bacterium has adapted itself to growth
within the normally bactericidal contents of the phagolysosome.
This requirement for the acidic conditions of the phagolysosome could provide, in part, for the extreme resistance of C.
burnetii to environmental conditions. This mechanism of
activation does not appear to be a general feature of obligate
intracellular parasites as demonstrated by the neutral pH
optima for metabolism by Rickettsia typhi and Chlamydia
psittaci. Of the substrates examined here, all were catabolized and/or incorporated better by C. burnetii under acidic
conditions than at neutrality. In addition, precursors of
both DNA and RNA were incorporated by C. burnetii at pH 4.5
in the presence of an energy source, thus implying the generation of a sufficient energy charge to drive macromolecular
synthesis in an axenic medium.

ACKNOWLEDGMENTS

We thank Earl Davis for his dedicated technical assistance
and Susan Smaus for secretarial preparation.

REFERENCES

1. Burton, P. R., Kordova, N., and Paretsky, D., Can. J.
    Microbiol. 17, 143 (1971).
2. Burton, P. R., Stueckeman, J., Welsh, R. M., and
    Paretsky, D., Infect. Immun. 21, 556 (1978).
3. McCaul, T. F., Hackstadt, T., and Williams, J. C., in
    "Rickettsiae and Rickettsial Diseases" (W. Burgdorfer and
    R. L. Anacker, eds.), p. . Academic Press, New York,
    (1981).
4. DeDuve, C., and Wattiaux, R., Ann. Rev. Physiol. 28,
    435 (1966).
5. Ohkuma, S., and Poole, B., Proc. Natl. Acad. Sci. U.S.A.
    75, 3327 (1978).
6. Goren, M. B., Ann. Rev. Microbiol. 31, 507 (1977).
7. Ormsbee, R. A., and Peacock, M. G., J. Bact. 88, 1205
    (1964).
8. Ormsbee, R. A., and Weiss, E., Science 142, 1077 (1963).
9. Weiss, E., Bact. Rev. 37, 259 (1973).
10. Paretsky, D., Zentralb. Bakteriol. Parasitenk.
    Infektionskr. Hyg. Abt. Orig. 206, 284 (1968).
11. Hackstadt, T., and Williams, J. C., Proc. Natl. Acad.
    Sci. U.S.A. (in press).
12. Ormsbee, R. A., and Peacock, M. G., Tissue Culture
    Association 2, 475 (1976).
13. Williams, J. C., Peacock, M. G., and McCaul, T. F.,
    Infect. Immun. (in press).
14. Weiss, E., Coolbaugh, J. C., and Williams, J. C., Appl.
    Microbiol. 30, 456 (1975).
15. Friis, R. R., J. Bact. 110, 706 (1972).
16. Coolbaugh, J. C., Progar, J. J., and Weiss, E., Infect.
    Immun. 14, 298 (1976).
17. Katz, J., and Wood, H. G., J. Biol. Chem. 238, 517
    (1963).
18. Ormsbee, R. A., Ann. Rev. Microbiol. 23, 275 (1969).
19. Meyer, W. H. III, and Wisseman, C. L., Abstr. Annu.
    Meeting of Amer. Soc. for Microbiol. (1980).
20. Chapman, A. G., Fall, L., and Atkinson, D. E., J. Bact.
    108, 1072 (1971).
21. Williams, J. C., and Weiss, E., J. Bact. 134, 884 (1978).

SUBCELLULAR COMPONENTS FROM <u>COXIELLA</u> <u>BURNETII</u> SYNTHESIZE COLIPHAGE PROTEIN[1]

John P. Donahue[1]
Herbert A. Thompson

Department of Microbiology
School of Medicine
West Virginia University
Morgantown, West Virginia

I. INTRODUCTION

The Protein Forming System (PFS) in free-living bacteria consists of ribonucleic acid polymerase, tRNA ligases, tRNAs, rRNAs, ribosomal proteins and translation factors. In free-living heterotrophs about 150 genes express these components, and the assembly of the entire unit into a functional system is coordinately and intricately controlled. Understanding of these relationships and their response to growth conditions provides an important central theme in bacterial physiology (1).

Studies of growth of obligate intracellular bacteria would also benefit from a fundamental knowledge of the occurrence, assembly and efficacy of their respective Protein Forming Systems. However, the component parts of the parasite PFS and its characteristics are not well defined. While it has generally been assumed that <u>Rickettsiae</u>, <u>Chlamydiae</u>, and <u>Coxiella</u> have at least some capacity for independent protein synthesis during their residence within host cells, few details are available concerning the assembly of their respective PF Systems, the genes which code for their expression and regulation, and the efficiency and fidelity of the assembled machinery during translation.

---

[1]Supported by grant #PCM 7903282 from the National Science Foundation.

441

To address these questions, we began a project intended to
define macromolecular synthesis and regulation in Coxiella
burnetii. The PFS of this organism has received some emphasis,
and the available information obtained from studies with cell-
free extracts have shown that 1. the organism possesses a very
active DNA-dependent RNA polymerase (2,3); 2. the organism has
typically prokaryote-like ribosomes (4,5) that translate synthetic polynucleotides (6-8); and 3. functions analogous to
those performed by bacterial elongation factors EF-Tu and
EF-G, and by phenylalanyl-tRNA ligase, are present in the
organism (7).

To begin, it was necessary to establish that the components and activities described before were representative of a
larger, complete protein synthesis apparatus. Evidence suggesting complete protein synthesis catalyzed by components
from C. burnetii has recently been obtained in this laboratory
(8). Utilizing extracts obtained by freeze-disruption of purified organisms, synthesis occurred only when exogenous synthetic polynucleotide or natural mRNA was added to incubations.
These extracts contained low concentrations of ribosomes in
the form of ribosomal subunits. The participation of these
subunits in protein synthesis required high amounts of magnesium (compared to conventional systems) and was inhibited by
chloramphenicol but not cycloheximide. When RNA from the positive strand coliphage Qβ was added to incubations containing
C. burnetii fractions, some of the polypeptides formed had a
molecular weight similar to that encoded by the Qβ coat
protein cistron (8).

In the present report, we provide evidence for a functional and complete ribosome cycle in the C. burnetii PFS.
Supplemented with bacteriophage Qβ RNA, components of protein
synthesis function such that the coat cistron of bacteriophage
RNA is translated repeatedly during incubations. Further, we
describe in detail the conditions (ionic, temperature, pH,
energy, and component concentrations) that are necessary for
optimal translation.

II. METHODS

Coxiella burnetii, Nine Mile Strain, Phase 1 was propagated in 6 day old embryonated chicken eggs, harvested and
purified as described (4,9). Escherichia coli Q13 was grown
and harvested as described (8). Bacteriophage Qβ (Miles
Laboratories) was propagated in E. coli C3000 as described
(8). Virus was recovered from culture fluids by ammonium sulfate precipitation and purified by differential and isopycnic
centrifugation as described (10). Qβ RNA was prepared by

phenol-chloroform extraction as described (8). This procedure routinely yielded homogeneous RNA with a molecular weight of 1.2 x 10[6] daltons. The preparation of ^{14}C-labelled Qβ coat protein was described elsewhere (8).

For the preparation of biosynthetically active subcellular extracts the method employed for cell disruption is important. The method used here for the preparation of extracts from C. burnetii and E. coli was a modification of the original Hughes Press as described by Eaton (11). The press consists of a cylinder block containing a 1 mm aperature at the bottom, a receiving-tube block and a piston that is forced through the center of the cylinder block by a hydraulic laboratory press (Carver: Summit, NJ). All parts of the press were milled from stainless steel. Bacterial cell pellets of purified E. coli or C. burnetii were suspended in twice their wet weight in TMKD buffer (0.01 M tris-HCl, pH 7.4, 0.01 M magnesium acetate, 0.05 M potassium acetate, 0.002 M dithiothreitol) and transferred to the cylinder block which had been prechilled to -85°C. The cell suspension was allowed to freeze. The piston was positioned in the cylinder block which was mounted on the receiving-tube block. This apparatus was then placed into the hydraulic press. A pressure of 10-15,000 psi was then exerted over the piston forcing the frozen bacterial cell suspension through the aperature into the receiving-tube block resulting in cell disruption. Disrupted C. burnetii or E. coli cells were then fractionated by differential centrifugation as described (8) except that S30 extracts from C. burnetii were dialyzed against TMKD buffer (4 hours at 4°C) without loss of activity, a finding contrary to our earlier observations (8). Both E. coli and C. burnetii extracts were stored at -85°C in aliquots. Although not routinely done, C. burnetii S30 fractions could be refrozen and thawed two or three times without loss of activity; aliquots remained stable for up to six months when stored at -85°C. Protein determinations were performed by the method of Bradford (12).

Optimal conditions for cell-free translation in E. coli and C. burnetii S30 extracts differ. Final concentrations of salts, buffer, energy compounds and amino acids were as follows for the E. coli system: 2 mM ATP, 0.27 mM GTP, 4 mM creatine phosphate, 60 μg/ml creatine phosphokinase, 10 mM magnesium acetate, 60 mM ammonium acetate, 67 mM tris-acetate pH 7.8, 1 mM dithiothreitol, 0.006 mM 1-leucine and 0.05 mM 19 unlabelled 1-amino acids. Final concentrations in the C. burnetii system were the same as in the E. coli system with the following exceptions: 1.3 mM ATP, 1.3 mM creatine phosphage, 20 μg/ml creatine phosphokinase and 13.3 mM magnesium acetate.

For the temperature study the above reactants, Qβ RNA (25 μg), ^{3}H-1-leucine (171 Ci mmol[-1], New England Nuclear) and either E. coli S30 (94 μg protein) or C. burnetii S30 (78 μg protein) extract were combined and incubated at the temperatures indicated. In the pH study, reactions containing E. coli S30 (187 μg protein) or C. burnetii S30 (63 μg protein) extract and Qβ RNA (40 μg) were incubated for 40 minutes at 34°C for the E. coli system and 37°C for the C. burnetii system. For reaction pHs of 6.6-7.6, the buffer used was 67 mM morpholinopropane-sulfonic acid-KOH; for reaction pHs of 7.9-8.6, the buffer was 67 mM tris-acetate. All other reaction component concentrations were as described above.

Reactions were terminated by the addition of 10% (w/v) TCA that contained 1 mg/ml leucine and heated to 90°C for 20 minutes. Protein precipitates were then filtered onto glass fiber filters, washed with 5% (w/v) TCA containing 1 mg/ml leucine, dried and assayed for radioactivity in Omnifluor-toluene scintillation cocktail. The efficiency of counting for tritium was 23-27%.

Reaction conditions for translation product analysis were the same as for the temperature study except that 0.006 mM leucine was omitted and reactions were incubated for 50 minutes at 34°C and 37°C for E. coli and C. burnetii respectively.

After protein synthesis incubations, reaction mixtures were incubated at 37°C for 15 minutes in 0.33 M NaOH and then protein precipitated by the addition of 0.4 vol of 25% (w/v) TCA. The protein precipitates were washed twice with 10% (w/v) TCA containing 1 mg/ml unlabelled leucine and once with acetone. The protein was suspended in buffer (0.05 M tris-HCl, pH 6.8) with 3% (w/v) sodium dodecyl sulfate (SDS), 3% (v/v) 2-mercaptoethanol, and 10% (v/v) glycerol and boiled for 5 minutes. After clarification, samples were layered into the sample wells of slab gels constructed with 5% acrylamide stacking portion above a 13% separating gel as described by Laemmli (13). Electrophoresis buffer was 0.05 M tris-0.38 M glycine, pH 8.2 with 0.1% (w/v) SDS. Proteins were electrophoresed at 10 mA constant current for 1 hr, followed by 15 mA for 3.5 hr or until the marker dye front was 1 cm from the end of the gel. Slab electrophoretograms were processed for fluorography as described (14). Fluorographs were developed with LKB Ultrafilm (LKB Instruments) for 7 days at -85°C.

III. RESULTS

It has been previously demonstrated that the addition of purified coliphage RNA to a C. burnetii cell-free system results in a 10-40 fold increase in amino acid incorporation. This protein synthetic activity was dependent on the addition of an energy source, ammonium and magnesium ions and possessed

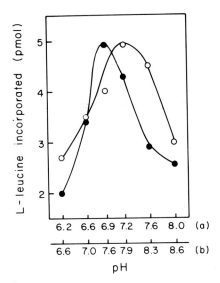

Fig. 1. Effect of pH on amino acid incorporation in E. coli (O) and C. burnetii (●) cell free systems directed by Qβ RNA. The number of pmols of ^{3}H-1-leucine incorporated were plotted versus the measured pH of the reaction mixtures after incubation (Scale a) and the pH of the added buffer prior to incubation (Scale b).

several characteristics typical of bacterial translation (8). In addition to specific cation and energy requirements, other factors which could be expected to affect the rate of protein synthesis are intracellular pH (15) and temperature (16). Cell-free synthetic systems should, therefore, be optimized for these parameters. The effect of pH upon the extent of incorporation in the E. coli and C. burnetii systems is compared in Figure 1. Both the pH of the buffered salts solution added to reactions (Scale b) and the pH determined after the reactions were run (Scale a - direct measurements) are shown; the pH values of the combined reactants were always lower than that of the buffer added. The optimum pH values for the C. burnetii and E. coli systems did not differ markedly since values of pH 6.9 and 7.2, respectively, were obtained. During temperature studies, it was found that the initial rate of protein synthesis in the E. coli system was greater than that of C. burnetii at all temperatures tested (Fig. 2A). However, the initial rate of the reaction was decreased sharply in the E. coli system when incubated at 40°C, whereas in the C. burnetii system the initial rate of reaction was highest at 40°C. Moreover, the full extents of the translation reactions

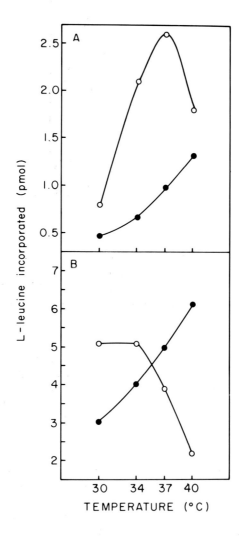

Fig. 2.   Effect of incubation temperature on the initial
rate (A) and final extent (B) of amino acid incorporation in
E. coli (O) and C. burnetii (●) cell-free systems directed by
Qβ RNA.   The number of pmols of leucine incorporated after 5
min (A, initial rates) and after 40 min (B, final reaction
extents) were plotted versus the reaction temperatures.

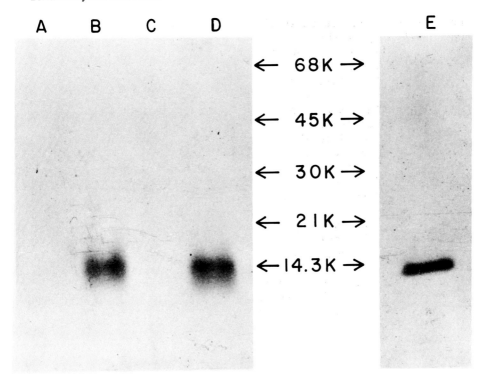

Fig. 3. Electrophoretic and fluorographic characterization of polypeptide products synthesized during cell-free translation of Qβ RNA. Lanes A and B, translation with C. burnetii extract; Lanes C and D, translation with E. coli extract. Lanes A and C represent incubations without added RNA. Lane E, ^{14}C-labelled Qβ coat protein, The molecular weight markers were detected by Coomassie Blue staining.

in the C. burnetii system (Fig. 2B) measured at 40 minutes, reflected the same temperature effect observed for the initial kinetics. By contrast, the extent of the reactions in the E. coli system were highest at 30°C and 34°C, whereas translation in the C. burnetii system is best at 37-40°C or higher. Other experiments (not shown) suggest that the optimal reaction rate and extent obtainable by the C. burnetii system occurs at 43-45°C; however, the quality of translation at those higher temperatures remains untested.

In all of the experiments described in the present work, the mRNA used was obtained from the positive strand RNA coliphage Qβ. This is a polycistronic mRNA that codes for four proteins. The molecular weights of these proteins are, in thousands of daltons: maturation, 41; coat, 14; synthetase

subunit, 64; coat readthrough, 36. In order to discover
which, if any, of these proteins were synthesized when C.
burnetii cell-free systems were "programmed" with Qβ RNA, the
contents of incubated reaction mixtures were extracted for
protein and then electrophoresed through sodium dodecyl sulfate-polyacrylamide gels as described in the methods section.
Molecular weight marker proteins were electrophoresed in a
separate lane. After electrophoresis, the slab gels were
fluorographed as described (14). Figure 3 shows the results
of fluorography and the positions of molecular weight markers.
When either E. coli or C. burnetii extracts were incubated
without added RNA and electrophoresed, no radioactive proteins
were detected (Fig. 3, lanes A and C, respectively). When Qβ
RNA was added to each of the two cell-free systems, both the
E. coli (lane B) and C. burnetii (lane D) cell-free systems
synthesized polypeptide that was approximately 13.5-14 K daltons in size. These polypeptides migrated the same distance
into the gel as did authentic Qβ coat protein (lane E), which
was labelled with ^{14}C-1-valine during coliphage Qβ infection
of E. coli C3000. Thus, the major protein made in either cell-
free system appears to be Qβ coat.

IV. DISCUSSION

     Previous work with the PFS in C. burnetii established the
presence of key enzymic functions and structures that would be
expected to be operational in the expression of its genetic
material (2-7). The results summarized in Table 1 which were
presented here and published elsewhere (8) demonstrate fairly
well the full characteristics and capabilities of that system.
Considering this information totally, two points of discussion
need to be focused.
     First, it is now apparent that the second half of the PFS
in C. burnetii, that concerning translation of mRNA, is present and functional, at least in vitro. Because the experiments presented herein utilized a natural mRNA and begin with
uncharged amino acids as precursors, the functions implied to
be present in C. burnetii are those of 1. aminoacylation of
tRNAs, 2. the binding of ribosomes or ribosomal subunits to an
initiation site on the mRNA, 3. binding of initiator tRNA to
the correctly positioned ribosome in response to an initiation
codon, 4. the binding of aminoacyl-tRNAs in response to the
universal genetic codons in the mRNA, and subsequent peptide
bond formation and translocation, and 5. recognition of termination signals with release of completed polypeptide. Moreover, data to be presented elsewhere shows that over one-half

Table 1.   Summary of the Characteristics of Qβ RNA Translation
in C. burnetii and E. coli Extracts

	C. burnetii	E. coli
Method of preparation		
sonication	–	+
freeze press	+	+
Optimum temperature	43–45°C	30–34°C
Optimum pH	6.9	7.2
Cation requirement[a]		
Mg^{+2}	12–14 mM	10–12 mM
NH_4^+	60 mM	60–70 mM
Cistron most frequently		
translated[b]	coat	coat
Translation efficiency[c]		
(ribosome transit time on Qβ coat protein)	3–4 min.	3–4 min.

[a]Data from Donahue and Thompson, 1980.
[b]Demonstrated by immune precipitation and electrophoresis.
 Data not shown, to be published elsewhere.
[c]Expressed as average time required for ribosome to translate
 Qβ coat cistron. Data not shown, to be published elsewhere.

of the polypeptide product synthesized during the C. burnetii
ribosome cycle is antigenically authentic. It is, therefore,
likely that the translation portion of the C. burnetii PFS is,
under the present conditions, reading faithfully a great majority of the codewords within the coat protein gene. Whether
or not the PFS isolated from C. burnetii is expressed solely
from the microbe's own genetic system is uncertain. It is
clear that this system is largely prokaryotic, because eukaryotic mRNAs are not translated and it is sensitive to chloramphenicol but not cycloheximide (8). Also, eukaryotic translation factors do not function with its ribosomes (7, and unpublished observations), but bacteriophage mRNAs are translated.
     Secondly, the establishment of this cell-free protein syn-
thesis system from C. burnetii should enable studies of gene

expression in the organism. This would be especially true if
mRNAs distinctly representative of the organism's various
physiological or morphological forms could be obtained
(Hackstadt and Williams, this volume; McCaul and Williams,
this volume). This would be especially valuable since so
little information on the genetics of this bacterium is available. In general, the utility of cell-free systems isolated
from various bacterial species has been limited because these
systems are often not well defined. In the present work,
efforts were made to optimize conditions so that rate, extent
and fidelity of translation were as good as reasonably possible. In our hands, the activity of the C. burnetii system
is equal or superior to that from E. coli Q13.

     It is presently difficult to assess the significance of
the several differences we have found between the C. burnetii
versus the E. coli cell-free systems. There are several minor
differences, but four major ones are worth noting. First, the
C. burnetii system requires an extremely high (17-20 mM) magnesium concentration for translation of synthetic poly-(U)
templates, but lower concentrations for translation of coliphage RNA (8). Second, the C. burnetii system translates
coliphage RNA very well at temperatures around 40°C or higher,
whereas E. coli components function poorly at these temperatures. Third, the C. burnetii system operates efficiently
with between one-fifth and one-third the ribosomes found
necessary for optimal function of the E. coli system. Fourth,
no endogenous mRNA activity has been found in C. burnetii
extracts, whereas such activity is evident in E. coli extracts,
and in those of most bacterial and animal cell-free systems.
Whether or not any of these observations are related to characteristics of the intact C. burnetii cell is unknown. However, the requirements for macromolecular synthesis in vitro
often reflect intracellular conditions. For example, cell-
free protein synthesis systems from halophilic bacteria require very high salt concentrations (17), and those from
thermophiles function best at 55-60°C (18). Further, the
intracellular concentration of ribosomes in the well-studied
heterotrophs E. coli and S. typhimurium has been demonstrated
to be directly proportional to their generation times (19);
since C. burnetii's generation time may be several-fold
greater, it would not be unexpected that it contained very few
ribosomes. On the other hand, C. burnetii is grown in eggs to
maximum yield, to the point of near embryo death, and for this
reason many of the C. burnetii cells isolated could be equivalent to stationary phase cells. It is well known that free-
living bacterial cells harvested beyond the log phase of the
culture are poorer in mRNA and ribosomes (20). Several of
these questions await further research for well-founded
answers.

REFERENCES

1. Maaløe, O., in "Biological Regulation and Development" (R. F. Goldberger, ed.) Vol. 1, p. 487. Plenum Press, New York, (1979).

2. Jones, F. Jr., and Paretsky, D., J. Bacteriol. 93, 1063 (1967).

3. Christian, R. G., and Paretsky, D., J. Bacteriol. 132, 841 (1977).

4. Thompson, H. A., Baca, O. G., and Paretsky, D., Biochem. J. 125, 365 (1971).

5. Baca, O. G., Hersh, R. T., and Paretsky, D., J. Bacteriol. 116, 441 (1973).

6. Mallavia, L. P. and Paretsky, D., J. Bacteriol. 93, 1479 (1967).

7. Baca, O. G., J. Bacteriol. 136, 429 (1978).

8. Donahue, J. P., and Thompson, H. A., J. Gen. Micro. 121, 293 (1980).

9. Paretsky, D., Downs, C. M., Consigli, R. A., and Joyce, B. K., J. Infect. Dis. 103, 6 (1958).

10. Webster, R. E., Engelhardt, D. L., Zinder, N. D., and Konigsberg, W., J. Mol. Biol. 29, 27 (1967).

11. Eaton, N. R., J. Bacteriol. 83, 1359 (1962).

12. Bradford, M. M., Anal. Biochem. 72, 248 (1976).

13. Laemmli, U. K., Nature 227, 680 (1970).

14. Bonner, W. M., and Laskey, R. A., Eur. J. Biochem. 46, 83 (1974).

15. Grainger, J. L., Winkler, M. M., Shen, S. S., and Steinhardt, R. A., Dev. Biol. 68, 396 (1979).

16. Stenesh, J., in "Extreme Environments: Mechanisms of Microbial Adaptation" (M. R. Heinrich, ed.) p. 85. Academic Press, New York, (1976).

17. Bayley, S. T., in "Extreme Environments: Mechanisms of Microbial Adaptation" (M. R. Heinrich, ed.) p. 119. Academic Press, New York, (1976).

18. Lodish, H. F., Nature 224, 867 (1969).

19. Kjeldgaard, N. O., and Kurland, C. G., J. Mol. Biol. 6, 341 (1963).

20. Forchhammer, J., and Kjeldgaard, N. O., J. Mol. Biol. 37, 245 (1968).

SOME MODULATING FACTORS OF TRANSCRIPTION IN Q FEVER

David Paretsky
Frank Gonzales

Department of Microbiology
University of Kansas
Lawrence, Kansas

I.   INTRODUCTION

Q fever is a rickettsiosis of world-wide incidence whose
epidemiology, immunology and gross clinical features have
been well studied. The pathobiochemistry of the disease is
far less understood. Q fever in guinea pigs is characterized
by early hepatic glycogen depletion due to inhibition of
uridine diphosphate glucose-glycogen transglucosulase (1-3).
There is a coincidental onset of a fatty-infiltrated liver
with a parallel increased concentration of cortisol and cAMP,
and a simultaneously stimulated synthesis of protein and RNA
(3,4). The latter phenomena suggested a search for regulatory
factors of transcription which are induced by the infection.
Ornithine decarboxylase is known to be induced during cellular
transitions from inactive to active states accompanied by
increased polyamine concentrations (5) so that these factors
might be implicated as modulators of DNA-dependent RNA polymerase activities.

II.   MATERIALS AND METHODS

A.   Organism

1.   Coxiella burnetii, phase I, Nine Mile strain, was
maintained in a yolk sac suspension from a first egg passage
of infected guinea pig spleens (1).

2. Guinea pigs. Hartley smooth-haired, white, male
guinea pigs, about 250 g., (Tumblebrook Farms, Scottsdale,
PA) were infected by intraperitoneal injection of 0.2 ml of a
20% infected yolk sac homogenate, $LD_{50} = 10^{-5}$. Animal weights
and temperatures were recorded daily. Because the peak of
pyrexia was usually at 84-96 hr., animals were sacrificed at
these times (1). The animals were exsanguinated and the
livers rapidly removed.

B. Enzyme Assays

1. Ornithine decarboxylase (ODC) and polyamine assays.
Livers were homogenized in 0.25 M sucrose/0.1 mM EDTA/1 mM
dithiothreitol to give a 5% suspension (w/v), and centrifuged
at 20,000 x g for 20 min. The supernatants were incubated in
the presence of 20 nmoles of L-ornithine + 30.4 nmoles of L-
$(1-^{14}C)$-ornithine, 46 mCi/mMole (New England Nuclear, Boston,
MA)1, in a final vol. of 0.2 ml (6). $^{14}CO_2$ liberated by ODC
was trapped and the radioactivity measured. Polyamines were
measured in a 10% liver homogenate deproteinized with 0.2 N
$HClO_4$. Polyamines were separated from amino acids by chromatography on Dowex 50, and reacted with dansyl chloride (7).
The dansylated derivatives were separated by thin layer
chromatography on silica gel plates (7). Quantitative measurements were made fluorimetrically, employing a scanning
densitometer (Kontes, Vineland, N.J.). Dansylated putrescine,
spermidine and spermine were used as standards.

2. Nuclei and RNA polymerases. Nuclei were prepared
from a 10% liver homogenate (w/v) in 2.2 M sucrose/0.25 mM
spermine/15 mM $MgCl_2$ by centrifuging at 11,200 x g, 35 min
(8). The nuclei were washed in 0.34 M sucrose/10 mM Tris
HCl, pH 7.9/1 mM dithiothreitol/0.1 mM p-methylphenylsulfonyl
fluoride to remove "free" RNA polymerases, leaving nuclei
with template-bound polymerases (9,10). RNA polymerase
activity was measured by incubating nuclei in the presence of
ATP, GTP, CTP and 0.5 µCi of 5-^{3}H-UTP, 20 Ci/mMole (New
England Nuclear, Boston, MA). Classes I, II and III were
discriminated on the basis of α-amanitin sensitivity (11).

3. Effect of alkaline phosphatase on transcription.
Alkaline phosphatase linked to agarose beads (Sigma Chem.
Co., St. Louis, MO) was reacted with uninfected guinea pig
liver crude RNA polymerase preparations for 20 min. at 22 C.
Buffer and agarose were substituted for phosphatase in control
vessels. After incubation, the agarose and agarose-linked
enzyme were removed by centrifuging, and the activitites of
the polymerases were measured.

TABLE 1. Ornithine Decarboxylase and Polyamines in Q fever

Hr post-infection	ODC[a] nmoles CO_2/ mg protein	pmoles/mg protein		
		Putrescine	Spermidine	Spermine
0	2.2	10.3	0.2	0.4
96	55.6	5.2	9.1	5.3

Analyses as described in text; 3 animals per normal and infected groups.

[a]ODC, ornithine decarboxylase.

TABLE 2. DNA-dependent RNA Polymerase Activity in Q fever

Hr post-infection	nmoles UTP incorporated per mg protein	percent distribution		
		Class I	Class II	Class III
0	1.97	31	62	7
96	5.79	47	52	1

Nuclei with engaged polymerases prepared and assayed as described in text; 3 animals per normal and infected groups.

TABLE 3. Effect of Alkaline Phosphatase on RNA Polymerase

Class	Pre-Pase	Post-Pase	% change
	^{3}H-UMP incorp, cpm/mg protein		
II	63,720	92,030	+13%
I + III	22,420	9,510	-58%

Conditions as described in text.

III.   RESULTS

Consistent with other observations (8) ODC activity rapidly increased, 25-fold at 4 days post-infection (Table 1). There were greater than 30-fold increases in spermidine, and spermine increased 10-fold at 4 days post-infection. Putrescine levels decreased at this time. In other work it was shown that the polyamines increased as early as day 1 post infection, with subsequent decrease at day 4 (8). Total RNA polymerase activities increased almost 3-fold at 4 days post infection, with the greatest increase, 1.5-fold, in class I polymerase (Table 2). This is consistent with observations that ribosomal RNA showed greatest increase of the RNA species during infection (4). When RNA polymerases were reacted with alkaline phosphatase, the class I + III group lost 58% of its activity, while class II was virtually unaffected (Table 3).

IV.   DISCUSSION

Induced ODC activity is a characteristic response in numerous instances of cell and organ transitions from quiescent to active states (5). This response is found in the present experiments. A frequent concomitant of this response is elevated polyamine concentrations, and Table 1 shows this to be the case in Q fever. Increased ODC activity and polyamine levels are accompanied by increased RNA polymerase activities, with an increased relative abundance of class I polymerase, confirming and extending previous observations (11). Although the biochemical significance of these correlations are not immediately known, when they are taken in context with other known correlates of Q fever, a model may be proposed for transcriptional regulation. It has been shown that hepatic cortisol concentrations increased during Q fever, from a 100% increment at 12 hr. post infection to 518% by 84 hr. post infection (4). The C. burnetii lipopolysaccharide also stimulated cortisol enhancement by 114% within 1 day post infection (12). cAMP likewise increased 100% within 84 hr post infection (13),and cAMP-independent nuclear protein kinase activity increased by 163% at 36 hr post infection (unpublished results). By 96 hr post-infection, this activity diminished to pre-infection levels (unpublished results).
We can propose a tentative set of coordinated mechanisms for the modulation of transcription during Q fever (Fig. 1). Cortisol and cAMP production are initially stimulated by the active infection, or by the lipopolysaccharide of C. burnetii.

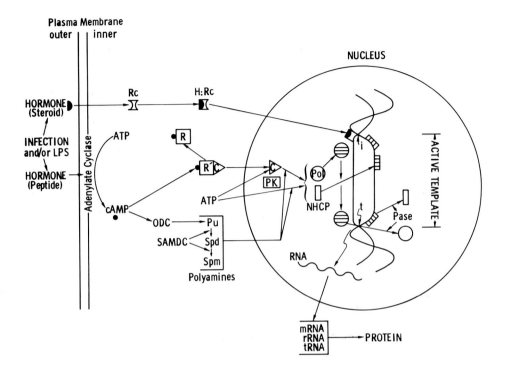

Fig. 1.   Rc, cortisol receptor protein; H:Rc, cortisol-receptor complex; R, regulatory subunit of cAMP-dependent protein kinase; c, catalytic subunit of cAMP-dependent protein kinase; ODC, ornithine decarboxylase; SAMDC, S-adenosylmethionine decarboxylase; Pu, Spd, Spm, putrescine, spermidine, spermine; PK, cAMP-independent protein kinase; O, θ, unphosphorylated and phosphorylated RNA polymerase; ◯, ⊜, NHCP, unphosphorylated and phosphorylated non-histone chromatin proteins; i, template initiation site for polymerase; t, template termination site for polymerase; Pase, nuclear phosphatase.

Cortisol is known to induce ODC and its putrescine product activates S-adenosyl methionine decarboxylase (5).   These two enzymes are directly involved in the synthesis of polyamines, which catalytically stimulate phosphorylation of class I RNA polymerase (14) via a cAMP-independent protein kinase (15) or a cAMP-dependent kinase.   The cortisol binds with its cytoplasmic receptor to form the cortisol:receptor complex.   The complex enters the nucleus, as proposed by others and complexes with the chromatin (16,17).   Non-histone chromatin

protein effectors are phosphorylated by a cAMP-dependent or
-independent protein kinase; the phosphorylated non-histone
chromatin protein together with the cortisol complex "activates" initiation sites on previously inactive DNA template
sites, resulting in increased transcription. On the basis of
experimental results it may be proposed that it is the rRNA
gene which is the more greatly activated (4,11). As the
infection runs its course nuclear alkaline phosphatases
dephosphorylate the modulator phosphorylated non-histone
chromatin proteins, including the polymerases (Table 3), and
the template is restored to its pre-infection condition.
Although some of the intermediate reactions in this model
have experimental support, the speculative steps await verification. While the proposed mechanisms will likely be
modified by ongoing work, the model should provide a basis
for future experiments to elucidate the modulating factors of
transcription during disease, and their mode of action.

ACKNOWLEDGMENTS

We thank K. Berquist and S. Drake for technical assistance. The work was supported by grants from the University
of Kansas General Research Committee, the University of
Kansas Biomedical Research Committee, and the National Science
Foundation, PCM76-11706.

REFERENCES

1. Paretsky, D., Downs, C. M., and Salmon, C. W. J.
    Bacteriol. 88, 137 (1964).
2. Paretsky, D., and Stueckemann, J. J. Bacteriol. 102,
    334 (1970).
3. Stueckemann, J., and Paretsky, D. J. Bacteriol. 106,
    920 (1971).
4. Thompson, H.A., and Paretsky, D. Infect. Immun. 7,
    718 (1973).
5. Jänne, J., Pösö, H., and Raina, A. Biochim. Biophys
    Acta. 473, 241 (1978).
6. Manen, C-A., and Russell, D. H. Biochem. Pharmacol.
    26, 2379 (1977).
7. Seiler, N., and Knödgen, B. J. Chromatog. 164, 155
    (1979).
8. Paretsky, D., Gonzales, F., and Berquist, K. J. Gen.
    Microbiol. in press.

9. Yu, F-L. Biochem. Biophys. Res. Commun. 64, 1107 (1975).
10. Lin, Y-C., Rose, K. M., and Jacob, S. T. Biochem. Biophys, Res. Commun. 72, 114 (1976).
11. Paretsky, D., and Anthes, M. L. J. Infect. Dis. 137, 486 (1978).
12. Baca, O. G., and Paretsky, D. Infect. Immun. 9, 939 (1974).
13. Becker, F., and Paretsky, D. Fed. Prod. 33, 1459 (1974).
14. Kuehn, G. D., Affolter, H. U., Atmar, V. J., Seebeck, T., Gubler, U., and Braun, R. Proc. Natl. Acad. Sci. USA 76, 2541 (1979).
15. Rose, K. M., and Jacob, S. T. J. Biol. Chem. 254, 10256 (1979).
16. O'Malley, B. W. and Means, A. R. Prog. Nucl. Acid. Res. 19, 403 (1976).
17. Spelsberg, T. C., Knowler, J., Boyd, P., Thrall, C., and Martin-Dani, G. J. Steroid Biochem. 11, 373 (1979).

RADIOLABELED POLYPEPTIDES OF RICKETTSIA
PROWAZEKII GROWN IN MICROCARRIER CELL CULTURES[1]

Edwin V. Oaks
Charles L. Wisseman, Jr.
Jonathan F. Smith

Department of Microbiology
University of Maryland School of Medicine
Baltimore, Maryland

I. INTRODUCTION

Polyacrylamide gel electrophoresis (PAGE) has been used by
several investigators to analyze the proteins of rickettsiae
within both the typhus and spotted fever groups (1-5). While
this technique has been successful in identifying members of
major rickettsial groups and distinguishing between individual
rickettsial species, it has not resolved differences between
strains of the same species that are detected by isoelectric
focusing (4). It is possible that additional strain differences exist which are not revealed by these techniques, but
which could be detected by the increased resolution and sensitivity afforded by two-dimensional (2-D) gel electrophoresis
using isotopically labeled rickettsial proteins.

In this report we describe a microcarrier bead cell
culture system which grows R. prowazekii to high titer and
allows the metabolic labeling of rickettsial polypeptides to
high specific activities. Analysis of labeled polypeptides

---
[1] Supported by Contract No. DADA 17-71-C-1007 with the
U.S. Army Medical Research and Development Command, Office of
the Surgeon General, Department of the Army, Washington, D.C.,
and also in part by the U.S. Public Health Service Training
Grant No. AI 00016.

from five R. prowazekii strains by PAGE and 2-D gel electrophoresis has revealed several strain differences, including
the major surface polypeptide of the attenuated E strain.

II. MATERIALS AND METHODS

A. Rickettsiae

The R. prowazekii strains used in this study included two
classic human isolates with long passage histories (Breinl and
E strains), two recent human isolates with short passage histories (Burundi X-16 and V-59) and a flying squirrel isolate
with a short passage history (strain GvF-12). More detailed
information about these strains can be found in a recent
report by Myers and Wisseman (6). Rickettsiae used to infect
L-cell cultures were prepared and stored as 20% yolk sac suspensions in brain heart infusion (BBL, Bioquest, Cockeysville,
MD).

B. Microcarrier Culture System

Cytodex (Pharmacia, Piscataway, NJ) microcarriers at a
concentration of 4 grams per liter were seeded with approximately 6×10^4 L-929 cells per ml. Spinner flasks containing
the culture were incubated at $37^{\circ}C$ in a 5% CO_2 atmosphere
until a subconfluent monolayer was present on each bead. A
half-strength modification of Dulbecco's medium (7) with
Earle's salts, 0.1% glucose and 5% fetal calf serum was used
throughout all cell culture procedures unless otherwise specified. The microcarrier culture was infected by the addition
of rickettsiae at a multiplicity of infection of 10 for 60
minutes at $34^{\circ}C$ to a reduced culture volume. The culture was
washed twice with fresh medium to terminate the infection
phase and finally incubated at $34^{\circ}C$ in a 5% CO_2 atmosphere.
Samples of the bead culture were monitored for rickettsial
growth (8) at 2, 24, 48 and 72 hours by centrifuging trypsinized cells onto glass slides (9) and then staining by the
method of Giménez (10).
    Under these conditions 85-95% of the cells contain
rickettsiae at 2 hours post-infection with approximately 4
organisms per infected cell. At 72 hours post-infection, when
there were greater than 50 rickettsiae per infected cell, the
rickettsiae were harvested by disruption of infected cells
(Omni-Mixer, Ivan Sorvall, Norwalk, CT) followed by differential centrifugation to remove the microcarriers and cell

debris. The rickettsiae were subsequently concentrated by
centrifugation at 20,000 x g for 30 minutes and purified on a
Renografin gradient (11).

C. Preparation of ^{3}H-Leucine Labeled Rickettsiae

The incorporation of radiolabeled amino acids into the
polypeptides of rickettsiae was accomplished under conditions
which minimized host-cell utilization of the label. Cycloheximide (1 µg/ml) (3) or emetine (1 µg/ml) was used to inhibit
specifically host-cell protein synthesis when there were
approximately 15 rickettsiae per infected cell. Twenty-four
hours following the addition of the inhibitor, the culture was
washed once and subsequently incubated in leucine-free Dulbecco's medium containing 3% dialyzed fetal calf serum (GIBCO,
Grand Island, NY), fresh inhibitor and 50 µCi/ml ^{3}H-leucine
(Swartz/Mann, Orangeburg NY). The culture was incubated for
an additional 18-24 hours at which time the isotopically
labeled rickettsiae were harvested and purified on Renografin
gradients. This system yielded 1-10 million acid precipitable
counts of purified rickettsiae from a single 25-ml bead
culture.

D. Iodination of R. prowazekii Surface Polypeptides

Surface-specific iodinations of R. prowazekii polypeptides
were catalyzed by 5 µg of 1, 3, 4, 6-tetrachloro - 3 α, 6 α -
diphenylglycoluril (Iodogen, Pierce Chemical Co., Rockford,
IL) plated onto the surface of a glass test tube (12).
Approximately 100 µg dry weight of Renografin purified R.
prowazekii, in 0.1 ml PBS, were added to the reaction vessel,
followed by 125 µCi of carrier-free Na^{125}I (Swartz/Mann). The
reaction was terminated after 10 minutes by transferring the
rickettsiae to another tube containing 25 µmol of carrier NaI
in PBS. The iodinated rickettsiae were concentrated by centrifugation and prepared for 2-D gel electrophoresis as
described below.

E. One and Two Dimensional Gel Electrophoresis

One dimensional PAGE in sodium dodecyl sulphate (SDS) was
conducted as described previously using a discontinuous slab
gel system (13). ^{3}H-labeled rickettsial preparations were

solubilized with hot sample buffer (13), placed in boiling
water for 2 minutes, and electrophoresed at constant voltage
(100 volts) for 14 hours.

[3]H-labeled R. prowazekii polypeptides to be separated by
2-D gel electrophoresis using a procedure modified from
O'Farrell (14) were solubilized at 4°C with 2% Triton X-100, 8
M urea, 2% ampholytes pH range 3-10 (Pharmacia, Piskataway,
NJ) and 5% beta-mercaptoethanol. The polypeptides were first
resolved according to isoelectric point on a flatbed polyacrylamide gel consisting of 5% acrylamide cross-linked with
bis-acrylamide, 2% Triton X-100, 8 M urea and 2.5% ampho-
lyte. Twenty-five watts constant power was applied for three
hours at 6°C, after which a surface electrode (Ingold
Electrodes Inc., Lexington, MA) was used to determine the pH
gradient (3.9-10). Individual sample tracts were prepared for
the second dimension according to O'Farrell (14). The second-
dimension gel was a discontinuous gradient slab gel composed
of 9-18% acrylamide cross-linked with N, N'-
diallytartardiamide. After electrophoresis, the gels were
fixed in 20% trichloroacetic acid and prepared for fluorography according to the procedure of Bonner and Laskey (15).

III.   RESULTS

A.   Polypeptide Analysis of R. prowazekii strains by PAGE

The polypeptides of five R. prowazekii strains metabolically labeled with ^{3}H-leucine are shown in Figure 1. Six
major polypeptides (3) of R. prowazekii are apparent as are
approximately 40 minor polypeptides. Identical polypeptide
profiles are present in the Breinl, Burundi and flying
squirrel strains. The E strain of R. prowazekii has a single
but reproducible major difference in its polypeptide profile
that has been resolved by the TRIS-SDS slab gel system employed. The #4 polypeptide, which is the major surface
protein (16, 17), migrates slightly faster than the #4 polypeptide of other R. prowazekii strains. Identification of the
E strain based on this major polypeptide difference can also
be accomplished by PAGE analysis of unlabeled rickettsiae
grown in either yolk sacs or in L-cells. The ability to
detect the E strain's characteristic polypeptide #4, while
other investigators have not been able to (4), is most likely
due to the increased resolution of the TRIS-SDS slab gels used
in these studies.

B. Polypeptide Analysis of R. prowazekii strains by
    2-D Gel Electrophoresis

Figure 2 is a 2-D gel fluorograph of the Burundi X-16
strain of R. prowazekii, which clearly shows separation of the
major typhus polypeptides. A one dimensional polypeptide profile of R. prowazekii (Burundi X-16) run in parallel is on the
extreme left side of the gel. This allows orientation and
identification of the polypeptides in the 2-D pattern. In
addition, specific identification of the #1 and #4 polypeptides was accomplished by 2-D analysis of rickettsial polypeptides iodinated by a surface specific reaction catalyzed by
Iodogen. The #1 and #4 polypeptides are predominantly labeled
by this technique and are readily identified on the 2-D
fingerprint, seen in Figure 3.

Although approximately 175 separate polypeptides were
revealed on longer exposures, close analysis of the 2-D
fingerprints indicates that the majority of ^{3}H-labeled polypeptides are similar for the Breinl, Burundi, and flying
squirrel strains. However, some polypeptides were found to be
unique for a particular strain. For example, the flying
squirrel strain has a polypeptide spot (gel not shown) at pH
7.2 and molecular weight 55,000 which is not found in the
other strains.

Analysis of 2-D polypeptide profiles of the virulent
Breinl (Fig. 4A) and attenuated E (Fig. 4B) strains of R.
prowazekii revealed several polypeptide differences.
Polypeptide spots B and C (Fig. 4A) are found only in the
Breinl strain, Burundi strains, and the flying squirrel
strain. Unique polypeptides of the avirulent E strain are
labeled D and E in Figure 4B. Also of interest is the
abundance of unresolved polypeptides in the E strain 2-D
gel. This might reflect an entire series of proteins with
very low isoelectric points or special properties of the E
strain proteins which render them insoluble in the first
dimensional electrophoresis under the conditions employed.

In the region of polypeptides 3 and 4, the large
horizontal tract indicates that these macromolecules have
charge heterogeneity. Carbamylation is an unlikely cause of
this effect since a "train" of spots is not evident, nor are
these basic proteins (18). The most likely explanation for
this unresolved material is carbohydrate association as
reported by Osterman and Eisemann (16).

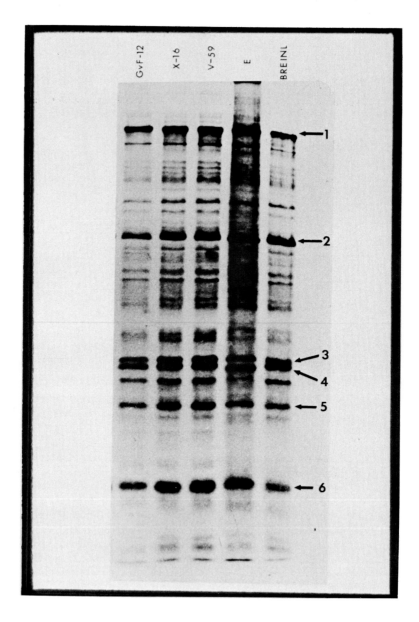

Fig. 1. Fluorograph of a discontinuous SDS-polyacrylamide
slab gel of the polypeptides from five R. prowazekii
strains. Approximately 50,000 acid precipitable counts of
each sample were applied to this gel. The six major
polypeptides are noted.

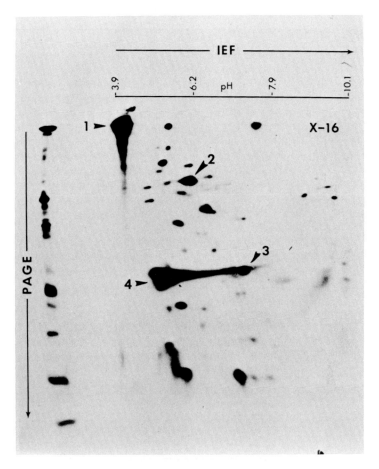

Fig. 2. 2D gel of R. prowazekii strain X-16 polypeptides. The major typhus polypeptides are identified on this 2
week exposure. A one-dimensional separation of the X-16
polypeptides is on the extreme left of the SDS-polyacrylamide
gel. The pH readings were determined at the end of the
electrofocusing run with a surface electrode.

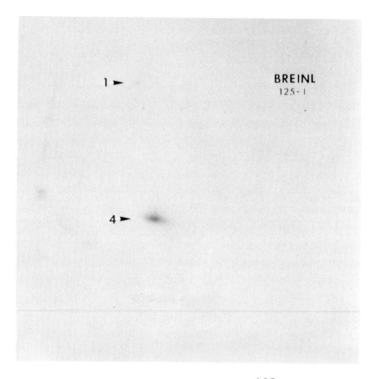

Fig. 3.   2-D gel electrophoresis of ^{125}I-labeled
polypeptides of R. prowazekii (Breinl strain). Polypeptides
#'s 1 and 4, which are predominantly labeled by the surface
specific iodination, are readily identified on this 2-D
fingerprint.

IV. DISCUSSION

    The growth of R. prowazekii in a microcarrier bead cell
culture system has allowed the production of a large quantity
of radiolabeled, purified rickettsiae with minimal cell culture reagents and equipment. Analysis of the labeled rickettsial proteins by 2-D gel electrophoresis resolved approximately 175 polypeptide species and has allowed the isoelectric
point determinations of specific polypeptides (see Table 1).
    The Breinl, Burundi and flying squirrel strains of epi-
demic typhus all show striking similarities by 2-D gel electrophoresis despite different sources of isolation and passage
histories. More importantly, the demonstration of differences

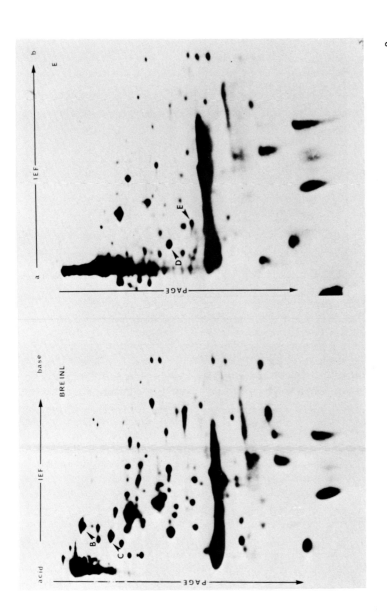

Fig. 4. 2-D gels of the Breinl and E strain run in parallel. Solubilized ³H-labeled rickettsial polypeptides for both strains were run on the same flatbed isoelectric focusing gel and in parallel in the 2nd dimension. Polypeptides B and C are unique to the virulent typhus strains, as are polypeptides D & E unique to the E strain.

in the polypeptides of the E strain, when compared to the
virulent strains, has been accomplished with the increased
resolution of the procedures used. In fact, positive identification of the E strain is now possible by SDS-PAGE. The
major polypeptide difference of the E strain is the lower
molecular weight polypeptide #4.

TABLE 1. Molecular Weights and Isoelectric Points of
Major R. prowazekii Polypeptides

POLYPEPTIDE	MOLECULAR WEIGHT[a]	ISOELECTRIC POINT[b]
1	138,000	4.1
2	64,500	5.9
3	32,000	7.3
4	31,000	5.0
5	24,000	N.D.[c]
6	15,000	N.D.

[a] = molecular weight determined by SDS-PAGE in 13% acrylamide
gels.
[b] = isoelectric points determined on flatbed analytical
isoelectric focusing gels with pH range of 3.9 - 10.
[c] = not determined.

Previous studies have attempted to find a clear difference
between the attenuated E strain and virulent strains of R.
prowazekii. Biochemical criteria, such as DNA homology (6),
specific enzymatic activities (4), and antigenic analysis (19)
have not revealed any marked differences. Only by isoelectric
focusing have minor polypeptides been shown to be characteristic of a particular epidemic typhus strain (4). Biological
phenomena, such as mouse toxicity (20), sheep erythrocyte
hemolysis (21), and plaque size (21), cannot distinguish the E
strain from the virulent Breinl strain. However, the ability
of the E strain to cause only mild disease in humans (22) and
its inability to survive in human macrophages in vitro (23)
clearly sets it apart from the virulent strains. The latter
two properties probably involve direct interactions between
the surfaces of the rickettsiae and the host. Surface structures, such as outer membrane proteins, which can differentiate between a virulent (Breinl) and attenuated (E) rickettsiae
would be likely candidates as the basis for attenuation.
Polypeptide #4 is one outer membrane protein that can clearly

distinguish the E strain from the virulent epidemic typhus
strains. The specific function of this major surface protein
of R. prowazekii and its role in virulence, immunogenicity,
toxicity, and other biological properties of rickettsiae
remain to be evaluated.

REFERENCES

1. Pedersen, C.E., Jr. and Walters, V.D., Life Sci. 22:583
    (1978).
2. Obijeski, J.F., Palmer, E.L. and Tzianabos, T.,
    Microbios. 11:61 (1974).
3. Eisemann, C.S. and Osterman, J.V., Infect. Immun. 14:155
    (1976).
4. Dasch, G.A., Samms, J.R. and Weiss, E., Infect. Immun.
    19:676 (1978).
5. Anacker, R.L., McCaul, T.F., Burgdorfer, W. and Gerloff,
    R.K., Infect. Immun. 27:468 (1980).
6. Myers, W.F. and Wisseman, C.L. Jr., Int. J. Syst.
    Bacteriol. 30:143 (1980).
7. Smith, J.D., Freeman, G., Vogt, M. and Dulbecco, R.,
    Virology 12:185, (1960).
8. Wisseman, C.L. Jr. and Waddell, A.D., Infect. Immun.
    11:1391 (1975).
9. Wisseman, C.L. Jr., Waddell, A.D. and Silverman, D.J.,
    Infect. Immun. 13:1749 (1976).
10. Gimenez, D.F., Stain Technol. 39:135 (1965).
11. Weiss, E., Coolbaugh, J.C. and Williams, J.C., Appl.
    Microbiol. 30:456 (1975).
12. Markwell, M.A. and Fox, C.F., Biochem. 17:4807 (1978).
13. Myers, W.F., Wisseman, C.L. Jr., Fiset, P., Oaks, E.V.
    and Smith, J.F., Infect. Immun. 26:976 (1979).
14. O'Farrell, P.H., J. Biol. Chem. 250:4007 (1975).
15. Bonner, W.M. and Laskey, R.A. Eur. J. Biochem. 46:83
    (1974).
16. Osterman, J.V. and Eisemann, C.S., Infect. Immun. 21:866
    (1978).
17. Smith, D.K. and Winkler, H.H., Infect. Immun. 29:831
    (1980).
18. Anderson, N.L. and Hickman, B.J., Anal. Biochem. 93:312
    (1979).
19. Bozeman, F.M., Masiello, S.A., Williams, M.S. and
    Elisberg, B.L., Nature (London) 255:545 (1975).
20. Perez Gallardo, F. and Fox, J.P., Am. J. Hyg. 48:6
    (1948).

21. Woodman, D.R., Weiss, E., Dasch, G.A., Bozeman, F.M., Infect. Immun. 16:853 (1977).
22. Fox, J.P., Amer. J. Pub. Health 45:1036 (1955).
23. Gambrill, M.R. and Wisseman, C.L. Jr., Infect. Immun. 8:519 (1973).

IODINATION OF <u>COXIELLA</u> <u>BURNETII</u> CELLS:
OPTIMAL CONDITIONS FOR THE IODINATION
OF EXPOSED SURFACE PROTEINS

Jim C. Williams

Laboratory of Microbial Structure and Function
Rocky Mountain Laboratories
Hamilton, Montana

I.   INTRODUCTION

The developmental cycle of <u>Coxiella</u> <u>burnetii</u>, the etio-
ogic agent of Q fever, consists of vegetative and sporogenic
differentiations during the intraphagolysosomal multiplication
of this Gram-variable bacterium (1). At least two morphological cell types, a large and small cell variant (LCV, SCV),
have been demonstrated (1). The cell wall of the SCV is
clearly different from the LCV (1, 2). However, both cells
are morphologically similar in that each possesses a cytoplasmic membrane(s), a peptidoglycan region and a limiting
outer membrane (2). Biochemically, muramic acid (3) and
diaminopimelic acid (DAP) (4) have been detected in the cell
walls of <u>C. burnetii</u> although the concentration of DAP was
lower than reported for Gram-negative bacteria (4). Lipopolysaccharide isolated from <u>C. burnetii</u> is similar in properties
to that of Gram-negative bacteria (5, 6). Although the amino
acid composition of cell walls has been investigated (3), no
reports have appeared on the surface proteins of <u>C. burnetii</u>.
Therefore, the many and unique functions of the outer membrane
of <u>C. burnetii</u> have prompted an investigation into the
membrane proteins associated with the cell wall.
    In this study the vectorial arrangement of the outer
membrane proteins of <u>C. burnetii</u> was investigated in a heterogenous population of large and small cell variants. Therefore, the optimal condition of labeling surface proteins by

the lactoperoxidase (LPOase)-catalyzed iodination of tyrosine
and histidine residues of proteins (7) was sought.

II. MATERIALS AND METHODS

A. Iodination Procedure

C. burnetii (9 Mile and Ohio Phase I strains) cells were
purified from the yolk sacs of fertile hens' eggs as previously described (8). Cells were extrinsically iodinated at room
temperature (20–22°C) with ^{125}I (carrier-free ^{125}I, 17 Ci/mg;
New England Nuclear, Boston, Mass.) as follows (7): i) C.
burnetii were purified while employing phosphate-buffered
saline sucrose (PBSS) as the diluent at pH 7.35 (8). Cells
were suspended in PBSS at the desired concentration employing
a standard curve which converts Klett units (A_{420}) to mg dry
weight, and direct rickettsial counts as previously described
(12, i.e., 3.78 X 10^{10} organisms = 1 mg dry weight of whole
cells). ii) The reaction mixture contained the following
components in a 2-ml volume: ^{125}I, ranging from 0.2 to 1.0
µCi per ml; KI, ranging from 0.05 to 30.05 µM; lactoperoxidase
(LPOase, Sigma Chemical Co., St. Louis, Mo.), ranging from 0
to 200 µg per ml; C. burnetii cells ranging from 0.5 to 4 mg
per ml; and H_2O_2. iii) Vectorial labeling was initiated by
adding 5 µl of 0.015% H_2O_2 (Matheson Coleman and Bell Manu-
facturing Chemists, Norwood, Ohio) per ml of reaction mixture
at time zero. Two more additions of H_2O_2 were made at 5 min
intervals. During the reaction the suspension was gently
shaken to keep the cells evenly suspended. The reaction was
terminated by diluting the suspensions with 20 ml of PBSS
at room temperature. Cells were then washed two times with
PBSS at 4°C by centrifugation at 12,100 x g for 30 min. The
final cell pellet was suspended in 2 ml of PBSS and 0.5 ml
aliquots were centrifuged in 1.5 ml Microfuge B tubes. The
supernatant was decanted and the pellet was frozen at -20°C.
Non-specific labeling of C. burnetii cells was monitored
in control reaction mixtures by deleting LPOase and/or H_2O_2.
Specific labeling was carried out in experiments designed to
determine the optimal KI and enzyme concentrations.

B. Analysis of Iodinated Surface Proteins of C. burnetii

Proteins of whole cell lysates were separated by polyacrylamide gel electrophoresis (PAGE) (12.5%) by slight modification of the method described by Laemmli (9) employing a

vertical slab apparatus (Model 221, BioRad Laboratories, Calif.). Molecular weight determinations were made by incorporating [^{14}C] methylated protein mixture (Amersham Corp., Arlington Heights, Ill.) ranging from 200,000 to 14,300 daltons into the polyacrylamide gel slab (10). Autoradiography was carried out by exposing dried gel slabs to XR-2 film (X-Omat R film, Kodak) for 24 to 48 hr. Processed film was scanned with a microdensitometer 3CS (Joyce-Loebl Division, Vicker Instruments, Inc., Mass.).

Labeled cells were fractionated in CHCl$_3$, methanol and NaCl (CMN) and 8.8% trichloroacetic acid (TCA) treatments as follows: i) Two hundred and fifty µl of cell suspension was added to a CMN solution containing 800 µl of CHCl$_3$, 400 µl of MeOH and 100 µl of 0.45 M NaCl in a glass screw-capped tube with a teflon-lined cap. The suspension was extracted overnight at 45°C and then centrifuged 480 x $\underline{g}$ for 20 min. The upper phase of MeOH, H$_2$O and NaCl was separated from the CHCl$_3$, and the distribution of radioactivity was determined. ii) TCA fractionation was carried out by adding 250 µl of sample to 200 µl of 20% TCA at room temperature. The sample was mixed with a vortex mixer and allowed to stand at room temperature for 50 min. The precipitate was pelleted in a Microfuge B for 5 min. The supernatant fraction (S1) was decanted and the pellet was washed with 400 µl of 10% TCA. After the second centrifugation the supernatant (S2) was decanted and the pellet (P2) was resuspended in 250 µl of sterile demineralized and distilled H$_2$O. The distribution of radioactivity was determined in the three samples.

III. RESULTS

A. Chemical Fractionation of ^{125}I-labeled $\underline{C}$. $\underline{burnetii}$

The distribution of radioactivity in TCA fractions S1, S2 and P2 were 35%, 3% and 62%, respectively. When ^{125}I-labeled whole cells of $\underline{C}$. $\underline{burnetii}$ were partitioned in CMN, 83% of the radioactivity was found in the methanol, water and NaCl phase, whereas 18% appeared in the CHCl$_3$ phase. A comparison of these fractions on SDS-PAGE indicated that all of the labeled components were in the methanol, water and NaCl phase.

B. Effect of Suspending Medium and KI Concentration on LPOase-Catalyzed Iodination of Surface Proteins of $\underline{C}$. $\underline{burnetii}$

$\underline{C}$. $\underline{burnetii}$ were suspended in PBSS or PBS and labeled with ^{125}I$^-$ in the respective diluents containing 1 mg of cells per

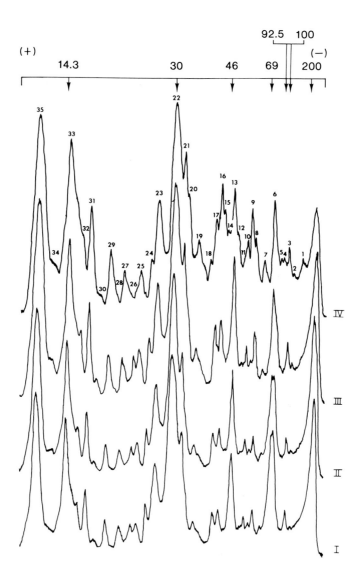

Fig. 1. Electropherogram of ^{125}I-labeled surface components of <u>Coxiella</u> <u>burnetii</u> employing phosphate-buffered
saline as diluent. I, II, III and IV are scans of autoradiographs of whole cells labeled in the presence of 0.05, 0.35,
3.05 and 30.05 µM KI, respectively. Molecular weight markers
are indicated at the top and should be multiplied by 10^3
daltons. Proteins are numbered 1 through 35.

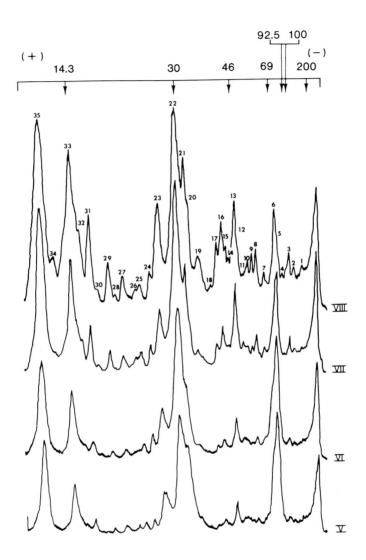

Fig. 2. Electropherogram of ^{125}I-labeled surface components of <u>Coxiella burnetii</u> employing phosphate-buffered saline plus 0.25 M sucrose as diluent. V, VI, VII and VIII are scans of autoradiographs of whole cells labeled in the presence of 0.05, 0.35, 3.05 and 30.05 µM KI, respectively. Molecular weight markers are indicated at the top and should be multiplied by 10^3 daltons. Proteins are numbered 1 through 35.

ml of reaction mixture, variable concentrations of KI ranging from 0.05 to 30.05 µM, and LPOase at 200 µg per ml of reaction mixture. At least 35 proteins were labeled with ^{125}I under these conditions (Fig. 1 and 2). The suspending medium and KI concentrations markedly influenced the number and intensity of proteins labeled with ^{125}I as determined from the intensity (or peak height) of each band on the XR-2 film, the KI concentration and diluent employed in the reaction mixture.

C. Effect of Changing Concentrations of KI, LPOase and H_2O_2 on Iodination of Surface Proteins of C. burnetii

Changing concentrations of unlabeled KI relative to the amount of ^{125}I greatly affected the efficiency of labeling of C. burnetii (Table I). Increasing the concentration of unlabeled KI from 0.05 to 0.35 µM increased the efficiency of labeling the whole cells (Table 1, cf tube No. 1 and 2). Whereas, increasing the concentration of unlabeled KI to 3.05 and 30.05 µM caused a decrease in radioactivity associated with the whole cells (Table 1, cf tube No. 3 and 4). This decrease in radioactivity paralleled the decrease in specific activity of the isotope and was expected since the efficiency of LPOase activity is enhanced with an increase in substrate

TABLE 1. Radioiodination of Viable C. burnetii Whole Cells

Tube No.	[KI], µM	LPOase (µg/ml)	H_2O_2	CPM/10 µl
		Components of the reaction mixture[a]		
1	0.05	200	+	39,030
2	0.35	200	+	55,672
3	3.05	200	+	24,200
4	30.05	200	+	3,443
5	3.05	0	+	523
6	3.05	2	+	20,220
7	3.05	20	+	24,421
8	3.05	200	+	24,040
9	3.05	200	−	3,974

[a]3.2 mg cells per ml reaction mixture.

concentration. More important, as the amount of KI was increased, there was an increase in the number of proteins
labeled by [125]I (Fig. 2, compare V, VI, VII and VIII). In
the absence of LPOase (Table 1, tube No. 5) no ^{125}I-labeled
component could be identified on SDS-PAGE (data not shown).
The concentration of LPOase required to label the exposed
protein was as little as 2 µg per ml (Table 1, tube numbers
6, 7, 8) in a reaction mixture with 3.2 mg of C. burnetii per
ml. In the absence of added H_2O_2, at least five proteins on
the cell surface were labeled (Table 1, tube No. 9, protein
profiles not shown).

D.   Standard Conditions for LPOase-Catalyzed [125]I Labeling of C. burnetii

The optimal conditions for labeling the exposed membrane
components of C. burnetii were arrived at by considering the
above results. In separate studies the optimal range of cells
was determined to be between 1-4 mg per ml of reaction mixture; whereas, the concentrations of KI, LPOase and H_2O_2 were
3.05 µM, 200 µg per ml and 0.225 X 10^{-3}% H_2O_2, respectively.
In the standard procedure the reaction was initiated at 20 to
22°C by adding 5 µl of 0.015% H_2O_2 per ml of reaction mixture
at t_0. Two more additions of H_2O_2 were carried out at t_5 and
t_{10} min. At t_{15} min, the reaction was terminated by diluting
the suspension 10-fold with PBSS. The cells were washed two
times with PBSS and cell pellets were frozen at -20°C.

IV.   DISCUSSION

The optimal conditions for labeling the surface proteins
of C. burnetii with ^{125}I by the LPOase method (7) have been
investigated. Since C. burnetii used in these experiments
were composed of a heterogenous population of LCV and SCV (1,
8), it is conceivable that both cell variants are labeled by
these procedures. Thus, the suspending medium for the purified organisms should maintain the morphological integrity of
each cell variant thereby assuring homogenous ^{125}I labeling
of surface proteins. Previous studies (8) have shown that
PBSS is preferred as a diluent during the purification of
viable C. burnetii from host components. PBSS induces slight
plasmolysis of the LCV, whereas the SCV was apparently not
affected (1, 8). Thus, surface labeling of C. burnetii cells
might be expected to be different for each of the cell
variants. Indeed, the cell walls of the LCV and SCV have

been shown to be different by ultrastructural analysis (2).
Differences between the surface proteins of the cell variants
are not known; therefore, the studies described herein are
representative of a mixed population of the two cell variants.

This study demonstrated that, at least, 35 surface pro-
teins were radioiodinated by the LPOase technique. Vectorial
iodination of the surface proteins was shown to be specific.
The radioactivity that was extracted into the $CHCl_3$ phase of
the CMN partition did not contain detectable proteins on SDS-
PAGE analysis. Also, components that were fractionated with
TCA into acid-soluble and acid-insoluble proteins showed SDS-
PAGE profiles similar to untreated whole cells.

Marked differences in intensity of bands on electropherograms were dependent upon the diluent and KI concentrations.
Plasmolysis of C. burnetii suspended in PBSS apparently buried
some proteins so that at low iodide concentrations (0.05 and
0.35 µM) these proteins were moderately labeled, whereas at
high iodide concentrations (3.05 and 30.05 µM) the proteins
were labeled more intensely, and in some cases new proteins
were radiolabeled. These data and the results of other investigations (11-18) suggest that the surface proteins were
labeled according to their i) accessibility, ii) relative
concentrations of tyrosine and/or histidine and iii) concentration of each protein on the surface of the cell. Therefore, a topographical relationship of the surface proteins
was estimated from the intensity of label on electropherograms,
thus separating the proteins into three classes (Fig. 1 and
2). Class I. Principal surface proteins (PSP) were highly
labeled at any concentration of iodide tested in either
diluent. These proteins are considered to be the most peripherally located. PSP were also the most concentrated as
determined by protein stained gels of whole cells (unpublished
results). Class II. Intermediate surface proteins (ISP)
were either embedded proteins or contained a low amount of
tyrosine and/or histidine residues. ISP were labeled with
increasing intensity which corresponded to the increase in
iodide concentration. The diluent also affects the labeling
profiles of ISP. For example, these proteins were more
efficiently labeled in PBS diluent, whereas upon increasing
the iodide concentration, the proteins were equally labeled.
Class III. Minor surface proteins (MSP) were poorly labeled
and apparently the least accessible as demonstrated by the
requirement for high iodide concentrations. Also, MSP
appeared to be buried since cells suspended in PBS were more
readily labeled than cells suspended in PBSS at low iodide
concentrations.

Surface proteins probably play dominant roles in the mosiac of antigenic determinants prominent on particular cells. The role of these components as antigenic components, in immunological recognition, as factors in the host-parasite interaction (i.e., complementary surface structures), as mediators of metabolic events and as virulence factors are not understood for Phase I C. burnetii. Phase II C. burnetii, which is generated by repeated passage in embryonated eggs (19), is a spontaneous mutant of C. burnetii, and it is not virulent for guinea pigs and mice. Preliminary studies employing Phase II C. burnetii have shown that this avirulent strain has retained only a few of the surface proteins of Phase I cells. Therefore, a comparison of the surface proteins of these two phases of the same strain of C. burnetii may lead to a better understanding of bacterial virulence.

V.   SUMMARY

A long range objective is the characterization of the membrane components unique to Coxiella burnetii cells. Iodination of C. burnetii cells was catalyzed in a mixture containing lactoperoxidase, iodide, phosphate-buffered saline (pH 7.3), sucrose, carrier-free ^{125}I, cells and H_2O_2. Vectorial labeling of membrane proteins was extensive over a KI concentration range from 0.05 to 30.05 μM. The optimal KI concentration was 3.05 μM at a cell concentration ranging from 1 to 4 mg dry weight per ml of reaction mixture. Cells were not labeled in the absence of lactoperoxidase, whereas some vectorial iodination occurred in the absence of added H_2O_2. Iodinated components were resolved by SDS-polyacrylamide gel electrophoresis into at least 35 components ranging in molecular weights from 150,000 to 11,800 daltons. At least eight principal surface proteins were observed, whereas numerous intermediate and minor proteins were noted. Vectorial labeling of several proteins by this technique indicates that the surface of C. burnetii cells is highly complex. An analysis of these surface components will help elucidate the nature of the interaction between C. burnetii, the host cell, and the immunologic apparatus of the infected host.

ACKNOWLEDGMENTS

The technical assistance of S. Stewart and the expert secretarial preparation of S. Smaus are gratefully acknowledged.

REFERENCES

1. McCaul, T. F., and Williams, J. C., J. Bact. (submitted).
2. McCaul, T. F., Hackstadt, T., and Williams, J. C., in
    "Rickettsiae and Rickettsial Diseases" (W. Burgdorfer and
    R. L. Anacker, eds.), p.   . Academic Press, New York,
    (1981).
3. Jerrells, J. R., Henrichs, D. J., and Mallavia, L. P.,
    Can. J. Microbiol. 20, 1465 (1974).
4. Myers, W. F., Ormsbee, R. A., Osterman, J. V., and
    Wisseman, C. L. Jr., Proc. Soc. Exp. Biol. Med. 125,
    459 (1967).
5. Baca, O. G., and Paretsky, D., Infect. Immun. 9, 939
    (1974).
6. Baca, O. G., and Paretsky, D., Infect. Immun. 9, 959
    (1974).
7. Morrison, M., in "Methods in Enzymology" (S. P. Colowick
    and N. O. Kaplan, eds.), Vol. XXXII, p. 103. Academic
    Press, New York, (1974).
8. Williams, J. C., Peacock, M. G., and McCaul, T. F.,
    Infect. Immun. (in press).
9. Laemmli, U. K., Nature 227, 680 (1970).
10. Swank, R. T., and Munkres, K. D., Anal. Biochem. 39,
    462 (1971).
11. Osterman, J. V., and Eisemann, C. S., Infect. Immun. 21,
    866 (1978).
12. Marchalonis, J. J., Cone, R. E., and Santer, V., Biochem.
    J. 124, 921 (1971).
13. Stanley, P., and Haslam, E. A., Virology 46, 764 (1971).
14. Sefton, B. M., Wickus, G. G., Burge, B. W., J. Virol.
    11, 730 (1973).
15. Moore, N. F., Kelley, J. M., and Wagner, R. R., Virology
    61, 292 (1974).
16. Tsai, C. M., Huang, C. C., and Canellakei, E. S.,
    Biochim. Biophys. Acta 332, 47 (1973).
17. Huang, C. C., Tsai, C. M., and Canellakei, E. S.,
    Biochim. Biophys. Acta 332, 59 (1973).
18. Morrison, M., and Bayse, G. S., Biochem. 9, 2995 (1970).
19. Stoker, M. G. P., and Fiset, P., Can. J. Microbiol. 2,
    310 (1956).

SEPARATION AND CHARACTERIZATION OF INNER
AND OUTER MEMBRANES OF THE PIERCE'S
DISEASE RICKETTSIA-LIKE BACTERIUM.[1]

William E. Kuriger
Norman W. Schaad

Department of Plant Pathology
University of Georgia
Georgia Experiment Station
Experiment, Georgia

I. INTRODUCTION

With the advent of culture media for the growth of some
plant rickettsia-like bacteria (RLB) (1), much can be learned
about the biochemistry and physiology of this group of plant
pathogens. Pierce's disease RLB, the causal agent of
Pierce's disease of grapes, alfalfa dwarf of alfalfa and
almond leaf scorch, is a gram-negative organism that is
catalase and oxidase positive (2) and which can use succinate
and citrate for growth, but not glucose (2). The outer
membrane (OM) of Pierce's disease RLB contains folds, or
ripples, which provide it with a distinct morphological
appearance (3). As viewed in sectioned material, the IM and
OM are separated by a periplasmic space, and both appear to
be of unit construction (3).
The IM and OM of Rickettsia prowazeki have been described
(4), and a comparison with those of gram-negative bacteria
presented. The OM of R. prowazeki was found to contain
2-Keto-3-deoxyoctonic acid (KDO) characteristic of other
gram-negative bacteria (5) (6). The structure of OM
preparations was found to resemble that of E. coli (7, 8) and

[1]Supported in part by USDA/SEA Competitive Grant
#5901-0410-9-0259-0 and Hatch 1228.

Salmonella (9). Like other gram-negative bacteria, succinate
dehydrogenase activity was associated with IM of R.
prowazeki, also. A unique characteristic of the membranes
of R. prowazeki was a molecular weight range of 20 to 130
Kdal for major proteins of the OM. However, no information
is available on the structure and functional properties of
membranes of a plant RLB.

    In an attempt to characterize the IM and OM of Pierce's
disease RLB, we separated membranes by a modified method of
Hancock and Nikaido (10). Linear 52-70% sucrose density
gradient centrifugation resulted in four bands, one light (L),
one intermediate (M), and two heavy (H_1 and H_2). SDH and KDO
analysis suggested the presence of IM in band L and OM in
bands H_1 and H_2. Band M contained a mixture of IM and OM.
Electron micrographs revealed a close similarity between
membranes of Pierce's disease bacterium and membranes of
other gram-negative bacteria, including R. prowazeki. On the
other hand, SDS-PAGE profiles of membranes of Pierce's disease
organism were much different from those of R. prowazeki.

II. MATERIAL AND METHODS

A. Culture and Growth of Pierce's Disease RLB

    Pierce's disease RLB, strain VP-5, originally isolated
from a grape vine in California was obtained from M. Davis
(Rutgers University, New Brunswick, NJ 08900). A culture was
maintained by weekly transfer to agar plates of PD 3 medium
(1), supplemented with potato starch instead of bovine serum
albumin. A liquid culture grown for 6-7 days at 28C was
used to seed 1.5 1 of PD 3 medium in 2.8 liter Fernbach
flasks. After 7-10 days growth on a rotary shaker at 28C,
cells were harvested by centrifugation at 12,100 x g for 20
minutes. Cells were resuspended in 10 mM N-2-hydroxyethyl
piperazine-N-2-ethanesulfonic acid, 2 mM ethylene-diamine
tetraacetic acid, pH 7.4 (HEPES-EDTA) and either used
immediately or stored frozen at -20C.

B. Membrane Isolation

    In initial experiments the methods of Smith and Winkler
were followed (4). Briefly, cells at a concentration of 1 gm
cell/20 ml HEPES-EDTA were broken in a French pressure cell
at 20,000 lb/in^2. Two passages through the pressure cell
were used. Whole cells were removed by centrifugation at

3,020 x g for 10 min and envelopes were obtained by
centrifugation for 3 h at 180,000 x g. The resulting pellets
from the second high speed centrifugation were homogenized in
HEPES-EDTA. 1 ml fractions (4-10 mg/ml protein) were layered
onto 41-55% or 41-70% step sucrose gradients and centrifuged
at 120,000 x g for 18 h at 4C.

Our modification of the above method, similar to the
method of Hancock and Nikaido (10), is as follows: to cells
suspended as above, 35 units each of DNase and RNase per ml
are added. After passage through a French pressure cell as
above, unbroken cells are removed by centrifuging at 12,100
x g for 10 minutes, and the supernatant fraction centrifuged
for 1 h at 195,000 x g to pellet envelopes. The envelopes
are suspended in HEPES-EDTA with a glass homogenizer and a
pasteur pipette. Protein concentrations are determined and
0.5 to 1.0 ml of envelopes containing 4-10 mg protein/ml
buffer layered onto 52, 58, 64, and 70% linear sucrose
gradients which are centrifuged at 120,000 x g for 18 h at 4C.

Gradient fractions (1.5 ml) or entire peaks are collected
using an ISCO gradient fraction collector, Model UA-5
monitor at 280 nm, and model 568 fraction collector.
Material from each band is pooled and dialysed at 4C for 24 h
with three to four changes of HEPES-EDTA. Membranes are
collected from dialyzed fractions by ultra filtration on
PM-30 membranes (Amicon, Danvers, MA 01923) or by centrifuging
at 195,000 x g for 1 h. Preparations were stored at -20C or
used fresh. For enzyme assays, unfrozen samples were
concentrated by high speed centrifugation and washed once
with HEPES-EDTA buffer. Densities of fractions were
estimated by measuring the sucrose concentration with a
Bausch & Lomb refractometer at 20C on 1 ml fractions of a
typical gradient.

C. Chemical and Enzyme Assays

Protein was determined by the method of Lowry (5).
Succinate dehydrogenase (SDH) activity was assayed by the
method of Kasahara and Amaku (11). Reaction mixtures
contained 50 mM Tris (tris(hydroxymethylaminomethane))-HCl
buffer pH 8.0, 4 mM KCN, 0.04 mM 2,6 dichlorophenol-indophenol
(DCPIP), 0.2 mM phenazine methosulfate, 30 mM potassium
succinate, and 100-200 μg membrane protein. Total volume was
3 ml. The 2-Keto-deoxyoctonic acid (KDO) content was
estimated by the thiobarbituric acid method (12). Each sample
was adjusted to contain approximately 200 μg membrane protein.
After the final reaction step, reactants were centrifuged at
5,090 x g for 10 minutes and chromogen extracted with an equal

volume of butanol acidified with 5% concentrated HCl (13).
Absorbance was measured at 552 and 508 nm to determine the
presence of residual sucrose (9). Concentration of KDO was
determined from a standard curve, or by using the micromolar
extinction coefficient of 19 (14).

D. SDS-Polyacrylamide Gel Electrophoresis
(SDS-PAGE)

SDS-PAGE was performed in vertical slab gels with a
Bio-Rad model 221 electrophoresis apparatus with the
discontinuous system of Laemmli (15). Stacking and separation
gels contained 3 and 10% acrylamide, respectively. Samples
were solubilized in sample buffer at 100 C for exactly 2 min.
Twenty µl of sample containing 800 µg protein/ml was applied
to each sample well and electrophoresis was performed at a
constant current of 12.5 ma for 3 to 3.5 h for a distance of
10 cm. Molecular weights were determined using a Bio-Rad low
molecular weight protein standard solution. The gels were
fixed in 5% TCA overnight and stained in pre-filtered 0.05%
coomassie blue R in methanol-acetic acid water (5:1:4) for 2 h
at room temperature.

E. Electron Microscopy

Preparations from gradient peaks were deposited on
parlodion-coated grids and stained with 2% aqueous uranyl
acetate for 2 minutes. Samples for sectioning were centrifuged at 195,000 x g for 1 h in Spinco type 40 polycarbonate
centrifuge tubes. The pelleted membranes were then fixed in
4% glutaraldehyde for 15 h, washed, and post-fixed in 2%
osmium tetroxide. The pellets were removed from the
centrifuge tubes, dehydrated in an alcohol series, and
embedded in Spurr's medium (6). Thin sections (silver to
gold) were stained in 2% aqueous uranyl acetate and 1% lead
citrate, and viewed under a Phillips 200 electron microscope
operated at 80 kV.

III. RESULTS

A. Sucrose Density Gradient Centrifugation

Initial attempts to separate inner and outer membranes
(OM) by using a 40-55% linear sucrose gradient following the
methods of Smith and Winkler (4) were unsuccessful. Most

membrane material sedimented to the bottom of the tubes under
these conditions. With a 40-70% linear sucrose gradient,
three major bands resulted, however, they were not well
separated, especially the two heavier bands. Chemical
analysis showed that each band contained moderate amounts of
SDH and KDO, suggesting an inadequate separation of IM and
OM. The use of DNase and RNase during membrane extraction
and a linear sucrose gradient of 52-70% resulted in four
major bands (Fig. 1). This method was deemed useful in the

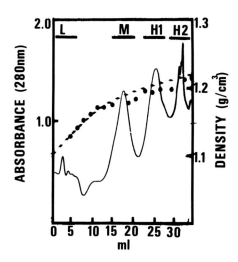

Fig. 1.   Separation of membranes of Pierce's disease
bacterium on 52-70% linear sucrose density gradients.
Gradients were centrifuged at 120,000 x g for 18 h at 4C.
Fractionation was monitored at 280 nm using a ISCO model
UA-5 absorbance monitor.   Densities on 1 ml fractions
measured with refractometer at 20C.

separation of membranes. The densities of bands L, M, H_1 and H_2 were 1.122, 1.179, 1.191 and 1.214 gm/cm^3, respectively (Table 1).

Analysis of the bands indicated that separation of IM and OM had been successful. Succinate dehydrogenase activity was highest in bands L and M, indicating the presence of IM (Table 1). The activity of this enzyme was much lower in band H_1 and decreased further in band H_2. In contrast, KDO was greatest in concentration in bands H_1 and H_2 and very low in band L. Band M contained a high KDO content, also, suggesting a mixture of IM and OM. Band H_2 contained less SDH than band H_1, but also less KDO/mg protein.

B. Electron Microscopy

Electron microscopy of negatively stained preparations revealed the presence of membrane structures in all bands. Membranes in band L were smaller in size than those in the other bands and were either fragmented or entire. Sectioned material from band H_1, high in OM, showed mostly uniform shaped bilaminar unit membrane structures predominating (Fig. 2).

TABLE 1. Distribution of Markers on Sucrose Gradients.

Gradient band	Density	Marker		
		Protein	KDO	Succinate Dyhydrogenase
L	1.122[a]	1.52[b]	1.6[c]	19[d]
M	1.179	2.88	6.6	23
H_1	1.191	3.64	8.8	11
H_2	1.214	1.20	6.0	6

[a] gm/cm^3
[b] mg/ml
[c] μg/mg protein
[d] μM/min/mg protein

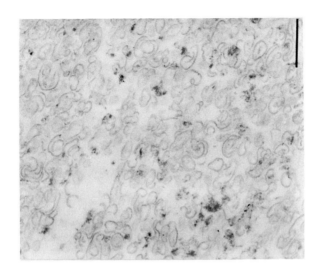

Fig. 2. Electronmicrograph of material from sucrose
gradient bands. Sample of gradient band H_1 was pelleted by
centrifugation at 195,000 x g, fixed in 4% glutaraldehyde,
washed, post-fixed in 2% osmium tetroxide, and embedded in
Spurr's medium (6).

C. SDS-Polyacrylamide Gel Electrophoresis

A total of three polypeptides could be considered "major"
polypeptides in membranes of Pierce's disease RLB. No major
polypeptides and only 6-8 "minor" polypeptides were observed
in the L band (Fig. 3, lane 1). Polypeptide profiles of the
M and H_1 bands were nearly undistinguishable (Fig. 3, lanes
2 and 3). Major polypeptides of the M and H_1 bands were
composed of 75, 71, and 18.5 kdal polypeptides in which the
75 and 71 kdal polypeptides predominated. Several minor
polypeptides were observed. Major polypeptides of the H_2
band were composed of 75 and 71, in which neither predominated
(Fig. 3, land 4). Eight-ten minor polypeptides were
observed in bands M, H_1 and H_2 with only minor differences
between bands.

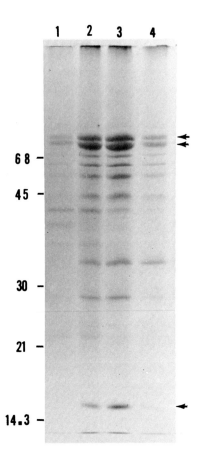

Fig. 3. Coomassie Brilliant blue-stained SDS-PAGE profile
of membrane fractions of Pierce's disease bacterium. The
fractions were prepared as described in Materials and Methods.
Electrophoresis was performed in vertical slab gels of 10%
polyacrylamide with the discontinuous system of Laemmli (15).
Each fraction preparation was solubilized in Laemmli sample
buffer for 2 min at 100 C. Samples were density gradient
bands (1) L, (2) M, (3) H_1, and (4) H_2. Numbers on the left
are molecular weight standards and arrows on right designate
a major polypeptide.

IV. DISCUSSION

The results reported here provide the first information on membrane analysis of plant RLB. Separation of IM and OM was accomplished with the use of DNase, RNase and a 52-70% linear sucrose gradient. Relatively pure preparations of both membrane fractions were obtained with this method. The presence of KDO was established in Pierce's disease RLB and used as a label of outer membrane. Succinate dehydrogenase was also present and used to detect IM. Electron microscopy of OM preparations showed the presence of a unit membrane structure in agreement with previous reports for Pierce's disease RLB (3) and similar to that reported for R. prowazeki (4) and gram-negative bacteria (7, 9).

The present study found that membranes of Pierce's disease RLB sedimented at lower densities than those reported for R. prowazeki (4), except for band H_2 which sedimented to a location similar to that of the heavy band reported by Smith and Winkler (4) (1.214 and 1.23 gm/cm^3, respectively). The contamination of IM with OM reported in preparations from R. prowazeki (4) was found in band M (1.179 gm/cm^3) but not in band L (1.122 gm/cm^3) in our study. Inner membranes of Pierce's disease RLB sedimented at a much lower density than the IM preparations of Smith and Winkler (4) (1.122 and 1.19 gm/cm^3, respectively). Whereas we observed four bands with Pierce's disease bacterium only three bands were observed with R. prowazeki (4). Centrifugation regimes and/or the use of DNase and RNase may be responsible for the different results. However, a structural difference in the membranes of the two organisms could be possible, also.

The polypeptide profile of SDS-PAGE of membranes of Pierce's disease bacterium is quite different from that of R. prowazeki (4). Rickettsia prowazeki contains 6 major polypeptides ranging in molecular weight from 16 to 135 kdal and numerous minor polypeptides. In contrast membranes of Pierce's disease RLB contain 3 major polypeptide ranging in molecular weight from 18.5 to 75 kdal and few minor polypeptides. None of the major polypeptides of membranes of these two organisms were of the same molecular weight. Whereas three major polypeptides were present in inner membranes of R. prowazeki (4), no major polypeptides were present in inner membranes of Pierce's disease RLB. The protein composition of membranes of Pierce's disease RLB indicates that plant RLB are significantly different than animal rickettsiae of similar size and morphology.

The methodology described here provides improved
procedures for separation of cytoplasmic and outer membranes
of rickettsiæ and plant RLB.

ACKNOWLEDGMENTS

We thank M. Davis for the original culture of Pierce's
disease RLB, strain VP-5, and J. C. Dianese for many helpful
discussions.

REFERENCES

1. Davis, M. J., Purcell, A. H., and Thomson, S. V.
    Science, 199, 75 (1978).
2. Davis, M. J. Ph.D. dissertation, University of
    California, Berkeley (1978).
3. Hopkins, D. L. Ann. Rev. Phytopathol., 17, 277 (1977).
4. Smith, D. K., and Winkler, H. H. J. Bacteriol., 137,
    963 (1979).
5. Lowry, O. H., Rosebrough, N. J., Farr, A. L., and
    Randall, R. J. J. Biol. Chem., 193, 265 (1951).
6. Spurr, A. R. J. Ultrastruct. Res., 26, 31 (1969).
7. Schnaitman, C. A. J. Bacteriol., 104, 890 (1970).
8. Schnaitman, C. A. J. Bacteriol., 104, 1404 (1970).
9. Osborn, M. J., Gander, J. E., Parisi, E., and Carson, J.
    J. Biol. Chem., 247, 3962 (1972).
10. Hancock, R. E. W., and Nikaido, H. J. Bacteriol., 136,
    381 (1978).
11. Kasahara, M. and Anraku, Y. J. Biochem., 76, 959
    (1974).
12. Weissbach, A., and Hurwitz, J. J. Biol. Chem., 234,
    705 (1959).
13. Scott, C. C. L., Makula, R. A., and Finnerty, W. R.
    J. Bacteriol., 127, 469 (1976).
14. Keleti, G., and Lederer, W. H. In "Handbook of
    Micromethods for Biological Sciences", (G. Keleti and
    W. H. Lederer, ed.), pp. 74. Van Nostrand-Reinhold Co.,
    New York (1974).
15. Laemmli, U. K. Nature (London), 227, 680 (1970).

SOME AUTONOMOUS ENZYMATIC REACTIONS
OF COXIELLA BURNETII IN THE INITIAL
PHASE OF PEPTIDOGLYCAN SYNTHESIS

Frank R. Gonzales
David Paretsky

Department of Microbiology
University of Kansas
Lawrence, Kansas

I.   INTRODUCTION

Coxiella burnetii is the rickettsia-like agent of Q
fever with a Gram negative-like cell wall containing glucosamine, muramic acid, and cell envelope containing a toxic
lipopolysaccharide (1-6). The cells have a typically
eubacterial trilaminar cell envelope with a dense intermediate layer, presumably peptidoglycan (7, 8). Although C.
burnetii has been shown to possess several host-independent
metabolic activities, there are no reports of peptidoglycan
synthesis by the organism (9,10). Peptidoglycan biosynthesis
requires perhaps 14 separate enzymatic steps from the glucose
precursor. Autonomous ability of C. burnetii to perform
aspects of this complex pathway leading to uridine sugar
intermediates was sought to help elucidate host-obligate
parasite relationships.

Abbreviations: CoA, Coenzyme A; UTP, uridine triphosphate; UDP, uridine diphosphate; DTT, dithiothreitol; EDTA,
ethylene diamine tetraacetate; PEP, phosphoenolpyruvate.
Enzymes nomenclature from, Dixon, M. and Webb, E.C. In
"Enzymes," 3rd ed., Academic Press, N.Y. (1979).

II. MATERIAL AND METHODS

A. Organism

Phase I C. burnetii (Nine Mile strain) was cultivated in antibiotic-free chicken eggs. Yolk sacs were aseptically removed and the rickettsiae were harvested and purified (11). Organisms were stored at -70 C until use.

B. Enzyme Preparation

Purified C. burnetii was suspended in 5 mM Hepes buffer, pH 7.5, to make 8-10% cell suspensions (w/v). Cells were disrupted in a French pressure cell (American Instrument Co., Silver Springs, MD) at 13,000 p.s.i. with at least 30% breakage. The extract was kept on ice and immediately used in enzyme assays.

C. Enzyme Assays

1. <u>L-Glutamine-D-fructose 6-phosphate Transaminidase</u>. Reaction mixtures contained fructose 6-phosphate, 50 mM; glutamine, 50 mM; dithithiothreitol (DTT), 5 mM; 0.3 ml rickettsial extract containing 0.2-1 mg protein; Hepes buffer (pH 7.5), 50 mM; in a final vol of 0.6 ml (12). Mixtures were incubated at 37 C for 30 min. The control was an identical reaction mixture acidified prior to the addition of the enzyme extract. Hexosamine was analyzed by the Benson modification of the Morgan-Elson reaction using glucosamine 6-phosphate as a standard (13). The lower limit of detection was 0.12 mM.

2. <u>D-Glucosamine-phosphate Acetyltransferase</u>. Mixtures contained glucosamine-6-phosphate, 5 mM; CoA, 0.1 mM; ATP, 20 mM; potassium acetate, 200 mM; $MgCl_2$, 10 mM; DTT, 5 mM; Hepes buffer (pH 7.5), 50 mM; 0.25 ml (12). Mixtures were incubated for 30 min at 37 C and the reaction was terminated by adding 0.05 ml of 80% trichloracetic acid. The control system was acidified prior to the enzyme addition. Analyses for hexosamines were made as described above except that N-acetylglucosamine-6-phosphate was used as a standard and the sensitivity of detection was 0.14 mM.

3. <u>CoA Acetyl Transferase</u>. The reaction mixture contained CoA, 0.15 mM; acetyl phosphate, 0.3 mM; EDTA, 1 mM; Tris buffer (pH 7.5), 50 mM; 0.3 ml extract, 0.4-1 mg protein,

in a final vol of 0.6 ml. Incubation time was 15 min at 30 C.
The control contained no acetyl phosphate. The free thiol
group of unreacted CoA was measured spectrophotometrically by
reaction with 90 nmole of dithio-bis-(2-nitrobenzoic acid)
(DTN) and the thionitrobenzoic acid released was measured
spectrophotometrically (E_{412}^{1M} = 13,600) (14,15). Acetyl-CoA
formation was proportional to the decrease in absorbance
relative to the control.

4. Acetate Kinase. Reaction mixtures contained ATP,
10 mM; potassium acetate, 100 mM; $MgCl_2$ 5 mM; CoA, 0.15 mM;
Tris buffer (pH 7.5), 50 mM; and extract containing 0.07-
0.91 mg protein in a final vol of 0.3 ml or 0.6 ml (16). The
mixtures were incubated for 20 min at 31 C. The control
contained no ATP. Analyses were performed using DTN as described above to measure the remaining free thiol groups
(14,15).

5. UDPacetylglucosamine Pyrophosphorylase. Reaction
mixtures consisted of [5-^{3}H]-UTP, 17 Ci/mmole (ICN Chemical
and Radioisotope, Irvine, CA), 20 µCi; N-acetylglucosamine-1-
phosphate, 2 mM; $MgCl_2$, 4 mM; KF, 4 mM; Tris buffer (pH 8.0),
30 mM; 0.08 ml extract, 0.27 mg protein, in a final vol of
0.20 ml (17,18). The mixtures were incubated at 37 C for
45 min, and the reaction terminated by the addition of 4 µl
of 12 N HCl. The control was acidified prior to the addition
of the cell extract. Protein was removed by centrifugation
and the supernatants were used for chromatography (19). Poly-
gram Cell 300-PEI thin layer plates (Brinkman Instruments
Inc., NY) were prewashed in absolute methanol, spotted with
5 µl of supernatant, and developed in 1.5 M LiCl:0.5 N HCOOH
(1:1) at 4 C. The uridine derivative was visualized with
ultraviolet light at 254 nm. The spot corresponding to
standard UDP-N-acetylglucosamine (R_f = 0.69) was scraped from
the plate as a fine powder, and placed in 3.0 ml of Omnifluor
scintillation cocktail (New England Nuclear Corp., Boston,
MA), and the radioactivity measured.

6. Phosphoenolpyruvate-UDPacetylglucosamine Transferase.
Reactions contained UDP-N-acetylglucosamine, 5 mM; [1-^{14}C]-
phosphoenolpyruvate, 13.3 mCi/mmole (Amersham Corp., Arlington Heights, IL), 0.84 mM; DTT, 2 mM; KF, 10 mM; Hepes buffer
(pH 7.5), 50 mM; 0.25 ml extract, 0.85 mg protein, in a final
vol of 0.50 ml (20,21). The mixture was incubated at 37 C
for 45 min and terminated by adding 10 µl 12 N HCl. Protein
was removed by centrifugation and the supernatants retained.
Pellets were extracted twice with 0.5 ml H_2O and all the
supernatants combined. Supernatants were adsorbed onto 50 mg
Norite A and the slurry was filtered; the charcoal was washed

with water to remove unreacted substrate. UDP-N-acetylglucosamine pyruvyl ether was eluted with 6 ml of 95% EtOH:0.2 N
NH_4OH (1:1). The eluate was taken to dryness by flash-vacuum
evaporation. The product was reconstituted in 2 ml of H_2O
and readsorbed on fresh Norite A. After washing 5 times with
25 ml of H_2O, the Norite was eluted with 10 ml of EtOH;NH_4OH
as above. Aliquots were removed and the radioactivity
measured.

7. <u>UTPacetylglucosamine Pyrophosphorylase Coupled with
Phosphoenolpyruvate-UDPacetylglucosamine Transferase</u>. Reactions contained UTP, 5 mM; N-acetylglucosamine-1-phosphate,
3 mM; $[1-^{14}C]$-PEP, 0.84 mM; DTT, 2 mM; KF, 10 mM; Hepes
buffer (pH 7.5), 50 mM; 0.25 ml extract, 0.85 mg protein, in
a final vol of 0.50 ml. The analyses were carried out as
described above.

8. <u>Protein</u>. Protein was measured by the Coomassie Blue
method using bovine serum albumin as a standard (12).

III. RESULTS

A. Glucosamine and N-acetylglucosamine

<u>C</u>. <u>burnetii</u> can form glucose-6-phosphate and fructose-6-
phosphate (23,24). The next steps in peptidoglycan synthesis
are formation of glucosamine-6-phosphate from fructose-6-
phosphate and glutamine, and N-acetylglucosamine-6-phosphate
from glucosamine-6-phosphate and acetyl-CoA (17,25). Repeated
efforts to demonstrate these reactions by <u>C</u>. <u>burnetii</u> were
unsuccessful, using sonicated <u>C</u>. <u>burnetii</u> as well as pressure-
disrupted cells. Parallel experiments were performed using
<u>E</u>. <u>coli</u> extracts. Both transamidase and transacetylase
activities were found in <u>E</u>. <u>coli</u>, showing that the assay
conditions used were satisfactory.
    Acetyl phosphate and acetyl-CoA synthesis of acetyl
donor compounds which are involved in formation of the
acetylated intermediates in peptidoglycan synthesis were
studied. Tables 1 and 2 show that <u>C</u>. <u>burnetii</u> extracts had
CoA acetyl transferase and acetate kinase activities, forming
acetyl phosphate and acetyl-CoA; both kinase and transferase
activities could be coupled in a reaction mixture containing
ATP and CoA.

TABLE 1.   CoA Acetyl Transferase Activity in C. burnetii
           CoA + Acetyl Phosphate $\rightleftharpoons$ Acetyl-CoA + P_i

| | Protein | | Acetyl-CoA formed | |
Expt.	mg	nmoles	nmoles/ mg protein	nmoles/mg protein/min
1	0.250	21	84	5.6
2	1.05	56	53	2.7
3	0.086	21	244	16

Reaction mixture vol. in expt. 3 was half that of expts. 1
and 2, but the reaction concentrations were the same. Conditions as described in text.

TABLE 2.   Acetate Kinase Coupled with CoA Acetyl Transferase
           in C. burnetii

   1. Acetate + ATP $\rightleftharpoons$ acetyl phosphate + ADP

   2. Acetyl phosphate + CoA $\rightleftharpoons$ acetyl-CoA + P_i

| | Protein | | Acetyl-CoA formed | |
Expt.	mg	nmoles	nmoles/ mg protein	nmoles/mg protein/min
1	0.074	25	338	17
2	0.91	33	36	2

Conditions as described in text.

TABLE 3.   UDPacetylglucosamine Pyrophosphorylase
           Activity in C. burnetii

   UTP + N-acetylglucosamine-1-phosphate $\rightleftharpoons$
   UDP-N-acetylglucosamine + PP_i

| | Protein | UDP-N-acetylglucosamine formed | |
Expt.	mg	cpm/mg protein	pmole/mg protein
1	0.28	40,143	1.1
2	0.27	611,941	17

Conditions as described in text.

TABLE 4.   Phosphoenolpyruvate-UDPacetylglucosamine
Transferase Activity in C. burnetii

Phosphoenolpyruvate + UDP-N-acetylglucosamine $\rightleftharpoons$
UDP-N-acetylglucosamine pyruvyl ether

	Protein mg	cpm above control	pmole/ mg protein
Control	0.85	0	0
Experimental	0.85	7,865	319

Conditions as described in text.

TABLE 5.   UDPacetylglucosamine Pyrophosphorylase Coupled with
Phosphoenolpyruvate-UDPacetylglucosamine Transferase
Activity in C. burnetii

UTP + N-acetylglucosamine-1-phosphate $\rightleftharpoons$
[UDP-N-acetylglucosamine + PP_i] + phosphenolpyruvate $\rightleftharpoons$
UDP-N-acetylglucosamine pyruvyl ether

	Protein mg	cpm above control	pmole/ mg protein
Control	0.85	0	0
Experimental	0.85	3,557	144

Conditions as described in text.

B.   Uridine Sugars

The first uridine sugar formed in peptidoglycan synthesis
is UDP-N-acetylglucosamine (UDP-NAG) from UTP and N-acetyl-
glucosamine-1-phosphate, mediated by UDPacetylglucosamine
pyrophosphorylase.   The presence of this enzyme was shown in
C. burnetii extracts (Table 3).   UDP-NAG reacted with phosphoenolpyruvate in the presence of phosphoenolpyruvate-
UDPacetylglucosamine transferase to form UDP-NAG-pyruvyl
ether (Table 4).   When UTP, N-acetylglucosamine-1-phosphate
and phosphoenolpyruvate were simultaneously incubated with C.
burnetii extracts, the reactions were coupled to form the
UDP-NAG-pyruvyl ether (Table 5).

IV. DISCUSSION

C. burnetii is an obligate intracellular parasite.
Little is known of the host's contributions to the organism's
biochemical requirements for growth and replication. It has
been proposed that the parasite has one or more biochemical
and/or physiological lesions responsible for the host-
dependency (9,10). Biochemical lesions may be represented by
the absence of critical catabolic or anabolic enzymes, or
coenzymes, or energy sources. Physiological lesions may
involve the cell envelope; defects in cell membrane or cell
wall structure could result in defective transport mechanisms,
in defective chemiosmotic-dependent reactions or in modified
resistance to environment. Cell-free extracts of C. burnetii
contain autonomous enzymes including nucleotide kinases
(26,27), protein and amino acid synthases (28-31), and glycolytic enzymes (23,24,32).

The chemical and ultrastructural composition of the C.
burnetii cell envelope resembles that of other Gram negative
organisms, with inner and outer membranes surrounding a dense
intermediate layer, presumed to be peptidoglycan (33). Semi-
purified cell walls contain N-acetylmuramic acid residues
(1), and cell envelopes contain hexosamines and several amino
acids (5). A purified lipopolysaccharide prepared from C.
burnetii resembled typical Gram-negative lipopolysaccharide
(2-4).

Peptidoglycan is a complex carbohydrate polymer unique
to procaryotes, requiring several enzymatic steps for synthesis (34-36). The complexity of peptidoglycan biosynthesis
raises the question, which intermediates in the pathway of
peptidoglycan synthesis are autonomously made by C. burnetii,
and which are contributed by the host cell? Initial reactions
in the cytoplasmic phase of peptidoglycan synthesis leading
to the formation of uridine sugars by C. burnetii are reported here. Phosphorylation of glucose to glucose-6-
phosphate (24) and its isomerization to fructose-6-phosphate
(23) were previously shown in cell-free preparations of C.
burnetii. In the present study, we could not demonstrate
the next step, the synthesis of glucosamine-6-phosphate from
exogenous glutamine and fructose-6-phosphate. Previous
experiments had implied the presence of acetate kinase and
CoA acetyl transferase in C. burnetii, but direct demonstra-
tions were not made (37). Results presented in this paper
(Tables 1 and 2) show that the cell-free preparations of C.
burnetii could phosphorylate acetate and then use the acetyl
phosphate to form acetyl-CoA, necessary in the formation of
N-acetylglucosamine-6-phosphate. Because acetyl-CoA is a
critical intermediate in many biochemical pathways, these

results could have important implications for the host-independent metabolism of C. burnetii. The acetylation of glutamine-6-phosphate by acetyl-CoA could not be demonstrated. Negative results are difficult to substantiate; repeated unsuccessful attempts to demonstrate rickettsial synthesis of glucosamine-6-phosphate and N-acetylglucosamine-6-phosphate could be due to insufficient sensitivity of the assay employed, or to the instability of transamidase and trans-acetylase in crude preparations (12). We may speculate that since several eucaryotic proteins have N-acetylglucosamine residues, these could be made available to the rickettsiae by hydrolase activities present in lysosomal vacuoles. C. burnetii proliferates in lysosomal vacuoles, wherein the released N-acetylglucosamine could become available for rickettsial peptidoglycan synthesis (38). This proposal would explain one aspect of host dependency by C. burnetii.

UDP-N-acetylglucosamine formation from UTP and N-acetylglucosamine-1-phosphate is mediated by UDP-acetylglucosamine pyrophosphorylase. C. burnetii can make UTP (26). The present report demonstrates the presence of the UDP-acetylglucosamine pyrophosphorylase in C. burnetii (Table 3), which forms the UDP-N-acetylglucosamine precursor of N-acetylglucosamine pyruvyl ether. This latter molecule is synthesized from UDP-N-acetylglucosamine and phosphenol-pyruvate. This reaction is mediated by C. burnetii in the presence of exogenous phosphoenolpyruvate and UDP-N-acetyl-glucosamine (Table 4). Furthermore, UDPacetylglucosamine pyrophosphorylase could be linked with phosphoenolpyruvate-UDPacetylglucosamine transferase to form UDP-N-acetylglucos-amine pyruvyl ether (Table 5).

V. SUMMARY

This paper shows that C. burnetii has the autonomous enzymatic capacities to form acetyl-CoA, UDP-N-acetylglucos-amine and UDP-N-acetylglucosamine pyruvyl ether, early steps in the cytoplasmic phase of peptidoglycan synthesis; autono-mous enzymatic glucosamine and N-acetylglucosamine synthesis could not be shown. If C. burnetii indeed lacks autonomous enzymes for making some of the other intermediates in the synthesis of the critical cell wall material, the cell would depend on the host to supply such metabolites, explaining one aspect of the organism's obligate parasitism.

ACKNOWLEDGMENTS

We thank J.M. Akagi for stimulating discussions and suggestions. The work was supported by grants from the University of Kansas General Research Committee, the University of Kansas Biomedical Research Committee, and the National Science Foundation, PCM76-11706.

REFERENCES

1. Allison, A. C., and Perkins, H. R. Nature. 188, 796 (1960).
2. Baca, O. G., and Paretsky, D. Infect. Immun. 9, 959 (1974).
3. Baca, O.G., and Paretsky, D. Infect. Immun. 9, 939 (1974).
4. Chan, M. L., McChesney, J., and Paretsky, D. Infect. Immun. 13, 21 (1976).
5. Jerrels, T. R., Hinrichs, D. J., and Mallavia, L. P. Can. J. Microbiol. 20, 1465 (1974).
6. Perkins, H. R., and Allison, A. C. J. Gen. Microbiol. 30, 469 (1963).
7. Anacker, R. L., Fukushi, K., Pickens, E. G., and Lackman, D. B. J. Bacteriol. 88, 1130 (1964).
8. Burton, P. R., Stueckemann, J., and Paretsky, D. J. Bacteriol. 122, 316 (1975).
9. Paretsky, D. Zentr. Bakteriol. Parasitenk. Abt. I., Orig. 206, 283 (1968).
10. Weiss, E. Bacteriol. Rev. 37, 259 (1973).
11. Thompson, H. A., and Paretsky, D. Infect. Immun. 7, 718 (1973).
12. Ghosh, S., and Roseman, S. In "Methods in Enzymology" (S.P. Colowick and N.O. Kaplan, eds.), Academic Press, N.Y. 5, 414 (1962).
13. Benson, R. L. Carbohydrate Res. 42, 192 (1975).
14. Alpers, D. H., Appel, S. H., and Tomkins, G. M. J. Biol. Chem. 240, 10 (1965).
15. Kredich, N. M., and Tomkins, G. M. J. Biol. Chem. 241, 4955 (1966).
16. Rose, I. A. In "Methods in Enzymology" (S.P. Colowick and N.O. Kaplan, eds.) Academic Press, N.Y. 1, 591 (1955).
17. Mayer, F. C., Bikel, I., and Hassid, W. Z. Plant Physiol. 43, 1097 (1968).

18. Strominger, J. L., and Smith, M. S. J. Biol. Chem. 234, 1822 (1959).
19. Randerath, K., and Randerath, E. J. Chromatogr. 16, 111 (1964).
20. Cassidy, P. J., and Kahan, F. M. Biochem. 12, 1364 (1973).
21. Venkateswaran, P. S., and Wu, H. C. J. Bacteriol. 110, 935 (1972).
22. Bradford, M. M. Analyt. Biochem. 72, 248 (1976).
23. McDonald, T. L., and Mallavia, L. J. Bacteriol. 107, 864 (1971).
24. Paretsky, D., Consigli, R. A., and Downs, C. M. J. Bacteriol. 83, 538 (1962).
25. Maley, F., Maley, G. F., and Lardy, H. A. J. Am. Chem. Soc. 78, 5303 (1956).
26. Christian, R. G., and Paretsky, D. J. Bacteriol. 132, 841 (1977).
27. Jones, F., Jr., and Paretsky, D. J. Bacteriol. 93, 1063 (1967).
28. Baca, O. G. J. Bacteriol. 136, 429 (1978).
29. Donahue, J. P., and Thompson, H. A. J. Gen. Microbiol. (1980) In Press.
30. Mallavia, L. P., and Paretsky, D. J. Bacteriol. 93, 1479 (1967).
31. Myers, W. F., and Paretsky, D. J. Bacteriol. 82, 761 (1961).
32. Consigli, R. A., and Paretsky, D. J. Bacteriol. 83, 206 (1962).
33. Burton, P. R., Stueckemann, J., Welsh, R. M., and Paretsky, D. Infect. Immun. 21, 556 (1978).
34. Fiedler, F., and Glaser, L. Biochim. Biophys. Acta. 300, 467 (1973).
35. Strominger, J. L. Fed. Proc. 21, 134 (1962).
36. Strominger, J. L., Park, J. T., and Thompson, R. E. J. Biol. Chem. 234, 3262 (1959).
37. Paretsky, D., Downs, C. M., Consigli, R. A., and Joyce, B.K. J. Infect. Dis. 103, 6 (1958).
38. Burton, P. R., Kordova, N., and Paretsky, D. Can. J. Microbiol. 17, 143 (1971).

HETEROGENEITY AMONG RICKETTSIA
TSUTSUGAMUSHI ISOLATES:
A PROTEIN ANALYSIS

Barbara Hanson
Charles L. Wisseman, Jr.[1]

School of Medicine
University of Maryland,
Baltimore, Maryland

I. INTRODUCTION

One of the hallmark characteristics of Rickettsia
tsutsugamushi is its heterogeneity with regard to both
virulence and serotype. Although 3 major prototype serotypes
(Karp, Gilliam, & Kato) have been recognized, several other
serotypes have been demonstrated as well, by the standard
techniques of complement fixation (CF), fluorescent antibody
assay (FA), cross-neutralization, and cross-vaccination (1-
7). R. tsutsugamushi strain variation has important practical
implications, because it interferes with the development of
permanent vaccine-induced and naturally-acquired resistance to
the disease of scrub typhus (8). It also raises questions
about the phenotypic stability of these organisms and the
natural forces which have exerted selective pressures on their
evolution and geographic spread (9, 10). The clarification of
all of these problems requires a coherent system for the
classification of R. tsutsugamushi strains.

[1] This study received support from Contract No. DADA 17-
71-C-1007 with the U. S. Army Medical Office of the Surgeon
General, Research and Development Command, Department of the
Army.

Rickettsial structural surfaces may be thought of as
antigen mosaics, and strains within a species may share
individual components of the mosaic to differing degrees.   The
extent of antigen sharing by R. tsutsugamushi serotypes is not
known, but group antigen activity is shared by at least the
Karp, Gilliam & Kato strains (11-13), and considerable
antigenic cross-reactivity among many serotypes has been
found.   The nature and number of group and unique antigens of
R. tsutsugamushi is undetermined.

Because of the probable existence of multiple antigens
within a strain which are not clearly distinguished by
classical serological procedures, and because critical strain
differences may occur in non-immunogenic sites, we have taken
a new approach to the problem of R. tsutsugamushi strain
variation, based on the examination of individual rickettsial
proteins, with a view toward understanding the molecular basis
of the heterogeneity described.

R. tsutsugamushi is not as amenable to a protein analysis
as are several other rickettsial species because scrub typhus
organisms are much more difficult to prepare in large quantity
and pure form.   Therefore, we have used a method which
requires only small numbers of unpurified organisms.   This
method was first used in our laboratory for the study of
Rickettsia prowazekii proteins by E. V. Oaks et al. (vide
infra, unpublished experiments) and it consists of sodium
dodecyl sulfate-polyacrylamide gel electrophoresis (SDS-PAGE)
of rickettsial proteins which have been radiolabeled in the
absence of significant host cell protein synthesis.   We also
have begun an analysis of scrub typhus rickettsial protein
antigens by SDS-PAGE of immunoprecipitated proteins.   This
presentation will describe our initial examination of the
proteins of 4 isolates of R. tsutsugamushi and of the major
protein antigens of one of the strains.

II.   METHODS

A.   Rickettsiae.

Three of the strains used, the 3 prototype serotypes
Karp, Gilliam, and Kato, have undergone 107, 143, and 45 egg
passages, respectively.   The 4th scrub typhus isolate
examined, designated JC472B, was obtained from an Indian
gerbil in Pakistan in the 1960's (9) and has been passaged 3
times in mice and 9 times in eggs.   It has been serotyped
unequivocally as Karp by FA and CF, using rabbit and guinea
pig sera, respectively, obtained 4 weeks after inoculation (9,

14). JC472B also resembles Karp in regard to virulence in outbred mice (Wisseman and Jones, unpublished experiments). In the present studies, the rickettsiae were prepared as yolk sac suspensions in brain heart infusion broth (BHI) for use as tissue culture inocula.

B. Radiolabeling of rickettsiae.

L cells were trypsinized from monolayer cultures in flasks, suspended in growth medium (Dulbecco's medium (GIBCO, Grand Island, NY) supplemented with 10% fetal calf serum (FCS)) and mixed either with a rickettsial yolk sac suspension at a final dilution of 1/8 in growth medium, or, for controls, with medium alone. This combination of L cells and rickettsiae represented a multiplicity of infection of 1-10 infectious particles/cell. After a 90 minute incubation with gentle mixing at 35°C, the cells were washed, plated in 60 mm plastic petri dishes or slide chambers (Lab-Tek Products, Naperville, IL) and incubated at 35°C in a humidified atmosphere of 5% CO_2 in air. The slide chamber cultures were fixed and stained with Giemsa at regular intervals to monitor the progress of the infection. Between 50 and 90% of the cells were infected initially, depending on the seed. By day 3, the cultures were considered to be moderately infected, with all cells infected and about 25 rickettsiae per cell. This was determined to be the best time to begin the labeling procedure, since it gave optimum ^{3}H-leucine incorporation with the 3 strains tested. We found that the same scrub typhus rickettsial polypeptide profiles were obtained regardless of whether the labeling procedure was begun on day 1, 2, or 3 after infection. The following protocol initially was developed for labeling epidemic typhus rickettsiae (E. V. Oaks et al., vide infra, unpublished experiments). On day 3 after infection, one or more antibiotics were added. For all labeling of rickettsiae, emetine (1 µg/ml, Boehringer Mannheim, W. Germany) was used to specifically inhibit host cell protein synthesis. In one experiment to be described, either chloramphenicol (20 µg/ml) or streptomycin (100 µg/ml) was used in addition to emetine. The antibiotics remained in the medium for the duration of the procedure. After about 18 hours, the growth medium was changed to leucine-free medium (MEM (Eagle), GIBCO) containing 3% dialyzed FCS and the desired antibiotics. After 4 more hours, this was removed, and fresh leucine-free medium containing FCS, antibiotics and 20-50 µCi/ml ^{3}H-leucine (65 Ci/mmole, Schwartz-Mann, Orangeburg, NY) was added. After continued incubation for 18-24 hours, the cells were scraped gently into the medium,

washed by low-speed centrifugation, resuspended in SPG (15) in
a volume equivalent to 1 ml per dish, quickly frozen in a dry
ice-ethanol bath and stored at -70°C.

C. SDS-PAGE.

SDS-PAGE was carried out in a standard Laemmli system
using 13% acrylamide: 0.52% DATD slab gels (16). Rapidly
thawed radiolabeled cell suspensions were concentrated 10-fold
by centrifugation at 12,800 x g to pellet rickettsiae, and
resuspended in hot sample buffer (2% SDS, 5% mercaptoethanol,
10% glycerol, 5 mM phosphate buffer, pH 7, and 5 µM
phenylmethylsulfonyl fluoride (PMSF)). The samples in the
buffer were held in a boiling water bath for 3 minutes before
application to the gels. After electrophoresis, the gels were
fixed in TCA and fluorographed by the method of Bonner and
Laskey (17). ^{14}C-labeled molecular weight marker proteins
were obtained from Amersham Searle (Des Plaines, IL).

D. Protein extraction.

Labeled cell suspensions were centrifuged to sediment the
rickettsiae. The pellets were resuspended in a half volume of
TX/DOC detergent solution, which consisted of 1% Triton X-100,
0.5% sodium deoxycholate, and 5 µM PMSF, and the mixtures were
held at 22°C for 1 hour and recentrifuged as above. The
supernatant fluids containing solubilized proteins were used
as antigen. Under these conditions, the TX/DOC extracted
about 45% of the TCA-precipitable counts in the rickettsial
suspension, and all rickettsial proteins detected by SDS-PAGE
were represented in the extracts (unpublished experiments).

E. Immunoprecipitation

The antigens in these protein extracts were immunoprecipitated by a standard procedure using Staphylococcus protein A
to separate the antibody-antigen complexes. Antisera were
prepared by hyperimmunizing rabbits with rickettsia-infected
mouse liver and spleen suspensions by W. T. Walsh. Labeled
cell extracts and antiserum were held together overnight at
4°C. An equal volume of Pansorbin (10.3% Staphylococcus
aureus cells, Calbiochem-Behring Corp., La Jolla, CA) then was
added to bind the immunoglobulin along with any complexed
antigen. After further incubation at 4°C for 30 minutes,
unbound molecules were separated from the bacterial cells by 3

washes. The antibody-antigen complexes bound to the washed
Pansorbin then were disrupted and removed from the final
bacterial pellet by resuspending it in 50 µl sample buffer,
holding in a boiling water bath for 3 minutes, and pelleting
the staphylococci once more. The supernatant fluid, which
contained the antigens which originally had been complexed
with antibody, was applied directly to the gels without
further treatment.

III.   RESULTS

A. SDS-PAGE of R. tsutsugamushi (Gilliam) and the effects of antibiotics

The gel profiles of R. tsutsugamushi (Gilliam)-infected
and uninfected L cells labeled with ^{3}H-leucine during various
antibiotic treatments are shown in Figure 1. In this
experiment, each lane of the gel received a tenth of the
contents of a single petri dish of cells. The first lane
contained extract from uninfected L cells which were treated
with emetine, an inhibitor of most eukaryotic, but not prokaryotic, protein synthesis. Emetine reduced ^{3}H-leucine
incorporation in these cells by about 90% (based on TCA-
precipitable counts), and no labeled bands appeared on the
gel. On the other hand, extracts from similarly treated
Gilliam-infected cells contained many radiolabeled polypeptide
bands (lane 2) whose emetine resistance implied they are
rickettsial. To further test the source of the labeled
proteins in these extracts, infected cells were treated with
chloramphenicol (a prokaryotic protein synthesis inhibitor)
along with the emetine (lane 3). There was substantial
reduction in all bands, supporting the conclusion that these
polypeptides are rickettsial. Significant amounts of the
60,000 dalton (60K) protein were synthesized in the presence
of chloramphenicol, but this protein is present in very large
amounts to start with, and its synthesis definitely was
reduced. (We know that this protein is rickettsial, because
it reacts with antirickettsial antibody, as will be shown
below.) Similar experiments testing the antibiotic effects on
the other scrub typhus strains yielded similar results.

The effect of streptomycin on the synthesis of
rickettsial proteins also was examined. R. tsutsugamushi is
relatively resistant to streptomycin, and, in fact, is sometimes grown in the presence of this antibiotic. The last lane
in Figure 1 shows, as expected, that rickettsial protein
synthesis was not grossly affected by streptomycin. However,

the synthesis of at least two bands appeared to be quantitatively altered (56K, 53K). The significance of this has not been determined yet.

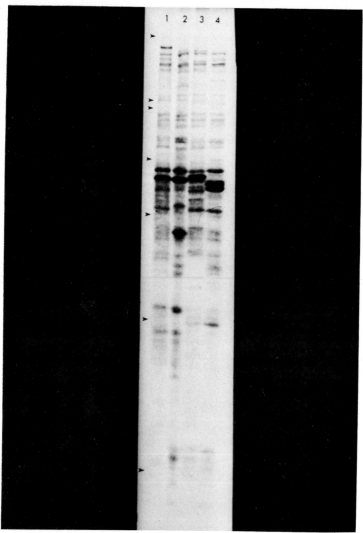

Fig. 1. SDS-PAGE of R. tsutsugamushi (Gilliam): outer lanes, molecular weight markers (myosin, 200K daltons; phosphorylase-b, 100K and 92.5K; bovine serum albumin, 69K; ovalbumin 46K; carbonic anhydrase, 30K; and lysozyme, 14.3K); lanes 1-4, emetine-treated L cells uninfected (lane 1), infected (lane 2), infected and also treated with chloramphenicol (20 µg/ml) (lane 3), or infected and also treated with streptomycin (100 µg/ml).

B.   SDS-PAGE of 4 Isolates of R. tsutsugamushi

Feeling confident that our procedures allowed us to label
rickettsial proteins exclusively, we compared the polypeptide
profiles of 3 prototype serotypes, Karp, Gilliam and Kato as
well as the "Karp-like" Pakistan isolate JC472B (Fig. 2). (In
an additional experiment not shown, the SDS-PAGE profile of a
plaque-purified seed of the Karp strain, kindly provided by
Dr. J.V. Osterman, was identical to that of our own Karp
seed.) The quantitatively major proteins of all 4 strains
fell in the molecular weight range of 56-63K. All 4 have predominant 63K bands, and Karp, Gilliam and JC472B have additional bands at 59-60K. Kato is most easily distinguished
from the others by its slightly lower molecular weight pair of
major bands at about 57K and 58K. Other prominent polypeptides in each strain are at the 48-49K position, the Karp band
appearing to migrate slightly more slowly than the others.
Despite certain similarities, comparison of the gel profiles
reveals that each of the four strains is unique. Particularly
important are the differences between Karp and JC472B. Even
though they were serotyped similarly by CF and FA, their
polypeptide profiles differ significantly.

C.   Immunoprecipitation of Rickettsial Proteins

SDS-PAGE of proteins from Karp-infected, emetine-treated
cells immunoprecipitated by homologous antiserum revealed
three major antigens with apparent molecular weights of 63K,
59K, and 49K (Fig. 3). The two heavier polypeptides also are
the most heavily labeled polypeptides of whole extracts (Fig.
2). Likewise, the major protein antigens in the Gilliam
strain had molecular weights of 63K, 60K, and 49K (not
shown). Several controls were done to establish that the
immunoprecipitated protein bands were specific for scrub
typhus rickettsiae. These included combinations of 1)
uninfected (non-antibiotic-treated) L cells and anti-Karp
antiserum, 2) infected cell extracts and normal rabbit serum,
and 3) infected cell extracts and no serum. All were negative
(Fig. 3).

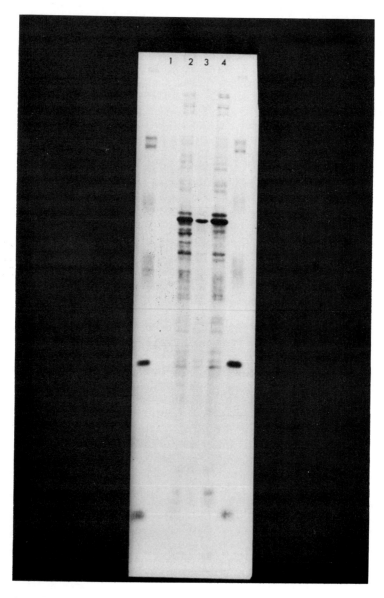

Fig. 2. SDS-PAGE of R. tsutsugamushi strains: arrows, molecular weight markers (see Fig. 1); lane 1, JC472B; lane 2, Karp; lane 3, Gilliam; lane 4, KATO.

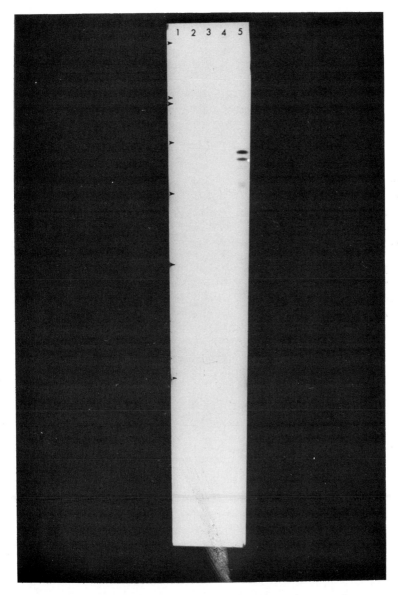

Fig. 3. SDS-PAGE of immunoprecipitated proteins.
Arrows, molecular weight markers (see Fig. 1), lane 1, 40,000
cpm uninfected cells treated with anti-Karp antiserum; lane 2,
40,000 cpm uninfected cells treated with normal rabbit serum;
lane 3, 18,000 cpm infected cells treated with TX/DOC only;
lane 5, 18,000 cpm infected cells treated with anti-Karp
antiserum.

IV. DISCUSSION

We have initiated this study, first, because we feel it
is important to be able to categorize definitively R.
tsutsugamushi isolates and, second, to understand the
molecular basis for the wide heterogeneity found within this
group of rickettsiae. The experiments reported here were
designed to determine the feasibility of our approach. We
have been able to analyze R. tsutsugamushi proteins by SDS-
PAGE for the first time, using only small quantities of
unpurified organisms. We can produce enough labeled scrub
typhus proteins in a single 60 mm petri dish for at least 10
electrophoresis runs. At the same time we have been able to
identify 3 major immunogenic polypeptides in R. tsutsugamushi
Karp and Gilliam extracts. We currently are determining if
these are outer membrane proteins, as seems likely from their
large quantity and strong immunogenicity. Hyperimmune sera
were used in the present studies so that the maximum number of
rickettsial immunogens would be detected. We now are applying
the technique of SDS-PAGE of immunoprecipitated rickettsial
proteins with more specific antisera to analyze the extent of
sharing of the individual antigenic polypeptides from various
scrub typhus strains and isolates.

In itself, SDS-PAGE analysis of rickettsial proteins
promises to be a useful method for strain identification. The
4 isolates tested so far could be distinguished easily from
each other by this technique. While it was expected that the
3 prototype serotypes (Karp, Gilliam, and Kato) would differ,
we thought that the polypeptide profile of the Pakistan
isolate JC472B might resemble that of the Karp strain, since
it had been serotyped as Karp-like by conventional methods (9,
14) and its virulence in outbred mice resembles that of the
Karp prototype strain (Wisseman and Jones, unpublished
experiments). Nevertheless, these two strains did exhibit
reproducible discrepancies in their protein patterns.
Although, of the 3 major Karp polypeptide antigens, 2 (63K,
60K) corresponded to major JC472B bands, it still isn't known
if they are antigenically identical. The third Karp major
protein immunogen, the 49K band, had no exact counterpart, but
JC472B did have a protein migrating just slightly faster, at
the 48K position. The relatedness of these 2 proteins
likewise remains undetermined. Although JC472B and Karp were
serotyped similarly, it remains possible that they have some
unique antigenic components whose presence was not detected by
standard CF or FA. On the other hand, the differences between
JC472B and Karp may occur entirely outside the realm of the
constituent antigenic determinants. In either case, we have

shown clearly that the two isolates are not identical. The
biological significance of their dissimilarities remains open
to further investigation. The potential significance of some
rickettsial differences not detected by standard serological
techniques and perhaps independent of antigenic makeup is
underscored by the finding of wide variations in virulence in
mice among several Pakistan isolates all serotyped as R.
tsutsugamushi (Karp) (Wisseman and Jones, unpublished). The
possibility that significant functional differences among
isolates may be attributed to non-antigen rickettsial
components emphasizes the importance of examining their total
polypeptide profiles as well as individual antigens. Our
results suggest that it may be possible to classify R.
tsutsugamushi isolates according to the electrophoretic
profiles of their composite proteins, as has been done
successfully with other bacteria.

V. SUMMARY

A preliminary examination of scrub typhus rickettsial
proteins and protein antigens has demonstrated the feasibility
of our approach to elucidating the molecular basis for the
wide biological variation encountered among Rickettsia
tsutsugamushi isolates. We have circumvented the difficulty
of obtaining large quantities of highly purified organisms by
preparing crude extracts of proteins from R. tsutsugamushi
which were labeled with ^{3}H-leucine during inhibition of host
cell protein synthesis. The labeled rickettsial proteins were
analyzed by SDS-polyacrylamide gel electrophoresis (SDS-PAGE)
and fluorography. Appropriate controls showed that this
method excluded detection of host cell proteins. SDS-PAGE
profiles of the Karp, Gilliam, and Kato strains of R. tsutsugamushi were remarkably different from each other. Moreover,
the polypeptide profile of the more recent isolate JC472B,
which had been classified serologically as "Karp-like," was
readily differentiated from that of the Karp strain, as well
as from Gilliam and Kato profiles, raising important questions
about the significance of standard serotyping techniques.
The major antigens of R. tsutsugamushi (Karp) were
determined by radioimmune precipitation, using hyperimmune
rabbit sera and fixed Staphylococci to separate the antigen-
antibody complexes from the non-reactive proteins. These
studies provide the foundation for an extensive analysis of R.
tsutsugamushi strain variation at a molecular level, in which
total polypeptide content, as well as individual protein
antigens, will be examined.

REFERENCES

1. Bengtson, I. A., Pub. Hlth. Rep. 60, 1483 (1945).
2. Bennett, B. L., Smadel, J. E., and Gauld, R. L., J.
    Immunol. 62, 453 (1949).
3. Fox, J. P., J. Immunol. 62, 341 (1949).
4. Elisberg, B. L., Needy, C. F., and Bozeman, F. M., in
    "Rickettsiae and Rickettsial Diseases" (J. Kazar, R. A.
    Ormsbee, and I. N. Tarasevich, eds.), p. 253. VEDA Publ.
    House of the Slovak Acad. Sci., Bratislava (1978).
5. Rights, F. L., Smadel, J. E., and Jackson, E. B., J. Exp.
    Med. 87, 339 (1948).
6. Shirai, A., Robinson, D. M., Brown, G. W., Gan, E., and
    Huxsoll, D. L., Jpn. J. Med. Sci. Biol. 32, 337 (1979).
7. Shishido, A., Jpn. J. Med. Sci. Biol. 17, 59 (1964).
8. Smadel, J. E., Ley, H. L. Jr., Diercks, F. H., Paterson, P.
    Y., Wisseman, C. L. Jr., and Traub, R., Amer. J. Trop.
    Med. Hyg. 1, 87 (1952).
9. Shirai, A., and Wisseman, C. L. Jr., Am. J. Trop. Med. Hyg.
    24, 145 (1975).
10. Traub, R., Wisseman, C. L. Jr., and Ahmed, N., Trans. Roy.
    Soc. Trop. Med. Hyg. 61, 23 (1967).
11. Kobayashi, Y., Nagai, K., and Tachibana, N., Am. J. Trop.
    Med. Hyg. 18, 942 (1969).
12. Shishido, A., and Hikita, M., Acta Virol. 12, 58 (1968).
13. Shishido, A., Hikita, M., Sato, T., and Kohno, S., J.
    Immunol. 103, 480 (1969).
14. Shirai, A., Ph.D. Dissertation, Univ. Md. Sch. Med. (1969).
15. Bovarnick, M. R., Miller, J. C., and Snyder, J. C., J. Bact.
    59, 509 (1950).
16. Myers, W. F., Wisseman, C. L. Jr., Fiset, P., Oaks, E. V.,
    and Smith, J. F., Infect. Immun. 26, 976 (1979).
17. Bonner, W. M., and Laskey, R. A., Eur. J. Biochem. 46, 83
    (1974).

ECOLOGY AND EPIDEMIOLOGY

EVOLUTIONARY AND BIOGEOGRAPHIC HISTORY AND THE PHYLOGENY OF VECTORS AND RESERVOIRS AS FACTORS IN THE TRANSMISSION OF DISEASES FROM OTHER ANIMALS TO MAN

Robert Traub[1]

Department of Microbiology
University of Maryland School of Medicine
Baltimore, Maryland

William L. Jellison[2]

There is a striking correlation between the position of a group of organisms on the tree of life and the numbers of specific infections which such animals transmit to man. This has been made clear by recent studies on the evolutionary and biogeographic history and phylogeny and interrelationships of ectoparasites like fleas and lice, and hosts such as rodents and other mammals. Nevertheless, there seems to have been remarkably few allusions to such conclusions in the literature. These factors are also far more important in the ecology and distribution of certain diseases than is generally realized. In this paper we will attempt to show: 1) how such a faunal approach, rather than a conventional one based primarily upon "nidality" or "landscape", has recently contributed notably to our understanding of the epidemiology, distribution and transmission of some of the zoonoses; 2) that the overwhelming majority of diseases contracted by humans from other animals, i.e., the zoonoses, are actually acquired from mammals that are higher on the evolutionary scale than is man, or belong to

[1] Supported by NIH grant AI-04242 and contract N00014-76-C-0393 with Office of Naval Research and Navy R & D Command.
[2] 504 South Third Street, Hamilton, Montana 59840

Orders that are more recently evolved, even though such mammals are frequently referred to as "the lower animals"; and 3) that the apparent exceptions (to item 2) are due to new and original contacts between the two groups, occurring in relatively recent times. Fourthly, we will suggest areas for future investigation, and will emphasize the rickettsioses because of the special interests of our audience.

BACKGROUND - THE FAUNAL APPROACH IN MEDICAL ECOLOGY

The characteristic occurrence of zoonoses like tick typhus, chigger-borne rickettsiosis (scrub typhus) and plague, in certain areas or habitats is well known, as is the association of these zoonoses with specific hosts or vectors. Pavlovsky formalized this concept in a highly useful manner with his theory of Natural Nidality of Transmissible Diseases (1). However, phylogenetic affiliations and the geological history of the vectors, hosts, and terrain may transcend nidality, as was shown by the successful quest for scrub typhus, tick typhus and tickborne viruses in geographic and ecological areas in Pakistan where their possible presence had not been suspected prior to such faunal analyses (2-7). This newer faunal approach, based on such ideas as the creation of "ecological islands" when the upthrust of the Himalayas rendered arid vast areas that had formerly been in forest, led to predictions, since verified, that zoonoses endemic in the mesic regions still exist in suitable minifoci scattered in the xeric zones of southwest and central Asia (7-8). These findings were based upon the observation that areas completely dissimilar in appearance can harbor a fauna with major elements in common. Equally contrary to the nidality concept was the discovery that what was apparently a homogeneous and continuous environment may contain faunal components that differ markedly, presumably depending upon the local geological history (4,9,10).
Data on epidemiology and on the zoogeography and taxonomic relationships of potential reservoirs of hemorrhagic fever with renal syndrome (HFRS) led us (11-13) to postulate 1) that this "Far Eastern" infection was intimately associated with certain Clethrionomys and Microtus voles; 2) the hemorrhagic fevers of eastern and northern Europe may be due to closely related, but surely not identical agents; 3) the infection may be endemic in areas wherever these particular species of voles occur, even in Europe, China, Japan and Alaska; 4) if Apodemus were the reservoir, then HFRS would be more widely distributed in Europe and Asia than was currently believed, but then it would be absent in the New World, where there are no native

murines; 5) if <u>Apodemus</u> became secondarily infected, then further geographical and ecological spread could be expected. Recent studies tend to support these ideas. The HFRS of northern Europe is related to that of the Far East (14,15) and the vole <u>Clethrionomys glareolus</u> is deeply involved. Cases have been found in China (16) and Japan (17) and the disease has "invaded the southern parts of the Korean Peninsula" (18). Some authorities (19) have assumed or inferred that the eastern and western forms of HFRS were the same, but antigenic differences have now been demonstrated (20). On the basis of data we have provided on the distribution of <u>Clethrionomys</u> and <u>Microtus</u>, Gajdusek (21) recently raised the question of whether HFRS may actually be present in North America, Great Britain or Iceland.

Faunal data along these lines were cited as evidence of transatlantic connections and faunal relationships among the southern continents, well before such ideas on continental drift became generally acceptable (9,22). It was also suggested that ancestral "hystrichomorph" rodents and platyrrhine (ceboid) monkeys emigrated in the Eocene by rafting from Africa to South America, and that such African–South American relationships may explain the occurrence of yellow fever and malaria on both continents (10). Dengue and yellow fever were therein regarded as sibling viruses, which would account for the absence of yellow fever in Asia.

CRITERIA AND DEFINITIONS

Because of discrepancies in the literature, it is necessary to explain our approach, and state our criteria for including some pathogens and deleting others.

The diseases and infections considered in this paper are restricted to those which are definitely believed to be acquired by man from other animals (zoonoses) or vice versa (anthroponoses), either directly or indirectly (as by a vector). Only major infections are included, and then only if actual passage from one Order of mammals to another actually occurs. We have deleted micro-organisms which are extremely widespread in nature, such as those occurring in soil, food and water, or living on the skin and mucous membranes, and/or which, as opportunistic or facultative agents, can cause disease in hosts whose mechanisms of immunity are impaired, e.g., the ubiquitous contaminative bacteria, etc., which have an exceptionally broad host-range, and which are so nonspecific that they cannot be said to be associated with any one group of hosts, even if they were deemed true pathogens. We have

not tallied organisms which otherwise meet the criteria but
are exceedingly rare in man or are known only from laboratory
cases, e.g., Bhanja virus. Also excluded are organisms which
are acquired by inhalation of soil contaminated with excreta
or secretions of infected hosts, e.g., histoplasmosis re bats
and birds; and melioidosis for rodents.

Escherichia coli, which is the cause of the most common
urinary infection in Homo and is frequently associated with
infant diarrheas, and is also responsible for much of the mas-
titis in cattle and abortion in sheep, is nevertheless excluded
because: 1) these diseases are not transmitted from one host
to the other, and 2) the organism is a natural inhabitant of
the soil and generally is a harmless intestinal parasite in
all these hosts. Also excluded are: Edwardsiella, Fusibac-
terium, Klebsiella pneumoniae, Pseudomonas such as P. aerugi-
nosa, and most of the atypical Mycobacterium, staphylococci,
most streptococci, most Salmonella, Yersinia enterocolitica,
certain fungal infections like aspergillosis, blastomycosis,
candidiasis, coccidioidomycosis, cryptococcosis, phaeohyphomy-
cosis and the mycetomas. On the other hand, we have included
Erysipelothrix despite its broad host range (e.g., mucus of
fish, seals) because most of the human cases (erysipeloid) are
from contact with swine or horses, and the agent is found in
the urine and feces of such hosts. Listeriosis is in a similar category.

To avoid weighting or bias, we have counted each of the
following as only a single entry: 1) the five species of
Clostridium that cause gas gangrene; 2) the three species of
Brucella involved in forms of brucellosis; 3) the many strains
of leptospirosis; 4) the California group; 5) the C-group
of viral infections; 6) the various tick-borne viral agents
like Langat virus which can cause encephalitis (although Central European tick-borne encephalitis is considered an entity);
7) the Actinomycetes and 8) Bacteroides infections. However,
the two rat-bite fevers are distinct diseases and are treated
as such, and because the ecology of the various arena viruses
appear to differ significantly, all are tallied. The ultimate
criterion was whether members of an Order or family of mammal
was a significant source of an infection, even if they were
not true reservoirs and even though an arthropod may serve as
the actual vector. The terms "reservoir" and "quasireservoir"
are used as per Traub et al., 1975 (23).

Mammals and birds of course can be of tremendous import in
the ecology of zoonoses by serving as critical hosts of the
cardinal vectors, even in instances where the arthropod-vector
may also be the true reservoir, as in the case of some tick-
borne infections (24,25), and, probably, scrub typhus (23).
The habits and range of the host may thus greatly affect the

geographical and ecological distribution of the infection, and
this is why rabbits and rodents respectively are listed (as
queried entries) regarding tick typhus and spotted fever in
the tables below. Otherwise the charts do not include entries
based solely on mammals as hosts for vectors. Because of severe constraints of space and time, we have not presented data
on metazoan parasites like flukes, nematodes and cestodes,
even though the observations tend to lead to the same general
conclusions presented here.

We have largely ignored observations based on susceptibility in experimental hosts because the available data are often
inadequate, confusing or irrelevant (23). What happens in the
laboratory when a host is given an overwhelming dose of a
pathogen by a special route (e.g., i.c.) may be completely
different from what happens in nature when an animal is inoculated with the same agent by a mosquito or flea. Under unusual conditions, as in captivity, many species of mammals can
atypically acquire diseases like tuberculosis, salmonellosis,
amebiasis, etc. Such reports have been excluded.

THE DEGREE OF SPECIALIZATION OF THE ORDERS OF MAMMALS

G. S. Miller (30) published a system for the Orders of
North American mammals in which the sequence was from the most
primitive to the most specialized or highly evolved, as follows: 1) Marsupialia; 2) Insectivora; 3) Chiroptera; 4) Carnivora; 5) Pinnipedia; 6) Primates; 7) Rodentia; 8) Lagomorpha;
9) Artiodactyla; 10) Perissodactyla; 11) Xenarthra; 12) Sirenia; and 13) Cetacea. Miller stated that the "term total of
specialization... denote(s) the sum of the physical modifica-
tions which any particular mammal or group of mammals is sup-
posed to have undergone during the course of its development
away from an assumed original or generalized stock. ... no
idea of 'excellence', 'efficiency', or their contraries is involved."

All subsequent systems of classification have followed
Miller insofar as concerns placing the primates below the rodents, lagomorphs (rabbits, pikas), artiodactylids (cattle,
swine, etc.) and perissodactylids (equines). Simpson's classification (26) followed these concepts and included Orders
from the Australian and other regions which Miller had not
considered. It has been accepted as standard throughout the
world (e.g., 27, 28) and we use it here, as outlined in
Table 1.

In interpreting this chart and such schemes of classification, it must be borne in mind that the evolution of mammals

did not proceed in a linear manner. The Artiodactyla and
Perissodactyla (and some others not considered) represent the
culmination of a divergence that occurred in the Triassic, ca.
210 m.y.a. The second line branched into two forks, one leading to the Marsupialia and the other to branches that eventually resulted in the Edentata, Pholidota, Lagomorpha, Rodentia,
Primates, Dermoptera, Chiroptera, Insectivora and Carnivora
(but not in that sequence) (29). For these reasons, in Table
1 we also indicate data on the known geological age or presumed time of origin for the pertinent categories, and will
speak of the infections of the more recently evolved and advanced or higher groups of mammals as compared to those of the
more ancient or primitive and lower groups, when discussing
transmission of zoonoses to man. It is thus important to
realize that even though the artiodactylids and perissodactylids are derived from a different line than the primates, they
nevertheless represent a much more recent evolutionary development than do the primates, and likewise are more "advanced"
in the sense employed by Miller.

TABLE 1.   The Orders of Mammals Arranged in Sequence from
           Most Primitive to Most Advanced, with Putative
           Dates of Origin for the Orders

Rank Order	Extant Examples	Approx.Age of Order M.Y.A.	Period
1. Monotremata	Echidna	180	L. Triassic
	Possums, kangaroos,	150-	U. Jurassic
2. Marsupialia	etc.	140	L. Cretaceous
3. Insectivora	Shrews, moles, etc.	80	Cretaceous
4. Dermoptera	Colugos,"Flying Lemurs"	62	Paleocene
5. Chiroptera	Bats	70	Cretaceous(?)
6. Primates	Lemurs,monkeys,man,etc.	70	Cretaceous
7. Edentata	Sloths, armadillos,etc.	60	Paleocene
8. Pholidota	Pangolins	60	Paleocene
9. Lagomorpha	Rabbits,hares,pika	67	Cretaceous
10. Rodentia	Rats,mice,squirrels,etc.	58	Paleocene
11. Cetacea	Whales	50	Eocene
12. Carnivora	Cats,dogs,civets, weasels,seals,etc.	70	Paleocene
13. Tubulidentata	Aardvarks	20?	Eocene
14. Probiscidea	Elephants, tapirs	42	Eocene
15. Hyracoidea	Hyrax	50	Eocene
16. Sirenia	Manatees	42	Eocene
17. Perissodactyla	Horses,tapirs,rhinoceros	58	Paleocene
18. Artiodactyla	Pigs,hippopotamus,deer, camels,cattle,goats	53	Eocene

That the primates (including man) are not at the apex of
the tree of life, except for the development of the brain, is
often overlooked or disregarded. Even very recent textbooks
and articles frequently allude to man's acquisition of diseases from the "lower animals", referring to cattle, sheep,
dogs, cats, etc., whereas the mammals that are really "lower"
are the marsupials, insectivorans and bats, and as we shall
see, they play only a very small role in the zoonoses. Of the
18 Orders of mammals listed in Table 1, we will discuss 10 as
sources of infection in man. The remainder, which are deleted
because of inadequate pertinent data, are the Monotremata,
Dermoptera, Pholidota, Cetacea, Tubulidentata, Probiscidea,
Hyracoidea, and Sirenia.

DATA AND OBSERVATIONS

A.   Infections Acquired by Man from
the Lower Forms of Life

It is patent that man does not acquire any specific diseases from the characteristic pathogens of plant, invertebrates or the cold-blooded vertebrates, although we have not
come across any such generalizations in the literature. None
of these forms of life are cited as sources of human disease
in the texts we have used as standard guides (31-38). The
only reference we have seen to a botanical disease occurring
in man was the humorous allusion of James Thurber to a relative who died of chestnut blight. It is true that a few
groups of agents can cause disease in both plants and animals,
e.g., Pseudomonas, but different species are involved, and the
plant pathogens apparently do not affect man or other animals.
It is highly unusual for a virus to be able to replicate in
both plants and animals, but a few, transmitted among plants
by leafhoppers, can do so (38), but are not known to be associated with disease in animals. Some plant diseases respond
favorably to certain of the antibiotics used in human medicine,
but even so, the premise that man and plants do not share diseases seems valid. The organisms that produce serious disease
or death in insects are so far removed from the human pathogens (in phylogeny and in effect) that they (e.g., Bacillus
thuringensis) are considered safe to use commercially as a
means of controlling insects. Of course, certain pathogens of
man are vectored by arthropods, or undergo part of their life
cycle in insects or ticks, etc., but presumably these are not
natural agents of disease in the arthropod itself. The rickettsiae of scrub typhus and tick typhus are not known to cause

disease in their regular vectors. Lice die if infected with
the rickettsiae of epidemic typhus, and the plague organism
kills Xenopsylla cheopis fleas, but these agents are acquired
from the reservoir host.

The few reported examples of human disease acquired from
the cold-blooded vertebrates, or of human pathogens occurring
in such hosts, do not meet our criteria of acceptance. Thus,
diseases due to certain contaminative, opportunistic bacteria,
e.g., Erysipelothrix and Listeria, have been traced to contact
with infected fish, and salmonellosis has been acquired from
handling pet turtles.

All of these forms of life are unquestionably far less
specialized than the primates, and they antedate the warm-
blooded vertebrates by eons. The separation of plants and
animals occurred near the dawn of life. Metazoan animals are
known from the Precambrian Era, ca. 670 m.y.a. (29). Vascular
plants date back to at least the Silurian Epoch (420 m.y.a.)
in the Paleozoic Era. Insects probably arose in the Devonian
(360 m.y.a.). The amphibians date to the Devonian, and the
first reptiles to the Pennsylvanian (300 m.y.a.). The cold-
blooded vertebrates are all Paleozoic in origin, but the roots
of the primates go back only to the Cretaceous (ca. 100 m.y.a.)
in the Mesozoic Era. The birds are very ancient, dating from
the Jurassic, ca. 150 m.y.a., and some of the living Orders of
birds, e.g., the cormorants and flamingos were present in the
Cretaceous, 70-100 m.y.a. (39).

The diseases that may be transmitted from birds to man are
shown in Table 2, but the only clear-cut examples are for
avian tuberculosis, ornithosis and Newcastle disease. The
precise role of birds in six of the viral diseases is unclear,
although various avian hosts may perhaps be the reservoirs or
quasireservoirs of some of the encephalitides. Man is not
known to be a regular source of disease to birds, but "fowl
pox" turned out to be influenza (35, 40). Strains of influenza
virus have been isolated from a variety of birds and mammals
but it is generally not clear which hosts were prime donors
and which recipients.

TABLE 2. Diseases Transmitted from Birds, Insectivora,
Chiroptera, and Lagomorpha, to Man

Rank	Age of Order[a]	Order/Class	Diseases
—	140	Birds (Aves)	Avian Tuberculosis Salmonellosis[b] Yersiniosis[b] Ornithosis Congo-Crimean Hemorrhagic Fever (?)[b] Equine Encephalitides (?) (R?) Japanese B Encephalitis (?)(R?) Murray Valley Encephalitis (?) (R?) Newcastle Disease Quaranfil Virus Disease (?) Russian Spring-Summer Encephalitis(?)[b]
3	80	Insectivora	Tick-Borne Encephalitis (?)
5	70	Chiroptera	Kyasanur Forest Disease (?) Rabies[b] Tacaribe Virus Infection (?)
9	67	Lagomorpha	Tularemia[b] Spotted Fever (?) Congo-Crimean Hemorrhagic Fever (?)

[a] = In millions of years
[b] = Several major sources. R = Reservoir.

The Marsupialia (opossums, kangaroos, etc.) is a primitive and ancient Order of mammals that arose in the Late Jurassic or Early Cretaceous, probably over 140 m.y.a. (10). The group is a very rich one - in Australia and South America there is a total of 15 families, 64 genera and 182 species of marsupials (10), but even so there are no diseases known for which these mammals are a major source of infection to man.

Table 2 also presents data on the Orders Insectivora, Chiroptera and Lagomorpha. The Insectivora (shrews, moles, hedgehogs, etc.) rank third from the bottom in both specialization and age, the Order having arisen in the Cretaceous (10). Shrews, moles and hedgehogs may perhaps serve as "maintenance hosts" for Russian spring-summer encephalitis (RSSE) because they sustain a relatively long viremia after experimental infection and may be common in endemic areas (41). The role of insectivorans as a source of disease for man is

probably relatively minor, since many other kinds of mammals
have been found naturally infected with the various agents
reported for these mammals.

The Chiroptera (bats) arose ca. 70 m.y.a. and are regarded
as being primitive in general despite their adaptations for a
winged existence (42). We have included rabies as a disease
significantly associated with bats because, although this infection has an exceedingly broad host-range, human cases of
rabies have apparently been contracted in bat caves as a result of airborne infection.

The Order Lagomorpha (rabbits, pikas) is more specialized
than the Marsupialia and Insectivora and ranks near the Rodentia but it is an ancient one, apparently having arisen in the
Cretaceous (43). There is an excellent and unexplained correlation in the distribution of the cottontail rabbit with
Rocky Mountain spotted fever (44), but the main importance of
the lagomorphs in human medicine is their role in tularemia as
a quasireservoir and direct source of infection. Congo-Crimean
hemorrhagic fever (CCHF) is included in the table on the basis
of data presented by Hoogstraal regarding hares (45). Like
the broad spectrum of rodents, rabbits can be the cause of an
occasional case of plague, but the lagomorphs do not qualify
for listing in this regard.

The Order Edentata merits mention because as many as 30%
of the armadillos tested in some parts of Louisiana have been
found infected with the agent of leprosy (37) and human cases
of leprosy occur in that state. Since actual transfer of the
infection from one host to the other has not been demonstrated,
and actual contact has not been reported, leprosy is not yet
considered a zoonosis (37). To ensure completeness, we are
including the association as a queried entry in the summation
(Table 7). Armadillos have also been found naturally infected
with the agents of spirochaetosis, leptospirosis and trypanosomiasis, but appear to be of little or no consequence in the
ecology of these zoonoses.

There are 25 diseases listed in Table 3 as occurring in
both man and other primates. Of these, influenza, infection
due to respiratory syncitial virus, and smallpox presumably
have man for the primary host. The primate sources of the majority are in doubt. All of the bacterial diseases occur in
one or more other groups of mammals.

The primates are believed to have originated in the Late
Cretaceous (29, 46). The monkey-branch separated from the
prosimians ca. 55-60 m.y.a., and the line of apes and man di-
verged from that of the Old World monkeys ca. 30-35 m.y.a.
The Hominidae (apes, baboons and man) apparently arose in the
Early Miocene, ca. 23 m.y.a. (46).

TABLE 3. Diseases Occurring in Both Man and Some Other
Primates. Rank: 6. Age of Order: 70 m.y.a.

Disease	From Man to Others	From Others to Man
Proteus infections	(?)——→	←——(?)
Salmonellosis	(?)——→	←——(?)
Shigellosis	(?)——→	←——(?)
Streptococcal infections	(?)——→	←——(?)
Tuberculosis	(?)——→	←——(?)
Amebiasis	(?)——→	←——(?)
Balantidiasis	(?)——→	←——(?)
Giardiasis	(?)——→	←——(?)
Plasmodium	(?)——→	←——(?)
B-Virus (Herpes simiae)		←——
Chikungunya fever	(?)——→	←——(?)
Dengue	(?)——→	←——(?)
Infectious hepatitis	(?)——→	←——(?)
Influenza	——→	
Kyasanur forest disease	(?)——→	←——(?)
Marburg disease		←——(?)
Measles	(?)——→	←——(?)
Pox virus of monkeys		←——
Respiratory syncytial virus	——→	
Semliki forest disease	(?)——→	←——(?)
Sindbis virus disease	(?)——→	←——(?)
Smallpox	——→	
SV40 papovavirus disease	(?)——→	←——(?)
Yellow fever	(?)——→	←——(?)
Zika virus disease	(?)——→	←——(?)

(?)——→ ; ←——(?) = Ultimate source in nature or role of
primate is unclear.

Rodents rank tenth in the scale of specialization listed
in Table 1, four levels above the primates. So far as known,
rodents do not acquire diseases from man, but as shown in
Table IV, there are 44 diseases (plus six queried entries)
which are presumably directly or indirectly contracted by man
from rodents. The rickettsial spectrum includes all of the
human rickettsioses, although 1) Q fever is probably more
closely associated with artiodactylids than with rodents; 2)
man still seems to be the main reservoir of epidemic typhus,
and the true part played by flying squirrels in the ecology of

TABLE 4.   Diseases of Man for Which Rodents Are Important
           Sources of Infection. Rank: 10. Age of Order:
           58 m.y.a.

Borreliosis[a]	Argentinian hemorrhagic fever
Leptospirosis[a]	Bolivian hemorrhagic fever
Listeriosis	Lassa fever
Plague	Lymphocytic choriomeningitis
Rat-bite fevers (2)	Six other arena viruses
Tularemia[a]	California-group infections
Yersiniosis	Central European tick-borne
	encephalitis
Babesiosis	C-group infections
Giardiasis[a]	Colorado tick fever
Cutaneous leishmaniasis[a]	Encephalomyocarditis
Muco-cutaneous leishmaniasis	Hemorrhagic fever with renal
Visceral leishmaniasis[a]	syndrome (Far Eastern)
neumocystis pneumonia (?)	Hemorrhagic fever with renal
Toxoplasmosis	syndrome (Scandinavian)
Trypanosomiasis (T. cruzi)	Kyasanur forest disease (?)[b]
	Louping Ill (?)[a]
Epidemic typhus (flying-	Omsk hemorrhagic fever (?)[b]
squirrel type)	Pneumonia virus of mice
Murine typhus	Powassan encephalitis[b]
Q fever[a]	Ross River virus (?)
Queensland tick typhus[b]	Russian spring-summer
Rickettsialpox[b]	encephalitis[b]
Scrub typhus (?)[b]	Tick-borne encephalitis[b]
Spotted fever[b]	Venezuelan equine
Tick typhus (other types)[b]	encephalomyelitis (?)

[a] = Several major sources.
[b] = Acarine vector may (also) be the reservoir.

Rickettsia prowazekii infection has yet to be determined; and
3) the vector ticks and mites may be the actual reservoirs
(through transovarial transmission) of the tick typhus complex,
scrub typhus and rickettsialpox, and the rodents may prove to
be negligible sources of rickettsiae for the vectors. This
last point may also apply to the tick-borne viruses so indicated in the table. We do not regard CCHF as rodent-borne and
do not consider trench fever a zoonosis.
   The Rodentia presumably arose in the Paleocene, ca. 58
m.y.a., in the New World (10, 46). The families Aplodontidae,
Ctenodactylida and Zapodidae, and the caviomorph rodents are
believed to be of Eocene age, ca. 46-50 m.y.a. and the

ancestral phiomorphs are perhaps Early Eocene (55 m.y.a.)
(10,47,48). The Cricetidae are somewhat younger, ca. 43 m.
y.a. (47). The Sciuridae apparently appeared in the Late
Oligocene, ca. 40 m.y.a. (49), and there is unanimity of
opinion that the Muridae is the youngest of all the families
of rodents. Simpson believed it arose in the Miocene (50).

Although the Carnivora rank as #12 in the sequence of specialization of mammals, and therefore are above the rodents,
they antedate the Rodentia by far, going back to the Paleocene
ca. 70 m.y.a. (10,51). The Canidae and Felidae are among
the oldest of the carnivorans ettant, and date from the Lower
Eocene, ca. 54 m.y.a. (op. cit.).

Among the 14 diseases listed in Table 5 as being transmitted from Carnivora to man, only cat-scratch disease is not
found in other Orders of mammals as well. In marked contrast
to what occurs in the other Orders which are major sources of
human disease, only two diseases of viral etiology are cited.
Man is not known to serve as a significant source of infection
to carnivorans.

TABLE 5. Diseases Transmitted from Carnivores and
          Perissodactylids to Man

CARNIVORA. Rank: 12. Age of Order: 70 m.y.a.	
Leptospirosis[a]	Chagas' Disease (T. cruzi)
Pasteurella multocida	Cutaneous leishmaniasis
infections	Toxoplasmosis
Rat-bite fevers (2)	Visceral leishmaniasis
Tuberculosis (?)	
Yersiniosis	Murray Valley encephalitis
	Rabies[a]
Blastomycosis	
Dermatophytoses[a]	Cat-scratch disease

PERISSODACTYLA. Rank: 17. Age of Order: 58 m.y.a.	
Anthrax	Central European tick-borne
Borreliosis	encephalitis (?)
Botulism	Equine encephalitides (?)
Corynebacteriosis	Horse pox
Erysipeloid	Vesicular stomatitis
Gas gangrene	
Glanders	Dermatophytoses[a]
Leptospirosis[a]	Sporotrichosis[a]
Listeriosis[a]	
Tetanus	

[a] = Several major sources.

Tuberculosis is listed in Table 5 because badgers have
been found naturally infected with bovine tuberculosis in
parts of England (52) and it has been assumed, perhaps inva-
lidly, that the badgers have been a source of infection to
dairy herds and thus to man.

Horses and their allies (Perissodactyla) are ranked 17th
on the evolutionary scale and hence are next to the highest
Order in development. They arose in the Paleocene, ca. 58
m.y.a. As shown in Table 5, there are 16 diseases which man
acquires from perissodactylids, even though horses and donkeys
are the only members with which man has much contact. Horse-
pox is not found in any other group of mammals. So far as
known, the perissodactylids do not acquire any diseases from
man.

The Order Artiodactyla, which includes cattle, goats,
sheep, swine, camels, llamas, reindeer, giraffes, hippopota-
mus, etc., is at the peak of the evolutionary tree insofar as
concerns degrees of specialization. The Order dates back
only to the Eocene, ca. 53 m.y.a.

There are 54 infections which man presumably acquires from
the artiodactylids. This is the highest figure for any category. Twenty-six of these diseases occur only in artiodactylids and man.

There are 52 diseases listed in Table 6 as one-way trans-
fers to humans. (Nairobi sheep disease is included on the
basis of human cases mentioned in 1980 by Hoogstraal & Valdez
(53)). In addition, cowpox, and perhaps influenza, can pass
in either direction. It is not yet definitely known (40)
whether man can acquire influenza from swine, etc., although
such claims have been made. The bulk of the infections in
Table 6 are acquired from cattle, sheep, goats and swine but
the Inkoo strain of California virus may be passed from reindeer to man, and camels may be a source of glanders, and
llamas of brucellosis. Artiodactylids may acquire rabies and
plague but they are not regarded as important sources of
those infections for man. There are only two diseases of man
that infect artiodactylids (i.e., cattle) in sufficient degree
to warrant inclusion, viz., tuberculosis caused by M. tuberculosis and infections caused by Group A Streptococcus, e.g.
S. pyogenes.

TABLE 6. Diseases of Man for Which Artiodactylids Are
Important Sources of Infection. Rank: 18.
Age of Order: 53 m.y.a.

Actinomycetes infections	Bovine pseudovesicular
Anthrax	stomatitis
Bacteroides infections	California-group viruses
Bordetella infection	Central European tick-borne
Borreliosis	encephalitis
Botulism	Cowpox[b]
Brucellosis	Congo-Crimean hemorrhagic fever
Campylobacteriosis	Dugbe virus disease
Corynebacteriosis	Equine encephalitides (?)
Erysipeloid	Foot and mouth disease
Fusobacterium infections	Influenza (?)[b](?)
Gas gangrene	Japanese B encephalitis
Glanders	Kemerovo virus disease
Leptospirosis	Louping Ill
Listeriosis	Nairobi sheep disease
Ornithosis (?)	Orf
Pasteurellosis	Pseudocowpox
Salmonellosis	Pseudorabies
Streptococcal infections	Rift Valley fever
Tetanus	Russian spring-summer
Tuberculosis (M. bovis)	encephalitis
Tuberculosis (M. avium)	Sendai virus infection
Vibriosis (s. str.)	Sheep pox
	Vaccinia
Babesiosis	Vesicular stomatitis
Sarcocystis[a]	Wadi Medani infection
Toxoplasmosis	Wesselbron virus disease
Trypanosomiasis (T.	
rhodesiense)	Dermatophytoses[a]
	Sporotrichosis[a]
Q fever[a]	

[a] = Several major sources.
[b] = Also passed in some degree from man to artiodactylids.

The data on the 10 Orders of mammals and the totals of the
122 infections acquired from them and from birds are summarized in Table 7, whence it can be seen that the artiodactylids are responsible for 54 (44%); the perissodactylids and
carnivorans for 16 each (13%); and the rodents for 50 (41%).
(Some of the infections may be acquired from more than one
group of host). These are the four Orders that are highest

TABLE 7. Summary: Numbers of Pertinent Major Infections
          Occurring in Both Man and Other Mammals and Birds

Rank	Age m.y.a.	Group	To man	From man	Both ways
18	50	Artiodactylids	50+(2?)	2	1+(1?)
17	56	Perissodactylids	14+(2?)	0	0
12	70	Carnivores	14+(1?)	0	0
10	30-60	Rodents	44+(6?)	0	0
9	67	Lagomorphs	1+(1?)	0	0
7	63	Edentates	0	(1?)	Same (?)
6	100	Other primates	3+(1?)	2	(19?)
5	70	Chiropterans	1+(2?)	0	0
	105	(Birds)	5+(6?)	(1?)	0
3	120	Insectivores	(1?)	0	0
2	130	Marsupials	0	0	0

Rank: #18 is highest in evolutionary sequence of mammals
       i.e., the most specialized; #2 = lowest of those
       considered.
Age: = Approximate date of origin of group expressed in
       millions of years ago.

in the scale of evolution among those considered and, except
for the Carnivora, are likewise the most recently evolved.
The 11 entries listed for birds constitute 9% of the total.
The numbers of infections derived from the other Orders of
mammals range from 0 to a maximum of 3 (2%). The two least
specialized Orders of mammals, the marsupials and insectivores,
account at most for a total of one such zoonosis. These animals antedate the primates by 20-30 million years.

Excluding the primates, where the available data cannot be
interpreted properly, there are 142 examples of transfer of
diseases from other mammals to man, including duplication
among the Orders. These represent 104 separate zoonoses. A
total of only four diseases (all different) are transmitted to
man by the Orders which are below the primates on the scale of
evolution. Thus, 96% of the total numbers of examples (147/
142) and 96% (100/104) of the diseases involve the higher
groups of mammals.

The tabulation clearly shows that these infections are
virtually all zoonoses, i.e., acquired by man from other animals, rather than vice versa. Among the top five Orders,
there are only two examples of diseases originating in man
(anthroponoses), plus one or two that may shuttle between man
and artiodactylids.

B.   Counterpart and Sibling Infections

Some groups or genera of microorganisms cause disease in both man and other mammals, but do not do so at the species level, i.e., no one species is pathogenic to both kinds of host. Thus, while Mycoplasma pneumoniae produces serious disease in man and M. myoides is responsible for pneumonia in cattle, the Mycoplasma are not even mentioned in leading text-books on zoonoses. Such pairs of organisms may very well be sibling species, both of which were derived from a common ancestor, or else one species may have been derived from the other, and adapted to the new host. In Table 8 are listed 15 sets of such allied or counterpart infections, caused by related organisms but usually occurring in diverse hosts. It is striking that 13 of the sets of counterpart infections include pathogens of artiodactylids (12 examples) or horses (one instance), and 14 involve zoonotic hosts that are higher on the evolutionary scale than the primates.

TABLE 8.   Some Possible "Counterpart" or "Sibling" Infec-
           tions Occurring in Man and Other Mammals

	Pathogenic Agent or Disease and Hosts		Main Zoonotic Host
Actinomyces israeli Actinomycosis. Man	A. bovis Lumpy Jaw Cattle		Cattle
Actinobacillus actinomycetemcomitans Man	A. lignieresi Cattle, etc.		Cattle
Bordetella pertussis Man	B. bronchisep- tica. Swine,Man	B. paraper- tussis. Man	Swine
Corynebacterium diphtheriae Diphtheria. Man	C. pyogenes Cattle, etc.		Artiodac- tylids
Haemophilus influenzae Influenza. Man	H. suis Swine		Swine
Mycobacterium tuberculosis Tuberculosis. Man	M. bovis Tuberculosis Cattle,Man,etc.	M. avium Tuberculosis Birds,Cattle, Man	Cattle
Mycobacterium leprae Leprosy. Man	M. lepraemurium Rat leprosy		Rats
Mycoplasma pneumoniae PPLO organisms Pneumonia. Man	M. myoides PPO Organisms Pneumonia. Cattle, etc.		Cattle
Salmonella typhi Typhoid. Man	S. enteriditis Salmonellosis Cattle, Man		Cattle
Streptococcus equi- similis Streptococcosis. Man	S. equi Streptococcosis Horses		Horses
Streptococcus pyogenes Man, etc.	S. agalactiae Bovine Mastitis		Cattle
Chlamydia trachomatis LGV., trachoma, etc. Man	C. psittaci Ornithosis Birds, Cattle, etc.		Birds, Cattle? Muskrats?
Herpes hominis Man	H. simiae (B-virus)		Monkeys
Measles Man	Canine Distemper Canids	Rinderpest Cattle	Cattle, Dogs
Creutzfeldt-Jakob disease. Man	Scrapie Sheep		Sheep

DISCUSSION

There can be no doubt that the overwhelming majority of
human infections acquired by man from other mammals are from
hosts that are either more specialized than man and/or more
recently evolved than the primates. How can this phenomenon
be explained? One obvious, possible answer is that the artiodactylids, etc., are the very mammals with which man is in
most intimate contact, i.e., the large number of zoonoses
merely reflect the degree and quantity of exposures by man to
cattle, sheep, dogs, rats, squirrels, etc. If this conjecture
were correct, then as corollaries, it would be expected that:
1) there must be little contact between man and the lower
Orders of mammals because there are so few zoonoses involving
marsupials, insectivorans and bats, etc., and 2) there would
be a large number of anthroponoses resulting from the heavy
exposure of man to cattle, horses, dogs, etc. Neither of
these are the case, casting doubt upon the basic premise.

People undoubtedly come into relatively greater contact
with livestock, commensal rodents, etc. - and their secretions
and excreta - than they do with moles, shrews or possums.
Nevertheless, there is greater exposure to marsupials and insectivorans than is generally appreciated. Thus, millions of
kangaroos are slaughtered annually in Australia for commercial
purposes, and a huge work-force is employed in that industry.
Possums are common in the countryside and suburbs in Latin
America, eastern North America, Australia and New Guinea, and
frequently enter, or even reside in domiciles. Some species
are often maintained as pets and the larger ones are hunted
for food. In Southeast Asia, Suncus shrews are common peri-
domestic pests in buildings, and in Africa other shrews frequently enter huts. The opportunity for the transfer of disease from Marsupialia and Insectivora to man certainly exists
then, but even so there are no significant reports of such
events. Occasionally natural infection with the agent of
scrub typhus or murine typhus is observed in shrews (7, 54),
or serological evidence of viral infection is noted in possums, but no firm data on transmission of disease to man exist.

If intensity of exposure were the critical item in the
zoonoses/anthroponoses interchange, then the 100 diseases acquired by man from the higher/more youthful Orders of mammals
would be matched by infection passing in the opposite direction. However, we have been able to find only two such clear-
cut examples (plus another two that travel readily in either
direction). The tremendous discrepancy cannot be ascribed to
insufficient knowledge about veterinary diseases. These animals have a surfeit of their own diseases, and it is extremely

unlikely that many of these could be misdiagnosed human pathogens. Similarly, epizootics among rodents have been sufficiently studied for us to know that they did not originate from
human sources.

The large size and extended home-range of artiodactylids,
perissodactylids and carnivorans are obviously important factors in their role as sources of infections in man. Such animals attract and feed more ticks and mosquitoes, etc., than do
small creatures like shrews and some marsupials, and those arthropods predominate regarding the number and gravity of disease transmitted to man. Nevertheless, size and territory per
se cannot be determinants regarding numbers of zoonoses transmitted because most rodents are small in size and all have
limited home-ranges, yet they are responsible for almost as
many zoonoses as the artiodactylids.

These observations support our long-held belief that man
acquires infections from artiodactylids, rodents, etc., because of evolutionary factors, i.e., those Orders represent
higher forms of life (55,56). Moreover, the passage of infection from one Order of non-primates to another likewise exhibit the same downwards trend. Thus, all 13 infections that
meet our criteria are transformed down the scale of evolution
and 11 of these are derived from artiodactylids, e.g., foot
and mouth disease, brucellosis, scrapie, etc., and are passed
to Insectivora, Rodentia or Carnivora (33-35). The main reservoir of tularemia seems to be the microtine rodents (10,
57), with rabbits and hares becoming secondarily infected.

Since the trend in the zoonoses is for the infection to
pass from higher Orders to man, it is easy to believe that in
the 13 of 15 counterpart infections which affect artiodactylids (12) or equines (1) and man, the human pathogen evolved
from the species affecting the hoofed animals. There are also
counterpart infections involving nonprimates, and these too
involve artiodactylids, e.g., eperythrozoonosis and babesio-
sis. Significantly, the more primitive rodents, such as the
aplodontids, ctenodactylids, phiomorphs, caviomorphs, etc.,
do not seem to serve as primary sources of infection to man,
in marked contrast to the higher, more recently evolved sciurids, microtines, and murids, etc. Epizootics of Argentinian
hemorrhagic fever in guinea pigs (caviomorphs), resulting from
contact with the cricetid reservoir Calomyscus (35) are in
accord with our concepts.

In our view, the principles of natural selection explain
why the exchange of diseases is so overwhelmingly in the direction towards the lower and more primitive groups. Thus,
during the eons of evolutionary history, the progenitors of
the various extant plants and animals had come to live in bal-
ance with their own microbial flora and pathogens and gradually

developed a natural resistance or native immunity to such
agents. As the plants and animals evolved further, they carried this natural resistance with them, and developed new and
superior immune mechanisms, and passed both to their progeny,
so that as new taxa arose, they were resistant to the diseases
of their forebears. However, their constituent microbial
flora and parasites were also being modified, and/or the hosts
were encountering new agents, either as the pathogens evolved
or as the hosts penetrated new areas. They thus must have
continually acquired, and coped with, new pathogens and diseases throughout their evolutionary history. Their relatives
down the scale often had no background exposure to such new
agents and possessed a defense-apparatus that in general was
less developed, and hence had no defenses against such organisms. In consequence the lower, older groups of mammals, for
example, are apt to be susceptible to the pathogens of the
higher, more recently evolved hosts, while the latter have
already developed the means to tolerate such agents, or are
doing so.

    This explanation may suffice for those mammals with a com-
mon line of descent, but what about the artiodactylids and perissodactylids, whose ancestors diverged in the Triassic from
the stem leading to the marsupials, primates, rodents, etc.?
Here, for 200 million years there have been no common ancestors to pass on comparable genetic material. However, the
same ultimate effect was apparently achieved by 1) the development, through these eons of genetic isolation, of an alien
flora of pathogens to which the primates, carnivorans, etc.,
could not develop natural immunity because of lack of contact,
and 2) the evolution of a highly advanced system of combating
infections, analogous to the concurrent development of greatly
specialized limbs, teeth, digestive systems, etc., so characteristic of the hoofed animals. Thus, all the groups of mammals at the top levels of the tree of life seem to be superi-
or to the lower Orders in their overall immunological responses and defense mechanisms against disease. The most advanced
Orders are therefore favored by two evolutionary developments:
1) a "natural" immunity, reflecting the past history of the
Order, which protects the species or family and 2) enhanced
immunological capabilities of the individual.

    Apparent exceptions to these principles really bolster our
hypothesis because they presumably represent contacts between
groups of animals that had not met in their previous evolutionary history and thus never had an opportunity to develop
resistance to one another's pathogens. For example, in central Asia, primitive cricetid rodents are believed to be the
natural reservoir of plague (7, 58), but murids and sciurids,
both higher groups, and which evolved elsewhere, have

penetrated the area and have sustained fatal epizootics of
plague. Rats and infected fleas, through the agency of man,
have since transported the disease to many parts of the world.
Ornithosis is another illustration. This infection has a very
broad host-range but is principally associated with avian
hosts. We believe it originated in psittacine birds (parrots,
etc.), a group native to the southern hemisphere, and that the
zoonosis and epizootic disease has been introduced into Europe,
northern Asia and North America, etc., and spread to local
susceptible hosts.

The types of laboratory hosts used in research support our
contention that phylogenetic and evolutionary status affect
the transmission of infections. Cattle, sheep, dogs and other
higher mammals are often used in studies on their own etiological agents, or in perfection of surgical techniques, or in
studies on basic physiology and immunity, or for production of
antisera or vaccines, etc. Costs and difficulties in handling
do not preclude their use in such investigations. These highly specialized mammals are of little value in studying agents
of hosts like primates, rodents and others down the scale because they are naturally resistant to such pathogens. For
example, unless specially treated, rats, mice, guinea pigs and
rabbits are of limited use in the primary isolation of human
pathogens (unless the species themselves suffer from the disease) whereas the lower primates, in contrast, are extremely
useful in this regard. The successful employment of rodents
generally entails special stratagems aimed at overcoming the
natural resistance of the host, e.g., using newborn mice or
specially-bred lines or strains like hairless mice; intra-
cerebral or intravenous inoculation; thymectomized or splenec-
tomized, radiated or chemically-treated hosts; use of tissue
cultures, including embryonic lines, etc. Analogous manipulations must be employed with rabbits, ferrets, etc. As
Burnet & White (39) aptly wrote, some viruses "can be per-
suaded to multiply in the mouse brain if inoculated there",
when emphasizing that there "are no viruses of man that are
'infectious' in the ordinary sense for mice..." (p. 58).

Where rodents are facile hosts for primary isolations,
etc., the species are of a more primitive stock than the affected host or is one which had not naturally encountered the
etiologic agent in its biogeographic history. Thus, laboratory mice (Mus) or gerbils are suitable for the isolation of
the rickettsiae of scrub typhus, an infection primordially
associated with the subgenus Rattus (Murinae) and their Leptotrombidium chiggers, but these experimental hosts originated
in nonendemic areas. The guinea pig is a caviomorph of ancient roots and South American origin, whereas the diseases

studied therewith were usually from other parts of the world, often involving higher forms of mammals.

It also seems significant that once a new agent is isolated and eventually becomes adapted to a laboratory animal, that host belongs to a group lower on the evolutionary scale. Examples include: kuru from man, then isolated in chimpanzees and later adapting to lower primates; scrapie, from sheep, to mice; mink encephalopathy to hamsters (59); canine distemper, from canids to hamsters and mice (33).

There of course are other factors besides evolution why the lower Orders are only of limited significance in the zoonoses. Degree of contact is one, small size and secretive habits are others. Shrews and other small hosts are infested by larval ticks rather than by nymphs and adults and therefore their ticks cannot have acquired an infection from an earlier feeding. Even so, there are limiting factors which can be ascribed to evolution and historical biogeography. Thus, there is a close correlation between the kinds of ectoparasites occurring on tetrapods and their evolutionary status and the geological period when the hosts first arose, and this extends to Class and Order (10). Mites constitute the only true ectoparasites on Amphibia (Paleozoic), but reptiles (later Paleozoic) have mites and ticks, while the birds (Jurassic) have mites, ticks, Mallophaga, certain Diptera and, secondarily, a few kinds of fleas. The mammals have a larger assortment, and the same trend is exhibited by the Orders and families. Lagomorphs and rodents have a richer fauna than the lower Orders; and in general the primitive rodents have fewer kinds of ectoparasites than do the more advanced groups. The kind of family of flea also depends upon where the characteristic hosts originated (10). Hosts arising before the Paleocene lack Anoplura; mammals arising in the northern hemisphere lack Amblyceran Mallophaga. Most kinds of cattle lack fleas, but all have a wealth of other kinds of ectoparasites and bloodsucking Diptera, etc.

Primitive hosts have primitive fleas and other ectoparasites and these are usually extremely host-specific; e.g., no genus of bat-flea has adapted to any other host, and this is virtually so in the Insectivora-fleas (10). Fleas characteristic of the lagomorphs and rodents, etc., tend to parasitize the tribe or subfamily of host with which they evolved. While they occasionally may switch to a higher type of host entering their area, only rarely do they transfer to a host lower down the evolutionary scale. There are very few rodent-fleas with relatives on Insectivora, for example. The Insectivora, which apparently arose in Asia, lack primary Anoplura, which originated in North America (10,60). Not only do the lower groups of mammals have fewer kinds of ectoparasites, but our extensive field experience leads us to believe they are infested by fewer individuals as well.

These points contribute to reduced capacity for the shrews, bats and marsupials to act as sources of zoonoses. Extreme host specificity means fewer contacts with infected rodents, which are such important hosts of infection, for instance. A limited fauna of ectoparasites entails a reduction in the number of species that could serve as potential vectors. Fewer individuals mean fewer vectors.

Even though little specific research has been done regarding anthroponoses among the lower animals, the number of human infections known to occur therein is impressive, viz. 11 in Insectivora, including leptospirosis, pasteurellosis, pseudotuberculosis, plague, etc. and 10 in Marsupialia, including spirochaetosis, leishmaniasis, trypanosomiasis, etc. (7,24, 34,35,40).

FAUNAL APPROACH AND FUTURE RESEARCH

Pertinent data on evolution, phylogeny and historical biogeography would continue to broaden our understanding of the zoonoses. The true epidemiological significance of the mammalian and avian hosts should be determined regarding those zoonoses where the vector serves as reservoir. This is particularly true in the tick typhus/spotted fever complex since some of the tick "vectors" are not as efficient as are the classical species regarding transovarial transmission of the agent. Even though the cottontail has a short period of rickettsemia in experimental infection of spotted fever, rabbits need further study in other respects, such as perhaps serving as a critical host for the precise vector (61) and thereby accounting for surprising gaps in the range of the infection. Was there tick typhus in Australia before the rabbit was introduced? What is the exact role of the tick in Queensland tick typhus, and is there a true vertebrate reservoir? Is there tick typhus in Indonesia, and if so, is it restricted to the habitat of the unique Sumatran rabbit? Similar questions can be asked about this rickettsiosis in South America.

Much remains to be learned about the ecology of rickettsialpox. If Mus musculus is the reservoir, what is the status of the wild outdoor forms of this mouse, now so common in many parts of the world, and what about the other species of Mus in Asia and Africa? What is the significance of the reported isolation of the agent in Korean Microtus? If the vector mite is also the reservoir, do rats play a part in the cycle, since they harbor this same mite in some areas?

One of the most fascinating and puzzling discoveries in rickettsiology is the realization that R. prowazekii occurs naturally in flying-squirrels in southeastern U.S. (62). Further, serological data suggests that some human cases of typhus are attributable to this agent (63). Since man was always assumed to be the reservoir of epidemic typhus, which is disseminated by human body-lice, urgent questions immediately spring to mind about the flying-squirrel association. Is natural infection limited to Glaucomys volans? Does it occur throughout the range of this rodent, e.g., Central America and northern Canada? What about G. sabrinus, whose range overlaps G. volans in certain areas but which is primarily a western form? Are flying-squirrel lice the vectors? What part do gray squirrels play in the cycle? They sometimes share the same tree, and are infested by some of the same fleas, mites and ticks, but preliminary data suggest lack of natural infection. Are the flying-squirrels in Asia and Europe, which may or may not be closely allied to Glaucomys, also naturally infected with R. prowazekii?

Where sought, scrub typhus has been demonstrated wherever chiggers related to Leptotrombidium (L.) deliense occur (7). Field teams from the University of Maryland School of Medicine have recently found new species of this group of chiggers on murines in the mountains of Ethiopia (unpubl. data), suggesting that R. tsutsugamushi may likewise be present. It is unclear whether or not this rickettsiosis occurs in Africa (7).

The faunal approach has broad application. Thus, a reviewer suggested that HFRS may occur in Australia but remains "unrecognized because it is so rare" (64). This is extremely unlikely as an endemic infection if indeed voles are the reservoir because the closest microtines are in northern Burma. Bell stated that "one of the peculiarities of tularemia is its strict holarctic distribution" (65). The infection ranges as far south as Mediterranean Africa, and Bell further observed that the "absence of the disease in South America, Australia and the great mass of Africa is puzzling." However, we believe that the occurrence of tularemia can readily be explained by the distribution of microtine voles, particularly Microtus, which we regard as the true reservoir. There is a species of Microtus in Libya, and since much of the adjoining desert is a relatively recent development, these voles probably ranged more widely in Mediterranean Africa in the past. There are no microtines in South America or the rest of Africa or Australia.

Because of the marked trend in zoonoses for passage to be down the evolutionary scale and because the higher animals tend to be resistant to infections of the lower groups, more

attention should be paid to using insectivorans and marsupials, bats and the lower primates as laboratory animals for the
primary isolation and study of etiological agents of man, artiodactylids, rodents, etc., instead of doing most of such
work in mice, rats, dogs, etc.

The evolutionary data also suggest that artiodactylids may
have greater utility in the development and production of vaccines than the record indicates. The concept of counterpart
or sibling infections may be particularly useful in this connection. For example, an attenuated vaccine against Mycoplasma myoides may prove safe and efficacious against M.
pneumoniae, or vice versa. The chlamydiae may also be ideal
candidates for such an approach. Greater use should be made
of arthropods and arthropod tissue-lines in studies on etiology and course of infection (66). Insect tissue cultures may
also prove useful in vaccine production.

The general hypothesis about the direction of the flow of
infection can also prove useful in planning or modifying cam-
paigns aimed at eradicating or controlling alleged reservoirs
of disease. Bovine tuberculosis in badgers in England may
have been acquired from diseased cattle instead of the other
way round, and there may have been no real justification for
the badger-extermination campaign that was launched there.

In conclusion, it appears that intensified research based
upon faunal and evolutionary concepts would be fruitful in a
variety of fields. Also, since man acquires 25-50 times as
many diseases from the higher groups of mammals than he passes
in that direction, the consequences of evolution evidently
preclude his following the biblical adage that it is better to
give than to receive.

SUMMARY

Studies on the evolution, phylogeny and historical biogeography of ectoparasites and their hosts indicate that the
overwhelming majority of diseases which man acquires from
other animals, i.e., the zoonoses, are actually contracted
from those Orders of mammals which are more highly specialized,
or more recently evolved, than man himself. Thus, 96% of 104
zoonoses listed for nonprimate mammals are acquired from artiodactylids (cattle, sheep, etc.), equines, carnivores, rodents
or lagomorphs (rabbits, etc.), all of which are higher on the
evolutionary scale than is man even though they are frequently
incorrectly designated as "lower animals". Only four zoonoses
are definitely associated with the primitive and ancient
Orders, Marsupialia, Insectivora and Chiroptera. None of the

true pathogens of plants, invertebrates, or cold-blooded vertebrates cause disease in humans, and there are but three
diseases for which birds are a major source for man.

Among "counterpart" or "sibling" infections in which one
species of pathogen affects only man and a second, closely
related species causes disease in nonprimate mammals, 13 of
14 involve hoofed animals. Enzootic diseases also generally
descend the evolutionary scale, e.g., 11 of 13 pass from artiodactylids to insectivorans and rodents. There are only
two acceptable examples of nonprimate diseases which are anthroponoses, i.e., originate in man, and affect the higher
Orders. This low number effectively seems to rule out the
degree of contact as the determining factor as to why the
vast bulk of zoonoses are contracted from the more advanced
mammals. Instead, we believe that by natural selection, the
higher Orders have become resistant to the pathogens of the
lower forms, either by racial or natural immunity or by the
evolution of superior defense mechanisms in general, or both.
Thus, the forebears of the greatly specialized groups gradually came into equilibrium with their flora of disease-agents
and passed their effective immune systems to their descendants
whereas the lower groups of mammals lack ancestral experience
with the commensals or pathogens of the higher groups. The
primates and lower Orders often cannot cope with such agents
when they come in contact with them. The few instances where
diseases ascend the evolutionary scale represent new experi-
ences due to introduction or extension of the range of a host
or pathogen.

Examples are cited where studies on evolution and historical biogeography, rather than "nidality" or "landscape features", led to predictions, later verified, of endemicity of
certain zoonoses in unexpected areas, habitats, or hosts,
e.g., scrub typhus and hemorrhagic fever with renal syndrome.
Suggestions are made regarding possible additional applications of this faunal approach, e.g., greater use of insectivores and marsupials in studies on etiological agents; the
utilization of artiodactylids in preparation of vaccine and
in studies on immunity.

ACKNOWLEDGMENTS

We are grateful to Helle Starcke of the Department at
Baltimore for editorial assistance and the typing of the manuscript and tables, and to the Rocky Mountain Laboratories,
NIAID, for the invitation to present this paper at the Conference.

REFERENCES

1. Pavlovsky, E. N., "Natural Nidality of Transmissible Diseases" (N. D. Levine, ed., Engl. Ed.). Univ. Illinois Press, Urbana, Ill. (1964).
2. Traub, R., Wisseman, C. L., Jr., and Nur Ahmad, Trans. Roy. Soc. Trop. Med. Hyg. 61, 23 (1967).
3. Traub, R., and Wisseman, C. L., Jr., Bull. WHO 39, 209 (1968).
4. Traub, R., and Wisseman, C. L., Jr., Bull. WHO 39, 219 (1968).
5. Robertson, R. G., Wisseman, C. L., Jr., and Traub, R., Amer. J. Epid. 92, 382 (1970).
6. Begum, F., Wisseman, C. L., Jr., and Traub, R., Amer. J. Epid. 92, 180 (1970).
7. Traub, R., and Wisseman, C. L., Jr., J. Med. Ent. 11, 237 (1974).
8. Kulagin, S. M., Tarasevich, I. V. Kudryashova, N. J., and Plotnikova, L. F., J. Hyg., Epid., Microb., Immunol. 12, 257 (1968).
9. Traub, R., Bull. Br. Mus. Nat. Hist. (Zool.) 23, 389 (1972).
10. Traub, R., in "Fleas" (R. Traub and H. Starcke, eds.), p. 93. A. A. Balkema, Rotterdam (1980).
11. Traub, R., Hertig, M. Lawrence, W. H., and Harriss, T. T., Amer. J. Hyg . 59, 291 (1954).
12. Commission on Hemorrhagic Fever, Reports to Armed Forces Epidemiological Board. Washington, D.C. (1951-54).
13. Traub, R. and Wisseman, C. L., Jr., J. Infect. Dis. 138, 267 (1978).
14. Svedmyr, A., Lee, H. W., Berglund, A., Hoorn, B., Nyström, K., and Gajdusek, D. C., The Lancet 8107, 100 (1979).
15. Brummer-Korvenkontio, M., Vaheri, A., Hovi, T., von Bonsdorff, C.-H., Vuorimies, J., Manni, T., Penttinen, K., Oker-Blom, N., and Lähdevirta, J., J. Infect. Dis. 141, 131, (1980).
16. Lee, P. W., Gibbs, C. J., Jr., Gajdusek, D. C., Hsiang, C. M., and Hsiung, G. D., The Lancet 8176, 1025 (1980).
17. Lee, H. W., Lee, P. W., Tamura, M., Tamura, T., and Okuno, Y., Biken J. 22, 41 (1979).
18. Lee, H. W., Paik, K. Z., Seong, I. W., and Baek, L. J., Korean J. Virol. 9, 1 (1979).
19. Casals, J., Henderson, B. E., Hoogstraal, H., Johnson, K. M., and Shelokov, A., J. Infect. Dis. 122, 437 (1970).
20. Svedmyr, A., Lee, P. W., Gajdusek, D. C., and Gibbs, C. J., Jr., The Lancet 8189, 315 (1980).

21. Gajdusek, D. C., 14th Pacific Sci. Congr., Moscow, p. 28 (1979).
22. Traub, R., J. Med. Ent. 9, 584 (1972).
23. Traub, R., Wisseman, C. L., Jr., Jones, M. R., and O'Keefe, J. J., Ann. N.Y. Acad. Sci. 266, 91 (1975).
24. Hoogstraal, H., Ann. Rev. Ent. 11, 261 (1966).
25. Hoogstraal, H., Ann. Rev. Ent. 12, 377 (1967).
26. Simpson, G. G., "The Principles of Classification and a Classification of Mammals", Bull. Amer. Mus. Nat. Hist., New York (1945).
27. Lord Rothschild, "A Classification of Living Animals", Longmans, London (1961).
28. Andersen, S., and Knox Jones, J., "Recent Mammals of the World", Ronald Press Co., New York (1967).
29. Valentine, J. W., Sci. Amer. 239, 140 (1978).
30. Miller, G. S., Jr., "List of North American Recent Mammals 1923". Smithson. Inst., U.S. Natl. Mus. Bull. 128, (1924).
31. Bisseru, B., "Diseases of Man Acquired from His Pets". J. B. Lippincott Co., Philadelphia (1967).
32. Boyd, R. F., and Marr, J. J., "Medical Microbiology". Little, Brown & Co., Boston (1980).
33. Bruner, D. W., and Gillespie, J. H., "Hagan's Infectious Diseases of Domestic Animals", 5th ed. Cornell Univ. Press, Ithaca, N.Y. (1966).
34. Davis, J. W., Karstad, L. H., and Trainer, D. O., "Infectious Diseases of Wild Animals". Iowa State Univ. Press, Ames, Iowa (1970).
35. Hubbert, W. T., McCulloch, W. F., and Schnurrenberger, P. R., "Diseases Transmitted from Animals to Man", 6th ed. Charles C Thomas, Springfield, Ill (1975).
36. Joklik, W. K., Willett, H. P., and Amos, D. B., "Zinsser Microbiology", 17th ed. Appleton-Century-Crofts, New York (1980).
37. Steele, J. H., "CRC Handbook Series in Zoonoses. Section A: Bacterial, Rickettsial, and Mycotic Diseases", Vol. I. CRC Press, Inc., Boca Raton, Fl. (1979).
38. Steele, J. H., "CRC Handbook Series in Zoonoses. Section A: Bacterial, Rickettsial, and Mycotic Diseases", Vol. II. CRC Press, Inc., Boca Raton, Fl. (1980).
39. Fairbridge, R. W. and Jablonski, D., "The Encyclopedia of Paleontology". Dowden, Hutchinson & Ross, Inc., Stroudsburg, Pa. (1979).
40. Burnet, M., and White, D. O., "Natural History of Infectious Disease", 4th ed. Cambridge Univ. Press, Cambridge, England (1972).
41. Nosek, I. I., Trans. 1st Internat. Theriol. Congr., Moscow, Vol. II (N-Z), p. 23 (1974).

42. Traub, R., in "Fleas" (R. Traub and H. Starcke, eds.), p. 44. A. A. Balkema, Rotterdam (1980).
43. Tobien, H., Trans. 1st Internat. Theriol. Congr., Moscow, Vol. II (N-Z), p. 238 (1974).
44. Jellison, W. L., U.S. Publ. Health Rep. 60, 958 (1945).
45. Hoogstraal, H., J. Med. Ent. 15, 307 (1979).
46. Szalay, F. S., and Delson, E., "Evolutionary History of the Primates". Academic Press, New York (1979).
47. Wood, A. E., Proc. Symp. N. Amer. Paleont. Conv. II, Milwaukee Publ. Mus. Spec. Publ. 2, 95 (1977).
48. Wood, A. E., J. Palaeont. Soc. India 20, 120 (1977).
49. Black, C. C., in "Evolutionary Biology" (T. Dobzhansky et al., eds.), p. 305. Appleton-Century-Crofts, New York (1972).
50. Simpson, G. G., Evolution 15, 431 (1961).
51. Kurten, B., "The Age of Mammals", Columbia Univ. Press, New York (1972).
52. Clarkson, E., Internat. Wildlife 10, 13 (1980).
53. Hoogstraal, H., and Valdez, R., Fieldiana Zool., N. Ser. 6, 1 (1980).
54. Traub, R., Wisseman, C. L., Jr., and Farhang-Azad, A., Trop. Dis. Bull. 75, 237 (1978).
55. Jellison, W. L., Proc. 9th Ann. Mtg. Internat. NW Conf. Dis. Nat. Commun. Man. Saskatchewan, p. 128 (1954).
56. Jellison, W. L., "Tularemia in North America 1930-1974". Print. Dept. Univ. Montana Found., Missoula, Mt. (1974).
57. Hopla, C. E., in "Fleas" (R. Traub and H. Starcke, eds.), p. 287. A. A. Balkema, Rotterdam (1980).
58. Kucheruk, V. V., in "Theoretical Questions of Natural Foci of Diseases" (B. Rosicky and K. Heyberger, eds.), p. 379. Publ. House Czech. Acad. Sci., Prague (1965).
59. Gibbs, C. J., Gajdusek, D. C., and Masters, C. L., in "Senile Dementia: a Biomedical Approach" (K. Nandy, ed.) p. 115. Elsevier, New York (1978).
60. Jellison, W. L., J. Mammal. 23, 245 (1942).
61. Jellison, W. L., J. Med. Ent. 9, 595 (1972).
62. Bozeman, F. M., Masiello, S. A., Williams, M. S., and Elisberg, B. L., Nature 255, 545 (1975).
63. McDade, J. E., Shepard, C. C., Redus, M. A., Newhouse, V. E., and Smith, J. D., Amer. J. Trop. Med. Hyg. 29, 277 (1980).
64. Anonymous, Book Review. Med. J. Austral., Jan 1, 3 (1972).
65. Bell, J. F., in "CRC Handbook Series in Zoonoses. Section A: Bacterial, Rickettsial, and Mycotic Diseases" (J. H. Steele, ed.), p. 161. CRC Press, Inc., Boca Raton, Fl. (1980).
66. Traub, R., Pacif. Insects 7, 21 (1965).

EPIDEMIOLOGY
OF ROCKY MOUNTAIN SPOTTED FEVER
1975-1979

Charles G. Helmick
William G. Winkler

Viral Diseases Division
Center for Infectious Diseases
Centers for Disease Control
Atlanta, Georgia

I. INTRODUCTION

Rocky Mountain spotted fever (RMSF) is one of the most commonly reported vector-borne diseases in the United States. There has been a steady increase in the number of reported cases since 1960. This report describes the surveillance system utilized by the Centers for Disease Control (CDC) to obtain data on cases of RMSF in the United States and presents results obtained through that surveillance for the years 1975-1979. Data for 1970-1974 were reported earlier (1).

II. SURVEILLANCE SYSTEM

Beginning about 1920, state health departments began collecting data on reported cases of RMSF. The number of reported cases rose steadily from about 200/year in the 1920's to about 500/year in the 1940's. Reported cases declined in the next decade reaching a nadir of 199 cases in 1959. Since then there has been a marked increase in reported cases (Fig 1). This increase in cases prompted CDC, in 1970, to establish a national RMSF reporting system.

Two distinct reporting systems have evolved. A weekly
reporting system of RMSF cases from the state health
departments to CDC provides only the number of cases
reported by the individual states each week. Cases are
reported to the state health department by physicians or
hospitals; the state cumulates numbers and sends them to
CDC once a week for inclusion in the Morbidity and Mortality Weekly Report (MMWR). Cases so reported may or may
not be supported by laboratory diagnosis.

The second reporting system utilizes a case report form
(CRF) which provides more information on cases including
epidemiologic, clinical, and laboratory data. This CRF
surveillance system is closely interrelated with the first
system, and most cases which are reported on the weekly
case counting surveillance system are now also reported on
the CRF surveillance system. Physicians, hospitals, or
other reporting sources which submit cases through the
case counting weekly surveillance system are asked to fill
out and submit a case report form. Case report forms are
submitted to CDC as cases occur, and these data are
cumulated yearly. The intermediate length form used in
1970-74 was replaced by 2 different case report forms for
1975-79: 1) a short form designed to increase case
reporting, which asks only age, sex, race, geographic
location, date of onset, and minimal other information;
and 2) a long form designed for reporting cases of special
interest, which provides extensive information on the
clinical course, laboratory data, diagnosis, treatment,
and epidemiologic features. In addition to the 2 case
report forms utilized by CDC, several states use modifi-
cations of these forms.

Beginning in 1977, a concerted effort was made to
insure that case report forms (long or short) be completed
on each case reported through the weekly surveillance
system. In 1975, CRF's were submitted on only 44% of
reported cases; by 1979 over 90% of reported cases were
supported by CRF's. In the period 1975-1979, a total of
5,067 cases were reported to CDC on the weekly case count
surveillance system; of these, 3,853 (76%) also had case
report forms submitted (see Table 1), compared with 55% in
1970-74. The data described in the remainder of this
report were obtained from the short CRFs for the years
1975-1979. These data have been updated from previously
published reports (2,3).

Table 1.   RMSF, 1975-1979,
Yearly Trends in Reporting and Fatalities

	1975	1976	1977	1978	1979	1975-1979
Total reported cases	844	934	1,153	1,063	1,070	5,067
Fatal cases (NCHS)[a]	29	41	43	30	NA[c]	
Death-to-case ratio	3.4	4.4	3.7	2.8		
CRFs submitted[b]	362	682	908	940	961	3,853
(% of total reported)	(43)	(73)	(79)	(88)	(90)	(76)
Fatal CRF cases	13	45	42	34	30	164
Death-to-case ratio	3.6	6.6	4.6	3.7	3.2	4.3

a   NCHS = National Center for Health Statistics
b   CRF = Case report form
c   NA = Not available

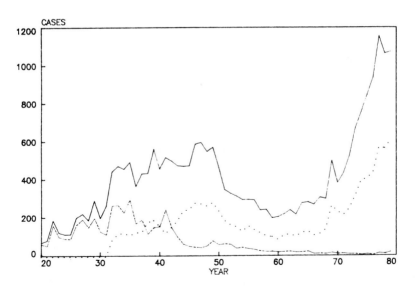

Fig. 1.   Reported RMSF cases by region, 1920-1979
_____ : Total U.S. cases; .....: South Atlantic cases;
_ _ _ _ _ _ _ : Mountain cases)

Table 2   RMSF,1975-1979,Yearly Trends in Diagnosis

	1975	1976	1977	1978	1979	Total
CRFs submitted[a]	362	682	908	940	961	3,853
Laboratory-confirmed CRFs (% of total CRFs)	117 (32)	447 (66)	540 (60)	534 (57)	507 (53)	2,145 (56)
% Confirmed by:[b]						
Complement fixation test	37	26	30	31	29	30
Weil-Felix agglut.	60	64	64	61	49	60
Other test	2	5	2	19	26	13

[a] CRF = Case report form
[b] Some cases were confirmed by more than one test

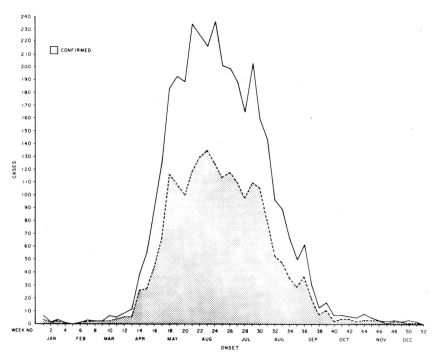

Fig. 2   Reported RMSF cases by week of onset,
United States, 1975-1979 (case report forms).

III. RESULTS AND DISCUSSION

A. Confirmed Cases

Of the 3,853 cases for which CRF's were submitted, 56%
(2,145) were laboratory confirmed (see Table 2) compared
to 51% in 1970-74. The following criteria were used for
laboratory confirmation:

      1. a compatible clinical illness,
 and 2. one of the following:
        a. a four-fold rise in antibody titer against
           spotted fever group antigen
        b. a single titer of:
           $\geq$1:16 by complement fixation
           $\geq$1:160 by Weil-Felix (OX-19) agglutination
           $\geq$1:8 by indirect fluorescent antibody test
        c. positive fluorescent antibody staining of
           tissue
        d. isolation of <u>Rickettsia</u> <u>rickettsii</u>

The most commonly used diagnostic tests were the Weil-
Felix (or Proteus OX-19) agglutination (60%) and the
complement-fixation (30%) tests, while 13% were confirmed
by other tests, generally the indirect fluorescent antibody test. Over the 5-year time span use of the
complement-fixation tests remained constant at about 30%,
while there was an increase in the use of more specific
tests, especially the indirect fluorescent antibody test
in 1978-79, and a decrease in use of the poorly specific
Weil-Felix test in 1979.
We compared laboratory-confirmed cases with cases
lacking laboratory confirmation to see if there were
epidemiologic differences between the two groups.
Unconfirmed cases had significantly more persons with "no
rash" than did confirmed cases. Unconfirmed cases also
tended to have more males and more whites, though the
difference was not significant. Age distribution, case
fatality rate, and week of onset were identical.

B. Seasonal Distribution

From Fig. 2 it is clear that the peak of RMSF cases
occurs in the spring and summer, with 97% of cases having
onset from week 13 to 39. This curve is consistent
whether one examined all reported cases or only laboratory-confirmed cases of RMSF, as in 1970-74.

Data from 1970-74 showed the epidemic curve to be
bimodal with peaks occurring in mid-May and again in
July. This was not seen in the increased number of cases
reported in 1975-79 data when cases for the U.S. as a
whole were examined. We are currently reexamining data to
determine if such bimodality might be seen in regions or
individual states.

C. Epidemiologic Aspects

As in 1970-74, RMSF remains a disease predominantly of
young people, though adults are being reported more and
more. Sixty percent of all cases were <20 years old (cf.
>66% in 1970-74), while 24% of cases were $\geq$30 years old
(cf. 17% in 1970-74). Examining incidence of RMSF shows a
sharp peak in the 5- to 9-year-old group, falling off to a
relatively low, stable incidence after age 20 (Fig. 3).

More cases were reported in males than females. The
male:female ratio was 1.66:1, slightly higher than for the
preceding 5 years (1970-74) when it was 1.56:1.

The racial composition of cases was unchanged from
1970-74, with whites accounting for 92% of cases, and
black or other races for 8%.

When age/sex/race groups were examined, the highest
incidence of RMSF infection was as follows (Fig. 3):

RACE	SEX	AGE (IN YRS.)	CASES/100,000/YEAR
White	Male	5-9	1.21
White	Female	5-9	.91
White	Male	10-19	.71
Black	Male	5-9	.69
White	Male	0-4	.60
White	Female	0-4	.53

Cases in the older adults (40-59 years) and blacks had a
higher rate of laboratory confirmation of cases than did
younger patients or whites. This may indicate underreporting of disease in older adults and blacks, since
better diagnosis of disease is not likely in these
atypical groups.

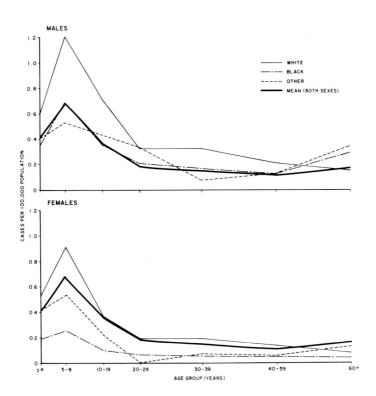

Fig. 3.   Reported average annual incidence
of RMSF, by age group, sex, and race,
United States, 1975-1979
(Case Report Forms; based on July 1, 1977,
estimate of resident U.S. population)

D.   Fatalities

The overall case fatality rate for CRFs in the 5-year
period 1975-79 was 4.3% (Table 1), comparing favorably
with the previous 5 years when the case fatality rate for
CRFs was 6.8%. This change reflects improved diagnosis/
reporting of non-fatal cases, since the actual number of
reported deaths rose in the second 5 years of reporting.
Again, the case fatality rate was seen to increase with
age. Whereas in the 0-29 year olds the case fatality rate
was 3.3%, in >30 year olds it was 7.5%. It is markedly
higher in blacks (13.0%) than in whites (3.9%). The group
at highest risk for death was blacks over 40 years old

(23.7%). The high case fatality rate in this group is
probably the result of 3 or more factors including: 1)
high case fatality rates in older persons, 2) underreporting of non-fatal cases in blacks, and 3) increased
misdiagnosis in blacks resulting in inadequate treatment.

E.   Geographic Distribution

    The geographic distribution has not changed signif-
icantly in recent years. In the 1920-1940's most cases of
RMSF were reported from the Western Mountain States but
since the 1940's, most cases have been reported in the
South Atlantic States (Fig. 1, Fig. 4).
    Cases of RMSF were reported during the 5-year period
(1975-79) in all states except Alaska, Hawaii, Maine, New
Hampshire, North Dakota, and Wisconsin. The highest
incidence of cases (>1/100,000/year) was reported in 8
states: NC (3.6), OK (2.7), SC (2.3), VA (2.2), TN (2.1),
MD (1.6), ARK (1.2), and GA (1.1); (see Fig. 5).

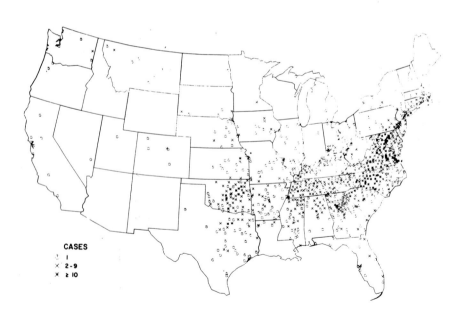

CASES
: 1
× 2 - 9
× ≥ 10

Fig. 4.   Reported RMSF cases, by county,
United States, 1975-1979 (case report form).

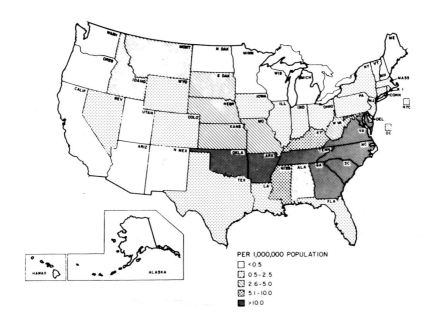

Fig. 5. Average annual incidence of RMSF
reported to CDC by state, United States, 1975-1979
(Based on July 1 estimated resident populations)

Comparison of reporting characteristics by region
showed that low incidence areas (<0.3/100,000/year) had a
higher percentage of reported cases supported by laboratory confirmation (67%) than did regions with high
incidence of infection (>1.0/100,000/year) where fewer
cases were laboratory confirmed (52%). This reflects a
greater reliance by physicians on clinical rather than
laboratory diagnosis in regions where the disease is more
frequent, which may or may not be legitimate. Low
incidence regions also showed a shift towards older ages
for cases; tended to use better diagnostic tests, i.e.,
complement fixation rather than Weil-Felix test; and
reported rash more often than did high incidence regions.
These differences may be due to geographical difference in
the disease, but it is more likely due to inclusion of
more non-RMSF cases in the high incidence regions.

F.   Rash

    Rash was reported in 82% of CRFs, down from 91% in
1970-74.   Those with no rash   constituted 9.5% (368) of
the total, compared with 3.6% (55) in 1970-74.   Among
cases without rash:

    1)   laboratory confirmation was less frequent than in
the overall population (51% vs. 56%), suggesting that
persons without RMSF are being diagnosed as RMSF, even
when they lack rash.
    2)   blacks were overrepresented (12.0% of cases
without rash vs. 6.2% of all cases), as in 1970-74,
emphasizing the difficulty in identifying a rash in
dark-skinned persons.
    3)   case fatality rates were lower than the overall
average (3.0% vs. 4.3%), in contrast to 1970-74, when the
fatality rate was higher (15% vs. 6.8%).   There is no
obvious reason for this change other than under/over-
reporting of non-rash RMSF cases.

IV. SUMMARY

    The incidence and number of reported cases of RMSF in
the U.S. have risen to record-setting highs since 1960,
and have only begun to level off in 1978 and 1979.   The
CDC's surveillance system has collected epidemiological
information on an increasing percentage of reported cases
since its start in 1970.   There has been a small rise in
laboratory confirmation of cases, and a trend towards
using more specific tests for confirmation.   The overall
fatality rate has dropped compared to 1970-74, but remains
relatively high for blacks and older adults.   Adults are
being reported more frequently, but race and sex
distribution is unchanged.   Rash is being reported less
frequently among cases than in 1970-74.

REFERENCES

1. Hattwick, M. A. W., O'Brien, R. J., and Hanson, B. F.,
    Ann. Intern. Med. 84, 732 (1976).
2. Center for Disease Control: Rickettsial Disease Surveil-
    lance Report No. 1, 1975-78, (1979).
3. D'Angelo, L. J., Winkler, W. G., and Bregman, D. J.,
    J. Infect. Dis. 138, 273 (1978).

GEOGRAPHIC DISTRIBUTION OF HUMAN CASES OF
ROCKY MOUNTAIN SPOTTED FEVER, INFECTED TICKS,
AND SEROPOSITIVE MAMMALS IN CONNECTICUT

Louis A. Magnarelli
John F. Anderson

Department of Entomology
The Connecticut Agricultural Experiment Station
New Haven, Connecticut

Willy Burgdorfer

Epidemiology Branch
Rocky Mountain Laboratories
Hamilton, Montana

I. INTRODUCTION

Dermacentor variabilis, the chief vector of Rickettsia
rickettsii for man in eastern United States is widely distributed in Connecticut (1). Concomitant with increased sub-
urbanization during the past 3 decades, D. variabilis and
Ixodes dammini have become abundant and a greater risk to
humans. Although previous studies suggested low level activity for spotted fever-group (SFG) rickettsiae in woodland
and deciduous forest-grassland transitional habitats (2),
there is increased evidence from clinical data of suspected
Rocky Mountain spotted fever (RMSF) cases, from tick/rickett-
sial surveillance, and from serologic studies of wildlife
that spotted fever rickettsiae may occur endemically at several sites in the state. This report presents the location
of suspected human cases of RMSF and the geographic distribution of infected ticks and seropositive mammals in Connecticut
and assesses the current status of the disease in this state.

RICKETTSIAE AND RICKETTSIAL DISEASES

559

II.   METHODS

   Clinical data on persons thought to have RMSF during
1965-1979 were provided by the Division of Preventable Diseases, Connecticut Department of Health and were examined to
determine possible sources and times of infection, whether
there was a history of tick exposure or bite, and whether
characteristic signs and symptoms occurred.   In clinically
compatible cases, laboratory confirmation was based on one or
more of the following criteria: a 4-fold rise in Weil-Felix
(WF) agglutinin titers in one or more of the Proteus OX series, a WF titer of $\geq$ 1:160 in a convalescent serum, presence
of a standard complement fixation (CF) test titer of $\geq$ 1:8,
or isolation of R. rickettsii.
   Adult ticks were obtained by (a) "flagging" vegetation
along trails or grasslands bordering deciduous forests, (b)
public referral, and by (c) examination of mammals.   Ticks
were screened for rickettsia-like organisms by the hemolymph
test (3) and if positive, were retested by direct immunofluorescence.   Tick tissues, which stained positively with high-
titered fluorescein isothiocyanate (FITC)-labeled rabbit antibody against R. rickettsii, were considered infected with
SFG rickettsiae.   Our conjugate did not distinguish R. rickettsii from other members of the SFG.   Isolations were made
by inoculating tick suspensions into laboratory meadow voles
(Microtus pennsylvanicus) or into Vero cell cultures (2,4).
   Medium and small-sized mammals were captured alive in
Tomahawk, Havahart, and Sherman traps, anesthetized, and
bled by cardiac puncture (2).   Sera were analyzed by a microagglutination (MA) test (5) or by indirect microimmunofluorescence (micro-IF) (6).   The rickettsial antigens used and
details on methodology will be reported elsewhere (7).   Antibody titers $\geq$ 1:8 in MA tests and $\geq$ 1:16 in micro-IF were
considered positive.

III.   RESULTS

A.   Human Cases

   Fifteen people (5 men, 3 women, and 7 children) may have
contracted RMSF at the following sites in Connecticut:
Bridgeport, Colchester, Darien, Deep River, East Haven, Lyme,
Madison (n=2), New Haven, Newtown (n=3), Oxford, Putnam, and
West Hartford (Figure 1).   Age distribution ranged from 2.5
to 48 years; illnesses occurred in March (n=1) , April (n=1),

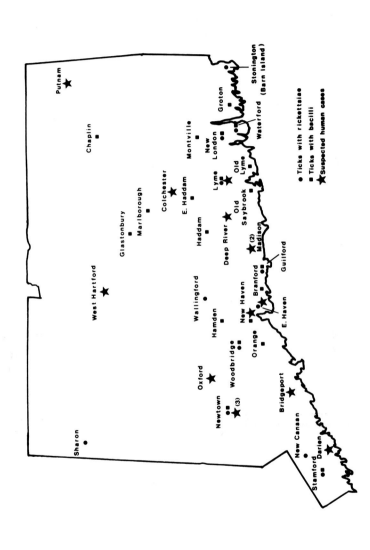

Fig. 1. Geographic distribution of suspected human cases of RMSF (1965-1979) and of D. variabilis infected with SFG rickettsiae or with unidentified bacilli in Connecticut, 1976-1979.

May (n=3), June (n=6), and July (n=4). History of tick exposure or bite was reported in 11 cases. All but one person
experienced high fever ($\geq$ 102°F), chills, severe headache,
myalgia, and macular or maculopapular rash at some time during the course of illness. One patient had no rash. Additional cases (4 with known tick bites) are reported for 8
persons who lived in Connecticut but who contracted RMSF in
other East Coast states. There were no deaths.

Serologic confirmation was made in 11 cases, and R. rickettsii was isolated from a person who had not been outside
of Connecticut for several weeks before onset of illness (7).
Test data were non-supportive in 3 cases and unavailable in
another. Significant WF agglutination and CF titers were reported for 10 (8 with $\geq$ 1:320) and 4 (2 with $\geq$ 1:16) people,
respectively; seropositivity was confirmed by 2 tests for 3
persons. With R. rickettsii antigens, MA titers of $\geq$ 1:32
and micro-IF (IgG) titers of $\geq$ 1:8192 provided additional
verification in 2 cases.

B. Infected Ticks

The following ticks were screened for SFG rickettsiae
during 1976-1979: Amblyomma americanum (n=1), D. albipictus
(n=285), D. variabilis (n=3331), I. cookei (n=56), I. den-
tatus (n=7), I. dammini (n=513), I. texanus (n=70), and
Rhipicephalus sanguineus (n=33). Rickettsia-like organisms
were recorded in hemocytes of 116 D. variabilis and 2 I. dammini. Direct immunofluorescence of duplicate hemolymph preparations indicated that 31 D. variabilis and 1 I. dammini
contained SFG rickettsiae. Fluorescent antibody (FA)-posi-
tive ticks were collected from coastal and inland areas, including the more northern regions (Figure 1). Rickettsia
montana was isolated from 4 D. variabilis collected at Woodbridge and Branford.

Eighty-five (73.3%) hemolymph test-positive D. variabilis contained long, bacterium-like organisms similar to the
unidentified bacilli previously described by Burgdorfer (3).
These rod-like organisms stained deeply with carbol basic
fuchsin, but in duplicate FA preparations, were totally
negative when treated with anti-R. rickettsii conjugate.
Bacilli-infected ticks were found throughout Connecticut,
including those areas where FA-positive specimens had been
collected and where suspected human cases are believed to
have originated.

TABLE 1. Prevalence and Titers of Microagglutination (MA) Seropositive Mammals Against R. rickettsii Antigens in Connecticut 1976–1979.

Animals	Total sera analyzed	No. (%) MA positive	No. with reciprocal MA titers of			
			8-16	24-48	64-128	>128
Beaver (Castor canadensis)	2	0				
Chipmunk (Tamias striatus)	17	0				
Eastern woodrat (Neotoma floridana)	1	1			1	
Gray squirrel (Sciurus carolinensis)	38	22 (57.9)	8	7	1	6
Meadow vole (Microtus pennsylvanicus)	5	0				
Mink (Mustela vison)	1	0				
Opossum (Didelphis virginiana)	20	0				
Rabbit (Sylvilagus floridanus)	2	0				
Raccoon (Procyon lotor)	192	48 (25.0)	10	10	12	16
Red squirrel (Tamiasciurus hudsonicus)	2	0				
Red back vole (Clethrionomys gapperi)	6	0				
Striped skunk (Mephitis mephitis)	3	0				
White-footed mouse (Peromyscus leucopus)	659	31 (4.7)	9	15	1	6
White-tailed deer (Odocoileus virginianus)	549	14 (2.6)	8	5		1
Woodchuck (Marmota monax)	10	1 (10.0)	1	1		
Totals	1507	117 (7.7)	35	38	15	29

C. Seropositive Mammals

MA tests detected antibodies in 48 of 192 raccoons, (Procyon lotor), 14 of 549 white-tailed deer (Odocoileus virginianus), 31 of 659 white-footed mice (Peromyscus leucopus), 22
of 38 gray squirrels (Sciurus carolinensis), one eastern wood-
rat, (Neotoma floridana), and one woodchuck (Marmota monax)
(Table 1). Although agglutinin titers ranged from 1:8 to 1:
1024, 71% were ≥ 1:24. Of the 197 raccoon sera tested by
micro-IF, 39 contained antibodies principally against R. rickettsii (1:64 to 1:32763) and 9 each reacted against R. montana (1:16 to 1:128) and the 369-C rickettsia (1:16 to 1:128).
Seropositive mammals were often found in the same areas
as rickettsiae-infected ticks. Their geographic distribution
(Figure 2) generally coincides with that of suspected human
cases of RMSF. Micro-IF test results suggest that raccoons
were exposed to different rickettsial agents in inland as
well as coastal regions; positive responses (≥ 1:128) to R.
rickettsii were noted for animals captured at Guilford, Lyme,
Newtown, Stonington (Barn Island), and Wallingford. Raccoons
from Branford, Cheshire, Guilford, and Newtown contained antibodies to R. montana, (≤ 1:128), whereas those from Cheshire, East Haddam, Guilford, West Hartford, and Woodbridge reacted at similar titers against the 369-C rickettsia.

IV. DISCUSSION

In spite of histories of tick exposure or bite, accurate
determination of the source of a spotted fever infection is
not always possible. People may travel great distances and
unknowingly may be carrying ticks, pets may transfer ticks
from outdoor settings to human dwellings and thereby increase
the chances for tick exposure and bite, or the onset of illness may be late and may make it difficult for a person to
accurately recall past events.
All 15 persons affected with RMSF referred to in this
paper are believed to have been infected in Connecticut.
Twelve were in the state several days before their exposure
to ticks and onset of illness, whereas the remainder had
been bitten by ticks in Connecticut and became ill within 5
days of their entry into neighboring states. Nevertheless,
clinical records were insufficient to define the areas endemic for spotted fever. Field investigations of tick and
mammal populations, however, provided valuable information
on rickettsial activity in areas where rickettsiae are
thought to be endemic. Based on these data, we feel that R.
rickettsii, the causative agent of spotted fever, is well

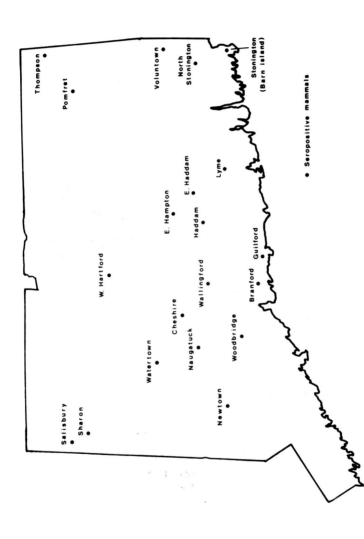

Fig. 2. Geographic distribution of seropositive mammals in Connecticut, 1976-1979.

established in tick populations at widely separated sites in Connecticut. At nearly all locations where persons may have contracted their illnesses, we found supportive evidence for the coexistence of rickettsiae-infected ticks and seropositive mammals. We realize, of course, that immunofluorescence of tick tissues and MA studies of mammalian sera can, at best, only indicate activity of SFG rickettsiae. These tests may be detecting R. montana, a species closely related to R. rickettsii (8,9), but apparently nonpathogenic to man and laboratory animals. Isolation efforts thus far have revealed R. montana infections in 4 D. variabilis (removed from dogs at Woodbridge and from a raccoon and an opossum at Branford) and the presence of a pathogenic strain of R. rickettsii in a person from West Hartford (7). Therefore, both organisms are endemic in Connecticut.

Micro-IF responses of raccoon sera to R. rickettsii and R. montana also suggest host exposure to these organisms at different locations in southern Connecticut. Nevertheless, the distribution of seropositive raccoons is not restricted to coastal areas where D. variabilis and I. dammini abound. Tick-infested raccoons are widespread in Connecticut, and wherever D. variabilis exists, there is potential for SFG rickettsial activity.

According to Cary et al. (10) and Anderson and Magnarelli (1), D. variabilis and I. dammini are abundant in southeastern Connecticut. Although rickettsiae-infected D. variabilis occurred at numerous sites, and serologic studies of mammals in this region indicated antibodies against SFG rickettsiae, only a single I. dammini was found infected with rickettsiae that stained by direct immunofluorescence. Because immature ticks of both species feed avidly on rodents (which may serve as reservoirs of rickettsial infection), it is unclear why more infected I. dammini have not been encountered.

The numbers of human cases, rickettsiae-infected ticks, and seropositive mammals recorded in Connecticut are generally much lower than those reported for other East Coast areas, such as Long Island, New York (11), the Tennessee Valley Region (12), and South Carolina (13,14). Although there is evidence suggesting that rickettsiae are endemic at widely separated sites in Connecticut, RMSF is still regarded as a rare human disease in this state.

V. SUMMARY

Information on clinical histories of persons thought to
have RMSF and data on the distribution of rickettsiae-infected ticks and seropositive mammals were compiled to determine
areas endemic for spotted fever in Connecticut. Human infections of RMSF may have originated at widely separated sites
in inland and coastal areas, but because clinical records
were often incomplete, foci could not be clearly defined.
Field studies on tick infectivity and seropositivity of mammals at these and other locations provided supportive evidence for widespread occurrence of SFG rickettsiae in D. variabilis, Sciurus carolinensis, Procyon lotor, Peromyscus
leucopus, and Odocoileus virginianus populations. Since results suggest that there are numerous foci for spotted fever
in Connecticut, the 15 human cases reported thus far during
1965-1979 are viewed as conservative estimates of rickettsial activity in the state.

ACKNOWLEDGMENTS

We are grateful to Carol Lemmon, Anthony Mavros, Ann
Whitney and Dan Walsh for their invaluable technical assistance and thank Paul Herig and other staff members of the
Connecticut Department of Environmental Protection (Wildlife
Unit) for their assistance in obtaining blood samples from
deer. Dr. Paul E. Waggoner and Malcolm T. Andrews helped
capture raccoons, and Dr. Cathryn Samples and Patricia Checko
of the Connecticut Department of Health provided clinical
information on suspected human cases of RMSF.

REFERENCES

1. Anderson, J.F., and Magnarelli, L.A., J. Med. Entomol.
   17, 314 (1980).
2. Magnarelli, L.A., Anderson, J.F., and Burgdorfer, W., Am.
   J. Epidemiol. 110, 148 (1979).
3. Burgdorfer, W., Am. J. Trop. Med. Hyg. 19, 1010 (1970).
4. Philip, R.N., and Casper, E.A., Am. J. Trop. Med. Hyg.
   (In Press).
5. Fiset, P., Ormsbee, R.A., Silberman, R., Peacock, M.,
   and Spielman, S.H., Acta Virol. 13, 60 (1969).
6. Philip, R.N., Casper, E.A., Ormsbee, R.A., Peacock, M.G.,
   and Burgdorfer, W., J. Clin. Microbiol. 3, 51 (1976).

7. Magnarelli, L.A., Anderson, J.F., Philip, R.N., Burg-
    dorfer, W., and Casper, E.A., Am. J. Trop. Med. Hyg. 30,
    (In Press, 1981).
8. Bell, E.J., Kohls, G.M., Stoenner, H.G., and Lackman,
    D.B., J. Immunol. 90, 770 (1963).
9. Lackman, D.B., Bell, E.J., Stoenner, H.G., and Pickens,
    E.G., Health Lab. Sci. 2, 135 (1965).
10. Carey, A.B., Krinsky, W.L., and Main, A.J., J. Med.
    Entomol. 17, 89 (1980).
11. Benach, J.L., White, D.J., Burgdorfer, W., Keelan, T.,
    Guirgis, S., and Altieri, R.H., Am. J. Epidemiol. 106,
    380 (1977).
12. Burgdorfer, W., Cooney, J.C., and Thomas, L.A., Am. J.
    Trop. Med. Hyg. 23, 109 (1974).
13. Burgdorfer, W., Adkins, T.R., Jr., and Priester, L.E.,
    Am. J. Trop. Med. Hyg. 24, 866 (1975).
14. Loving, S.M., Smith, A.B., DiSalvo, A.F., and Burgdor-
    fer, W., Am. J. Trop. Med. Hyg. 27, 1255 (1978).

ROCKY MOUNTAIN SPOTTED FEVER IN MARYLAND. SEROSURVEY
OF DOGS. PRELIMINARY REPORT.

P. Fiset
C. L. Wisseman, Jr.
A. Farhang-Azad

Department of Microbiology
School of Medicine
University of Maryland

H. R. Fischman

Department of Epidemiology
School of Hygiene and Public Health
Johns Hopkins University

D. Sorley
J. Horman

Communicable Diseases Division
Maryland Department of Health and Mental Hygiene

I. INTRODUCTION

A collaborative study of the epidemiology of Rocky
Mountain spotted fever and the ecology of Rickettsia
rickettsii in Maryland is currently underway. The project has
several facets: increased surveillance of cases of RMSF;
serosurvey of dogs in areas of low and high endemicity;
surveillance of ticks from humans, dogs, small mammals and the
environment, in areas of low and high endemicity, for the
presence of rickettsiae of the spotted fever group by the
hemolymph test (1); isolation and characterization of
rickettsiae from cases of RMSF and from ticks. The various
aspects of the project are in different stages of progress.

The present report is limited to preliminary results of a serosurvey of dogs. The purpose of this part of the study is to gain further information on the role of the dog in the epidemiology of RMSF and the ecology of R. rickettsii.

II. MATERIALS AND METHODS

Dog sera. Two hundred and eighty-eight (288) sera were obtained from animal hospitals and veterinary clinics from various areas in Maryland between February and April 1980 at a time when little tick activity was evident.

One hundred and fifty-six (156) blood samples were obtained on filter paper (Wisseman, in preparation) from various animal shelters and veterinary clinics between April and August 1980. This sampling was carried out at the same time as ticks were collected from the dogs. The results of the tick survey will be reported elsewhere.

Forty-five sera were obtained from the National Institutes of Health Animal Center, Poolesville, Maryland, courtesy of Dr. Nathan Jackson. These animals were bred and maintained under optimal conditions and were known to be free of ectoparasites.

Serial bleedings were also obtained from two dogs suspected of having been infected with RMSF rickettsia.

Serological procedures. The sera were tested by indirect immunofluorescence (IFA) according to a modification (Wisseman, unpublished) of the procedure of Bozeman and Elisberg (2). Primary chick embryo fibroblast cultures infected with R. rickettsii were used as antigen. The infected cultures are treated in such a way that all the rickettsial antigens are preserved. Such preparations are broadly reactive, are excellent for screening purposes but do not discriminate between the members of the spotted fever group.

All sera were screened at a dilution of 1:40 and all positives were titrated to end-point.

III. RESULTS

The 45 dog sera obtained from the NIH Animal Center in Poolesville, Md. were all negative (titers of <1:40).

Forty-six of 288 sera (16%) obtained from various veterinary clinics and animal hospitals were positive with titers ranging from 1:40 to 1:10240 (Table 1). Twenty-three of 156 (14.7%) blood samples obtained on filter paper were positive with titers varying from 1:40 to 1:10240 (Table 1).

The incidence of positive dogs ranged from 4.5% in Carroll County to 28% in Talbot County (Table 2).

The high titers (1:5120 - 1:10240) led us to believe, at first, that they were indicative of very recent infections. Recent infections, however, were difficult to explain with sera obtained in mid-winter at a time when no <u>Dermacentor variabilis</u> activity could be suspected. A possible answer was obtained when two dogs were identified as having had RMSF.

The first dog became ill within two weeks before his owner developed RMSF. Serum obtained from the dog approximately six weeks after onset of its illness had an IFA titer of 1:40960. A month later the titer was 1:20480 and ten months later, 1:2560

The second dog was seen by a veterinarian for anorexia, abdominal pain, generalized myalgia and mild ataxia of a few days duration. When examined by the veterinarian it had a temperature of 104.3. Tetracycline was administered. Within 48 hours the temperature was back to normal and the animal showed marked improvement. Tetracycline was continued for a week. Although this dog was not associated with a human case of RMSF, the veterinarian suspected it might have had the infection. Blood drawn approximately three weeks after onset of illness had an IFA titer of 1:40960. Eight and a half months later the titer was still 1:10240.

TABLE 1. Indirect Immunofluorescence Titers against
<u>R. rickettsii</u> in Dogs in Maryland

Titer	Sera	Filter Paper Eluates	Total
< 1:40	242	133	375
1:40	9	10	19
1:80	13	2	15
1:160	5	1	6
1:320	6	3	9
1:640	4	3	7
1:1280	5	2	7
1:2560	--	1	1
1:5120	3	--	3
1:10240	1	1	2
Total	288	156	444

TABLE 2. Serosurvey of Dogs in Selected Counties in Maryland

Counties	Sera	Filter Paper Eluates	Total
Talbot	19/50[a] (38%)	10/52 (19.2%)	29/102 28.4%)
Anne Arundel	4/23 (17.4%)	4/21 (19%)	8/44 (18%)
Calvert	2/25 (8.0%)	2/10 (20%)	4/35 (11.4%)
Frederick	7/29 (24%)	3/24 (12.5%)	10/53 (18.8%)
Carroll	---	1/22 (4.5%)	1/22 (4.5%)
Howard	4/43 (9.3%)	0/4 ---	4/47 (8.5%)
Harford	7/59 (11.9%)	1/9 (11.1%)	8/68 (11.7%)
Baltimore	3/59 (5.1%)	2/14 (14.3%)	5/73 (6.8%)
Total	46/288 (16.0%)	23/156 (14.7%)	69/444 (15.5%)

[a] Number positive/number tested.

IV. DISCUSSION

The observation that D. variabilis was the main if not the sole vector of R. rickettsii in the Eastern United States also implicated the dog as an important link in transmission to man. The question as to whether the dog serves as a mere mechanical carrier bringing infected ticks in proximity to man or whether it plays a more active role as a source of infection for ticks is still unanswered.

As early as 1933 Badger (3) clearly demonstrated that dogs infected either by intraperitoneal injection or by infected ticks developed a rickettsemia that could be detected between the 4th and 10th day after infection. He also noted that most dogs failed to show any sign of illness. Keenan et al. (4, 5) on the other hand, showed that the intravenous injection of large inocula ($>10^5$ GPID$_{50}$) could kill dogs, whereas smaller doses resulted either in mild illness (10^4 GPID$_{50}$) or no illness (10^2 GPID$_{50}$).

Under natural conditions infections of dogs are probably quite mild and usually go unrecognized. Over the years there have been a few reports of confirmed infections in dogs associated with human cases of RMSF (6, 7, 8). To our knowledge there is only one published report of primary infections of dogs without association with human cases (9).

Our preliminary results do not allow us to conclude that the dog is an important host in the maintenance of R. rickettsii in nature. However, since the dog is known to become rickettsemic (3, 4, 5, 8, 10) the possibility definitely exists that it may be responsible for infecting ticks under natural conditions (7). There is no doubt, as suggested by Feng et al. (8), that the dog can serve as a sensitive indicator for the detection of foci of RMSF.

ACKNOWLEDGMENTS

Supported by NIAID Contract No. NO1-AI-92622. We wish to acknowledge the excellent assistance of J. Stephen Dumler, Janet Friedman and Cecilia Queen.

REFERENCES

1. Burgdorfer, W., Am. J. Trop. Med. Hyg. 19, 1010 (1970).
2. Elisberg, B. L., and Bozeman, F. L., Arch. Inst. Pasteur, Tunis 43, 193 (1966).
3. Badger, L. F., Pub. Health Rep. 48, 791 (1933).
4. Keenan, K. P., Buhles, W. C., Jr., Huxsoll, D. L., Williams, R. G., and Hildebrandt, P. K., Am. J. Vet. Res. 38, 851 (1977).
5. Keenan, K. P., Buhles, W. C., Jr., Huxsoll, D. L., Williams, R. G., Hildebrandt, P. K., Campbell, J. M., and Stephenson, E. H., J. Infect. Dis. 135, 911 (1977).
6. Shepard, C. C., and Topping, N. H., J. Infect. Dis. 78, 63 (1946).
7. Sexton, D. J., Burgdorfer, W., Thomas, L., and Norment, B. R., Am. J. Epidemiol. 103, 192 (1976).

8. Feng, W. F., Murray, E. S., Rosenberg, G. E., Spielman,
    J. M., and Waner, J. L., J. Clin. Microbiol. 10, 322
    (1979).
9. Lissman, B. A., and Benach, J. L., J.A.V.M.A. 176, 994
    (1980).
10. Burgdorfer, W., Brinton, L. P., Krinsky, W. L., and
    Philip, R. N., in "Rickettsiae and Rickettsial Diseases",
    (J. Kazar, R. A. Ormsbee, and I. N. Tarasevich, eds.),
    p. 307. Veda, Bratislava, (1978).

ECOLOGY OF TICK-BORNE AGENTS IN CALIFORNIA.
II. FURTHER OBSERVATIONS ON RICKETTSIAE

Robert S. Lane

Department of Entomological Sciences
University of California
Berkeley, California

Robert N. Philip
Elizabeth A. Casper

Epidemiology Branch
Rocky Mountain Laboratories
Hamilton, Montana

I.   INTRODUCTION

Fourteen of 25 laboratory-confirmed cases of Rocky Mountain spotted fever (RMsf) acquired in California from 1954-79
were contracted in San Francisco Bay area or coastal counties
from San Diego in the south to Sonoma in the north.   Since
the classic tick vector of RMsf in western U.S., Dermacentor
andersoni, is absent in this part of the state, and the
vector-pathogen-host relationships had been little studied,
an intensive survey of potential tick vectors and mammalian
hosts of rickettsiae was begun there in 1974 (1).   Isolates
of spotted fever group (SFG) rickettsiae were recovered in
guinea pigs or Vero cell cultures from 3 pools of D. occidentalis collected by flagging chaparral and from a single pool
of Haemaphysalis leporispalustris taken from a black-tailed
jack rabbit.
    A follow-up study was undertaken in 1979 to determine
what species of rickettsiae occur in 3 ixodid tick species
that bite man in western California (2).   Eighty-five isolates

of SFG rickettsiae were recovered in Vero cell cultures and
typed by microimmunofluorescence (micro-IF). They comprised
4 distinct but homogeneous serotypes, 2 of which were obtained
only from D. occidentalis, and one each only from D. variabilis and Ixodes pacificus, respectively. Most strains from D.
occidentalis possessed the serologic characteristics of Rickettsia rhipicephali (3), but 3 were similar to, yet distinguishable from, R. rickettsii and are representatives of an
unclassified serotype referred to as 364D (4). Both isolates
from D. variabilis resembled the unclassified 369C serotype
previously shown to be associated with this species and D.
andersoni elsewhere in the U.S. (5). The isolate from I.
pacificus was similar to SFG organisms recovered from this
tick in western Oregon, the prototype of which is the Tilla-
mook strain (6).

In 1980, the latter study was extended to encompass other
ticks such as D. andersoni from northeastern California and
species that rarely bite man but are considered important in
maintaining rickettsiae in nature. Additional material of
species examined previously also was obtained from widely
scattered localities chiefly in western counties including
areas where 2 confirmed cases of RMsf were presumably contracted in 1979. The purpose of this report is to summarize
results of our 1980 field and laboratory studies and their
public health implications.

II. MATERIALS AND METHODS

A. Sampling Locations

Ticks were collected from 12 areas in 11 counties from 12
March to 23 July 1980 as follows: 13 km ESE of Lower Lake,
Lake Co., 7 May; Ash Creek Campground, Lassen Co., 24 April;
Coast Guard Light Station area, Point Bonita, Marin Co., 13
March; University of California, Hopland Field Station (UCHFS),
Mendocino Co., 1 April, 29 April, 19 June, 16 July, and 22-23
July; areas within ca. 2.4 km NW, SW, and S of Fee Reservoir,
Modoc Co., 23 April; Hackamore, Modoc Co., 24-25 April, Lytle
Canyon, San Bernardino Co., 21 April; Vandenberg Air Force
Base, Santa Barbara Co., 3 June; ca. 3.2 km N of Anderson,
Shasta Co., 20 May; 2.4 km SSE Annapolis, Sonoma Co., 12
March; Del Puerto Canyon, Stanislaus Co., 13 April; and ca.
3.2 km NNW Santa Paula, Ventura Co., 3 May.
The major vegetational type by locality consisted of
chaparral (Lake, Mendocino in part, San Bernardino, and Ven-
tura counties), oak woodland or woodland-grass (Mendocino in

part and Stanislaus counties), coniferous forest (Sonoma Co.),
coastal strand/northern coastal scrub (Marin Co.), or pine/
juniper woodland interspersed with sagebrush scrub (Lassen
and Modoc counties). The plant communities of sampling sites
in Santa Barbara and Shasta counties were insufficiently
characterized.

Details of climate and environment at the UCHFS are given
by Pitt and Heady (7) and Lane et al. (1).

B. Tick Collections

Approximately 79% of all ixodid ticks were collected by
flagging vegetation or by removing them from man (unattached)
or vegetation by hand. H. leporispalustris and D. parumapertus were taken from black-tailed jack rabbits, Lepus californicus, 11 adults of D. variabilis were obtained from a coyote,
Canis latrans, and 8 nymphs of I. pacificus were removed from
a western fence lizard, Sceloporus occidentalis. Ornithodoros coriaceus was collected from bedding areas of Columbian
black-tailed deer, Odocoileus hemionus columbianus, in chaparral or woodland-grass vegetational types with dry ice-
baited enamelware pans sunk in the ground, or by hand following attraction to dry ice or man.

All ticks were identified to life stage and species, and
kept alive in plastic containers with snap-on lids that generally had a 9:1 mixture of plaster-of-Paris and charcoal at
the bottom. The containers were placed inside sealed plastic
bags with damp paper toweling and stored in darkness until
they were sent to the Rocky Mountain Laboratories (RML) for
testing.

C. Laboratory Studies

At RML, each tick was examined for rickettsia-like organisms by hemolymph test (HT) according to a modification (5)
of the method of Burgdorfer (8). Hemolymph, acetone-fixed to
microscope slides, was first stained with a conjugate of
fluorescein-labeled antibody prepared in rabbits against R.
rickettsii, R strain and examined for SFG immunofluorescence.
The coverslips were then removed, the slides were washed in
tap water and restained by the method of Gimènez (9), and re-
examined. Immediately after hemolymph was obtained, ticks
were frozen and stored individually at -65°C.

Isolation of rickettsiae was attempted from ticks containing hemocyte-associated rickettsia-like organisms and all
H. leporispalustris ticks by previously described methods (5,

10). Serotyping of isolates was accomplished in micro-IF
tests (4).

III. RESULTS

In total, 1,065 ticks representing 1 argasid and 6 ixodid
species were examined by HT. The number and percentage of
ticks tested by species were as follows: D. occidentalis, 381
(35.8%); I. pacificus, 286 (26.9%); H. leporispalustris, 193
(18.1%); D. variabilis, 89 (8.4%); D. andersoni, 64 (6.0%); O.
coriaceus, 51 (4.8%); and D. parumapertus, 1 (0.1%). Of these,
181 ticks were HT-positive (Tables 1-2), i.e., hemocyte-associated, typical coccobacillary, or fine bacillary organisms
were observed in Giménez-stained hemolymph.

HT-positive ticks were collected from 7 counties and from
every county wherein at least 26 individuals were examined.
One or more ticks of all species except O. coriaceus were HT-
positive. The percentage HT-positive by species, in descend-
ing rank, was: D. parumapertus, 100%; H. leporispalustris,
51.3%; D. occidentalis, 15.0%; D. variabilis, 13.5%; D. andersoni, 4.7%; and I. pacificus, 3.1%. The highest percentages
of HT-positive ticks were detected among those taken from 5
jack rabbits at the UCHFS (Table 2). Hemocyte-associated
coccobacillary or fine bacillary organisms were observed in 99
(52.1%) of 190 H. leporispalustris. Additionally, bacilli
were noted in the only D. parumapertus found on these animals.
High infection rates also were detected among D. occidentalis
ticks from San Bernardino (30.8%) and Lake (21.4%) counties,
and among D. variabilis ticks (15.4%) from Ventura Co. (Table
1).

A total of 443 ticks of 2 species was collected from areas
where 2 cases of RMsf were presumably contracted in 1979. Six
(2.9%) of 210 I. pacificus taken from 1 site and 47 (20.2%) of
233 D. occidentalis from both localities were HT-positive
(Table 1).

Sixty-four isolates belonging to 6 serotypes were recovered in Vero cell cultures from 5 tick species (Tables 1-2).
All isolates were obtained from HT-positive ticks except 2
strains of the unclassified 369C-like serotype from H. leporispalustris. Isolates from D. occidentalis included 27 strains
typed as R. rhipicephali, 16 as 364D, 2 as 369C, and 2 as both
R. rhipicephali and 369C. All but 3 isolates from this tick
were from Lake and San Bernardino counties. Eight strains of
369C were obtained from D. variabilis collected in Ventura Co.,
and an isolate distinguishable from all known serotypes was
recovered from D. parumapertus in Mendocino Co. I. pacificus
from Sonoma Co. yielded 2 strains of the unclassified

Table 1. California Tick Survey for Rickettsiae, 1980. Results of Hemolymph Tests, Isolation Attempts, and Serotyping in Various Counties by Species.

County	Tick species	Number examined	HT-positive[a] no.	HT-positive[a] %	Number isolates	Serotypes[b] 364D	Serotypes[b] rhip	Serotypes[b] 369C	Serotypes[b] Tilla
Lake[c]	D. occidentalis	215	46	21.4	36[d]	8	27	3	
Lassen	D. andersoni	6	0	0	0				
	D. occidentalis	5	0	0	0				
Marin	D. occidentalis	80	0	0	0				
	I. pacificus	68	3	4.4	0				
Mendocino	I. pacificus	8	0	0	0				
	O. coriaceus	51	0	0	0				
Modoc	D. andersoni	58	3	5.2	0				
	H. leporispalustris	3	0	0	0				
San Bernardino	D. occidentalis	26	8	30.8	8	6	2		
Santa Barbara	D. variabilis	11	0	0	0				
Shasta	D. occidentalis	9	0	0	0				
Sonoma[c]	D. occidentalis	18	1	5.6	1			1	
	I. pacificus	210	6	2.9	2				
Stanislaus	D. occidentalis	7	0	0	0				
Ventura	D. occidentalis	21	2	9.5	2	2			
	D. variabilis	78	12	15.4	8			8	2
Total	All species	874	81	9.3	57	16	29	12	2

[a]HT-positive = hemolymph test-positive.
[b]Serotypes: 364D = Unclassified 364D-like isolates; rhip = R. rhipicephali-like isolates; 369C = Unclassified 369C-like isolates; Tilla = Unclassified Tillamook-like isolates.
[c]Rocky Mountain spotted fever case area.
[d]Two isolates each typed both as R. rhipicephali-like and 369C-like.

579

Table 2. California Tick Survey for Rickettsiae, 1980. Results of Hemolymph Tests, Isolation Attempts, and Serotyping among Ticks Collected from Lepus californicus, Mendocino County.

Hare number	Tick species	Number examined	HT-positive coccobacilli no.	%	HT-positive bacilli no.	%	Number isolates	Serotypes[a] cana	369C	Other
500	H. leporispalustris	8	0	0	6	75.0	0			
501	H. leporispalustris	37	5	13.5	17	45.9	1	1[b]		
	D. parumapertus	1	0	0	1	100.0	1			1[c]
502	H. leporispalustris	41	0	0	19	46.3	3		3	
503	H. leporispalustris	71	1	1.4	38	53.5	2		2	
504	H. leporispalustris	33	1	3.0	12	36.4	0			
Total	All species	191	7	3.7	93	48.7	7	1	5	1

[a] Serotypes: cana = R. canada-like isolates; 369C = 369C-like isolates.

[b] This isolate was obtained from 1 of the 5 ticks with hemocyte-associated coccobacilli.

[c] This isolate was distinctive from all known serotypes.

Tillamook-like serotype. Lastly, 5 strains of 369C and a
rickettsia of the typhus group resembling R. canada were
obtained from H. leporispalustris in Mendocino Co.

Isolations from ticks collected in areas where RMsf cases
apparently were acquired included 8 strains of 364D, 25 of
R. rhipicephali, 2 of 369C, and 2 as both R. rhipicephali and
369C, all from D. occidentalis, and the 2 strains of the
Tillamook-like agent from I. pacificus (Table 1).

IV. DISCUSSION

In western California, 4 serologically distinct kinds of
rickettsiae occur in D. occidentalis, D. variabilis, and I.
pacificus, the 3 principal ixodid ticks that bite man in this
region. The recent findings of Philip et al. (2) of an association of R. rhipicephali and the unclassified 364D agent
with D. occidentalis, and the unclassified 369C and Tillamook-
like agents with D. variabilis and I. pacificus, respectively,
were reconfirmed in this study.

Isolates of 364D-like organisms have been obtained only
from D. occidentalis ticks in California (2,4,11, E.J. Bell,
unpublished). These strains are serologically homogeneous and
closely related to, but as a group distinguishable from,
classical strains of R. rickettsii from the Rocky Mountain
region and eastern U.S. We isolated this rickettsia from
adult ticks collected in Lake, San Bernardino, and Ventura
counties, which brings to 5 the number of counties wherein
364D has been found and to 21 the total number of isolates of
this serotype that we have identified. Isolates of this serotype typically are of low virulence for guinea pigs and meadow
voles, give rise to well-defined target-like plaques and round
cell-type cytopathic changes in Vero cells, and kill 5-day
chick embryos 4 to 5 days after yolk sac inoculation of low
dilutions of low-passage Vero-cell seed (2). Limited serologic evidence suggests that 364D may cause human illness, as
discussed below.

R. rhipicephali, recently proposed as a new species belonging to the SFG (3), has been found in Rhipicephalus sanguineus and D. variabilis from southeastern states, in D.
andersoni from western Montana (5), and in D. occidentalis
from California (2) and Oregon (J. Cory, pers. commun.). In
California, infected ticks have been obtained from Humboldt,
Lake, Mendocino, Monterey, San Bernardino, and San Diego counties. Isolation rates from 1,041 D. occidentalis flagged from
vegetation in these counties averaged 10.4% and ranged from
1.9% in San Diego to 21.9% in Mendocino (2, present study).
Due to the generally high infection rates of this tick with R.
rhipicephali throughout western California and the low inci-

dence of RMsf in the state, it seems unlikely that this rickettsia is pathogenic for man. This presumption is consistent
with observations that the 4 R. rhipicephali-like isolates
that have been examined, which include 2 from this study, are
nonpathogenic for guinea pigs, meadow voles, and chick embryos
(2).

Recovery of 369C-like isolates from D. occidentalis and H.
leporispalustris, which rarely bites man, is the first documented association of this serotype with these ticks. Isolates also were obtained from 10 of 80 D. variabilis adults
taken from vegetation in Monterey (2) and Ventura counties.
At RML, sera from patients with tick-related illnesses have
been tested routinely against this serotype. Although most
patients with RMsf develop cross-reacting antibodies to 369C,
no evidence has been obtained which suggests that this organism causes human disease.

The unclassified Tillamook-like serotype associated with
I. pacificus from Monterey (2) and Sonoma counties is typically nonpathogenic for both guinea pigs and laboratory mice
but highly virulent for chick embryos. There is no evidence
that this organism infects humans, but this possibility should
be investigated further because it is present in a tick that
avidly bites man in an area known to be endemic for RMsf.

Surprisingly, a coccobacillus isolated from H. leporispalustris removed from L. californicus at the UCHFS was serologically similar to R. canada. Four other H. leporispalustris
ticks from hare number 501 also were HT-positive for coccobacilli (Table 2), but bacterial contamination precluded their
recovery in Vero cell cultures. R. canada was originally
recovered from H. leporispalustris ticks taken from an indicator domestic rabbit near Richmond, Ontario, Canada (12) and
has not been found again until perhaps the present study.

Discovery of a R. canada-like strain in California demonstrates that the Canadian isolate is not an aberrant rickettsia, and its occurrence in the same tick species from such
distant localities suggests that migratory birds may be involved in its transmission cycle. Clifford et al. (13) have
shown that migratory birds may be important in disseminating
ticks harboring rickettsial agents in the eastern U.S. They
isolated a strain of R. rickettsii and obtained serologic evidence that an unknown typhus-group organism was present in H.
leporispalustris ticks removed from migratory birds. Burgdorfer (14) showed that R. canada produced rickettsemia of 10
days duration after inoculation into baby chicks and suggested
that this rickettsia may be maintained in a bird-tick cycle.

In 1980, the presumed sites of infection in Sonoma and
Lake counties of 2 confirmed cases of RMsf with onsets in July
and September 1979 were visited. At the former site, ticks
were collected from grasses along an old lumber road in a

coniferous forest and, at the latter, they were flagged from
brush near the cabin where the patient had slept and from
brush surrounding a meadow where his hunting party had killed
a deer.

Antibody absorption tests of convalescent-phase sera provided indirect evidence that the infecting organism in both
cases resembled 364D (R.W. Emmons et al., unpublished data).
In Lake Co., 8 strains of 364D were obtained from D. occidentalis from both the cabin and deer areas, whereas in Sonoma
Co., no 364D-like rickettsiae were isolated from either the
few D. occidentalis or the many I. pacificus ticks examined
(Table 1). The preponderance of I. pacificus at the Sonoma
Co. site undoubtedly reflected ecologic conditions and seasonal factors at the time of sampling.

Besides the fact that 364D-like strains have been recovered only from D. occidentalis, the importance of this tick as
the likely vector is supported by numerous records of it from
man, its widespread occurrence throughout California except in
the southeastern desert and parts of the Central Valley, and
collection records of adults for every month of the year (D.P.
Furman, pers. commun.). However, proof that any of the tick-
borne rickettsiae cause human infection or illness must await
their recovery both from man and the tick vectors that bite
him.

Finally, it is notable that in California no strains of
typical R. rickettsii were isolated from 6,429 ticks (9 spp.)
tested since 1974 (1, 2, present study). However, insufficient numbers of D. andersoni and D. variabilis were tested to
exclude the possibility that R. rickettsii may be associated
with these ticks.

V. SUMMARY

In California, 1,065 ticks representing 1 argasid and 6
ixodid species from 11 counties were examined for rickettsia-
like organisms by hemolymph test (HT) in 1980. Of these, 181
ixodids (6 spp.) from 7 counties were HT-positive. Sixty-four
isolates of rickettsiae were recovered in Vero cell cultures
from Dermacentor occidentalis, D. parumapertus, D. variabilis,
Haemaphysalis leporispalustris, and Ixodes pacificus. These
comprised 6 serotypes, 5 of which belonged to the spotted
fever group (Rickettsia rhipicephali and 4 unclassified serotypes) and one to the typhus group (R. canada-like). Among
these, only the unclassified 364D serotype, associated solely
with D. occidentalis, is suspect as a cause of human illness
in this state.

ACKNOWLEDGMENTS

The following persons are gratefully acknowledged for contributing ticks or for permission to collect material from properties under their supervision: J.R. Anderson, J.R. Clover, R.E. Doty, J.M. Dusch, G. Grodhaus, H.N. Johnson, M. Lucchesi, A. McGowan, A.H. Murphy, B.C. Nelson, M.A. Thompson, and E.I. Schlinger. D.P. Furman and R.W. Emmons are thanked for permission to cite previously unpublished data.

REFERENCES

1. Lane, R.S., Emmons, R.W., Dondero, D.V., and Nelson, B.C., Am. J. Trop. Med. Hyg. 30 (in press).
2. Philip, R.N., Lane, R.S., and Casper, E.A., Am. J. Trop. Med. Hyg. 30 (in press).
3. Burgdorfer, W., Brinton, L.P., Krinsky, W.L., and Philip, R.N., in "Proceedings of the 2nd International Symposium on Rickettsiae and Rickettsial Diseases" (J. Kazar, R.A. Ormsbee, and I.N. Tarasevich, eds.), p. 307. VEDA, Bratislava (1978).
4. Philip, R.N., Casper, E.A., Burgdorfer, W., Gerloff, R.K., Hughes, L.E., and Bell, E.J., J. Immunol. 121, 1961 (1978).
5. Philip, R.N., and Casper, E.A., Am. J. Trop. Med. Hyg. 30 (in press).
6. Hughes, L.E., Clifford, C.M., Gresbrink, R., Thomas, L.A., and Keirans, J.E., Am. J. Trop. Med. Hyg. 25, 513 (1976).
7. Pitt, M.D., and Heady, H.F., Ecology 59, 336 (1978).
8. Burgdorfer, W., Am. J. Trop. Med. Hyg. 19, 1010 (1979).
9. Gimènez, D.F., Stain Technol. 39, 135 (1964).
10. Cory, J., Yunker, C.E., Ormsbee, R.A., Peacock, M., Meibos, H., and Tallent, G., Appl. Microbiol. 27, 1157 (1974).
11. Cory, J., Yunker, C.E., Howarth, J.A., Hokama, Y., Hughes, L.E., Thomas, L.A., and Clifford, C.M., Acta virol. 19, 443 (1975).
12. McKiel, J.A., Bell, E.J., and Lackman, D.B., Can. J. Microbiol. 13, 503 (1967).
13. Clifford, C.M., Sonenshine, D.E., Atwood, E.L., Robbins, C.S., and Hughes, L.E., Am. J. Trop. Med. Hyg. 18, 1057 (1969).
14. Burgdorfer, W., J. Hyg. Epidemiol. Microbiol. Immunol. 12, 26 (1968).

NONPATHOGENIC RICKETTSIAE IN DERMACENTOR ANDERSONI: A LIMITING FACTOR FOR THE DISTRIBUTION OF RICKETTSIA RICKETTSII

Willy Burgdorfer
Stanley F. Hayes
Anthony J. Mavros

Epidemiology Branch
Rocky Mountain Laboratories
Hamilton, Montana

I. INTRODUCTION

In the Bitterroot Valley of western Montana, most cases of spotted fever have occurred among residents on the west side or among persons exposed to and bitten by ticks from the west side of the Valley. Many people, on the other hand, have been bitten by east side ticks but few contracted spotted fever and for most of these, a possible contact with west side ticks could not be ruled out. Similarly, spotted fever rickettsiae virulent for guinea pigs have with one exception (1) never been recovered from ticks collected on the east side of the Bitterroot.

This phenomenon of disease focality has been the subject of numerous speculations and investigations, none of which has ever led to a reasonable explanation.

Recently, we initiated a project to explore the possibility that genetically determined variations among Dermacentor andersoni in its susceptibility to virulent Rickettsia rickettsii may be responsible for the situation on the east side of the Bitterroot Valley. To secure large quantities of supposedly "normal" ticks, larval progeny of several females from the east side of the valley were fed on male guinea pigs. Although none of these hosts developed fever, some had low titers of antibodies to R. rickettsii when tested 30 days later by microagglutination or complement fixation tests. This suggested that larvae of some tick females were infected with an ovarially acquired rickettsia that was not detected by hemolymph testing parental females. Subsequent dissection and examination of hemolymph test-negative females revealed in large percentages of ticks a spotted fever-group rickettsia whose distribution in tick tissues was limited to the posterior lobes of the midgut, small intestine, occasionally also to the anterior parts of the malpighian tubules, and to the ovary. It is the purpose of this paper to describe this agent, tentatively referred to as "East side agent", and to present preliminary data incriminating it as an important factor for preventing introduction and distribution of virulent R. rickettsii on the east side of the Bitterroot Valley.

II. MATERIALS AND METHODS

To determine the prevalence of D. andersoni with limited rickettsial infections, adults were collected by flagging in several drainages of the Sapphire Mountains on the east side of the Bitterroot Valley. As control, collections were made also on the Valley's west side. All ticks were first subjected to the hemolymph test (2) to eliminate those with generalized infection by rickettsiae or bacilluslike organisms. Hemolymph test-negative females and, to a lesser extent, also males were then dissected individually and smears from each tissue were stained either by the Giménez method (3) or with fluorescein isothiocyanate-labelled antibodies to R. rickettsii and were examined microscopically. To determine pathogenicity of the East side agent for male meadow voles (Microtus pennsylvanicus) and guinea pigs, infected ovaries of several ticks were triturated individually in 2.0 ml of cold brain heart infusion (BHI) broth, and 0.25 to 0.5 ml of the suspensions were injected intraperitoneally into each of 4 voles and 2 guinea pigs. Infections and development of antibodies in voles were evaluated as described previously (4). Rectal temperatures of guinea pigs were recorded for 14 days. Thirty days after inoculation, the guinea pigs were bled and their sera were tested for microagglutinating (MA) and complement fixing (CF) antibodies to spotted fever-group rickettsiae. Limited attempts were also made to isolate the East side agent in embryonated hens' eggs and in cell cultures. Infected ovaries were triturated in cold BHI and aliquots of 0.25 to 0.5 ml were injected into the yolk sac of 5-day-old embryos or into monolayers of Vero cells (5). To identify ultrastructural morphology of the East side agent, ovarial and midgut tissues of infected ticks were processed as previously described (6) and were examined with a Hitachi 11 EU electron microscope at 75 kV.

Finally, interactions between the East side agent and virulent R. rickettsii were determined by feeding larval progeny of ticks infected with the East side agent on rickettsemic guinea pigs that had been inoculated with 0.5 ml of a yolk sac suspension containing 10^3 egg LD_{50} of virulent R. rickettsii. After they had dropped and developed to nymphs, the ticks were fed on susceptible or immunized guinea pigs. Resulting females were eventually fed and mated to obtain filial generations. Throughout developmental stages of challenged ticks, presence of R. rickettsii was monitored microscopically as well as by injection into male guinea pigs.

III. RESULTS

A. Prevalence and Microscopic Characterization of the East Side Agent

Surprisingly large numbers of ticks collected in the Sapphire Mountain range on the east side of the Bitterroot were found to harbor the East side agent. In areas such as Daly Creek or Skalkaho Game Reserve, it was not unusual to find up to 80 percent of ticks infected. The same organism was encountered also on the west side of the valley, but the percentages of infected ticks were considerably lower (8-16%).

In adult ticks, the East side agent exhibited limited distribution. In females, it occurred to varying degree in the ovarial tissues, the posterior lobes of midgut diverticula, and in the small intestine. Occasionally, it was also detected in malpighian tubules near the connection with the rectal ampule. In male ticks, only the posterior diverticula of the midgut and the small intestine have been found infected. A more widespread distribution including tissues of salivary glands has been noted in some, but not all, ovarially infected larvae. Nymphal ticks, however, exhibited rickettsial distribution characteristic for adults.

The East side agent stains well by Giménez' method. In smears of ovarial tissues of freshly molted females, it appears as a dark-pink, well-outlined rickettsia of rather uniform morphology. Only occasionally, longer, thicker, and curved organisms are seen. In fasting ticks, morphology of the organism is characterized by pleomorphism that varies from typical oval and lanceolate, rickettsialike forms to thick and club-shaped or irregularly curved, short-to-long filamentous and thread-like forms (Fig. 1). Growth occurs intracellularly; intranuclear parasitism has not as yet been seen.

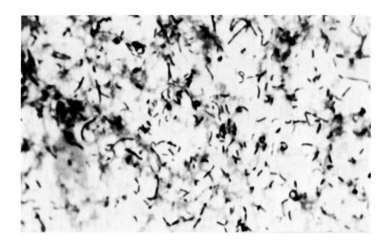

Fig. 1. East side agent in smear of ovarial tissues of
D. andersoni collected from the east side of Bitterroot Valley
Giménez stain。 1,100X

When stained with FITC labelled anti-R. rickettsii conjugates, the East side agent exhibits complete but mild fluorescence that can be readily differentiated from the brilliant
fluorescence of R. rickettsii (Fig. 2).
     Ultrastructurally, the organism cannot be distinguished
from R. rickettsii. Its cytoplasm consists of ground substance, uniformly dense in organisms of ovarial tissues but
electronlucent in those of midgut (Fig. 3).

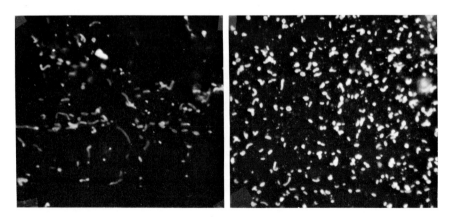

Fig. 2. Direct fluorescent antibody staining of East side
agent (on the left) and of R. rickettsii (on the right) with
anti-R. rickettsii conjugate. 1,100X

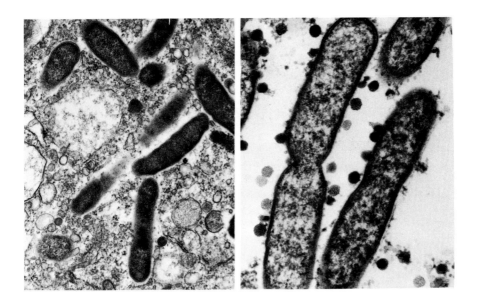

Fig. 3. Electron micrograph of East side agent in ovarial
tissue (on the left 21,000X) and in midgut epithelium (on the
right 47,000X) of D. andersoni.

B. Pathogenicity for Laboratory Animals
and Isolation Attempts

The East side agent is nonpathogenic for male meadow
voles, i.e., intraperitoneal injection of infected ovarial
tissues caused neither splenomegaly nor microscopically detectable infections in tunica vaginalis. Similar injections
into guinea pigs elicited 1 to 2 days of fever (39.8) but no
other clinical manifestations. Both guinea pigs and meadow
voles responded to such injections with CF (1:128) and MA
(1:32) antibodies to R. rickettsii but were not immune when
challenged with 100 egg LD$_{50}$ of a virulent strain of this
agent.

Guinea pigs fed on by large numbers of larval ticks derived from infected females occasionally developed low titered
(1:16) CF and MA antibodies to spotted fever antigens.

All attempts to isolate the organism in chick embryos or
cell cultures have been unsuccessful.

590

Rickettsiae and Rickettsial Diseases

C. Interactions between East Side Agent and Virulent R. rickettsii

The larval ticks used for these experiments were derived from two females (2 and 31) that transmitted the East side agent to 98 and 94 percent of filial ticks, respectively. Upon challenge with virulent R. rickettsii by feeding the larvae on rickettsemic guinea pigs, both lines when tested as nymphs showed 100 percent infection rates for the spotted fever agent. Transmission experiments in which 10 pools of 5 to 10 challenged nymphs per line were placed on susceptible guinea pigs resulted in infections typical of virulent spotted fever in all test animals. After these nymphs had molted to adults, 10 females of each line were dissected and their tissues were examined microscopically. Nine females of line 2 and 8 of line 31 had intense infections by R. rickettsii in all tissues except the ovaries which proved to be heavily infected with the East side agent. The remaining three females showed generalized R. rickettsii infections including the ovaries. Two of these females were negative and one only mildly positive for the East side agent.

Ten additional females from line 2, and 8 from line 31, all hemolymph test-positive for R. rickettsii, were then allowed to feed and mate on guinea pigs and after dropping were placed individually into vials for oviposition. After deposition of several hundred eggs, the females were dissected and their tissues were examined microscopically. Similarly, 10 eggs randomly selected from each female were smeared, stained by FA and examined for rickettsiae. Seven females from line 2 and 4 from line 31 failed to transmit R. rickettsii via eggs; their ovarial tissues and eggs were heavily infected with the East side agent. On the other hand, 7 females - 3 from line 2 and 4 from line 31 - oviposited eggs of which either all or at least some were infected with R. rickettsii. Those females that transmitted R. rickettsii to all eggs examined were negative for the East side agent; the others were rather mildly infected for both the East side agent and R. rickettsii.

IV. DISCUSSION

Presence of bacterialike microorganisms in certain tissues of the wood tick, D. andersoni, has been the subject of many investigations, and there is no doubt that the East side agent discussed in this study has been encountered before. However, identification with a previously described organism is not possible because in-depth studies on the nature of these organisms and on their relationship(s) to the spotted fever agent, R. rickettsii, are not available. Ricketts, as early as 1909, described a bacillus-like pleomorphic organism in tissues and eggs of ticks that produced spotted fever. However, morphologically indistinguishable forms in "normal ticks" provided doubts whether the organisms he saw were the cause of the disease (7). Wolbach also detected the presence in ticks, especially in eggs, of rodlike microorganisms that were nonpathogenic for guinea pigs. According to him, these organisms "may occur together with the spotted fever parasite" (8).

Three bacillus-like organisms for which the names, Bacillus rickettsiformis, B. pseudoxerosis, and B. equidistans were proposed, were isolated on special media by Noguchi from ticks collected in the Bitterroot Valley (9). These organisms were nonpathogenic for laboratory animals and immunologically were not related to the spotted fever agent. B. rickettsiformis, on the other hand, was said to be transmitted ovarially by ticks whose ovarial tissues were heavily infected.

Of particular interest in regard to the present study are observations by Parker and Spencer (10) who found rickettsial infections limited to the reproductive tissues of 36 of 100 D. andersoni (sex not stated) from the east side of the Bitterroot Valley. Injection of the viscera into guinea pigs did not produce spotted fever and none of the test animals was immune to subsequent challenge with virulent R. rickettsii.

A rickettsialike organism from a laboratory colony of D. andersoni was isolated in embryonated hens' eggs by Steinhaus (11). This rickettsia for which the name Rickettsia dermacentrophila was proposed occurred most abundantly in the epithelial cells of the intestinal diverticula, although occasionally it was found throughout the tick. It was maintained transstadially as well as transovarially and was nonpathogenic for laboratory animals and various rodent hosts.

In recent years, several spotted fever-group agents related to but distinct from R. rickettsii have been found associated with the wood tick, D. andersoni (12, 13). These rickettsiae are also relatively nonpathogenic for guinea pigs but differ from the East side agent in that they produce in ticks a generalized infection that involves all tissues including hemolymph. The relationship of the East side agent to these rickettsiae remains to be established. A certain degree of relatedness, however, is indicated by FA staining reactions with anti-R. rickettsii conjugates and by the serologic responses of guinea pigs that had been injected with suspensions containing the East side agent, or were fed on by infected larval ticks.

Both the prevalence of infected D. andersoni on the east
side of the Bitterroot Valley and the limited distribution of
the East side agent in the tick cannot be explained at this
time. One may only speculate that hundreds or thousands of
years ago, virulent spotted fever rickettsiae were present
also in the Sapphire mountains, and that these rickettsiae as
a result of changes in antigenic makeup had become avirulent
for host animals and eventually also nonpathogenic for their
tick vector. It appears that they lost their invasiveness
for certain tick tissues but manage to survive in organs occupied by the wolbachia-like symbiotes, i.e., in ovary, posterior lobes of the midgut, and in small intestine. Massive
development in ovarial tissues leads to transovarial infection - the only mechanism by which the East side agent is
maintained.

Inability of virulent R. rickettsii to invade ovarial
tissues harboring the East side agent is a typical example of
"interference" known to occur among many animal, plant, and
bacterial viruses. Although the mechanism(s) of this phenomenon in our case has not been clarified and is the subject
of a separate study, it appears that development of R.
rickettsii does not take place in epithelial and germinative
ovarial cells that are infected with the East side agent.
Lack of transovarial infection with R. rickettsii is convincing evidence of this phenomenon. However, since intensity of
infection with the East side agent may vary from tick to tick,
so does the percentage of R. rickettsii-infected oviposited
eggs. A more detailed quantitative analysis of this subject
is in progress.

Interference of somewhat different nature between nonvirulent and virulent spotted fever rickettsiae has been reported by Price (14) who found that 80 to 90 percent of
guinea pigs infected intraperitoneally with a strain of low
virulence of R. rickettsii were protected against a simultaneous injection of a virulent strain provided the low virulent strain was given in about 10 to 30 times the concentration of the virulent strain. The author speculated that animals simultaneously fed on by ticks infected with R. rickettsii of low and high virulence may be protected against the
virulent strain. Interference in ticks observed in our present study may have far more important implications in explaining the epidemiology of spotted fever. Indeed, it may
provide a logical answer to the questions why in certain localities such as the east side of the Bitterroot Valley virulent strains of R. rickettsii are rare or have never been
established.

Finally, it should be mentioned that interactions similar to those reported for the East side agent and R. rickettsii have been obtained in our laboratory (Burgdorfer et al. - unpublished data) between the nonvirulent serotypes of R. montana and R. rhipicephali on one hand, and virulent R. rickettsii, on the other. The results and their epidemiological significance will be reported elsewhere.

V.   SUMMARY

Up to 80 percent of D. andersoni from the east side of the Bitterroot Valley contained a spotted fever-group rickettsia with limited distribution to the posterior lobes of midgut, small intestine, occasionally also to anterior portions of malpighian tubules, and to ovary. The organism referred to as "East side agent" appears to be ovarially transmitted to larval ticks where it may invade tissues of salivary glands. In nymphs and adults, however, it exhibits a strong organotropism for the tissues cited above.

The East side agent is nonpathogenic for guinea pigs and meadow voles (Microtus pennsylvanicus) but elicits low titers of antibodies to spotted fever antigens. Ultrastructurally it cannot be distinguished from R. rickettsii. Although D. andersoni harboring the rickettsia occur on both sides of the Bitterroot, the prevalence on the east side is considerably higher. In such infected ticks, virulent R. rickettsii cannot become established in the ovarial tissues and therefore is not passed via eggs. This interference phenomenon appears to be an important factor responsible for limiting the distribution of virulent R. rickettsii.

REFERENCES

1.   Philip, C. B., Pub. Health Rep. 74, 595 (1959).
2.   Burgdorfer, W., Am. J. Trop. Med. Hyg. 19, 1010 (1970).
3.   Giménez, D. F., Stain Technol. 39, 135 (1964).
4.   Burgdorfer, W., Cooney, J. C., and Thomas, L. A., Am. J. Trop. Med. Hyg. 23, 109 (1974).
5.   Cory, J., Yunker, C. E., Ormsbee, R. A., Peacock, M., Meibos, H., and Tallent, G., Appl. Microbiol. 27, 1157 (1974).
6.   Hayes, S. F., and Burgdorfer, W., J. Bact. 137, 605 (1979).
7.   Ricketts, H. T., Med. Record 76, 843 (1909).

8. Wolbach, S. B., J. Med. Res. 41, 1–197 (1919).

9. Noguchi, H., J. Exp. Med. Res. 43, 515 (1926).

10. Parker, R. R., and Spencer, R. R., Pub. Health Rep. 41, 461 (1926).

11. Steinhaus, E. A., Pub. Health Rep. 57, 1375 (1942).

12. Philip, R. N., Casper, E. A., Burgdorfer, W., Gerloff, R. K., Hughes, L. E., and Bell, E. J., J. Immunol. 121, 1961 (1978).

13. Philip, R. N., and Casper, E. A., Am. J. Trop. Med. Hyg. (In press).

14. Price, W. H., Proc. Soc. Exper. Med. 82, 180 (1953).

A NEW SPOTTED FEVER GROUP RICKETTSIA FROM THE
LONE STAR TICK, <u>AMBLYOMMA AMERICANUM</u>

Willy Burgdorfer
Stanley F. Hayes
Leo A. Thomas

Epidemiology Branch
Rocky Mountain Laboratories
Hamilton, Montana

Jay L. Lancaster, Jr.

Department of Entomology
University of Arkansas
Division of Agriculture
Fayetteville, Arkansas

I. INTRODUCTION

Tick rickettsial surveys conducted in Tennessee (1) and
South Carolina (2) revealed spotted fever group rickettsiae
in 16 (16.6%) of 96 and 64 (11.7%) of 545 lone star ticks,
<u>Amblyomma</u> <u>americanum</u>. Even greater prevalence of infected
ticks has since been recorded in Arkansas where in areas surrounding Fayetteville, 194 (41.9%) of <u>A</u>. <u>americanum</u> taken off
animals or vegetation were infected with similar agents.
Characterization of isolates from the various regions has
shown that the rickettsiae are identical. The prototype isolate used in this study is referred to as WB-8-2 and originated from a tick collected off vegetation in Tennessee (1).
Certain of its properties have been reported in an analysis
of similarities and differences of isolates of spotted fever-
group rickettsiae (3). However, the present study is far
more complete and shows that the WB-8-2 agent represents a
new rickettsia of the spotted fever group.

RICKETTSIAE AND RICKETTSIAL DISEASES

II. MATERIALS AND METHODS

Morphologic appearance and development of the WB-8-2 rickettsia in A. americanum were determined microscopically. For this purpose, hemolymph test-positive ticks were dissected and their tissues were smeared and stained by Giménez (4) or by fluorescent antibody conjugates against Rickettsia rickettsii (5).

Passage of the WB-8-2 rickettsia via eggs to progeny of infected females was evaluated by microscopic examination of Giménez-stained smears prepared from various developmental stages including eggs, larvae, nymphs, and adults of the filial generation.

For electron microscopic studies, tissues of infected ticks were treated as outlined previously (6) and were examined with a Hitachi HU-11E electron microscope at 75 kV.

Isolation of the WB-8-2 rickettsia was attempted by injecting hemolymph of adult ticks into primary chick embryo tissue cultures (7). These ticks represented the first filial generation of naturally infected A. americanum females. Attempts were also made to establish rickettsial growth in embryonated hens' eggs by injecting via yolk sac aliquots of 0.25 ml of brain-heart-infusion broth suspensions containing triturated infected chick-embryo fibroblasts.

Pathogenicity of the WB-8-2 rickettsia was determined for male meadow voles (Microtus pennsylvanicus) and guinea pigs (Hartley strain) either by feeding infected ticks on these animals or by injecting intraperitoneally 0.25 to 0.5 ml of suspensions containing triturated infected ticks or cell cultures (8).

Serologic responses of guinea pigs were determined by complement fixation (CF) and those of voles by microagglutination (MA) (9) tests against antigens prepared from the spotted fever agent, R. rickettsii. In addition, suspensions of cell culture-grown WB-8-2 rickettsiae were inoculated intravenously into Swiss mice (RML strain) whose sera subsequently were tested by microimmunofluorescence (10) against a battery of rickettsial agents including R. rickettsii (Sawtooth ♀2), R. montana (M 5-6), R. rhipicephali (3-7-♀6), R. parkeri (Alabama-1974), R. conorii (Simko), and R. akari (No. 29 Am RP).

III. RESULTS

A. Characterization and Development of
WB-8-2 in Ticks

When stained by Giménez, the WB-8-2 rickettsia in hemocytes and tissues of infected A. americanum appears as a light
to dark-pink, well-outlined round to oval organism that often
occurs in pairs. Bacillary or lanceolate forms are rare unless the tick has been starved for long periods. Infection
of hemocytes is generally mild and often may involve less than
10 percent of cells with seldom more than 5 to 10 organisms
per cell (Fig. 1). Although all tick tissues are infected,
the degree of rickettsial development is generally mild with
ovary and malpighian tubules being more heavily infected than
other organs. There is transstadial and transovarial passage
of the WB-8-2 rickettsia, but filial infection rates vary between 30 to 100 percent depending on the intensity of rickettsial development in ovarial tissues.

When treated with anti-R. rickettsii conjugates, the
WB-8-2 organism fluoresces moderately and in complete fashion,
i.e., the entire organism shows a rather uniform reaction
(Fig. 2).

Electron microscopy of WB-8-2 shows a mean length and
width of 1.41 and 0.68 μm, respectively. As illustrated in

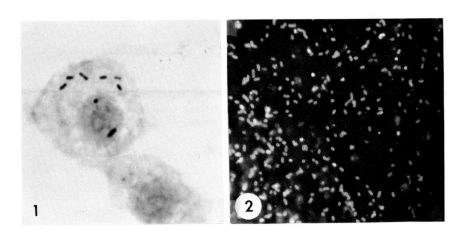

Figs. 1 and 2. WB-8-2 rickettsia in tissues of A. americanum. Figure 1 illustrates organisms in a hemocyte (Giménez
stain, 1,100X). Figure 2 shows appearance of WB-8-2 in smear
of ovary (fluorescent antibody stain, 1,100X).

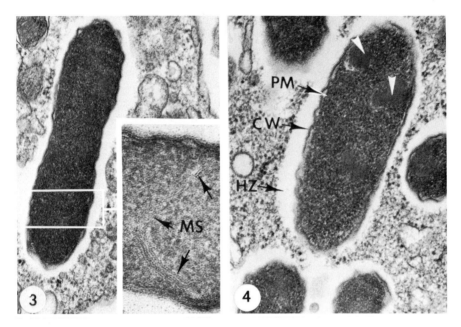

Figs. 3 and 4. Micrographs of WB-8-2 in tick tissues.
Figure 3 shows a darkstained rickettsia (45,000X). Arrows in
insert point toward mesosomal structures (120,000X). Figure
4 illustrates electron-lucent rickettsia with inclusion bodies
(arrows). HZ = halo zone; CW = cell wall; PM = plasma membrane.

Figures 3 and 4, the organism is surrounded by a prominent
halo zone (HZ) or slime-layer and possesses the quadra- or
trilaminar cell wall (CW) characteristic of spotted fever-
group rickettsiae. The cell wall varies from rigid to sinuous
and contains an osmophilic inner mucoprotein layer (5-9 nm), a
middle, less osmophilic lipopolysaccharide layer (3-4 nm), and
an outer osmophilic layer (2.5 - 3.5 nm). Associated with
the cell wall is a poorly osmophilic and usually ill-defined
bead-like microcapsular layer (8-10 nm).
    Internally and immediately adjacent to the cell wall is a
variable periplasmic space bordered by a plasma membrane (PM)
of typical unit membrane construction (7-10 nm in width).
This membrane in many organisms is in close contact with the
cell wall. It envelopes a cytoplasm that contains tightly
packed prominent ribosomes. As seen in Figure 4, there are
also rickettsiae with somewhat electron-lucent cytoplasm
that contains randomly-dispersed, prominent ribosomes and

fine amorphous ground substance. These organisms occur along
with the darker stained rickettsiae in the same cells.

Crystalline inclusion bodies as pictured in Figure 4 are
regularly present. In addition, mesosomal or membranelike
structures are seen to traverse the width of the rickettsiae.
Occasionally these structures encompass the dense, fine-
grained material of the crystalline inclusion bodies (Fig. 3).

B. Isolation of the WB-8-2 Rickettsia in Tissue Culture and Embryonated Hens' Eggs

The WB-8-2 rickettsia could readily be isolated in primary chick embryo culture where it produced plaques that were
somewhat turbid and averaged 1.7 to 2.0 mm in diameter. Also
successful was the cultivation in embryonated hens' eggs but
only after inoculation of infected culture suspensions. Death
of chick embryos occurred from days 5 to 7 after inoculation.
Rickettsial growth in yolk sac tissues was generally mild and
remained so even after 15 serial passages of infected eggs.

C. Pathogenicity of the WB-8-2 Rickettsia for Laboratory Animals

Male guinea pigs fed on by pools of up to 50 infected A.
americanum, or injected with suspensions of infected ticks or
cell cultures did not develop elevated temperatures or other
clinical manifestations. Meadow voles also were not adversely
affected by tick feeding or injection of triturates of infected ticks. However, transient rickettsial infections were
occasionally noted in tunica vaginalis after injection of suspensions of infected chick embryo fibroblasts. Repeated
attempts to maintain such infections by passage into normal
voles failed. Neither guinea pigs nor voles developed CF or
MA antibodies to R. rickettsii.

The results of the microimmunofluorescence testing of sera
of Swiss mice inoculated with suspensions of infected chick
embryo fibroblasts are summarized in Table 1. They indicate
high homologous titers and practically no cross reactions with
any of six other spotted fever-group serotypes.

TABLE 1.   Identification of WB-8-2 in Microimmunofluorescence of Mouse Sera

Antisera	Antigens WB-8-2[a] (16)	R. rickettsii (15)	R. montana (9)	R. rhipicephali (12)	R. parkeri (75)	R. conorii (2)	R. akari (8)
WB-8-2 (16)	4096[b]	16	0	0	0	0	tr[c]
R. rickettsii (15)	16	512	tr	8	32	32	0
R. montana (9)	0	0	512	16	0	0	0
R. rhipicephali (12)	0	128	32	2048	64	64	tr
R. parkeri (75)	8	64	tr	8	2048	256	0
R. conorii (2)	0	32	0	tr	128	1024	0
R. akari (8)	0	64	32	64	128	128	32,768

[a]Figures in parentheses denote code numbers of rickettsial strains.
[b]Serum dilution endpoint.
[c]Trace of reaction at 1:4 dilution.

IV.   DISCUSSION

Our findings suggest that the WB-8-2 rickettsia present
in large percentages of A. americanum from Arkansas, South
Carolina, and Tennessee represents a hitherto undescribed,
new spotted fever-group serotype. Its association with the
lone star tick is not a recent one but has gone unnoticed by
earlier investigators because the rickettsia is nonpathogenic
for guinea pigs which, prior to the application of the hemolymph test, were the most often used means for detection of
rickettsial infections in ticks.
    The WB-8-2 rickettsia appears to be nonpathogenic also
for man. Since 1973, 14 of 24 persons from whom infected A.
americanum had been removed provided epidemiological follow-
up information. None of these individuals experienced fever
headache or rash after removal of the tick (2; 11). Indeed,
if the WB-8-2 rickettsia were the cause of human illness,
case incidence in areas like Arkansas where 41.9 percent of
A. americanum were found to carry this agent would likely be
extremely high, especially in view of the fact that man is
readily attacked by all developmental stages of this tick.

Relatedness of the WB-8-2 rickettsia to the spotted fever
group is indicated, not only by staining reactions with conjugates against R. rickettsii, but also by more sophisticated
biochemical methods (3). Thus, the molar percentage of guanine plus cytosine (G + C) of the rickettsia's DNA proved to
be similar to that of the other spotted fever-group rickettsiae. On the other hand, there were significant differences
between its protein profile and those of virulent R. rickettsii as determined by sodium dodecyl sulfate-polyacrylamide
gel electrophoresis (SDS-PAGE).

Like most spotted fever-group rickettsiae, the WB-8-2
organism produced generalized infection of all tissues in its
tick vector, A. americanum. However, the degree of infection
unlike that for R. rickettsii, R. montana, and R. rhipicephali in their respective vectors is characteristically
mild.

Morphologically, the WB-8-2 rickettsia differs from the
above-mentioned tick-borne agents in that most organisms are
diplo-elliptical. Its ultrastructure is similar to that of
other spotted fever-group rickettsiae except that its cytoplasm shows a characteristically dense matrix and often contains crystalline inclusions of unknown nature.

A. americanum has long been known (12, 13) to be an efficient experimental vector of R. rickettsii, and there have
been isolations in guinea pigs of rickettsiae, possibly R.
rickettsii, from ticks collected off vegetation or animals in
the immediate surroundings of spotted fever patients (13).
However, to the best of our knowledge, this tick has never
been proven to be a natural vector of spotted fever. Parker
and associates (13) examined in guinea pigs some 5,000 larval,
nymphal, and adult ticks from Texas, Oklahoma, Arkansas, and
Missouri without obtaining convincing evidence of spotted
fever infections. In our own studies, we examined 1,700 A.
americanum without encountering R. rickettsii. Five hundred
forty-five of these came from areas near Fayetteville,
Arkansas, where numerous spotted fever cases had occurred. Our
present consensus is that these cases resulted from bites of
the American dog tick, Dermacentor variabilis.

V.   SUMMARY

A hitherto undescribed rickettsia was found in up to 42
percent of field-collected lone star ticks, A. americanum.
Based on fluorescent antibody staining reactions, the organism
appears to be related to the spotted fever group. In its tick
host, the rickettsia, referred to as WB-8-2, invades all

tissues but, in general, produces a mild to moderate infection
except in the ovary where it may be abundant and from where
it is passed via eggs to as many as 100 percent of progeny.
The organism grows well in avian cell cultures but very poorly
in embryonated hens' eggs that nevertheless die from 5 to 7
days after inoculation. The WB-8-2 rickettsia is nonpathogenic for guinea pigs. In male meadow voles (Microtus pennsylvanicus) it produces microscopically detectable mild and
transient infections in tunica vaginalis but only after inoculation of heavily infected tissue culture suspensions.
Epidemiological evidence suggests that this rickettsia is nonpathogenic for man.

REFERENCES

1. Burgdorfer, W., Cooney, J. C., and Thomas, L. A., Am.
    J. Trop. Med. Hyg. 23, 109 (1974).
2. Burgdorfer, W., Atkins, T. R., Jr., and Priester, L. E.,
    Am. J. Trop. Med. Hyg. 24, 866 (1975).
3. Anacker, R. L., McCaul, T. F., Burgdorfer, W., and
    Gerloff, R. K., Infect. Immun. 27, 468 (1980).
4. Giménez, D. F., Stain Technol., 39, 135 (1964).
5. Peacock, M., Burgdorfer, W., and Ormsbee, R. A., Infect.
    Immun., 3, 355 (1971).
6. Hayes, S. F., and Burgdorfer, W., J. Bact. 137, 605
    (1979).
7. Wike, D. A., and Burgdorfer, W., Infect. Immun. 6, 736
    (1972).
8. Burgdorfer, W., Ormsbee, R. A., Schmidt, M. L., and
    Hoogstraal, H., Bull. WHO 48, 563 (1973).
9. Fiset, P., Ormsbee, R. A., Silberman, R., Peacock, M.,
    and Spielman, S. H., Acta Virol. 13, 60 (1969).
10. Philip, R. N., Casper, E. A., Burgdorfer, W., Gerloff,
    R. K., Hughes, L. E., and Bell, E. J., J. Immunol. 121,
    1961 (1978).
11. Loving, S. M., Smith, A. B., DiSalvo, A. F., and
    Burgdorfer, W., Am. J. Trop. Med. Hyg. 27, 1255 (1978).
12. Maver, M. B., J. Infect. Dis. 8, 327 (1911).
13. Parker, R. R., Kohls, G. M., and Steinhaus, E. A., Pub.
    Health Rep. 58, 721 (1943).

ANALYSIS OF A CHEMICAL CONTROL STUDY
FOR <u>DERMACENTOR</u> <u>VARIABILIS</u>

Dennis J. White

New York State Department of Health
Saranac Lake, New York

Jorge L. Benach

New York State Department of Health
Stony Brook, New York

Laurel A. Smith
Soo P. Ouyang

Department of Applied Mathematics
State University of New York
Stony Brook, New York

I. INTRODUCTION

Cases of Rocky Mountain spotted fever (RMsf) reported in the United States and in New York State have increased in number dramatically since 1970 (1-2). The mean number of cases per year in the United States from 1960-1970 was 290, and since 1970, this has increased to a mean of 822 cases per year. Similarly, in New York from 1960-1970, there was a mean of 7 RMsf cases per year, and since 1970 this has increased to 26 cases per year. A peak in disease incidence occurred in 1977 for both the United States (1153 cases) and New York (40 cases). Within New York State, over 80% of the reported cases occur in Nassau and Suffolk counties of Long Island. The remaining cases are represented most often by visitors to Long Island who were bitten by an infected tick and later had the disease diagnosed

elsewhere at his/her permanent residence. The rapid increase
of RMsf cases on Long Island has stimulated local and state public health agencies to vigorously promote a public awareness
campaign (3). In addition to printed pamphlets, radio announce-
ments and television news clips, widely read local newspapers
frequently publicized information concerning disease occurrence,
symptoms, case histories, tick biology, etc. Subsequent demands
for control of ticks prompted local and state governmental representatives to actively promote a tick and RMsf control program. In 1976, state senators and assemblymen passed legis-
lation mandating a tick and RMsf control program to be instituted by the New York State Department of Health (NYSDH).

II. METHODS

    In order to establish locations and obtain descriptions of
infected tick foci on Long Island, we used a two-front approach.
In addition to performing the hemolymph test (4) on all acquired
tick specimens to determine the presence of the typical pleomorphic rickettsiae of the spotted fever group (5-6), we also
received information concerning all confirmed and most presumptive RMsf cases in New York. After we had confirmed the
presence of rickettsiae at the designated foci, the state health
department was then able to conduct limited applications of
insecticides on an experimental basis. Since Dermacentor
variabilis (Say) often congregates on roadside edges or pathways (7), chemical applications could be effectively applied by
a mist blower which produces droplets greater than 50 μ. The
NYSDH purchased a Buffalo Turbine mist blower and a heavy-duty
pick up truck to haul the equipment.
    Recent local environmental legislation and court actions on
Long Island precluded the use of some insecticides and acari-
cides already labeled for area tick control. Therefore, it
became necessary to increase the choice of chemicals that could
be available for area control of D. variabilis that did not
exhibit a pronounced residual activity (8-9). Field applications of chemicals not specifically labeled for area control
of D. variabilis were made possible by experimental use permits
issued by the New York State Department of Environmental
Conservation (NYSDEC) as per Part 172 of the Federal Insecticide,
Fungicide and Rodenticide Act of 1972.

---

[1]Acarina:Ixodidae

Laboratory tests were designed to assess the susceptibility of 10–20 day old D. variabilis larvae to various dilutions of propoxur, naled, chlorpyrifos, ronnel or pyrethrins with piperonyl butoxide by a modified treated surface technique (10). Adults were exposed to the same emulsifiable insecticides and acephate by topical applications of $1\,\mu$l aliquots of the diluted insecticide. Probit analyses were conducted on all LD_{50} data derived from the bioassay experiments (11). Field trials were subsequently performed with all 6 chemicals against caged adult ticks to determine efficacy data under field conditions. Additional field trials with emulsifiable naled were conducted to determine a spraying regimen for seasonal control of D. variabilis. Nine 0.5 ha plots were selected, based on vegetational characteristics and tick density. Three mist applications of naled (168g Dibrom/ha) at 4 wk intervals were scheduled over a 3 month season to more fully determine the effect of regular applications on the questing tick population. Data derived from these experiments were subjected to exploratory data analysis, simple, and multiple regression statistical techniques.

III. RESULTS AND DISCUSSION

Data derived from the probit analyses indicated that naled was more toxic to larvae than the remaining selected compounds. Topical application experiments on adults indicated that naled and chlorpyrifos may have a high potential for an area tick control program. The field trial experiments confirmed the finding that naled was relatively more toxic to D. variabilis than other compounds and could be applied at a dose acceptable to the NYSDEC, and still prove to be a highly effective acaricide. Recommendations were established for county vector control programs using concentrations of all six chemicals indicated in Table 1. Local vector control programs could apply any sequence of these chemicals over a typical adult season with a definite preference for naled, due to its short persistence under field conditions and its effective acaricidal activity. The Chevron Chemical Company obtained a 24(c) local use registration for area control of D. variabilis in New York State based on our experimentation.

Since ticks may happen to be at the base of some vegetation or otherwise be protected from the effects of one particular chemical application, it would be desirable to expose that tick population to repeated applications so that chances of tick exposure to the acaricide are enhanced. Data derived from the experiments designed to determine the proper frequency of naled

Table 1. Chemicals and concentrations to be used for the control of Dermacentor variabilis on Long Island, New York.

Manufacturer	Chemical	Field Concentration a.i.	Amount Technical In-gredient/Acre	Amount Formulated Material/Acre
Chevron	Orthene 75% acephate 75% O,S-Dimethyl acetylphos-phoroamidethioate	6.0%	1.5 lbs.	2 lbs.
Chevron	Dibrom 8 naled 58% 1,2-dibromo-2,2-dichloro-ethyl dimethyl phosphate	0.4%	0.1 lb.	0.17 lbs.
Chemagro	Baygon 1.5 propoxur 2-(1-methylethoxy)phenol methyl carbamate 13.9%	1.1%	0.28 lbs.	2 lbs.
Dow	Korlan 24E ronnel 24% O,O-dimethyl O-(2,4,5-trichloro-phenyl)phosphorothioate	0.75%	0.187 lbs.	0.78 lbs.
Dow	*Dursban 2E chlorpyrifos 24% O,O-Diethyl O-(3,5,6-trichloro-2-pyridyl)phosphorothioate	0.25%	0.056 lbs.	0.23 lbs.
FMC	Pyrenone Pyrethrins 1%	0.1%	0.03 gal.	0.3 gal.

* Dursban M may be considered = 41% chlorpyrifos

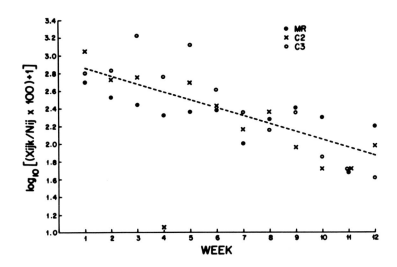

Fig. 1. Decrease of questing tick populations at 3 control plots from week 1-12. X = no. of ticks; N = no. of 10 m subplots.

applications are illustrated in Figures 1-3. Regression analyses of data derived from weekly drags at 3 control plots provided an estimate of questing ticks that would be expected to be present at a plot during any given week during the adult season. Data indicate that there existed a 20% decay in tick numbers from week to week during that season on those representative plots. However, since all blocks of plots were homogeneously structured, the same rate can be assigned to each block, i.e. treated or non-treated. The normalized and transformed raw data were subjected to simple regression, which then allowed a reassignment of the expected population counts to what can be referred to as the tick threshold value. In other words, any figure above this threshold value (at point 0.0 in Fig. 2 and 3) indicates a population of ticks in excess of the expected value, and conversely, a figure below this value indicates fewer ticks than what was expected for that particular week.

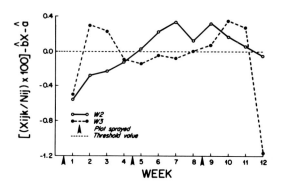

Fig. 2.   Effect of spraying water on tick populations at 2 plots.

Applications of water to 2 plots during weeks 1, 5 and 9 had no observable effect on the questing tick population, since population data points hover near the 0.0 expected value and no increase or decrease in tick numbers can be seen just after the water treatment (Fig. 2). In comparison, applications of naled on three plots produced a very distinct effect on the tick populations (Fig. 3). Three plots were sprayed once during week 1, resulting (through exploratory data analysis) in an 82% reduction in tick numbers. Immediately afterwards, ticks gradually increased in number back to the threshold value and eventually exceeded that figure. Two plots (D2, D3) were sprayed twice at weeks 1 and 5 resulting in a 95% reduction in tick numbers after the second application. Within two weeks, tick numbers then just exceeded the threshold value. This period also coincided with peak adult tick activity on Long Island. During week 9, one plot (D3) was sprayed for the third time, resulting in a 96% reduction of tick numbers at that plot.

IV. SUMMARY

The 4-week interval between sprays allowed a resurgence of tick numbers soon after application of such a non-residual chemical as naled. Since chlorpyrifos and propoxur exhibit

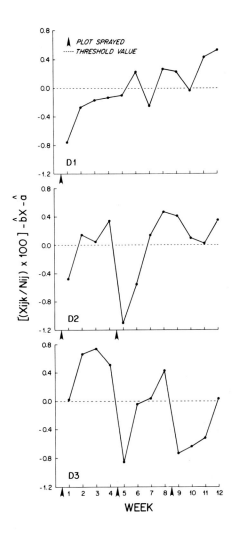

Fig. 3. Effect of spraying naled once (D1), twice (D2) and three times (D3) on tick populations at 3 plots at 4-wk intervals.

longer residual activity, which under certain circumstances may pose a threat to the fragile water supply of Long Island, local or county legislative or health boards may not approve their application. In addition, the cost of effective applications of pyrethrins with piperonyl butoxide is out of the range of most local budgets. Therefore, we recommend that

efforts to control D. variabilis in infected foci on Long
Island include at least 3 (preferably 4) applications of
emulsifiable naled at 3 week intervals. This application
frequency can reduce the number of questing ticks by up to
96-97%, and thereby minimize the potential transmission of
pathogenic rickettsiae by Dermacentor variabilis.

REFERENCES

1. Anonymous. Morbidity and Mortality Weekly Report. 29, 213.
    (1980).
2. Anonymous. New York State Department of Health Records,
    Albany, NY.
3. Benach, J.L., White, D.J., Burgdorfer, W., Keelan, T.,
    Guirgis, S., and Altieri, R.H. Am. J. Epidemiol. 106, 380.
    (1977).
4. Burgdorfer, W. Am. J. Trop. Med. Hyg. 19, 1010. (1970).
5. Ormsbee, R., Peacock, M., Philip, R., Casper, E., Plorde,
    J., Gabre-Kidan, T., and Wright, L. Am. J. Epidemiol.
    108, 53. (1978).
6. Philip, R.N., Casper, E.R., Burgdorfer, W., Gerloff, R.K.,
    Hughes, L.E., and Bell, E.J. J. Immunol. 121, 1961. (1978).
7. Smith, C.N., Cole, M.M., and Gouck, H.K. U.S. Dep. Agric.
    Tech. Bull. 905. (1946).
8. Collins, D., and Nardy, R. New York State Museum Circular
    No. 26. (1951).
9. Mount, G.A., Pierce, N.W., and Lofgren, C.S. J. Econ.
    Entomol. 64, 262. (1971).
10. Hansens, E.J. J. Econ. Entomol. 49, 281. (1956).
11. Finney, D. Probit Analysis - a statistical treatment of
    the sigmoid response curve. 2nd edit. Cambridge at the
    University Press. (1964).

AN EXAMPLE OF GEOGRAPHIC CLUSTERING OF
DERMACENTOR VARIABILIS ADULTS INFECTED WITH
RICKETTSIAE OF THE SPOTTED FEVER GROUP

Jorge L. Benach

State of New York Department of Health
State University of New York at Stony Brook
Stony Brook, New York

Laurel A. Smith

Department of Applied Mathematics
State University of New York at Stony Brook
Stony Brook, New York

Dennis J. White

State of New York Department of Health
Saranac Lake, New York

I. INTRODUCTION

Rocky Mountain spotted fever (RMSF) cases are well-known to
occur in defined clusters. In Long Island, New York, human
cases of RMSF occur predominantly, but not exclusively, within
a 3-mile belt from the shoreline (1). While populations of
Dermacentor variabilis are abundant and seemingly continuous in
the shoreline belts, human cases and evidence of infection in
ticks are not, suggesting a clustering tendency.
   D. variabilis adults do not show migratory tendencies (2,3)
and dispersal of this species may be host-associated (4,5).
Successful completion of subadult blood meals can produce
piecemeal dispersal in small areas according to the territorial
range of the rodent hosts. Dispersal of adults is probably
achieved by the more widely-ranging larger mammals, with

RICKETTSIAE AND RICKETTSIAL DISEASES

concomitant dispersal of infection. Transovarial transmission of rickettsiae (6) may be responsible for appearance of new foci after dispersal of successful females. Thus, these dispersal factors provide evidence to suggest that a cluster or foci of infection is subject to change.

Disappearance of infected foci may be due to an intrinsic but unknown limiting factor in the host-parasite-vector cycle. Disappearance may also be the result of successful dispersal of all infected adult ticks from an area. Collection of ticks for study can also contribute to focal disappearance since a tick used for hemolymph test (7) cannot be returned to the environment.

In their classic series of studies, Sonenshine and co-workers (3-5,8,9) have made extensive use of statistics and analytical inferences as essential adjuncts to the study of ticks in the environment. The development of the hemolymph test has made it possible to examine large numbers of ticks (1,10-13) for the presence of rickettsiae rapidly and accurately.

In this study, adult D. variabilis were collected from defined linear plots, tested for the presence of rickettsiae, and the results quantified in order to answer three questions: 1) is the proportion of infected adult D. variabilis uniform in a given area, 2) is there any evidence of clustering of infected ticks within a given area, and 3) is there any evidence of clustering of infected ticks in time and space within the same area?

II. MATERIALS AND METHODS

Two sites (Plot A, Plot B) were selected from RMSF endemic areas in eastern Long Island. The sites were essentially packed sand linear paths (mean width of approximately 2 to 3 meters). Predominant vegetation consisted of dune grass (Ammophila brevigulata) interspersed with strands of choke cherry (Prunus spp.), wild rose (Rosa spp.), poison ivy (Rhus toxicocodendron), and bayberry (Family Myriacaceae). Each plot measured 220 linear meters; plot A ran in an almost straight north-south axis and plot B in a slightly NE-SE axis; both plots began on a paved road and ended at the base of primary sand dunes on the Atlantic Ocean.

Each plot was divided into 10 meter sectors. Ticks were collected weekly for 16 weeks (April 28th-August 11th) by dragging a white flannel cloth ($1m^2$) over the edge vegetation. Both the eastern and western edges of each plot were sampled; therefore, in each plot there were 44 sectors. In plot A, ticks were collected from each sector and tested for the presence of rickettsiae by the hemolymph technique. The hemolymph test provides for the identification of group specific rickettsiae. Our references to infected ticks throughout the study are thus to infection with rickettsiae of the spotted fever group. In plot B, ticks were collected and returned to the sector after counting and used as a control for measuring the population decline.

The hypothesis of uniformity was tested using a chi-square test (14). Spatial clustering was studied by the use of a non-parametric test for clustering. The changing patterns of clustering across time were investigated using linear regression (14).

III.   RESULTS AND DISCUSSION

Tick populations in both plots: there were 1,387 ticks collected in plot A, and 3,932 ticks collected and released in plot B during the entire study period. It should be noted, however, that many ticks in plot B may have been counted more than once. Figure 1 shows the transformed tick counts (log of actual tick counts + 1) for the 16 weeks of the study for both plots A and B. Numbers of ticks increased in both plots during the first 5 weeks of the study (May), followed by declines during the succeeding weeks. Linear regression for the last 11 weeks (period of population decline) gave a log count slope of -0.40 for plot A, and a log count slope of -0.29 for plot B. The 95% confidence intervals for these slopes correspond to weekly declines of 27-39% for the plot A tick counts and to weekly declines of 16-34% for the plot B tick counts. Population declines in plot A began earlier and produced lower counts for the whole season than in plot B. The decline in ticks in plot B was consistent with that found in other studies involving Long Island tick populations (15).

Uniformity of infected ticks in Plot A: total number of ticks captured in plot A for the 16-week period are given in Table 1, and per sector in Figure 2. There were 31 sectors (out of a total of 44) where no infected ticks were found; 13 sectors produced at least one infected tick. A chi-square test showed a highly significant deviation from the overall infection rate of 4.6% over all sectors ($X^2=220.1$, 43 degrees of freedom, p <0.01). The predominant contribution to the larger X^2 value was provided by a few sectors with large numbers of infected ticks.

Clustering of infected ticks in Plot A: for the purpose of analysis, the 44 sectors (22 East and 22 West) were divided into three groups: 1) 31 sectors where no infected ticks were found, 2) 5 sectors where only a single tick was found during the entire study period, and 3) 8 sectors where more than two

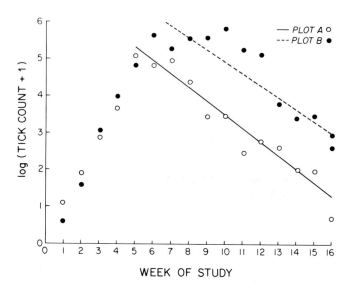

Fig. 1. Linear regression for log (tick counts +1) of number of ticks captured and tested for the presence of rickettsiae in Plot A, and ticks captured, counted and released in Plot B for 16-week study. Fitted regression lines for the last 11 weeks of the study showing population declines.

infected ticks were found. The assumption for the three groups is that a single infected tick per sector may have occurred by chance whereas finding two or more infected ticks per sector is more suggestive of a common source. Each sector (except 1 and 22) had two adjacent neighbors, therefore, an analysis for spatial clustering had to involve pairs of sectors rather than independent sectors alone. Thus, a clustering model is based on whether neighboring pairs of sectors across the plot (east and west) had more infected ticks than any pair of sectors chosen at random. For the clustering analysis, a pair of sectors was scored according to how similar the infected tick counts were: a score of 0 reflected the greatest similarity: either both sectors had two or more infected ticks, or both sectors had exactly one infected tick, or neither sector had any infected ticks. A score of 1 reflected partial similarity: one sector of the pair had only one infected tick and the other sector of the pair had either none or two or more infected ticks. A score of 2 reflected the least similarity: two or more

TABLE 1.   Total Number of Ticks, Number and Percent of
Infected Ticks Captured in Plot A by Week of Collection

MONTH	WEEK NUMBER	TOTAL NO. TICKS CAUGHT	NUMBER AND % INFECTED	
April	1	4	NONE	
May	2	9	1	(11.1%)
	3	37	1	(2.7%)
	4	100	2	(2.0%)
	5	249	24	(9.6%)
June	6	334	9	(3.8%)
	7	271	11	(4.1%)
	8	149	4	(2.6%)
	9	60	4	(6.7%)
	10	72	4	(5.1%)
July	11	21	NONE	
	12	32	NONE	
	13	20	5	(25.0%)
	14	14	NONE	
August	15	13	NONE	
	16	2	NONE	
TOTAL		1,387	65	(4.6%)

infected ticks in one sector of the pair and no infected ticks
in the other sector of the pair. Neighboring pairs of sectors
showed more similarity (lower mean scores) than pairs of sectors
chosen at random. The mean score for adjacent pairs of sectors,
same side of the plot, was 0.43; the mean score for cross-plot
neighboring pairs of sectors was 0.41. A mean score of 0.72
was obtained when all 946 possible pairs of sectors were considered (44x43/2=946). Standardized normal deviates (Z scores)
for adjacent pairs was -2.29 (p <0.05) and for across-plot
pairs was -1.77 (p <0.10) demonstrating that neighboring pairs
show significantly greater similarity than pairs chosen at random. A study on the testing of significance for geographic
clusters of disease (16) has shown that the type of nonpara-
metric analysis used here is conservative in its estimations of
significance particularly in cases where the geographic pattern
is visually obvious (Fig. 2).

   Clustering of infected ticks in plot A over time: in the
weekly testing for the presence of rickettsiae, infected ticks
were more likely to appear in or near sectors where there had
been infected ticks the week before. Since ticks collected

TABLE 2. Standardized Regression Coefficients for Predicting the Number of Infected Ticks

Predictor from previous week	Week predicted						
	4	5	6	7	8	9	10
No. caught, same sector	0.021	0.027	-0.018	0.006	0.044	0.283	-0.088
No. infected, same sector	-0.023	0.713[a]	0.195	0.680[a]	0.603[a]	-0.392	0.309
No. infected adjacent sector	0.478[b]	0.263[b]	0.710[a]	0.321[a]	0.227[c]	0.699[a]	0.308
No. infected, across plot sector	-0.015	0.128	0.131	0.198[c]	-0.848[a]	0.121	-0.075
No. infected, diagonal sector	-0.027	0.177[c]	-0.186	0.268[b]	0.692[a]	-0.474[b]	-0.079
Total No. Infected	2	24	9	11	4	4	4

[a] $p < 0.001$, [b] $p < 0.01$, [c] $p < 0.05$.

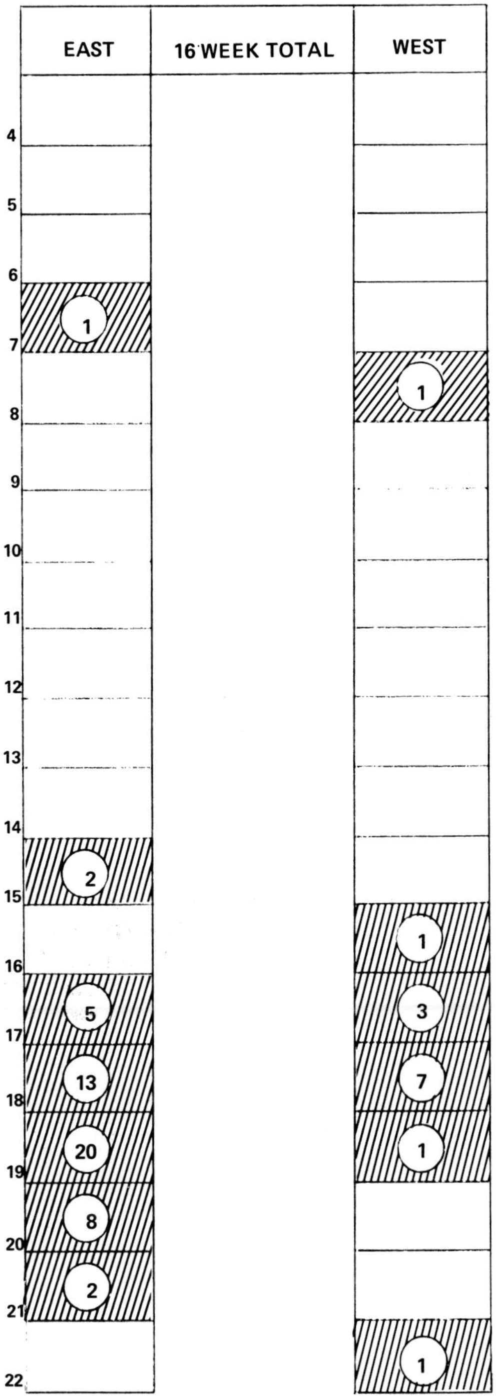

Fig. 2. Schematic representation of locations where the total of infected ticks were found in the 16 week period in study in Plot A. (Sectors 1 to 3 omitted.)

each week were not returned to the plot, recurrence of infected ticks in approximately the same sector suggests a common source. In this analysis, five possible predictors of the numbers of infected ticks in a given sector during the current week were considered (Table 2). Standardized regression coefficients for predicting the number of infected ticks during the following week are shown for 5 predictors in Table 2. The most consistent predictors were the number of infected ticks in the same sector and the number of infected ticks in adjacent sectors. These results are based on very small numbers of observations (small number of infected ticks) and thus must be interpreted with caution. They do, however, offer more detailed support of the clustering patterns observed during the entire season. This analysis shows that infected ticks are significantly more likely to appear in the same sectors where infected ticks had been previously collected, or in adjacent sectors. Fluctuations in the weekly infection rates were within the assumptions of binomial sampling from a population with an infection rate of approximately 5%. Again, since ticks were removed from the plot on a weekly basis, the clustering pattern in space as well as in time is strongly suggestive of a common source. We suggest that the cluster of infected ticks may be composed of transovarially infected siblings; alternatively, the cluster may be composed of ticks which acquired the infection from common rickettsemic rodents as subadults.

IV.   SUMMARY

An example of visual and statistical evidence has been provided to show that adult _D. variabilis_ infected with rickettsiae of the spotted fever group are not uniformly distributed in a given area, that geographic clustering of infected ticks can exist, and that clustering can occur in space as well as in time.

ACKNOWLEDGMENT

We wish to gratefully acknowledge all the help that Dr. Willy Burgdorfer has generously given us over the last few years.

REFERENCES

1. Benach, J. L., White, D. J., Burgdorfer, W., Keelan, T., Guirgis, S., and Altieri, R. H., Am. J. Epidemiol. 106, 380 (1977).
2. Smith, C. N., Cole, M. N., and Gouck, H. K., United States Department of Agriculture Technical Bulletin 905 (1946).
3. Sonenshine, D. E., Atwood, E. L., and Lamb, J. T., Ann. Entomol. Soc. Am. 59, 1234 (1966).
4. Sonenshine, D. E., and Stout, J., J. Med. Entomol. 5, 49 (1968).
5. Sonenshine, D. E., Ann. Entomol. Soc. Am. 66, 44 (1973).
6. Burgdorfer, W., and Brinton, L. P., Ann. New York Acad. Sci. 266, 61 (1975).
7. Burgdorfer, W., Am. J. Trop. Med. Hyg. 19, 1010 (1970).
8. Sonenshine, D. E., Ann. Entomol. Soc. Am. 65, 1164 (1972).
9. Sonenshine, D. E., and Stout, I. J., Ann. Entomol. Soc. Am. 61, 679 (1968).
10. Burgdorfer, W., Cooney, J. C., and Thomas, L. A., Am. J. Trop. Med. Hyg. 23, 109 (1974).
11. Burgdorfer, W., Adkins, T. R., Jr., and Priester, L. E., Am. J. Trop. Med. Hyg. 25, 866 (1975).
12. Magnarelli, L. A., Anderson, J. F., and Burgdorfer, W., Am. J. Epidemiol. 110, 148 (1979).
13. Linnemann, C. C., Jr., Schaeffer, A. E., Burgdorfer, W., Hutchinson, L., and Philip, R. N., Am. J. Epidemiol. 111, 31 (1980).
14. Snedecor, G. W., and Cochran, W. G., "Statistical Methods". Iowa State University Press, Ames, Iowa (1967).
15. White, D. J., Smith, L. A., and Benach, J. L., J. New York Entomol. Soc. In press. (1981)
16. Ohno, Y., Aoki, K., and Aoki, N., Int. J. Epidemiol. 8, 273 (1979).

GENETIC STATES POSSIBLY ASSOCIATED
WITH ENHANCED SEVERITY OF ROCKY
MOUNTAIN SPOTTED FEVER

David H. Walker[1]
Henry N. Kirkman[2]

Departments of Pathology[1] and Pediatrics[2]
University of North Carolina
Chapel Hill, North Carolina

Peter H. Wittenberg

Department of Pathology
Gaston Memorial Hospital
Gastonia, North Carolina

I.   INTRODUCTION

Previous studies of the epidemiology of Rocky Mountain
spotted fever (RMSF) have documented an increased fatality-
to-case ratio in American blacks, particularly black males
(1). It has been suggested that difficulty in recognition of
the rash in darkly pigmented skin and less access to good
health care were possible explanations for this high fatali-
ty-to-case ratio. However, the nearly identical mortality
rates for black and white females in the age group 15-44 years
(5.0% and 4.4% respectively) contrasts with strikingly different fatality rates for males in that age group (6.8% for
whites and 18.3% for blacks) (1). These data suggest minimal importance of skin pigmentation and socioeconomic status
and fit the hypothesis of a sex-linked recessive genetic condition that is found predominantly in the black race. Such a
condition is glucose-6-phosphate dehydrogenase (G6PD) deficiency, which is present in 12% of American black males but is
much less common in American whites or in black females (2).

G6PD A⁻, the variant of G6PD-deficient black males, moves
faster than the normal enzyme (G6PD B) on electrophoresis.
Another variant, G6PD A, is present in 17-20% of American
black males and is similar to G6PD A⁻ on electrophoresis.   It
is accompanied by essentially normal activity.

Two cases of rickettsial infection have been reported previously with acute renal failure and G6PD deficiency (3).   If
G6PD deficiency is the principal reason for the higher fata-
lity-to-case ratio in black males, then the frequency of G6PD
deficiency in black males with severe RMSF should be several
times greater than the expected frequency of 12%. Our findings on 10 black males support that supposition at a significance level of 0.024.   Because death is a major criterion for
severity of RMSF, the necessity for G6PD phenotyping of
stored, postmortem samples can be anticipated.   Stored samples from 15 white males, who also had RMSF, served to document that neither the deficiency nor electrophoretic phenotype of G6PD was an artifact of storage.

II. MATERIALS AND METHODS

Samples were available from 25 males who had been diagnosed as having Rocky Mountain spotted fever (Table 1).
Freshly drawn, heparinized blood was obtained from two con-
valescing black males. All other samples consisted of liver,
clotted blood, or red cells that had been stored at -70°C
from 1 month to 9 years. The frozen samples were thawed,
then sterilized by passage through a pair of Millipore filters: a prefilter to remove coarse particles and a 0.22 μm
filter to retain rickettsiae. Some samples required preliminary homogenization with several volumes of water in a Potter
Elvehjem homogenizer at 0°C. Electrophoresis on cellulose
acetate allowed the electrophoretic phenotype of the G6PD to
be determined (4). Activities of 6-phosphogluconate dehydrogenase (6PGD) and G6PD were measured by the method of Glock
and McLean (2). A unit of each enzyme was defined as the
activity that generates one μmole of product per minute at
25°C.

Clinical records from each of these black patients were
reviewed for clinical, laboratory, and histopathologic data.
Severe RMSF was defined in this study as fatal or complicated
by acute renal failure, coma, seizures, multiple focal neurologic signs, or severe coagulopathy.

TABLE 1. Results of Measurements of Activity and Electrophoresis of G6PD from Red Blood Cells

Subjects[a]	Activity (μMoles/min/g Hb)			Electrophoretic phenotype	Conclusion (G6PD type)
	G6PD	6PGD	G6PD/6PGD		
I – 1[b]	0.531	4.074	0.130	A⁻ or A	A⁻
I – 2	0.677	3.433	0.197	A⁻ or A	A⁻
I – 3	2.567	2.132	1.204	A⁻ or A	A⁻
I – 4	1.025	4.966	0.206	A⁻ or A	A⁻
I – 5	3.412	2.172	1.571	A⁻ or A	A
I – 6	4.633	3.667	1.263	B	B
I – 7[b]	3.039	2.795	1.087	B	B
I – 8[b]	1.143	4.800	0.238	A⁻ or A	A⁻
II – mean	3.679	3.239	1.127	B	B
II – S. D.	1.527	1.120	0.258	–	–
III – mean[b]	4.311	3.400	1.287	B	B
III – S. D.	0.253	0.415	0.197	–	–

[a]Group I consists of 10 black males with severe RMSF. For 2 of these, G6PD studies were possible only on liver. Both were G6PD B by electrophoresis. Group II consists of 15 white males with RMSF. For 2 of these, also, G6PD studies were possible only on liver and both were G6PD B by electrophoresis. Group III consists of 7 healthy white men without RMSF.

[b]Fresh hemolysates.

A case of fatal RMSF in an 11 year old black male with
sickle cell trait is reported with data obtained from review
of the clinical record, autopsy protocol, microscopic slides,
and immunofluorescence microscopy for R. rickettsii on autopsy tissues.

III. RESULTS

A. Investigation of Glucose-6-Phosphate Dehydrogenase
and RMSF

Table 1 shows the G6PD activity, 6-phosphogluconate dehydrogenase activity (6PGD) and ratio of G6PD activity to
6PGD activity for each black male with severe RMSF. Also
shown are the means and standard deviations of the same
activities for 13 white males with RMSF and for seven normal
white men without RMSF. The mean activities with the frozen
samples were slightly less than the corresponding means of
the fresh hemolysates from the seven normal white men. Six
of these hemolysates were electrophoretically G6PD A or G6PD
A⁻. One sample of frozen blood was not usable. It had a
brown color, very low activities of both dehydrogenases, and
slurred bands of hemoglobin and G6PD on electrophoresis.
Blood was unavailable from 3 other males. Frozen liver was
available from these 4 males (2 black, 2 white), however;
and the electrophoretic pattern of their G6PD was normal.
As a consequence, the G6PD phenotype of all 25 males could
be identified (Table 2).

TABLE 2. Numbers of Males, by G6PD Phenotype

| | | Normal Activity | | Deficient Activity |
Group	Description	G6PD B	G6PD A	G6PD A⁻
I	Black, severe RMSF	4	2	4
II	White, RMSF	15	0	0
III	White, healthy	7	0	0

By the Fisher exact test (5), the difference in occurrence of G6PD A⁻ between black and white males was significant (P = 0.017). Similarly, a binomial expansion revealed
that the proportion of G6PD A⁻ subjects among black males
(4/10) exceeded the expected proportion (2) of 0.12 at a
significance level of P = 0.024. On the other hand, the
proportion of G6PD A males (2/10) was not significantly different from the expected proportion (2).

All ten cases of RMSF studied in black males were classified as severe. Two of the G6PD deficient cases died of fulminant RMSF. Brief clinical summaries of three of the G6PD-
deficient cases follow.

Case 1.

A 65 year old black man was transferred to North Carolina
Memorial Hospital on August 3, 1978 because of oliguria, fever, and undiagnosed multisystem disease. He had been a
working tobacco farmer until four days before transfer, when
he experienced the sudden onset of nausea, vomiting, fever,
and myalgias. Two days later he was admitted to another hospital. Laboratory data included hematocrit 33%; BUN 48 mg/
dl, creatinine 2.7 mg/dl, and total bilirubin 2.6 mg/dl. The
two-day hospital course was remarkable for sequential development of projectile vomiting, oliguria, anuria, and obtundation. No rash was observed before transfer.

On admission to North Carolina Memorial Hospital, a petechial macular rash was noted on the abdomen, trunk, and proxi-
mal extremities. Over the next four hours the rash became
confluent, macular, non-blanching, reticular purpura with involvement of the scrotum and sparing of palms and soles. On
admission, the BUN was 95 mg/dl, creatinine 9.9 mg/dl, total
bilirubin 11.9 mg/dl, hematocrit 34%, and SGPT 139 U/l (normal range 7-29). The platelet count was 25,000/µl, prothrom-
bin time 15.6 sec (control 11.8), partial thromboplastin time
82.6 sec (control 59.6), and fibrinogen 206 mg/dl (normal
range 200-400). Urine contained renal tubular casts, 30 WBC/
high power field, >50 RBC/high power field, sodium 75 mEq/l,
and osmolality 301 mosm. Chest roentgenogram revealed no ab-
normality; however, bilateral diffuse interstitial infiltrates were noted eight hours later. From Swan-Ganz measurements the pulmonary artery pressure was 37/18 mm Hg, mean 27
mm Hg, and pulmonary capillary wedge pressure was 10 mm Hg,
thus documenting noncardiogenic pulmonary edema. Treatment
included penicillin G, chloramphenicol, tobramycin, methyl-
prednisolone, and hydrocortisone. Death occurred eleven
hours after admission and five days after onset of illness.

A skin biopsy examined by specific direct immunofluorescence revealed large numbers of <u>Rickettsia</u> <u>rickettsii</u>, which were also isolated by inoculation of guinea pigs. Observations at necropsy were disseminated thrombonecrotic vasculitis with massive rickettsial burden and minimal leukocytic reaction.

Case 2

A 13 year old black male was transferred to North Carolina Memorial Hospital after three days of hospitalization with unexplained fever. Onset of fever and malaise was noted nine days before transfer. On the second day of fever, his local physician treated him with ampicillin, but the patient continued to have high fever, chills, delirium, and anorexia. On the sixth day of fever he was admitted to his local hospital with hematocrit 35%, normal platelets, and WBC 13,400/µl. He was treated initially with ampicillin and sulfamethoxozole and subsequently also with cephalosporin and glucocorticoid.

On transfer he had edema, weakness, fever, orthostatic hypotension, a macular petechial rash involving palms and soles, and myalgia. Laboratory data included hematocrit 24%, platelets 195,000/µl, serum sodium 125/mEq/1, BUN 65 mg/dl, creatinine 3.0 mg/dl, SGPT 88 U/1, SGOT 473 U/1, CPK 2049 U/1, coagulation times moderatly prolonged, <u>Proteus</u> OX19 agglutination titer 1:640, and skin biopsy immunofluorescent demonstration of <u>R. rickettsii</u>. The hospital course included seven days of fever following onset of treatment with intravenous chloramphenicol. Complications were acute renal failure and hemolysis with hematocrit 16% and undetectible haptoglobin. Follow-up examinations after discharge revealed an apparently complete recovery.

Case 3

An eight year old black male was admitted to the hospital after five days of illness. Symptoms of fever and periumbilical abdominal pain brought the patient to his physician on the second day of illness. Treatment with penicillin and ampicillin were without effect. The fever continued, and delirium was noted on day four of illness. On the day of death he had a hematocrit of 33%, 3 nucleated RBC/100 WBC, platelets 43,000/µl, prolonged coagulation times, and hyponatremia. His course included generalized seizures, obtundation, shock, purpura of extremities including palms and soles, terminal treatment with phenobarbital and chloramphenicol, and death

early on the sixth day of symptoms. R. rickettsii was isolated by inoculation of guinea pigs. Autopsy revealed minimal leukocytic response to generalized vascular injury.

    B. Case Study of Sickle Cell Trait and RMSF

    An 11 year old black male had been in good health until
one week prior to admission when he developed fever. Three
days later he was seen in the emergency room at Gaston Memorial Hospital, where he was felt to have a viral syndrome with
fever, headache, abdominal pain, and an episode each of vomiting and diarrhea. Laboratory data were hemoglobin 12.6 gm/dl,
hematocrit 36.7%, and white blood cell count 11,600 cells/µl
with 86% neutrophils, 2% bands, and 12% lymphocytes. Over the
following three days at home he experienced vomiting and periumbilical and leg pain. A tick was seen crawling on the patient during this interval. On the day before admission, he
was examined in a physician's office and was treated with penicillin for a presumed streptococcal infection. Throat culture and mono spot test from that visit were nondiagnostic.
    Because he appeared worse the next day, he was admitted to
the hospital. Physical examination revealed temperature 39.3°
C, pulse 88/min, respirations 28/min, blood pressure 92/62 mm
Hg, abdominal tenderness, tender hepatomegaly, and pain on
movement of the fifth digit of the right hand. Admission laboratory data included WBC count 10,500/µl with 49% neutrophils,
33% bands, 4% metamyelocytes, 10% lymphocytes, and 4% monocytes, platelet count 39,500/µl, partial thromboplastin time
41.4 sec (control 27.6 sec), fibrinogen 102 mg/dl, serum sodium 125 mEq/l, serum potassium 5.1 mEq/l, serum chloride 86
mEq/l, and blood urea nitrogen 40 mgm/dl. Further laboratory
evaluation revealed extensive hepatic involvement with SGOT
3410 (normal 11-38), LDH 4680 (normal 100-190), and serum
total bilirubin 4.8 mg/dl (normal 0-1.5). On the second hospital day hypoalbuminemia (2.9 gm/dl) and progressive hyper-
bilirubinemia (12.6 mg/dl) were documented. Treatment with
intravenous chloramphenicol was given for the possibility of
RMSF; however, the patient did not respond. Death occurred
two days after admission.
    At autopsy there was a diffuse macular rash which was most
prominent on the extremities and the palms and plantar surface
of the feet. Vascular demarcation of ischemic zones were noted on the hand and foot. The liver was enlarged and contained
many small infarcts. Likewise, there was splenomegaly with
multiple prominent splenic infarcts. The lungs were diffusely
edematous and contained multifocal infarcts. Sickled intra-

vascular erythrocytes were observed, and hemoglobin electrophoresis demonstrated 40% S hemoglobin, 57% A_1 hemoglobin, and
3% A_2 hemoglobin. R. rickettsii was identified in tissues
postmortem by direct immunofluorescence.

IV. DISCUSSION

     This small series of cases of severe RMSF in black Ameri-
can males suggests an association between severity and G6PD
deficiency. Activities of both dehydrogenases decay slowly
at -70°C, but reliable identification of G6PD (A⁻) deficiency
was indicated by the finding that low activities of G6PD, relative to 6-phosphogluconate dehydrogenase activities, were:
present only in samples from black males; accompanied by the
expected G6PD A⁻ electrophoretic phenotype; and present in
the two samples of fresh blood and in another with the least
storage time at -70°C.
     Three alternative interpretations can be given to this
preliminary evidence that G6PD deficiency may be dispropor-
tionately represented in black males with severe forms of
Rocky Mountain spotted fever: 1) A drug-induced hemolysis
occurs in G6PD-deficient males during their course of treatment with large doses of tetracycline or chloramphenicol. 2)
The greater severity is a result of some other adverse interaction between G6PD deficiency and the rickettsial infection,
eg., increased rickettsial burden due to enhanced replication
or defective host defense, greater tendency to thrombosis, or
hemolysis due to rickettsial interaction with the erythrocytic
membrane. 3) The association is false, representing only an
unusual result of sampling. The P value (0.024) seems sufficiently low, however, to justify a request that other investigators also look for this association. Some urgency exists
for distinguishing among possibilities 1 through 3. If 1 is
valid, the antibiotic treatment of G6PD-deficient patients
will need to be modified. If 2 or 3 is valid, such modification might only increase the fatality rate from Rocky Mountain spotted fever. The authors welcome collaboration in a
prospective study of black males with severe Rocky Mountain
spotted fever.
     Although it is accepted that sickle cell trait is a gen-
erally benign condition and carries the expectancy of a normal
lifespan (6,7), the case reported herein documents pathologic
lesions which are not expected in fatal RMSF. Extensive infarcts of lung, spleen, and liver indicate severe antemortem
ischemic injury and suggest that the observed sickled erythro-

cytes may have occluded the vascular supply to the irregularly
distributed microinfarcts. In contrast, the presence of sickled erythrocytes without necrosis, a commonly observed postmortem state in sickle cell trait individuals, would not
necessarily indicate premortem sickling. Thrombosis was not
a prominent feature. Further investigation of black patients
with RMSF is needed to determine whether or not this autosomal genetic state (hemoglobin AS), which is present in 8%
of American blacks, predisposes to a severe course of RMSF.

That an unknown number of rapidly fatal summer deaths in
black males may be due to fulminant RMSF and go undiagnosed
is emphasized by Cases 1 and 3. Fulminant RMSF was originally defined by Parker as an attack with fatality within 3-5
days of onset of symptoms, either no rash or spots rapidly
coalescing to form large ecchymotic blotches, and early evidence of involvement of the central nervous system (8). The
patients died before developing antibodies to rickettsiae or
generating the characteristic leukocytic response to the vascular injury. The only previously documented case of fulminant RMSF in which the pathologic lesions have been reported
was in a 14 year old black male whose autopsy findings were
similar to Case 1 (9). Only rickettsial isolation or immunofluorescent demonstration of the etiologic agent (10,11) af-
fords a definitive diagnosis in such cases.

The mortality rate has been reported previously to be as
high as 28.1% in black males in the age group 0-9 years (1).
This fact and the results of the present study emphasize the
need for special care in the approach to febrile disease in
black males between April and September, especially in the
southeastern United States. Management should include screening for G6PD deficiency, attempt to establish history of tick
exposure, collection of bacterial cultures appropriate to the
individual patient, and early treatment with tetracycline or
chloramphenicol prior to onset of a rash. Ultimately, G6PD-
deficient persons may represent a target population for an effective vaccine against RMSF.

ACKNOWLEDGMENTS

The authors wish to acknowledge the assistance of Dr.
Joseph E. McDade in providing materials from many of the patients studied, of Dr. Harvey Hamrick in providing the diagnostic specimen for one case, and of Mrs. Jennie Lu Hollander
in preparation of the manuscript.

REFERENCES

1. Hattwick, M. A. W., O'Brien, R. J., and Hanson, B. F.,
    Ann. Intern. Med. 84, 732 (1976).
2. Report of a WHO Scientific Group. "Standardization of
    Procedures for the Study of Glucose-6-Phosphate Dehydro-
    genase", WHO Techn. Rep. Ser., No. 366 (1967).
3. Whelton, A., Donadio, J. V., Jr., and Elisberg, B. L.,
    Ann. Intern. Med. 69, 323 (1968).
4. Migeon, B. R., and Kennedy, J. F. Am. J. Hum. Genet. 27,
    233 (1975).
5. Fisher, R. A., in "Statistical Methods for Research
    Workers", (11th Ed. Rev.), Hafner Publishing Co., New
    York (1950).
6. Sears, D. A., Am. J. Med. 64, 1021 (1978).
7. Report of a WHO Scientific Group. "Haemoglobinopathies
    and Allied Disorders." WHO Tech. Rep. Ser., No. 338
    (1966).
8. Parker, R. R., J. A. M. A. 110, 1185 (1938).
9. Moon, J. H., and Silverberg, S. G., Va. Med. Monthly 98,
    271 (1971).
10. Woodward, T. E., Pedersen, C. E., Jr., Oster, C. N., Bag-
    ley, L. R., Romberger, J., and Snyder, M. J. J. Infect.
    Dis. 134, 297 (1976).
11. Walker, D. H., Cain, B. G., and Olmstead, P. M., Am. J.
    Clin. Path. 69, 619 (1978).

GAS-LIQUID CHROMATOGRAPHY OF ACUTE-PHASE SERUM AS A TECHNIQUE FOR EARLY DIAGNOSIS OF RICKETTSIAL DISEASES

Joseph E. McDade
David E. Wells
John B. Brooks
Cynthia C. Alley

Centers for Disease Control
Atlanta, Georgia

I. INTRODUCTION

Although there have been significant improvements in recent years in the techniques for diagnosis of rickettsial diseases (1-6), there still is no procedure which will consistently provide an accurate diagnosis early enough to insure that every patient receives prompt antimicrobial therapy. Because most of these techniques are based on serologic principles, the usual approach to improving diagnosis has been to devise methods which will enhance a given antigen-antibody reaction (5,6). Recently, however, we explored an alternate approach to the diagnosis of rickettsial diseases, namely, gas-liquid chromatography of acute-phase sera. Gas-liquid chromatography has been used extensively in recent years for the diagnosis of infectious diseases (7) as well as for certain metabolic disorders (8), but heretofore has not been used for the diagnosis of rickettsial illnesses. In our studies we used frequency-pulsed electron capture gas-liquid chromatography (FPEC-GLC) to analyze the sera from patients with Rocky Mountain spotted fever, epidemic typhus, and tick typhus infections for the presence of organic acids, amines, and alcohols. This report presents the results of these analyses.

II.   METHODS

Sera were selected from among specimens that had been sent to the Center for Disease Control (CDC) from 1978 through 1980 for testing with rickettsial antigens. They had been stored at -20°C from the time they were tested until they were used in this study. In all, acute-phase sera from 19 patients with a documented history of rickettsial illness were selected for study, including 15 patients with Rocky Mountain spotted fever (RMSF), two with epidemic typhus, and two with tick typhus. Serum specimens from 10 healthy employees of CDC were included in the study as controls.

Fatty acids, amines, hydroxy acids, and alcohols were extracted from sera and esterified to form electron-capturing derivatives by using methods published previously (9,10). Two microliters of the derivatized extracts were analyzed on a Perkin-Elmer Model 3920 gas chromatograph under column conditions described elsewhere (11). For TCE esters, the instruments were programmed from 100°C to 265°C at 4°C/min. HFBA esters were held at 90°C for 8 min, then the temperature was raised to 265°C at 4°C/min. In all analyses the final temperature was maintained for 30 min. Whenever possible, compounds were tentatively identified by comparing their relative retention times with those of standards.

III.   RESULTS

In comparing the FPEC-GLC profiles of serum extracts, we looked for qualitative differences, large quantitative differences, and differences in peak ratios. Generally speaking, the hydroxy acid profiles and carboxylic acid profiles of the various rickettsial sera were similar, although there were both qualitative and quantitative differences. Figure 1 illustrates the hydroxy acid profile of serum from one of the epidemic typhus patients and the corresponding profile of serum from a normal individual. Peak 6 is the internal standard, 2-hydroxyisovaleric acid. Selected peaks are blackened to facilitate comparisons among the various rickettsial sera. The hydroxy acid profiles of sera from the epidemic typhus patients (Fig. 1A) were qualitatively different from those obtained with serum from normal individuals (Fig. 1B) in that the typhus sera contained peaks 8, 12, 21, 31, 34, 35 and 41, which were not present in normal sera. There were also large quantitative differences in the amounts of peak 4, 14, 19, 20,

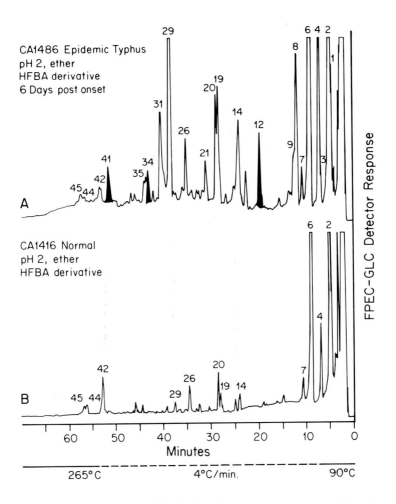

Fig. 1. Frequency-pulsed electron capture gas–liquid chromatography (FPEC–GLC) chromatograms of heptafluorobutyric anhydride–ethanol (HFBA) derivatives prepared from acidic ethyl ether extracts (after acidic and basic extraction with chloroform) of an acute-phase serum specimen from a typhus patient and of a normal serum.

and 29 in normal vs. epidemic typhus sera. As with the epidemic typhus sera, the hydroxy acid profiles of sera from persons with RMSF or tick typhus infections (Fig. 2) also had relatively high levels of peaks 4, 8, 14, 19, 29, 34, and 35. Differences among the hydroxy acid profiles of the various rickettsial sera included the following: (a) the tick typhus sera had high concentrations (i.e., above full scale) of

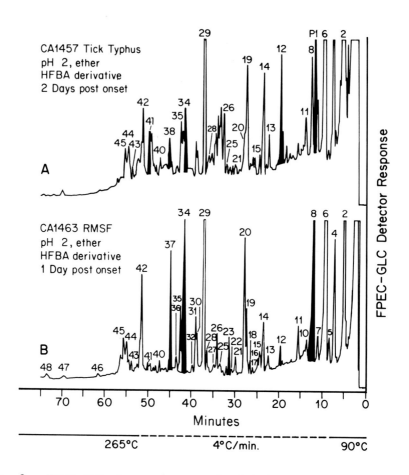

Fig. 2.   FPEC-GLC chromatograms of HFBA derivatives prepared from ethyl ether extracts (after acidic and basic extraction with chloroform) of acute-phase serum specimens from patients with disease as indicated. For an explanation of derivatives, see Fig. 1.

peak Pl, whereas epidemic typhus sera did not have this peak and most of the spotted fever sera contained little (i.e., below 1/4 scale), if any, of peak Pl; (b) tick typhus sera had peak 38, which was missing in spotted fever and epidemic typhus sera; (c) only spotted fever sera had peak 37; (d) there were large differences in the concentrations of peak 34; and (e) tick typhus and epidemic typhus sera had higher levels of peaks 12 and 41 than did the spotted fever sera.

The carboxylic acid profiles of the acute-phase rickettsial sera are illustrated in Figures 3 and 4. Compared to normal serum (Fig. 3B), serum from epidemic typhus patients (Fig. 3A) had elevated levels of the following carboxylic acids: C2, iso-C4, iso-C5, C6, C8, phenylacetic acid (PAA), C10, C12, C14, C16:1, C18:1, and C18. C7 is the internal standard, heptanoic acid. Spotted fever and tick typhus sera also had elevated levels of many carboxylic acids (Fig. 4). Differences in the carboxylic acid profiles of the various rickettsial sera were as follows: (a) both tick typhus serum specimens and several RMSF sera contained substantial levels of arachidonic acid (C20:4), whereas the amount of arachidonic acid in the epidemic typhus sera did not exceed the levels found in the controls; (b) the ratio of C12 to C10 was near unity in epidemic typhus and RMSF sera, but was considerably greater than one with tick typhus sera; (c) the concentration of PAA was much higher in spotted fever sera than in the other rickettsial specimens; (d) both spotted fever and tick typhus sera contained two compounds (peaks P3 and P4) not found in the other sera; and (e) only spotted fever sera had peak P5. The large peak (P2) located at 24 min in both the RMSF and tick typhus sera was not identified, but it had a relative retention time similar to that of aspirin.

Relatively few amines were observed in the rickettsial sera, and consistent profiles were not observed (data not shown).

IV. DISCUSSION

The study was part of a larger investigation (12) designed to assess the relative value of gas-liquid chromatography as a technique for distinguishing RMSF from clinically similar illnesses. Because the study was retrospective in nature, it had several limitations: (a) the number of specimens that could be studied was limited because few sera were available in the amount needed for testing (2 ml); (b) complete clinical histories usually were not available; (c) the patients had not been treated uniformly; and (d) serum specimens had been collected at various times after onset of illness. Despite these difficulties, there was remarkable uniformity in the hydroxy acid and carboxylic acid FPEC-GLC profiles of all the rickettsial sera. Only a limited number of epidemic typhus and tick typhus sera were tested, however, and additional specimens from such patients need to be examined to verify our preliminary findings.

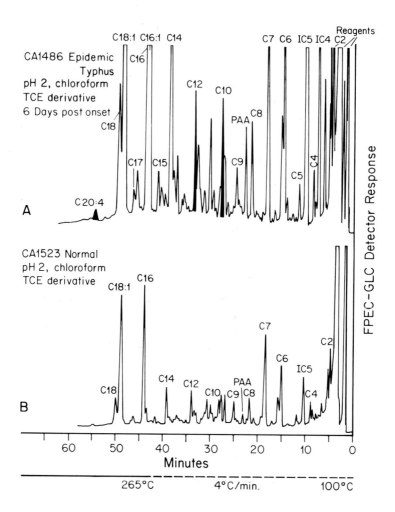

Fig. 3. FPEC-GLC chromatogram of trichloroethanol-HFBA (TCE) derivatives prepared from acidic chloroform extracts from an acute-phase sera from a typhus patient. The letter C followed by a number indicates a saturated straight chain carboxylic acid, with the number of carbon atoms indicated by the number. The letter I indicates the iso form of the acid, and the use of a colon between two numbers indicates unsaturation. The letter P next to a number indicates an unidentified compound. PAA is phenylacetic acid.

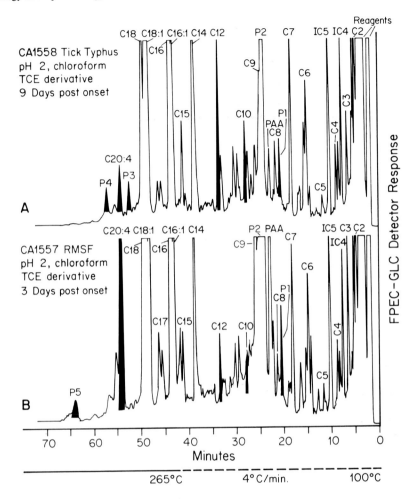

Fig. 4. FPEC-GLC chromatograms of TCE-HFBA derivatives
prepared from acidic chloroform extracts of acute-phase sera
from patients with disease as indicated. For an explanation
of abbreviations and peak designations see Figs. 1 and 3.

With RMSF patients, typical hydroxy acid and carboxylic
acid profiles were observed in specimens collected as early
as 1 day after onset of illness, and in most instances the
acute-phase sera did not contain significant levels of anti-
rickettsial antibodies when tested by either the IFA or CF
techniques (data not shown). Because the results of our
other studies (12) suggest that the respective hydroxy acid

and carboxylic acid profiles of sera from patients with
chickenpox, rubella, rubeola, enterovirus infections, and
meningococcal meningitis are also characteristic, GLC of acute-
phase serum specimens may prove to be a useful tool for
differentiating RMSF from clinically similar illnesses.
Obviously, much more data needs to be accumulated to assess
the relative sensitivity, specificity, reproducibility and
practicality of this procedure.

We tentatively identified many of the carboxylic acids
in patients' sera by comparing their retention times with
standards, but we were unable to identify most of the hydroxy
acids with available standards. We intend to use mass
spectrometry to identify selected compounds in the sera of
spotted fever patients. Once the structures of key compounds
are known, they could possibly be synthesized and used as
standards in future analyses. Further, the role of such
compounds in the infectious process could then be evaluated
under experimental conditions. For example, it is well
known that fatty acids have profound effects on immunocompetent
cells (13) and a recent report showed that the A series of
prostaglandins have antiviral activity (14), but it is not
known if these acids play a role in immunity to rickettsial
infections. It would be of interest to know if the compounds
found in patients' sera are mediators of infection, pathology,
and immunity, or if they are secondary to these processes.
Finally, although the source of the acids in patient sera is
not known with certainty, available information suggests that
they are not structural components of the rickettsiae:
analyses of the fatty acids of purified rickettsiae indicate
that relatively few fatty acids, namely C15, C16:1, and C18:1,
are found in significant quantities in these organisms (15).

V.   SUMMARY

Studies were conducted to determine if frequency-pulsed
electron capture gas-liquid chromatography (FPEC-GLC) of
acute-phase sera is a suitable technique for early diagnosis
of certain rickettsial diseases. The acid profiles of the
rickettsial sera were different from the corresponding profiles detected in earlier studies of sera from patients with
rubella, rubeola, chickenpox, meningococcal meningitis and
enterovirus infections. The fact that the typical rickettsial
profile was observed in sera collected as early as 1 day after
onset of illness suggests that gas-liquid chromatography
of serum may be a useful technique for early diagnosis of
rickettsial diseases.

REFERENCES

1. Newhouse, V.F., Shepard, C.C., Redus, M.D., Tzianabos, T., and McDade, J.E., Am. J. Trop. Med. Hyg., 28, 387 (1979).
2. Philip, R.N., Casper, E.A., MacCormack, J.N., Sexton, D.J., Thomas, L.A., Anacker, R.L., Burgdorfer, W., and Vick, S., Am. J. Epidemiol., 105, 56 (1977).
3. Woodward, T.E., Pedersen, C.E., Jr., Oster, C.N., Bagley, L.R., Romberger, J., and Snyder, M.J., J. Infect. Dis., 134, 297 (1976).
4. Walker, D.H., Cain, B.G., and Olmstead, P.M., Am. J. Clin. Pathol., 69, 619 (1978).
5. Halle, S., Dasch, G.A., and Weiss, E., J. Clin. Microbiol., 6, 101 (1977).
6. Dasch, G.A., Halle, S., and Bourgeois, A.L., J. Clin. Microbiol., 9, 38 (1979).
7. Larsson, L. and Mårdh, P-A., Acta Pathol. Microbiol. Scand., Sect. B, Suppl. 259, 5 (1977).
8. Jellum, E., J. Chromatogr., 143, 427 (1977).
9. Craven, R.B., Brooks, J.B., Edman, D.C., Converse, J.D., Greenlee, J., Schlossberg, D., Furlow, T., Gwaltney, J.M., Jr., and Miner, W.F., J. Clin. Microbiol., 6, 27 (1977).
10. Alley, C.C., Brooks, J.B., and Choudhary, G., Anal. Chem., 48, 387 (1976).
11. Brooks, J.B., Craven, R.B., Schlossberg, D., Alley, C.C., and Pitts, F.M., J. Clin. Microbiol., 8, 203 (1978).
12. Brooks, J.B., McDade, J.E., Alley, C.C., and Edman, D.C., J. Clin. Microbiol. (In Press.)
13. Meade, C.J. and Mertin, J., Adv. Lipid Res., 16, 127 (1978).
14. Santoro, M.G., Benedetto, A., Carruba, G., Goraci, E., and Jaffe, B.M., Science, 209, 1032 (1980).
15. Winkler, H.H. and Miller, E.T., J. Bacteriol., 136, 175 (1978).

INDEX